Modalities for Therapeutic Intervention

FIFTH EDITION

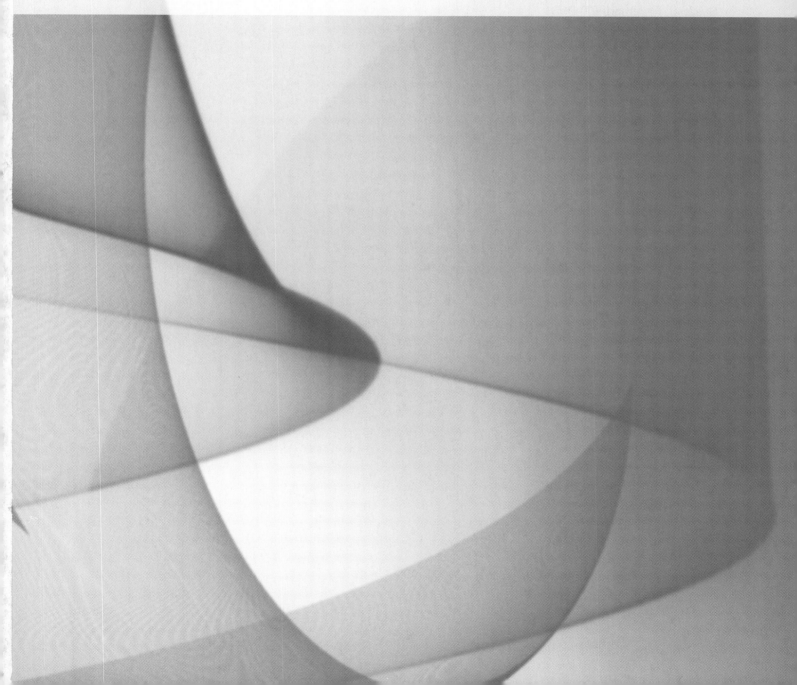

Contemporary Perspectives in Rehabilitation

CPR

Steven L. Wolf, PT, PhD, FAPTA, Editor-in-Chief

Fundamentals of Musculoskeletal Imaging, 3rd Edition
Lynn N. McKinnis, PT, OCS

Pharmacology in Rehabilitation, 4th Edition
Charles D. Ciccone, PT, PhD

Wound Healing: Alternatives in Management, 4th Edition
Joseph M. McCulloch, PT, PhD, CWS, and Luther C. Kloth, PT, MS, CWS, FAPTA

Vestibular Rehabilitation, 3rd Edition
Susan J. Herdman, PT, PhD

Spinal Cord Injury Rehabilitation
Edelle Field-Fote, PT, PhD

Modalities for Therapeutic Intervention

FIFTH EDITION

Previously titled Thermal Agents in Rehabilitation, editions 1, 2, and 3

Susan L. Michlovitz, PT, PhD, CHT

Adjunct Associate Professor, Rehabilitation Medicine, Columbia University, New York, NY

Associate Clinical Professor, Faculty of Rehabilitation Science

McMaster University, Hamilton, Ontario

Professor, Rocky Mountain University of Health Professions, Provo, UT

James W. Bellew, PT, EdD

Associate Professor, Krannert School of Physical Therapy

University of Indianapolis

Indianapolis, IN

Thomas P. Nolan Jr., PT, DPT, OCS

Associate Professor, School of Health Sciences

The Richard Stockton College of New Jersey

Pomona, NJ

 F.A. Davis Company • Philadelphia

F.A. Davis Company
1915 Arch Street
Philadelphia, PA 19103
www.fadavis.com

Copyright © 2012 by F.A. Davis Company

Printed in the United States of America

Last digit indicates print number: 10 9 8 7 6 5 4 3

Acquisitions Editor: Melissa Duffield
Manager of Content Development: George W. Lang
Developmental Editor: Susan R. Williams
Art and Design Manager: Carolyn O'Brien

As new scientific information becomes available through basic and clinical research, recommended treatments and drug therapies undergo changes. The author(s) and publisher have done everything possible to make this book accurate, up to date, and in accord with accepted standards at the time of publication. The author(s), editors, and publisher are not responsible for errors or omissions or for consequences from application of the book, and make no warranty, expressed or implied, in regard to the contents of the book. Any practice described in this book should be applied by the reader in accordance with professional standards of care used in regard to the unique circumstances that may apply in each situation. The reader is advised always to check product information (package inserts) for changes and new information regarding dose and contraindications before administering any drug. Caution is especially urged when using new or infrequently ordered drugs.

Library of Congress Cataloging-in-Publication Data

Modalities for therapeutic intervention / [edited by] Susan L. Michlovitz, James W. Bellew, Thomas P. Nolan Jr. – 5th ed.
  p. ; cm.
 Includes bibliographical references and index.
 ISBN-13: 978-0-8036-2391-0
 ISBN-10: 0-8036-2391-7
 1. Physical therapy. 2. Medical rehabilitation. I. Michlovitz, Susan L. II. Bellew, James W. III. Nolan, Thomas, 1955–
[DNLM: 1. Physical Therapy Modalities. 2. Wounds and Injuries—rehabilitation. WB 460]
 RM700.M63 2012
 615.8'32—dc22

2012006044

I would like to dedicate this edition to the students, clinicians, and faculty who have supported and had faith in this project since 1986.
— *Sue Michlovitz*

To my wife Mary Helen and daughters Kate and Caroline . . . quite simply, you are my everything.
— *Jim Bellew*

To my wife, Diana, and children, Tommy and Jennifer, for their love, support, and enthusiasm as we hurtle through life together.
— *Tom Nolan*

Foreword

"Thou dost make possible things not so held
Communicat'st with dreams."
(William Shakespeare, *The Winter's Tale*, act 1, scene 1)

At a time when the "possibility" of optimally integrating information about the importance of modalities into practice has become obscured by the myriad of other course material that must be addressed within constraining curricula, Sue Michlovitz and Tom Nolan have added Jim Bellew to their team to create a "dream" that not only inspires appreciation for the value of modalities but empowers the topic through contemporary, creative, and precise presentation of content. Indeed, as Sue Michlovitz has noted, the idea for a book on thermal agents was born nearly 30 years ago. Coincidently, this fifth edition of her initial efforts marks not only the 25th anniversary of this text but the quarter century mark since the birth of the *Contemporary Perspectives in Rehabilitation* series.

During that time and particularly within the past decade, what we teach and how we practice within the purview of the "academic health professions" (a contemporary name that is gaining popularity over the more obtuse term, "allied health professions"), continues to change dynamically. Such change is driven by profoundly varied health-care reimbursement policies and by an exponential growth in knowledge. Information availability and expansion are most difficult to capture, even for the keenest of web browser connoisseurs. The importance of tracking information lies in creating interdisciplinary collaborations on the one hand and contemporizing new data on the other. For example, at the recent Physical Therapy and Society (PASS) meeting, an external perspective of the physical therapy profession was offered by experts in at least 20 different content areas including: consumers, engineers, basic scientists, technology advocates, health lawyers, stem cell researchers, health care, practitioners,

physicians, virtual practice advocates, innovative media experts, nurses, instrumentation designers, bioethicists, and federal agency employees. They concluded that physical therapists must position themselves to develop and provide leadership in testing and applications of new technologies and approaches that optimize health-care delivery and that best practices be defined and defended as a vehicle for stemming the tide of constricting rehabilitation services. The recommendations emerging from PASS were endorsed unanimously by the American Physical Therapy House of Delegates.

Such introspection and its embedded prognostication are compatible with the intent of *Modalities for Therapeutic Intervention* (5th edition). Students, clinicians, and educators are encouraged to read Dr. Michlovitz's Preface to this edition and to absorb the content regarding "How to Use This Book." The philosophy underlying the reformulation of content is in synchrony with the direction in which rehabilitation health-care delivery is headed, while defining the "possibilities" for best practice usage of modalities. The message is clear. Given the need to rethink and retool how we inform our present and future clinicians, there is an undeniable need to integrate the use of modalities within the context of specific clinical diagnoses and symptomatology. In fact, Michlovitz, Bellew, and Nolan delineate curricular areas and courses in which components of this book can be best used. The point is clear and inescapable—modality usage is important, evidence for successful applications abound, and the notion of isolating modalities as a separate entity disconnected from the realities of comprehensive treatment is no longer a viable option.

Accordingly, the possibility which to some may still appear as a dream advocates for total integration of modalities within the context of core courses governed by evidence and documentation. In fact, each chapter is laced with multiple "key points," which for some students might be interpreted as the proverbial "what or why do I need to know this," clinical decision making examples, invaluable tips for documentation, and clinical controversies. The evolution of this text has come a long way since its creation. The book is now expanded from its original 317 pages and 12 chapters to 512 pages, 16 chapters, 13 contributors, and 10 reviewers. Sue Michlovitz has highlighted some of the newest components to this edition in the Preface. The text provides a comprehensive Introduction and then reviews all modalities relevant to contemporary practice. The importance and practicality of modalities, particularly neuromuscular electrical stimulation and functional electrical stimulation as they pertain to treatment of musculoskeletal and neurological disorders, pain symptoms and promotion of tissue healing are extraordinary.

Given the realities underlying best assimilation of new information, the anticipated glut of knowledge governing molecular science, bioengineering, and genomics that are filtering into rehabilitation professional curricula, the possibility of integrating information within problem-based learning can no longer be held as a dream. Perhaps when this text is reviewed after another 25 years, we can conclude that *Modalities for Therapeutic Intervention* (5th edition) heralded the endorsement of comprehensive, integrative evidence-based learning within rehabilitation curricula.

Steven L. Wolf, Ph.D., PT, FAPTA, FAHA
Editor-in Chief, Contemporary Perspectives in Rehabilitation Series
Atlanta, Georgia
May 2011

Preface to the Fifth Edition

Close to three decades ago, the first edition of *Thermal Agents in Rehabilitation* was a concept in development. At the time, I felt there was a need to teach "modalities" and write about them in a way that emphasized clinical decision-making for selection and application of these techniques. Emphasis prior to this time was on the "circuitry" and mechanistic steps in application. Of course, these latter points are important for safe and effective application, but effective use of modalities depends on a foundational understanding of the physiological effects and potential for healing. The first three editions were well received and used throughout the United States and Canada for entry-level PT courses. For the 4th edition, Dr. Tom Nolan joined in the venture as we repurposed the text to include aspects of electrotherapy.

Since the fourth edition was published, there has been increasing scrutiny of all techniques used in rehabilitation, with more and more evidence suggesting that what was "standard practice" for years may not have the efficacy once expected by the clinicians using those techniques. From this we have learned that modalities should be carefully selected for their intended effect to complement and enhance functional recovery.

In this fifth edition, Dr. Jim Bellew joins us for a new generation of how we present and teach concepts of modalities. Together, we optimistically look forward to improved and supported use of therapeutic modalities. Included in this revision is expanded content with special features that include:

1. Case scenarios incorporated throughout the text to enhance application of basic principles.
2. "Key Points" to indicate clinically important content and tips.
3. "Clinical Controversies" to discuss areas of misunderstanding or disagreement.
4. Expanded discussion of the principles and applications of electrotherapy.
5. Updated evidence from the research literature.
6. Discussion and applications of clinical EMG biofeedback.
7. A new chapter dedicated to clinical electroneuromyography examination.

The reader is encouraged to use the foundational materials in this text to supplement their knowledge base with new research as it appears. Practice and use with these techniques may be modified or expanded based upon new research findings.

Susan L. Michlovitz, PhD, PT, CHT

Preface to the First Edition

Thermal agents are used in physical therapy and rehabilitation to reduce pain, to enhance healing, and to improve motion. The physical therapist should have a solid foundation in the normal physiologic control of the cardiovascular and neuromuscular systems prior to using an agent that can alter the function of these structures. In addition, a background in the physiology of healing mechanisms and of pain serves as a basis for the rationale of using thermal agents.

Often, the decision to include a thermal agent in a therapy plan or to have the thermal agent be the sole treatment rendered (as in the case of the frequently used "hot packs and ultrasound combination" for back pain) is based on empirical evidence. The purpose of this book is to provide the reader with the underlying rationale for selection of an agent to be included in a therapy program, based on (1) the known physiologic and physical effects of that agent; (2) the safety and use of the heat/cold agent, given the conditions and limitations of the patient's dysfunction; and (3) the therapeutic goals for that particular patient. The authors have been asked to review critically the literature available that documents the efficacy and effectiveness of each thermal agent. A problem-solving approach to the use of thermal agents is stressed throughout the text.

The primary audience for this text is the physical therapist. The student will gain a solid foundation in thermal agents, the clinician will strengthen his or her perspective of thermal agents, and the researcher is given information that will provide ideas for clinical studies on thermal agents. Athletic trainers and other professionals who use thermal agents in their practice should find this text of value.

The text is in three parts. Part I, Foundations for the Use of Thermal Agents, includes information from basic and medical sciences that can serve as a framework for the choice to include thermal agents in a rehabilitation program. A discussion of the proposed mechanisms by which heat and cold can alter inflammation, healing, and pain is included in these chapters.

Part II of the text, Instrumentation: Methods and Application, incorporates concepts of equipment selection, operation and maintenance, and clinical application. The leading chapter in this part is on instrumentation principles and serves to introduce concepts of equipment circuitry and safety as applied to equipment used for thermal therapy. Physical therapists have become responsible for product purchase and making recommendations about products through the expansion of consultation services, private practices, sports medicine clinics, extended care facilities, and home health care. Therefore, we must be prepared to engage in dialogue with manufacturers, product distributors, and other colleagues about the safety and quality of these products. To this end, some practical suggestions are provided in Chapter 3 to assist with purchase decisions.

Chapters 4 though 8 discuss the operation and application of heat and cold agents. Numerous principles of clinical decision making are included within each chapter. There are certain principles inherent to all agent applications: (1) The patient must be evaluated and treatment goals established; (2) contraindications to treatment must be known; and (3) the safe and effective use of equipment must be understood.

Chapter 9, on low-power laser, deviates somewhat from the overall theme of thermal agents. Low-power laser is not expected to produce an increase in tissue temperature, so its effects could not be attributed to thermal mechanisms. Therefore, this cannot be categorized as a thermal agent. However, I believe this topic is worthy of inclusion in this text because (1) the indications for its use overlap those of thermal agents; (2) laser is a form of non-ionizing radiation, as are diathermy and ultrasound, which are used for pain reduction and tissue healing; and (3) laser would most likely be included in a physical therapy student curriculum in the coursework that includes thermal agents. At the time of this writing (summer 1985), low-power laser is still considered by the U.S. Food and Drug Administration as an investigational device. Only carefully designed clinical studies will help determine the laser's clinical efficacy—perhaps contributing to the body of knowledge needed to change the laser's status from an investigational to an accepted therapeutic product.

Part III, Clinical Decision Making, is designed to assist the student and clinician in integrating basic concepts that have been presented throughout the entire book, emphasizing problem solving and evaluation.

Much information has been published in the medical literature on the effects or clinical results of heat and cold application. Oftentimes, the therapist is called upon to justify the use of a certain modality. A careful review of the research literature may be necessary to provide an explanation for treatment.

There are many areas that require further investigation. For example, contrast baths (alternating heat and cold) are often used in sports medicine clinics. But a careful review of the literature reveals that only scanty information supports the use of contrast baths for any patient population. It is important for the clinician to be able to interpret accurately and to apply the methods and results that are presented in the literature. The inclusion of a chapter (Chapter 10) on techniques for reviewing the literature and establishing a paradigm for clinical studies of thermal agents provides the clinician with such a background on which to build.

Chapters 11 and 12 are devoted to specific patient populations in which thermal agents are commonly used. The chapter on sports medicine is representative of a population with a known cause of injury and predictable course of recovery. The majority of these patients are otherwise healthy. On the other hand, the chapter on rheumatic disease presents a model for a patient population that can be expected to have chronic recurrent—sometimes progressive—dysfunction associated with systemic manifestations.

An appendix is included: temperature conversion scales (this text uses the centigrade scale).

Susan L. Michlovitz, PhD, PT, CHT

Acknowledgments

It is not possible to produce a modalities text without the support of folks who sell and distribute such equipment. Thank you to Rich Silverstein of RAS Medical Systems, Inc. (Old Tappan, NJ) for providing us with much of the equipment we used in our photo shoots and to our photographer, Mark Lozier of Mark Lozier Photography (Cherry Hill, NJ) for providing us with clear and precise images. Many thanks to the crew at FA Davis, Melissa Duffield and George Lang, for working with us and keeping us on an even track through this project, and to our developmental editor, Susan Williams, of the Williams Company, Ltd. Thanks to the following Richard Stockton College physical therapy students for participating as models for the photo shoot: Jamie Umstetter, Brandon Dooley, Kavita Patel, and Matthew Romen, and to Sarah Monath for providing illustrations for figures in Chapter 6.

Biographies

Sue Michlovitz

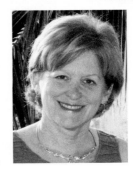

Sue Michlovitz, PT, PhD, CHT, has a physical therapy private practice, Cayuga Hand Therapy PT, in Ithaca, NY. Her clinical interests in hand therapy include arthritis, trauma, and disorders affecting the wrist. Dr. Michlovitz is an Adjunct Associate Professor, Rehabilitation Medicine, Columbia University, where she teaches in the Doctorate of Physical Therapy Program; an Associate Clinical Professor, Faculty of Rehabilitation Science, McMaster University, Hamilton, Ontario; and Professor, Rocky Mountain University of Health Professions, Provo, UT. Before moving to Ithaca in 2005, she was Professor, Department of Physical Therapy, Temple University, Philadelphia. Her published research has been in determining the effectiveness of therapy interventions and in reliability and validity of examination techniques, mostly related to hand and upper extremity conditions.

Dr. Michlovitz has extensive experience in teaching therapists at the American Physical Therapy Association (APTA) Combined Sections Meetings, American Society of Hand Therapists (ASHT) and American Association for Hand Surgery (AAHS) Annual Meetings, and the International Federation for Societies of Hand Therapists. She is assistant editor for Clinical Commentaries, *Journal of Hand Therapy*, and she serves on the editorial boards of *Hand* and *Techniques in Hand & Upper Extremity Surgery*.

Her volunteer outreach work is spent with Guatemala Healing Hands Foundation for teaching and patient care in Guatemala City. She lives in Ithaca, NY, with her husband, Paul Velleman, their bassett hound-beagle, Mr. Baxter, and a somewhat calico cat named Shayna. She is a wanna-be photojournalist.

James W. Bellew

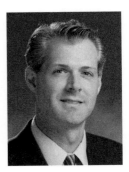

James W. Bellew, PT, EdD, is Associate Professor of Physical Therapy in the Krannert School of Physical Therapy at the University of Indianapolis. Dr. Bellew received his entry-level Bachelor of Science degree in Physical Therapy from Marquette University. After several years of clinical practice in Milwaukee, he received a Master of Science degree in Physical Therapy and Doctor of Education degree in Exercise Physiology, both from the University of Kentucky. His research encompasses the use of electrotherapeutic waveforms, muscle physiology, and control of balance in older adults. Dr. Bellew has published more than 50 peer-reviewed scientific manuscripts and abstracts in the areas of exercise training, balance, and muscle physiology. He teaches in the areas of clinical medicine, therapeutic modalities, and human physiology. He has previously served as a manuscript reviewer for *Archives of Physical Medicine and Rehabilitation, Physiotherapy Theory and Research, Journal of Pediatric Physical Therapy, Journal of Geriatric Physical Therapy, Journal of Women's Health Physical Therapy, Journal of Aging and Physical Activity,* and *Clinical Anatomy.* He is a regular presenter and speaker at APTA's Combined Sections Meetings and is routinely sought nationally and internationally for consultation regarding clinical applications of electrotherapeutic agents. He is a member of the APTA and specialty sections on Orthopedics and Clinical Electrophysiology and Wound Management. Dr. Bellew resides with his family in Indianapolis and maintains a regular clinical practice at St. Francis Hospital Outpatient Services.

Thomas P. Nolan Jr.

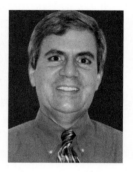

Thomas Patrick Nolan Jr., PT, DPT, OCS, is Associate Professor of Physical Therapy at Richard Stockton College of New Jersey. Dr. Nolan received his BS in Physical Therapy from New York University and his MS and DPT in Physical Therapy from Temple University. He is a certified orthopedic specialist (OCS) through the American Board of Physical Therapy Specialties. At Stockton College, Dr. Nolan teaches physical modalities and electrotherapy, kinesiology of the spine, musculoskeletal physical therapy for neck and back pain, and pharmacology. He is also the coordinator of physical therapy continuing education courses at Stockton College. His clinical practice is primarily with the Virtua Health Care System in southern New Jersey. He is a member of the American Physical Therapy Association, including the New Jersey Chapter, Clinical Electrophysiology and Wound Management Section, and the Orthopaedic Section. Tom lives in Marlton, NJ, where he enjoys running, playing volleyball, reading, hiking, camping, and spending time with his family.

Contributors

C. Scott Bickel, PT, PhD
Assistant Professor, Department of Physical Therapy
University of Alabama at Birmingham
Birmingham, Alabama

Elaine L. Bukowski,
PT, DPT, (D) ABDA Emeritus
Professor and Director, Department of Physical
Therapy
School of Health Sciences
Richard Stockton College of New Jersey
Pomona, New Jersey

Enrico M. Dellagatta, PT, MEd, DPT
Maple Leaf Physical Therapy
Hammonton, New Jersey

Stacie J. Fruth, PT, DHS
Associate Professor, Krannert School of Physical
Therapy
University of Indianapolis
Indianapolis, Indiana

Chris M. Gregory, PT, PhD
Assistant Professor, Department of Health Sciences
and Research
College of Health Professions
Medical University of South Carolina

Charles Hazle, PT, MS, PhD
Associate Professor, Center for Excellence in Rural
Health
University of Kentucky
Hazard, Kentucky

Therese E. Johnston, PT, PhD, MBA
Assistant Professor, Physical Therapy
University of the Sciences
Philadelphia, Pennsylvania

Ellen Lowe, PT, MHS
Professor, Department of Physical Therapy
Arizona School of Health Sciences
Mesa, Arizona

Ed Mahoney, PT, DPT, CWS
Assistant Professor
Louisiana State University Health Sciences Center
Shreveport, Louisiana

Arthur J. Nitz, PT, PhD
Professor
University of Kentucky
Lexington, Kentucky

Stephanie Petterson, PT, PhD
Adjunct Assistant Professor, Columbia University
Regional Clinical Director, Sports Physical Therapy of
New York
New York, New York

Sandy Rennie, PT, PhD
Director and Associate Professor, School of
Physiotherapy
Dalhousie University
Halifax, Nova Scotia

Karen J. Sparrow, PT, PhD
Former Director, Transitional DPT Program
Virginia Commonwealth University Medical Center
Richmond, Virginia

Reviewers

Karen W. Albaugh, PT, DPT, MPH, CWS
Assistant Professor, Department of Physical Therapy
Neumann University
Aston, Pennsylvania

Clarence Chan, PT, DPT
Associate Professor, Department of Health Sciences
LaGuardia Community College, City University of
New York
Long Island City, New York

John DeWitt, PT, DPT, SCS, ATC
Assistant Clinical Professor, Division of Physical
Therapy
The Ohio State University
Columbus, Ohio

Burke Gurney, PT, PhD
Associate Professor, Orthopaedics and Rehabilitation
Department
University of New Mexico
Albuquerque, New Mexico

John Steven Halle, PT, PhD, ECS
Chair and Associate Dean, School of Physical Therapy
Belmont University
Nashville, Tennessee

M. Alysia Mastrangelo, PT, PhD
Associate Professor, Department of Physical Therapy
Richard Stockton College of New Jersey
Pomona, New Jersey

James T. Mills, III, PT, MS, ECS, OCS
Major, Command and General Staff College Inter-
Agency Fellowship Program
Department of Veterans Affairs
Washington, D.C.

Carey Rothschild, PT, DPT, OCS, CSCS
Instructor, Department of Health Professions
University of Central Florida
Orlando, Florida

Wayne B. Scott, PT, PhD
Assistant Professor, Department of Physical Therapy
Husson University
Bangor, Maine

Andrew J Starsky, PT, BSEE, PhD
Clinical Assistant Professor, Department of Physical
Therapy
Marquette University
Milwaukee, Wisconsin

Contents

SECTION III CLINICAL APPLICATIONS OF MODALITIES 279

How to Use This Book

Therapeutic Modalities as a Curricular Thread

Traditional classroom and lab-based education in the principles and administration of therapeutic modalities has remained a cornerstone in educational programs within the rehabilitation sciences. The history and evolution of the clinical rehabilitation sciences have shown that certain areas of practice, such as electrical stimulation for denervated muscle or ultraviolet treatment for psoriasis, have waned whereas other areas of clinical practice, such as integumentary or wound care and oncology, have grown immensely over the past few decades. Consequently, curricular content has accordingly undergone continual change and updating. This flux of curricular content reflects the advancement of scientific discovery and application and the mounting rise of literature to bolster evidence-based practice. The fact that curricular content given to principles and applications of therapeutic modalities has remained pervasive in educational programs within the rehabilitation sciences substantiates the continued contribution of this area of practice to the more encompassing patient management model.

Although principles and applications of therapeutic modalities remain foundational content in most programs in the rehabilitative sciences, this content is far too often insular or taught apart from other curricular content, such as orthopedics and neurologic rehabilitation, integumentary care, patient management, and other areas. This is wholly ironic because therapeutic modalities represent a group of interventions used to augment or supplement interventions taught in these course areas. Many areas of rehabilitative science, such as orthopedics or neurologic rehabilitation, are taught with strategic course sequencing with content increasing accordingly in more advanced courses. However, content in therapeutic modalities often exists in a single "how to" course or, worse yet, a smaller part of a single course. Few educational programs sequence curricular content in therapeutic modalities in a progressive manner. Rather, therapeutic modalities are often taught separate from the interventions they complement. For example, orthopedic or musculoskeletal courses include instruction in rehabilitation following surgical repair of the anterior cruciate ligament. Incorporation of the use of therapeutic modalities, such as neuromuscular electrical stimulation, biofeedback, or cryotherapy, reflects the reality of clinical care and better represents the complete patient management model than teaching these elements in a separated or disengaged manner. Because therapeutic modalities are too frequently taught in isolation, students receive a limited "one-time" exposure. It is our intention that this book be used not only in the primary therapeutic modalities course but also in courses where therapeutic modalities supplement or complement the interventions taught in those content-specific course areas, such as orthopedics, neurologic rehabilitation, and others.

At risk is clinical competency when therapeutic modalities are taught in isolation with little to no carry-through in the curriculum to relate or connect therapeutic modalities to those conditions or impairments for which they are advocated. It is our suggestion that the content of this book be used throughout the curriculum where therapeutic modalities offer adjunctive interventions. By maintaining continuity throughout the curriculum between therapeutic modalities and the specific clinical areas of their supported application, a curricular thread is created, thereby improving clinical decision-making skills and competency.

The table on the next page represents specific chapter content in this text and the potential curricular areas where use of therapeutic modalities are part of common clinical practice. It is our belief that the content of this text may be threaded or cross-referenced across the curriculum to reinforce the supplementary role that is offered by therapeutic modalities.

Susan L. Michlovitz, PT, PhD, CHT
James W. Bellew, PT, EdD
Thomas P. Nolan Jr. PT, DPT, OCS

CHAPTER CONTENT	RELATED CURRICULAR AREAS
Therapeutic modalities for:	*Cross-referenced courses:*
Flexibility/ROM Thermotherapy (Chapter 3) Ultrasound (Chapter 4) Hydrotherapy (Chapter 5) Traction (Chapter 7)	Orthopedics, Neurological Rehabilitation, Therapeutic Exercise, Kinesiology, Integumentary for US and Hydrotherapy
Strengthening NMES (Chapters 9, 10, 11) Biofeedback (Chapter 11)	Orthopedics, Therapeutic Exercise, Exercise Science/Physiology, Neurological Rehabilitation
Neuromuscular Reeducation FES (Chapters 9, 10, 12) Biofeedback (Chapter 11)	Neurological Rehabilitation, Orthopedics
Pain Modulation Cryotherapy and thermotherapy (Chapters 2, 3) Ultrasound (Chapter 4) Hydrotherapy (Chapter 5) LASER and diathermy (Chapter 6) Traction (Chapter 7) Electrotherapy (Chapters 9, 10, 13) Alternative modalities (Chapter 15)	Orthopedics, Integumentary
Tissue Healing Electrotherapy (Chapters 10, 14) Hydrotherapy (Chapter 5) Cryotherapy and thermotherapy (Chapters 2, 3) Ultrasound (Chapter 4) Compression (Chapter 8) Alternative modalities (Chapter 15)	Orthopedics, Neurological Rehabilitation, Integumentary, Pharmacology
Neurodiagnostics EMG and NCV (Chapter 16)	Orthopedics, Neurological Rehabilitation

Introduction

Chapter 1
Therapeutic Modalities
A Role in the Patient Care Management Model

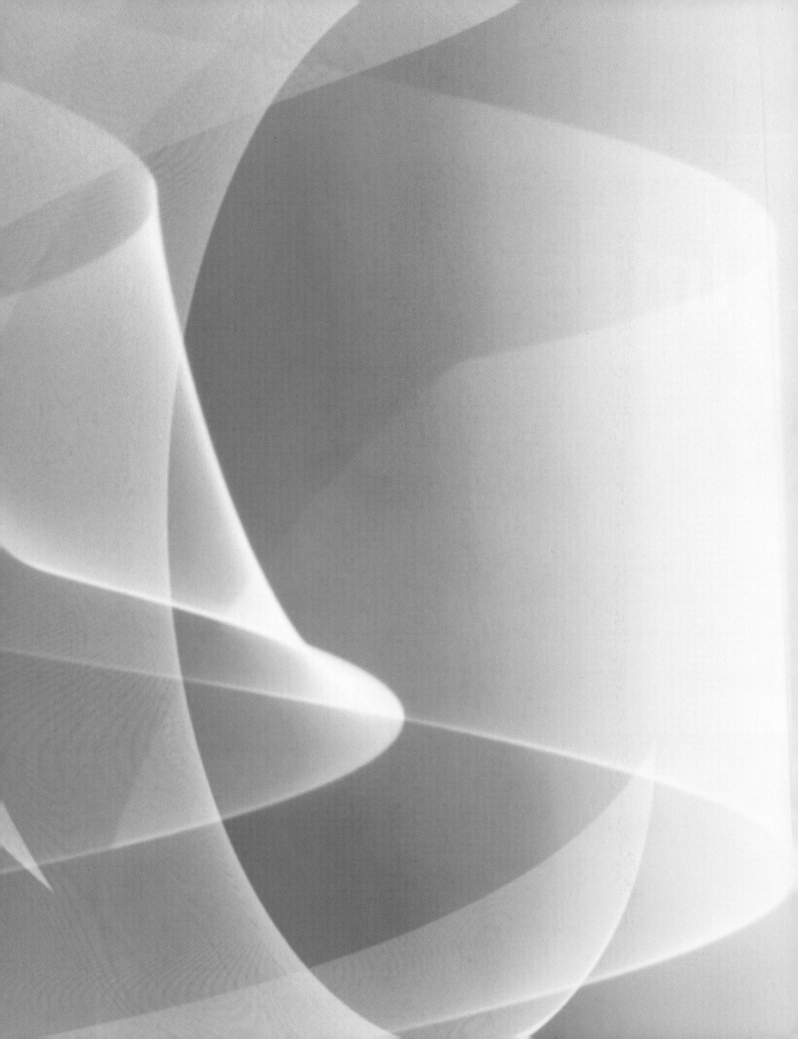

Therapeutic Modalities
A Role in the Patient Care Management Model

James W. Bellew, PT, EdD | Susan L. Michlovitz, PT, PhD, CHT

Way to go! You just completed a thorough examination of a patient who sustained a left knee injury with suspected damage to the medial collateral ligament. You selected accurate clinical testing tools, applied critical thinking in differentiating findings, and documented the patient's impairments and disabilities. You found (1) decreased passive and active range of motion into flexion secondary, in part, to wearing a long leg immobilizer for the past 10 days; (2) three-centimeter greater swelling around the joint center compared to the uninvolved side; (3) decreased strength and ability to volitionally contract the quadriceps femoris; and (4) pain rated at 6 out of 10 with palpation of the medial joint line of the knee.

So what's next? You need to identify an intervention strategy to address these findings of the examination and the patient history—and this might be the most challenging part. Which limitation of body function or impairment do you work with first? What do you choose to do? Do you choose a therapeutic modality? How do you decide? What information do you use in your decision-making process? Do you do what you have seen other clinicians do? Do you do something that you have experience with and are comfortable with? Do you choose an intervention based on convenience for the patient, for you, or for your clinical environment? Does cost of time and money play a role in your decision-making? What about evidence in the literature to support your choice? When do you decide to switch from one choice to another? What do you plan to do in the first few weeks of rehabilitation versus the latter weeks? What are your patient's goals and expectations?

These questions and others represent the basis of *clinical decision-making*. Competency with clinical decision-making is the basis for effective patient outcomes and attainment of goals.

Therapeutic Modalities: Roles in Rehabilitation

Therapeutic modalities represent the administration of thermal, mechanical, electromagnetic, and light energies for a specific therapeutic effect (to decrease pain, increase range of motion, improve tissue healing, or improve muscle recruitment). Therapeutic modalities have long been part of rehabilitation and complement other elements of the more comprehensive therapy plan, such as therapeutic exercise (strengthening, stretching, neuromuscular re-education, balance), manual therapy (joint and tissue mobilization, manipulation), and patient education (body mechanics, postural retraining, home exercise program, risk reduction).

KEY POINT! The terms *therapeutic modalities* and *physical agents* are often used interchangeably to describe a wide array of treatments and interventions used by therapists to provide a variety of therapeutic benefits. The term *physical agents* reflects the use of physical energies such as thermal, mechanical, electromagnetic, or light but fails to include the purpose or intention of their application. The term *therapeutic modalities,* as used throughout this text, more appropriately reflects the ability of these interventions to provide therapeutic benefits in the patient care management model.

For the patient just evaluated, cold therapy and compression may be used initially to limit the swelling and pain as the patient begins the early phases of rehabilitation. Ultrasound or heat therapy may be applied to improve elasticity of the medial collateral ligament and joint capsular structures prior to beginning range-of-motion (ROM) activities after the swelling has subsided. Electrical stimulation may be used to increase activation and volitional recruitment of the quadriceps muscle until the patient can effectively contract the muscle and begin additional activities. All of these options are viable, but you may not choose all of them! While the effectiveness of each of these treatments will vary between patients, the practitioner is challenged to identify which patients are more likely to respond to a specific intervention. In this manner, sound clinical decision-making involves the practitioner considering or judging the probability or likelihood that a given intervention will help a given patient.

Clinical decision-making can therefore be thought of as the process of using information, experience, and judgments to decide which clinical interventions will most likely improve the problems identified in the examination. The bottom line is this: When identifying and establishing an intervention plan, the focus should be on selecting interventions that will most likely achieve positive results or outcomes—both quantitative and qualitative. When judiciously selected and applied, therapeutic modalities may play a significant role in successful patient care.

We are often challenged by patients who have multiple impairments and dysfunctions. Our role as experts in rehabilitation is to identify and skillfully provide interventions to address these impairments, thus providing optimal recovery of function. Even when facing a seemingly uncomplicated patient case whose therapy plan is clear, the emergence of confounding variables often impacts the execution of the initial plan of care. Imagine this happening during therapy: Your patient, who has decreased ROM and strength, is unable to complete the appropriate therapeutic activities to address ROM and strength because of underlying pain, or your patient has significant swelling of the knee and is unable to effectively contract the quadriceps secondary to effusion inhibition. While increasing ROM and strength or volitional muscle recruitment are obvious goals in the plan of care, attention may first need to be given to decreasing the pain or reducing the effusion to help the patient continue with the therapy plan. In their assessment of how therapeutic modalities affect muscle inhibition following knee joint effusion, Hopkins et al.[1] reported that effusion-induced inhibition of the quadriceps was temporarily suspended with application of cold or transcutaneous electrical nerve stimulation (TENS), noting a near complete reversal of quadriceps inhibition. This finding provides a rationale for using therapeutic modalities as complements to the therapy plan.

KEY POINT! In many patient cases, therapeutic modalities may be used to attenuate or overcome factors that hinder continuation of the therapy plan. This emphasizes the role that therapeutic modalities play.

Modalities as Part of the Comprehensive Plan

Therapeutic modalities have long been used in rehabilitation, and history of their use is well documented. With advancing technology and scientific discovery has come the evolution and emergence of newer modalities that add to the spectrum of interventional strategies and that enhance their role in rehabilitation. Use of therapeutic modalities has been and will remain a cornerstone to rehabilitation for joint and soft tissue injury, acute and chronic pain, and impaired muscle function. Whether used only during specific phases of rehabilitation or throughout the entire rehab program, therapeutic modalities represent a group of interventions that are adjunctive components of a more comprehensive therapy plan. Figure 1-1 depicts the complementary role therapeutic modalities play in the complete intervention plan.

Clinicians should review current evidence when therapeutic modalities are considered as adjuncts for an intervention plan. Many techniques in common use have not been studied, which has led to scientific inquiry addressing the efficacy of many therapeutic modalities. However, it should be noted that many studies examining the effectiveness of therapeutic modalities often assess their efficacy when used alone or in isolation—separate from and counter to the supplementary role that we and the APTA advocate.

KEY POINT! The American Physical Therapy Association's (APTA's) position statement on the use of therapeutic modalities states that "without documentation that justifies the necessity of the exclusive use of physical agents, the use of physical agents, in the absence of other skilled therapeutic or educational intervention, should not be considered physical therapy."[2] This statement reflects the standpoint from which we, the authors of this text, attempt to present the use and administration of and evidence for therapeutic modalities as supplementary, not stand-alone, therapy.

Types of Therapeutic Modalities

Therapeutic modalities are generally categorized as *thermal* (heat and cold), *electromagnetic* (electrotherapy, diathermy, ultraviolet and infrared light), or *mechanical* (traction and compression). These modalities are used to increase the probability of a specific therapeutic effect (e.g., decreased pain, increased range of motion, tissue healing, or improved muscle recruitment). Therapeutic modalities may be procedural, in-clinic interventions, such as ultrasound, or they may be home-based interventions, such as ice packs or continuous, low-level heat wraps; these serve to enhance additional therapeutic interventions identified in the more extensive plan of care, such as range of motion or muscle strengthening.

KEY POINT! The term *therapeutic modality* can imply a *type* of energy used by the modality, a specific *range* of that energy, or the *method* of application of that modality.

Remember the impairments you found in your evaluation of the patient with a suspected knee injury—decreased range of motion, decreased strength, pain, and swelling? These are just a few of the many problems therapeutic modalities may be used for, but again, in conjunction with other interventions. In this manner,

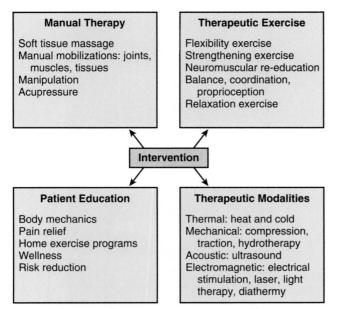

Manual Therapy	Therapeutic Exercise
Soft tissue massage Manual mobilizations: joints, muscles, tissues Manipulation Acupressure	Flexibility exercise Strengthening exercise Neuromuscular re-education Balance, coordination, proprioception Relaxation exercise

Intervention

Patient Education	Therapeutic Modalities
Body mechanics Pain relief Home exercise programs Wellness Risk reduction	Thermal: heat and cold Mechanical: compression, traction, hydrotherapy Acoustic: ultrasound Electromagnetic: electrical stimulation, laser, light therapy, diathermy

Fig 1•1 Therapeutic modalities represent a diverse group of interventions that add to and complement other therapies that are part of the comprehensive rehabilitation plan.

therapeutic modalities are used to increase the chances that certain clinical outcomes are realized.

The term *therapeutic modality* can have several meanings and is variable based on the context in which the term is used. For example, ultrasound represents both a *form* of energy (i.e., sound energy) and a specific *range* of energy (i.e., greater than 20,000 Hz). By convention, ultrasound has come to represent a *method* or means of delivering a therapeutic modality. It is prudent to be as specific as possible regarding the administration of a modality. When applying ultrasound, for example, it is recommended that the specific frequency used (i.e., 1 MHz or 3.3 MHz) be documented in addition to documenting the form of energy applied (i.e., ultrasound).

KEY POINT! Human hearing can detect sound frequencies ranging from approximately 15,000 to 20,000 Hz. Thus, *ultrasound* is named for the frequency range above human hearing.

Thermal Modalities: Cold and Heat

Cryotherapy

Cryotherapy (i.e., cold therapy) is the use of cold to induce the therapeutic and physiological responses that result from a decrease in tissue temperature. Therapeutic application of cold will result in reduced blood flow and tissue metabolism—physiological responses used to decrease bleeding and acute inflammation following injury or tissue disruption. The application of cold also results in a reduction in pain as the threshold for pain perception is elevated, thereby desensitizing peripheral afferent nociceptors.[3] Collectively, reducing swelling and pain may permit patients to complete the other components of the therapy plan, again reinforcing the supplementary role of modalities.

Therapeutic cold can be applied using ice, cold water, cold gel-filled packs, or vapocoolant sprays. Cold packs and ice packs are the most common and familiar applications of therapeutic cold (Fig. 1-2). Ice packs can easily be made at home and used as part of the patient's home program. Commercially made cold packs often contain a gel-like substance that allows the cold pack to mold to the affected body part. Cold water may provide therapeutic benefit and may be applied as cool whirlpool, cold water baths, or added to ice packs to create a slushy ice-water mixture that can be molded to the body part.

In addition, larger pieces of ice held in the hand may be used to provide an ice massage (Fig. 1-3) or may be used as an "ice pop" (Fig. 1-4). Also used to reduce tissue temperature are topical, or vapocoolant, sprays (such as Spray and Stretch) that result in rapid, superficial, and short-lived tissue cooling by means of evaporation.

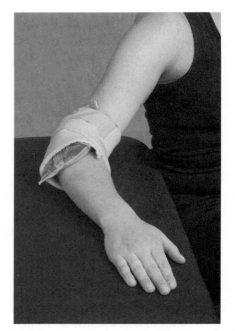

Fig 1•2 Cold therapy can be applied by use of gel or ice packs.

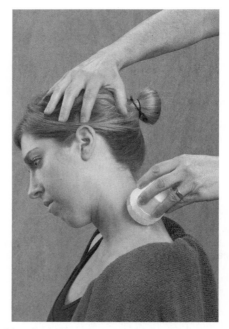

Fig 1•3 Handheld ice cups provide cold therapy during an ice massage.

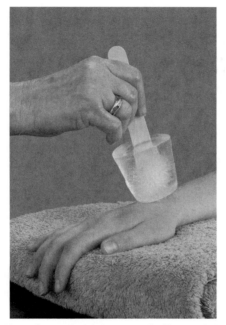

Fig 1•4 Use of handheld "ice pops" offers quick and efficient cold therapy to many areas where cold packs may be less effective.

Which application of therapeutic cold is most appropriate and most effective will depend on several factors, including but not limited to the size of the affected area, the depth of the tissues to be treated, the patient's tolerance to cold, and whether the application will occur in the clinic or at home. More extensive descriptions of cryotherapy and therapeutic use of cold are found in Chapter 2.

Thermotherapy

The therapeutic application of heat provides a variety of benefits that augment the comprehensive therapy plan. Application of heat may facilitate tissue healing; relax skeletal muscles and decrease spasms; decrease pain; promote an increase in blood flow; and prepare joints, capsular structures, muscles, and other soft tissues for stretching, mobilization, and exercise.[4-7]

Heat can be applied in many forms and through various mediums. Warm water as used in a bath or whirlpool has long been used in rehabilitation and can easily be used at home. Use of heat packs, both in-clinic and at home, have led to the commercial production of single-use heat wraps that can be placed on various body regions (Fig. 1-5). Heat may also be delivered through the use of light, sound, and electromagnetic

energies. The warmth of the sun's rays is a well-known example of heat transfer via ultraviolet energy. Shortwave diathermy can provide therapeutic heat through the use of electromagnetic energy, and acoustical or sound energy from ultrasound can be used to increase tissue temperature. Warm water and hot packs are used to raise tissue temperature in the skin and the superficial subcutaneous tissues, whereas continuous-wave ultrasound and shortwave diathermy are better suited to raising temperature is deeper tissues (up to 5 cm in depth). Selection of the appropriate form of therapeutic heat will depend on several factors, including the area to be treated, the depth of the tissues to be heated, the patient's tolerance to heat, the patient's medical history, and the interventions to be used that are complemented by therapeutic heat. More extensive detail on therapeutic heat and its application is presented in Chapter 3.

Electromagnetic Modalities

Electrotherapy

Electrical currents are used for a wide variety of therapeutic benefits and for an equally wide variety of needs. General therapeutic benefits of electrotherapy may include strengthening and relaxing skeletal muscle, decreasing pain, facilitating neuromuscular reeducation, augmenting range of motion, attenuating disuse atrophy, promoting tissue and wound healing, reducing edema,

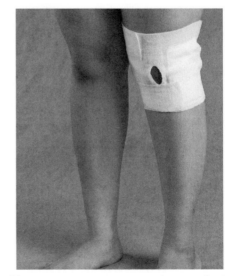

Fig 1•5 Heat wraps are an easy and convenient source of heat therapy.

increasing local blood flow, and delivering medicinal ions transdermally. The robust and wide-ranging therapeutic benefits of electrotherapy are derived from the selection of specific parameters of electrical currents such as amplitude, duration, and frequency.

Fundamental to most applications of electrical stimulation is the depolarization, or activation, of peripheral nerves. Use of TENS to decrease perception of pain is one of the most widely recognized applications of electrotherapy and its clinical effects have been extensively researched.[8–10] Activation of skeletal muscle is used for increasing strength (known as *neuromuscular electrical stimulation,* or NMES), or for restoring or improving use of skeletal muscle during functional activities such as walking (known as *functional electrical stimulation,* or FES; Fig. 1-6). Research continues to delineate the benefits of electrotherapy for actuation of skeletal muscle.[11,12]

Use of certain electrotherapeutic currents have also demonstrated specific and unique effects on cell populations found in wounds and healing tissues.[13–16] Iontophoresis is the use of electrical current to facilitate the delivery of specific drugs and ions to reduce tissue inflammation, decrease local pain, reduce calcium deposits, and reduce scar restrictions. More extensive descriptions of the principles and applications of electrotherapy are presented in Chapters 9 and 10.

Electromagnetic radiation is used for a variety of therapeutic benefits, both thermal and nonthermal. Classified according to the specific frequency of the electromagnetic wave, therapeutic electromagnetic radiation includes shortwave diathermy (SWD), infrared radiation (IR), and ultraviolet (UVA and UVB) radiation. Continuous shortwave diathermy and infrared are used to increase tissue temperature. IR increases temperature more in superficial tissues while SWD heats both superficial and deep tissues (Fig. 1-7). The therapeutic benefits of tissue heating complement soft tissue and joint mobilization,[17,18] muscle activation,[19] flexibility,[17] tissue healing,[20] and pain modulation.[19,21]

SWD has primarily been used as a thermal modality. Nonthermal benefits of therapeutic electromagnetic radiation (e.g., UVA and UVB and pulsed diathermy) remain somewhat unclear but are thought to affect activity at the cellular level, perhaps by altering permeability of the semipermeable phospholipid bilayer, enhancing metabolic activity of the cell and production of adenosine triphosphate (ATP), or altering the activity of membrane-bound cell proteins.[20] More detailed descriptions of the therapeutic benefits and applications of electromagnetic energy are provided in Chapter 6.

Mechanical Modalities

Compression

Force, either of a compressive or distractive nature, may be used for therapeutic benefit during rehabilitation. Compressive force may come from application of wraps, stockings, or garments. Compression may also

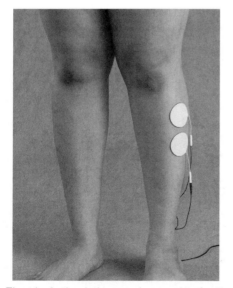

Fig 1•6 Electrical stimulation can be used to facilitate functional activities. Stimulation of the anterior tibialis in patients with impaired activation can assist in dorsiflexion of the ankle during gait.

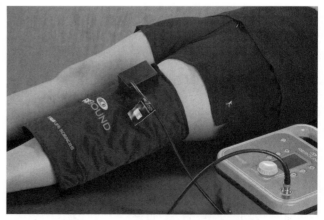

Fig 1•7 Diathermy provides heating of deep tissues and may precede stretching or other ROM activities.

come from compression pumps and even from water via the hydrostatic pressure created when a body part is submerged in water. Compression techniques are applied to prevent, attenuate, or reverse swelling that may follow soft tissue injury or compromise the circulatory system, or they may be applied to alter formation of scar tissue during the proliferation and maturation phase of scarring. The principal mechanism underlying the use of compression for the management of edema is an increase in applied external compression on the body or body part to increase hydrostatic pressure in the interstitial space. By increasing hydrostatic pressure of the interstitial space, a counterpressure is directed at the outflow of fluid from the compromised vessels, thereby reducing the accumulation of fluid in the interstitial space. Compression may also be used during the formation and modeling of scar tissue (e.g., following burn injury) to minimize scar formation and reduce hypertrophic scarring. Unlike collagen synthesis, which requires oxygen, collagen lysis does not require oxygen, therefore compression can be used to limit scar formation while not affecting scar lysis[22] (Fig. 1-8).

Traction

Mechanical or manual traction is the application of distractive forces to lessen or reduce compression on a structure and is most commonly associated with spinal traction (Fig. 1-9). By separating or reducing compression of adjacent segments, such as joints, or reducing pressure on anatomical structures, such as nerves, blood vessels, and joint capsules, traction may be used to decrease pain, increase range of motion, improve functional ability, increase blood flow, and reduce muscle guarding. Manual therapy, exercises for muscle strengthening and retraining, and neural mobilization are often incorporated in conjunction with traction as part of a patient's care plan.[23–26] Devices are available that allow the patient to perform traction at home as part of a comprehensive rehabilitation program. Chapter 7 details the therapeutic benefits and clinical application of traction, along with the controversies of proposed effects of these techniques.

Clinical Applications of Therapeutic Modalities

Modulation of Pain

Pain may be the most common symptom leading patients to seek medical intervention. The unique experiences of pain among individuals make this a challenging alteration in body function to manage. The neurobiophysiology of pain generation, transmission, and perception is well described in other sources, and all academic programs in rehabilitation sciences contain curricular content given to the description of pain.[27,28]

Early discussions of pain modulation centered on interrupting the ascending pathways of pain (i.e., blocking the transmission of pain along the nerve pathways to more central centers). Widely recognized as the "gate control" theory of pain, this theory described a relationship between painful sensory input carried by small myelinated A-delta and unmyelinated C fibers

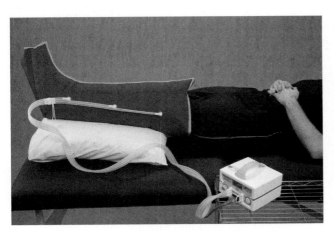

Fig 1•8 Compression can be used to limit or reduce swelling that often follows soft tissue damage.

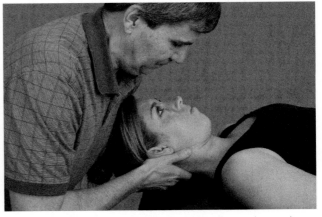

Fig 1•9 Manual or mechanical traction is used to reduce the compression on a structure, such as a joint, nerve, or tissue. Both clinical and home-based forms of traction are used for therapeutic benefit.

versus larger diameter and myelinated A-beta nerve fibers.[29] According to this theory, noxious stimuli carried by A-delta and C fibers are blocked by sensory input along A-beta fibers. Logically, then, efforts to treat pain are often directed at stimulating the large A-beta fibers through various means. Electrical stimulation targeting large afferent nerve fibers is common to rehabilitation, as is the use of ultrasound, cold, heat, diathermy, and other treatments to decrease or modulate noxious sensory input.

Understanding the neurobiophysiology of pain generation, transmission, and perception has grown immensely since the origination of the gate control theory. For a more detailed description of the neurobiophysiology of pain, the reader is directed to other resources.[28]

KEY POINT! The attention given to the gate control theory of pain in the late 1960s and early 1970s spurred tremendous growth and development of handheld electrical stimulators designed to provide electrical stimuli to A-beta fibers. This period is considered the birth of TENS and other devices to deliver such currents.

Modulating pain is undoubtedly a central focus of rehabilitation, both in the initial stages and throughout the therapy plan. Because the presence of pain may limit or even preclude rehabilitative efforts to restore or increase function, attempts to decrease pain often coincide with or even precede efforts toward restoring function. Following the initial injury, for example, soft tissue insult may result in a cascade of inflammatory and reparative physiological events manifesting in pain. Swelling secondary to vascular damage may result in compression of nearby structures, and chemical irritants associated with injury (e.g., bradykinin, PGE1, PGE2) may be released; both of these result in the generation and transmission of pain. Use of therapeutic modalities such as cold and compression in the initial stages following injury can reduce swelling and limit production and accumulation of pain-associated chemicals, thereby reducing the patient's perception of pain. This initial reduction of pain can then allow the patient to initiate activities as part of the larger therapy plan (Fig. 1-10).

In the later stages of rehabilitation, therapeutic modalities such as ultrasound may be used to

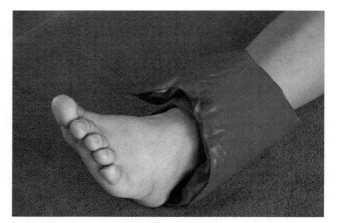

Fig 1•10 Cold therapy is often used during the initial stages of injury to decrease swelling and pain. The reduction of pain and swelling may allow the completion of other activities of the rehab plan.

facilitate formation and organization of collagen when administered right before soft tissue mobilization and flexibility exercises. Likewise, muscle weakness and lack of neuromuscular coordination have been associated with dysfunctional movement patterns, and practitioners commonly acknowledge that pain may result from these dysfunctional movement patterns. Electrical stimulation and electromyographic (EMG) biofeedback can be used to increase muscular strength and coordination, thus addressing the underlying factors related to the movement dysfunction.

To reduce pain, therapeutic modalities may act locally at the site of injury and inflammation to limit the local chemical irritants; this positively impacts the perception of pain by reducing or attenuating the initial creation and generation of pain. (The local effects of therapeutic modalities on tissue's response to injury are addressed in chapters throughout this text and are a strong focus of Chapter 14.) The activity and direction of the migration of specific cells associated with the healing response of tissues, such as neutrophils and macrophages, can be influenced by applying therapeutic modalities such as electrical stimulation. This is further evidence of the enhanced effect on healing that can be harnessed with the use of therapeutic modalities.[15,16,30]

KEY POINT! Modalities are used to improve or ameliorate alterations in body function, such as loss of range of motion, pain, and other tissue damage.

Alteration of Skeletal Muscle Performance: Facilitation and Inhibition

Therapeutic modalities can be used both directly and indirectly to influence the activity and performance of skeletal muscle to increase or decrease levels of muscle activation for therapeutic benefit. Direct applications of therapeutic modalities to facilitate skeletal muscle performance may occur, for example, by using electrical stimulation to depolarize peripheral nerves in order to recruit more motor units. A patient with decreased ability to contract the quadriceps after knee surgery may demonstrate increased muscle recruitment following application of electrical stimulation.

Neuromuscular electrical stimulation (NMES) and functional electrical stimulation (FES) are used to increase strength, endurance, and functional use of skeletal muscle for a variety of therapeutic purposes. More recent evidence shows that NMES directly increases the volume or total number of motor units recruited and the duration those motor units are activated; these are both fundamental to the positive adaptations underlying gains in strength seen with NMES.[31] Facilitation of skeletal muscle in patients with compromised ability to activate specific muscles or muscle groups can be used to assist in functional activities such as retraining gait; increasing function of the upper extremity and hand; improving range of motion; decreasing spasticity; and exercising to prevent muscle atrophy, cardiorespiratory decline, and bone degradation[32–34] (Fig. 1-11).

Modalities such as heat, cold, or electrical stimulation may also be used to directly inhibit, or decrease, skeletal muscle activity. By decreasing motor nerve conduction velocity and sympathetic activity in the injured muscles, modalities can play a large role in rehabilitating skeletal muscle. For example, a patient with hyperactivity of skeletal muscle following acute trauma from a whiplash injury may benefit from application of electrical stimulation to decrease muscular activity in the involved muscles, thus permitting range-of-motion activities (Fig. 1-12).

Modalities can also act indirectly on skeletal muscle, resulting in increased or decreased activation. By decreasing pain, therapeutic modalities may act indirectly on muscle and result in increased muscle performance. For example, a patient with subacute lumbar

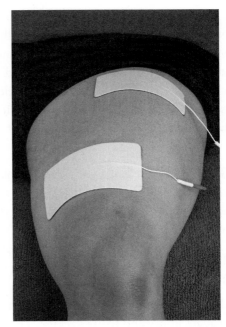

Fig 1•11 Neuromuscular electrical stimulation is used to increase strength, prevent or limit atrophy, and reeducate muscles. Electrical stimulation alters the manner in which muscle is activated providing a stimulus for positive adaptation.

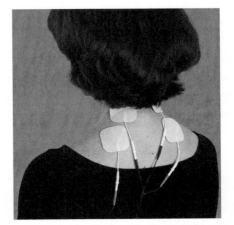

Fig 1•12 Electrical stimulation can be used to decrease the excitability or hyperactivity of skeletal muscle following injury.

radiculopathy (e.g., low back injury with radiating pain due to nerve irritation) resulting from a lifting injury may report decreased pain after administration of cold modalities. This may allow the patient to complete stabilization exercises that he or she was otherwise unable to perform because of pain. Cold application may also act indirectly on muscle activity by decreasing the synaptic activity of peripheral sensory nerves; this, in turn, may elevate the pain threshold, potentially allowing improved skeletal muscle activation secondary to decreased pain. Likewise, altering either blood flow to the muscle or cell membrane transport in muscle tissues via ultrasound, diathermy, cold or heat modalities may indirectly facilitate improved performance of skeletal muscle.

KEY POINT! If you cannot explain the physiological and clinical reasoning for using the therapeutic modality you select, then perhaps you should not be using the technique!

Decreasing Inflammation and Facilitating Tissue Healing

Use of therapeutic modalities often is recommended following acute injury and tissue damage. The primary goals at this point are to minimize inflammation and promote the most expedient and effective healing process. While it is critical to keep in mind that the *inflammatory stage* is the beginning of the process of tissue healing, use of therapeutic modalities can facilitate and augment progression through the stages of healing so as to provide expedient yet effective healing (Table 1-1).

Cold therapy has long been a standard treatment for the inflammation that occurs in the first several days following acute injury. Cold therapy can decrease local blood flow and metabolic activity in the involved tissues. This provides support for using cold modalities in

the period following injury when vascular increases in permeability and the resultant swelling are likely. The analgesic effect of cold modalities also offers palliative benefit to the patient after injury. Use of electrical stimulation or compression to minimize leakage of large blood proteins from damaged vessels and to limit agglutination of proteins in the interstitial space can minimize duration and residual effects of the inflammatory phase.

The *proliferation stage* follows the onset of the acute inflammatory stage and is characterized by the production, organization, and infiltration of collagen at the site of tissue damage. Collagen serves to repair damaged tissue and represents the first stages in the formation of new tissue. Cells involved in the healing process, such as macrophages and neutrophils, demonstrate unique and specific behaviors as they migrate to the site of tissue repair.[13,16] Bloodborne proteins such as fibrinogen and fibronectin aggregate in the involved area, acting to reinforce collagen in the injured tissue. Modalities such as superficial heat, ultrasound, and diathermy can facilitate and enhance local blood flow and cellular activity, thereby promoting the proliferation, or repair, of the damaged tissue.

The third and final stage of tissue healing is the *maturation stage*. This stage is characterized by the modeling, remodeling, organization, and maturation of collagen into new tissue and may last from several days to years. Therapeutic modalities such as ultrasound are commonly used to influence the maturation and organization of collagen. Heating collagen tissue by applying ultrasound complements stretching and mobilization of newly formed, maturing collagen. This heat-and-stretch aids in restoring functional integrity to the newly formed and repaired tissue.

Increasing Tissue Extensibility: Flexibility and Range of Motion (ROM)

Efficiency of functional movement depends on flexibility, and because disuse, immobilization, and detraining can negatively impact flexibility, rehabilitation often focuses on maintaining and restoring flexibility. Flexibility in tissue is largely related to the amount, organization, and extensibility of collagen—the primary protein imparting integrity to connective tissue.[35]

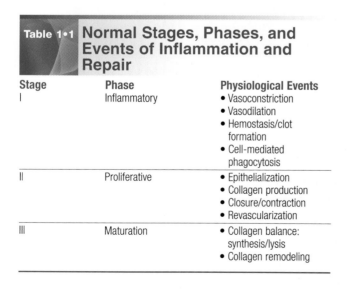

Table 1•1	Normal Stages, Phases, and Events of Inflammation and Repair	
Stage	**Phase**	**Physiological Events**
I	Inflammatory	• Vasoconstriction • Vasodilation • Hemostasis/clot formation • Cell-mediated phagocytosis
II	Proliferative	• Epithelialization • Collagen production • Closure/contraction • Revascularization
III	Maturation	• Collagen balance: synthesis/lysis • Collagen remodeling

Decreased extensibility and organization of collagen can lead to decreased flexibility and can therefore impair function. This decreased extensibility may persist and perhaps worsen unless the tissues can be exercised through full ROM activities.

Intervention aimed at improving or increasing flexibility must address the viscoelastic and remodeling properties of collagen. These properties are enhanced by elevating tissue temperature; therefore, heating of collagen facilitates elongation and deformation of collagen fibers to result in sustained or lasting gains in flexibility. These changes support the rationale for heat as an effective and appropriate modality. Heating delivered to connective tissues by modalities such as hot packs, continuous wave ultrasound, and continuous shortwave diathermy complement stretching, mobilization, and other techniques and remodel connective tissue (Fig. 1-13). Further description of the use and effect of heat is presented in Chapter 3, and interventions for loss of motion are presented in Chapter 13.

KEY POINT! The reparative processes of tissue healing are dependent on the production, organization, and maturation of collagen. Collagen is the most abundant protein in the body and has a tensile strength approaching that of steel. It is collagen that imparts strength to the newly formed tissue.[36,37]

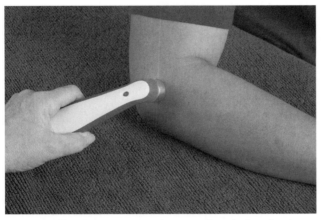

Fig 1•13 Continuous wave ultrasound and other heat modalities can be used to increase tissue temperature. Decreased pain, increased tissue extensibility, and increased blood flow follow tissue heating and provide therapeutic benefit.

Assessing Clinical Effectiveness of Modalities

Use of therapeutic modalities augments other interventions, increasing the probability that the collective effect of the therapies will result in the desired outcomes. Consequently, use of therapeutic modalities has remained a key element of rehabilitation.[38] Of late, however, therapeutic modalities have been scrutinized in regards to outcome measures, the most common being modulation or alleviation of pain.[10,20,39] While scrutiny and examination of efficacy are warranted for all elements of the intervention plan, much of the scrutiny given to therapeutic modalities has failed to assess them in their role as complementary interventions. This point is reflected in a 2009 Cochrane Review by Walsh et al.[39] that examined and ultimately criticized the efficacy of TENS in acute pain. Randomized controlled trials of adults with acute pain (injuries that were less than 12 weeks old) were included only if they examined TENS given as the sole treatment. To assess therapeutic modalities separate from the other interventions they complement is contrary to the position of the American Physical Therapy Association and these authors.

Studies, data, and recent statements have imposed a negative viewpoint regarding the efficacy of TENS in the role of pain modulation. These studies and statements have often assessed effectiveness using more quantitative methods such as pain scales, overlooking qualitative measures of improvement in quality of life and functional ability, reduction in the use of pharmacological agents, or simply patient satisfaction. Examining or assessing the efficacy of therapeutic modalities outside the context of their complementary role assumes they have the inherent ability to induce the desired effect when used in isolation, which is inconsistent with the fundamental use of therapeutic modalities.

Recent Cochrane Reviews examining the effectiveness of TENS have concluded that such studies are often plagued by heterogeneity in design, outcomes, chronic pain conditions, TENS treatments, and methodological quality. Reporting of methods and results for analgesic outcomes were largely inconsistent across studies and were generally poor, making meta-analysis infeasible.[9,10]

Examinations of this nature have not demonstrated so much that therapeutic modalities are ineffective as much as they have demonstrated that research examining the effects may be ineffective and problematic. Effectiveness of therapeutic modalities must be considered in the context of their intended use—as adjuncts to other elements of the therapy plan of care. To examine the efficacy of modalities when used separately from the interventions they supplement is unfair. It also trivializes the adjunctive skill of application and coordination with other therapeutic interventions that skilled practitioners use when selecting and applying therapeutic modalities. Use of therapeutic modalities in unskilled, inexperienced hands and, more importantly, in isolation from other elements of rehabilitation is like placing a scalpel in the hands of a novice versus the hands of a skilled surgeon—the probability of a successful outcome is inherently reduced.

KEY POINT! Study of the efficacy of therapeutic modalities has not so much shown lack of efficacy for therapeutic modalities as much as lack of quality research performed on therapeutic modalities.

Using the Right Outcomes?

So what can we use as appropriate measures to assess the effectiveness of therapeutic modalities? This can greatly determine the attitudes and beliefs associated with clinical use of these therapies. If we use inappropriate measurements or match techniques with the wrong diagnoses or stages of healing, we are more likely to conclude that the modality is ineffective. If we do use appropriate measures, we are more apt to expand our understanding of when and to whom the modality is most appropriate.

There must also be consideration of whether a specific measure of effectiveness is appropriate for all patients or whether the effectiveness of a modality be measured differently for different patients based on the specific clinical presentation. For example, consider the following two patients: The first patient has cervical pain while sitting at work and the second has pain in the knee following surgery. As noted previously, the amount of pain and the location is often measured and used to assess efficacy of therapeutic modalities. But pain may be the sole dysfunction for one patient whereas for another patient it may be an anticipated consequence of some additional factor, such as surgery. For these examples, it must be considered whether measurement of pain in and of itself is the best indicator of effectiveness for a given therapeutic modality. Perhaps the answer is yes for the first patient, where pain is the primary clinical complaint, and no for the second patient, where pain is an expected consequence and part of the rehabilitation process. In other words, the measure used to assess a modality should consider the role, relevance, or significance of the variable to be evaluated.

KEY POINT! Academic preparation and experience are fundamental factors related to successful patient management; however, individuality and differences between patients will always influence the probability that a specific intervention will yield effective outcomes. This simply reflects nature and the natural differences between people. To what extent these can influence our clinical decision-making is questionable and likely equally variable.

The enigmatic nature of pain makes measurement precarious, and the effectiveness of interventions to address pain is equally precarious. Pain scales, ratings, and so on, are used, and each practitioner likely has a preferred method of assessing pain. However, pain is often assessed in a quantitative manner such as a 1 to 10 scale or a 10 cm line, and while necessary, these fail to consider qualitative matters such as functional ability with pain, quality of life, and so on.

Perhaps, then, assessment of clinical effectiveness of therapeutic modalities should be considered in the larger picture of the patient's overall outcome. For example, pain is an expected part of the clinical course for many patients. Simply assessing the effectiveness of modalities for pain during periods when pain is expected to be present or elevated (i.e., in the acute stages of injury) may yield less favorable attitudes toward modalities than if pain is assessed in terms of what functional improvements were made when pain was attenuated or decreased, permitting other aspects of the therapy plan.

Practitioners are encouraged to assess the efficacy of therapeutic modalities when used with other components of the more comprehensive therapy plan. Many variables or methods of assessing effectiveness of therapeutic modalities are available. The astute practitioner will select measures that clearly reflect the expected or anticipated physiological effect of a therapeutic modality. Table 1-2 presents a variety of outcome measures

Table 1•2 **Measures Used to Assess Effectiveness of Therapeutic Modalities**

Measurement	Clinical Presentation	Therapeutic Modality	Rationale
Girth; circumference; volumetrics	Swelling	Cryotherapy	Cold can reduce swelling and inflammation
		Compression	Compression can decrease edema and swelling
Goniometric measures	Decreased ROM, flexibility	Thermotherapy	Superficial heating of tissue prior to stretching can increase ROM
		Diathermy	Continuous wave diathermy can increase tissue temperature to allow for increased elasticity of tissue
		Ultrasound	Thermal ultrasound can increase tissue temperature to allow for increased elasticity of tissue
Strength tests (MMT, dynamometry)	Decreased strength	Neuromuscular electrical stimulation	Electrical stimulation can enhance volitional muscle activation
		Biofeedback	Biofeedback can augment volitional activation of muscle
Tests of function (balance, jump height)	Decreased functional ability	Variable	Therapeutic modalities can help increase function
Tissue healing (closure time, wound depth)	Compromised integumentary	Electrical stimulation	Monophasic current can increase rate of healing
Pain (VAS scales)	Pain	Cryotherapy	Application of cold can reduce pain
		Thermotherapy	Application of heat can reduce pain
		Ultrasound	Acoustic energy can decrease pain
		Electrotherapy	Electrical stimulation can attenuate pain

associated with the use of modalities and the physiological rationale for their use.

Overview of Contraindications and Precautions

If a technique can have a positive effect, there is also potential for it to cause harm. For example, a correct dosage of aspirin may relieve a headache, but too much may cause gastric bleeding. The same principles of dosage and treatment selection apply to modalities. Clinical decision-making involves the judgment and determination of whether to use specific techniques and must consider the probability that the modality will result in a favorable response. In addition, the practitioner must decide if the patient's history or current status present any factors or risks that may render a specific therapeutic modality harmful or disadvantageous to the patient's well-being.

Contraindications are conditions or factors of a patient that make using a specific modality inadvisable. Contraindications are against (or contra-) the usual indication to use a specific therapeutic modality. This may be due to an increased risk of an adverse effect or undesired outcome such as use of mechanical traction to the cervical spine in a patient with spinal instability or the use of cryotherapy in a patient with compromised circulation in the area to be treated.

Precautions present a somewhat different aspect to clinical decision-making. While not outright contraindications, precautions are those findings, circumstances, or factors presented by a patient that require special consideration. Practitioners need to assess the risks and potential benefits prior to applying a specific therapeutic modality. For example, use of ice packs over bony areas presents a precaution due to the decreased tissue and blood flow in the treatment area.

The following sections detail the most common contraindications or precautions that practitioners are likely to encounter.

Compromised, Impaired, or Diminished Sensation

Safe administration of most therapeutic modalities requires that the patient have the ability to feel the treatment so that proper adjustments in temperature, intensity, time, position, etc may be made to allow for optimal therapeutic benefit while minimizing risk for tissue injury. In most cases, compromised or impaired sensation presents a precaution but may become a contraindication in certain patients.

Compromised, Impaired, or Diminished Cognition or Communication

Proper and safe administration of therapeutic modalities requires communication and feedback between the patient and the practitioner. An impaired ability to recognize or communicate the associated sensation of many modalities makes diminished cognition or impaired communication a precaution.

Electronic Implants: Pacemakers, Cardioverter Defibrillators, Phrenic Nerve Stimulators, and Pain Pumps

Administration of therapeutic modalities that deliver electrical or electromagnetic energy near implanted or external electrical devices worn by the patient requires special consideration and are largely considered a contraindication by most practitioners. This is mainly due to the potential for the energy emitted by the modality to interfere with the functioning of the electronic device. Application of other modalities such as hot and cold packs, compression, and traction may potentially be used in patients with electronic implants but should at least be considered precautions.

Pregnancy

Pregnancy is widely considered a contraindication to the use of modalities if the energies delivered may reach the low back, abdominal, and pelvic areas. This is largely due to the potential and unknown effect on fetal development.

Presence of Cancer

Cancer in the area of modality application is considered a contraindication primarily if the therapeutic energy delivered has the potential to alter metabolic activity or blood flow in or around the area of the cancerous tissue. These factors are associated with accelerated cell growth and are to be avoided because of the risk of proliferating cancerous cell growth. While electrical stimulation has been used to manage cancer-related pain, this has largely been given during palliative care in late-stage cancer, and evidence is equivocal.[8,40–42]

Clinical Controversy

There continues to be a lack of consensus as to whether a history of cancer versus the presence of cancer remains a contraindication for some modality applications. Because cancerous cells can metastasize and go undetected for periods of time, there is no clear answer. Thus, there is no point at which a history of cancer should not be considered at least a precaution, if not a contraindication.

Closing Comments from the Authors

This text is written for and directed at those practitioners who recognize the proper role of therapeutic modalities and understand and embrace their role in the larger continuum of the intervention plan. The authors of this text encourage the use and application of therapeutic modalities within the context of their biophysical properties. In this textbook we address each modality in this manner. It is imperative and mandatory that clinicians recognize how therapeutic modalities can complement their skills in the interventions used in comprehensive patient management. Scrutiny and further examination of therapeutic applications are warranted and encouraged, but only when done so in a manner consistent to actual clinical use and in a way that considers and incorporates qualitative measures of improvement or effectiveness.

REFERENCES

1. Hopkins J, Ingersoll C, Edwards J, et al. Cryotherapy and TENS decrease arthrogenic muscle inhibition of the vastus medialis following knee joint effusion. *J Athl Train.* 2002;37:25–32.
2. American Physical Therapy Association. Position statement on exclusive use of physical agents/modalities. HOD P06-95-29-18: 1995.
3. Algafly A, George K. The effect of cryotherapy on nerve conduction velocity, pain threshold, and pain tolerance. *Br J Sports Med.* 2007;41:365–369.
4. Baker R, Bell G. The effect of therapeutic modalities on blood flow in the human calf. *J Orthop Sports Phys Ther.* 1991;13(23):23–27.
5. Halvorsen G. Therapeutic heat and cold for athletic injuries. *Phys Sports Med.* 1990;18:87.
6. Leung M, Cheing GJ. Effects of deep and superficial heating in the management of frozen shoulder. *Rehabil Med.* 2008;40:145–150.
7. Robertson V, Ward A, Jung P. The effect of heat on tissue extensibility: a comparison of deep and superficial heating. *Arch Phys Med Rehabil.* 2005;86:819–825.

8. Berkovitch M, Waller A. *Treating Pain with Transcutaneous Electrical Nerve Stimulation (TENS)*. Oxford: Oxford University Press; 2005:1–6.

9. Khadilkar A, Odebiyi D, Brosseau L, Wells G. Transcutaneous electrical nerve stimulation (TENS) versus placebo for chronic low-back pain. Cochrane Database of Systematic Reviews: Art. No.: CD003008. DOI: 10.1002/14651858.CD003008.pub3.; 2008.

10. Nnoaham K, Kumbang J. Transcutaneous electrical nerve stimulation (TENS) for chronic pain. Cochrane Database of Systematic Reviews (Issue 3): Art. No.: CD003222. DOI: 10.1002/14651858.CD003222.pub2., 2008.

11. Gregory C, Bickel C. Recruitment patterns in human skeletal muscle during electrical stimulation. *Phys Ther.* 2005;85(4):358–364.

12. Gregory C, Dixon W, Bickel C. Impact of varying pulse frequency and duration on muscle torque production and fatigue. *Muscle Nerve.* 2007;35(4):504–509.

13. Nuccitelli R. A role for endogenous electrical fields in wound healing. *Curr Top Dev Biol.* 2003;58:1–27.

14. Petrofsky J, Schwab E, Lo T, Cuneo M, Kim J, et al. Effects of electrical stimulation on skin blood flow in controls and in and around stage III and IV wounds in hairy and non-hairy skin. *Med Sci Monit.* 2005;11:309–316.

15. Raja K, Garcia M, Isseroff R. Wound re-epithelialization: modulating keratinocyte migration in wound healing. *Front Biosci.* 2007;12:2849–2868.

16. Zhao M, Song B, Pu J, et al. Electrical signals control wound healing through phosphatidylinositol-3-OH kinase-y and PTEN. *Nature.* 2006;442:457–460.

17. Draper D, Castro J, Feland B, Schulthies S, Eggett D. Shortwave diathermy and prolonged stretching increase hamstring flexibility more than prolonged stretching alone. *J Orthop Sports Phys Ther.* 2004;34:13–20.

18. Peres S, Draper D, Knight K, Ricard M. Pulsed shortwave diathermy and prolonged long-duration stretching increase dorsiflexion range of motion more than identical stretching without diathermy. *J Athl Train.* 2002;37:43–50.

19. Cetin N, Aytar A, Atalay A, Akman M. Comparing hot pack, short-wave diathermy, ultrasound, and TENS on isokinetic strength, pain, and functional status of women with osteoarthritic knees: a single-blind, randomized, controlled trial. *Am J Phys Med Rehab.* 2008;86:443–451.

20. Hill J, Lewis M, Mills P, Kielty C. Pulsed short-wave diathermy effects on human fibroblast proliferation. *Arch Phys Med Rehabil.* 2002;83:832–836.

21. Laufer Y, Porat R, Nahir A. Effect of pulsed short-wave diathermy on pain and function of subjects with osteoarthritis of the knee: a placebo-controlled double-blind clinical trial. *Clin Rehabil.* 2005;19:255–263.

22. Sherwood L. *Human Physiology: From Cells to Systems.* 7th ed. Belmont, CA: Brooks/Cole; 2010:78–83.

23. Child J, Cleland J, Elliott J, et al. Neck pain: Clinical practice guidelines linked to the International Classification of Functioning, Disability, and Health from the Orthopedic Section of the American Physical Therapy Association. *J Orthop Sports Phys Ther.* 2008;38(9):A1–A34.

24. Cleland J, Fritz J, JM W, Heath R. Predictors of short-term outcome in people with a clinical diagnosis of cervical radiculopathy. *Phys Ther.* 2007;87(12):1619–1632.

25. Cleland J, Whitman J, Fritz J, Palmer J. Manual physical therapy, cervical traction, and strengthening exercises in patients with cervical radiculopathy: a case series. *J Orthop Sports Phys Ther.* 2005;35(12):802–811.

26. Waldrop M. Diagnosis and treatment of cervical radiculopathy using a clinical prediction rule and a multimodal intervention approach: a case series. *J Orthop Sports Phys Ther.* 2006;36(2):152–159.

27. McMahon S, Koltzenberg M. *Textbook of Pain.* 5th ed. Edinburgh: Churchill Livingstone; 2006.

28. Sluka K. *Mechanisms and Management of Pain for the Physical Therapist.* Seattle: International Association for the Study of Pain; 2009:394.

29. Melzack R, Wall P. Pain mechanisms: a new theory. *Science.* 1965;150:971–978.

30. McCaig C, Rajnicek A, Song B, Zhao M. Controlling cell behavior electrically: current views and future potential. *Physiol Rev.* 2005;85:943–978.

31. Gregory C, Bickel C. Recruitment patterns in human skeletal muscle during electrical stimulation. *Phys Ther.* 2005;84(5):358–364.

32. Kamper D, Yasukawa A, Barrett K, Gaebler-Spira D. Effects of neuromuscular electrical stimulation treatment of cerebral palsy on potential impairment mechanisms: a pilot study. *Pediatr Phys Ther.* 2006;18:31–38.

33. Maenpaa H, Jaakkola R, Sandstrom M, von Wendt L. Does microcurrent stimulation increase the range of movement of ankle dorsiflexion in children with cerebral palsy? *Disabil Rehabil.* 2004;26:669–677.

34. Vaz D, Mancini M, da Fonseca S, et al. Effects of strength training aided by electrical stimulation on wrist muscle characteristics and hand function of children with hemiplegic cerebral palsy. *Phys Occup Ther Pediatr.* 2008;28:309–325.

35. Calliet R. *Soft Tissue Pain and Disability.* 2nd ed. Philadelphia: FA Davis; 1988.

36. Simkin P. *Primer on the Rheumatic Diseases.* 9th ed. Atlanta: Arthritis Foundation; 1988.

37. Widmann F. *Pathobiology: How Disease Happens.* Boston: Little Brown; 1978.

38. Wong R, Schumann B, Townsend R, Phelps C, Robertson V. A survey of therapeutic ultrasound use by physical therapists who are orthopaedic certified specialists. *Phys Ther.* 2007;87(8):986–1001.

39. Walsh D, Howe T, Johnson M, Sluka K. Transcutaneous electrical nerve stimulation for acute pain. Cochrane Database of Systematic Reviews (2): Art. No.: CD006142. DOI: 10.1002/14651858.CD006142.pub2.; 2009.

40. Filshie J, Thompson J. *Acupuncture and TENS.* Oxford: Oxford University Press; 2000:188–223.

41. Robb K, Newham D, Williams J. Transcutaneous electrical nerve stimulation vs. transcutaneous spinal electroanalgesia for chronic pain associated with breast cancer treatments. *J Pain Symptom Manage.* 2007;33:410–419.

42. Robb K, Oxberry S, Bennett M, Johnson M, et al. A Cochrane Systematic Review of transcutaneous electrical nerve stimulation for cancer pain. *J Pain Symptom Manage.* 2009;37(4):746–753.

Modalities

chapter 2

Cold Therapy

Stacie J. Fruth, PT, DHS | Susan L. Michlovitz, PT, PhD, CHT

The use of cold as a therapeutic agent has a long history, beginning in Egypt around 2500 BC.[1] However, the use of cold for injury management and rehabilitation did not become prevalent until the 1950s and 1960s.[2–4] While many technological advances have been made in the realm of therapeutic modalities in the past century, the use of cold (water, ice, or gel) remains one of the most effective and least expensive modes of acute injury and pain management.

Cryotherapy, defined as the use of cold modalities for therapeutic purposes, is used as a first-aid measure after trauma and as an adjunctive tool in the rehabilitation of musculoskeletal and neuromuscular dysfunctions. The basis for cryotherapy is grounded in the physiological responses to a decrease in tissue temperature. Cold decreases blood flow and tissue metabolism, thus decreasing bleeding and acute inflammation immediately or soon after injury or surgery. Muscle spasms and tightness from myofascial trigger points can be diminished, allowing for greater ease of motion. Cold can elevate a patient's pain threshold, facilitating ease of exercises with less discomfort. Muscle force production can also be temporarily altered with tissue cooling.

Cold can be easily applied through a variety of means, including cold packs, ice massages, cool baths, vapocoolant sprays, and cold compression devices. Caution should be taken, though, to avoid undue exposure to cold in persons with cold-hypersensitivity conditions, impaired circulation, or hypertension. This chapter includes discussions on the physical principles, biophysical responses, and clinical applications of cold therapy modalities. The use of cryotherapy for ablative surgery, a topic that often appears in electronic database searches for literature on cold therapy, is beyond the scope of practice in rehabilitation and is not included in this chapter. Chapters 13 and 14 include discussions of the use of cold therapy for pain control and tissue inflammation.

Physical Principles

Cooling is accomplished by *removing* or *abstracting* heat from an object, rather than by *adding* cold. Therefore, when a therapeutic cooling agent is applied, the temperature of the skin and underlying tissues is lowered by abstracting heat from the body (Fig. 2-1). The principal modes of energy transfer used for therapeutic cooling include conduction, convection, and evaporation (Table 2-1).

Conduction

Conduction is the transfer of heat by direct interaction of the molecules in the warmer area with those in the cooler area. Internal energy is gained by the slower-moving, cooler particles from the more rapidly moving, warmer particles.[5] The most common conductive methods of cooling in rehabilitation are placing ice or cold packs over an area, immersing a distal extremity in cool or cold water, or applying an ice-water-filled cuff (with manual or automatic recirculation of the water) around the affected area. With these cooling agents, the body part comes in direct contact with the cold source,

Table 2•1	Methods of Energy Transfer with Cold Modalities		
	Conduction	Convection	Evaporation
Cold or ice packs	✔		
Ice massage	✔		
Vapocoolant sprays			✔
Controlled-cold units	✔		
Cool or cold immersion	✔	✔ (with agitation of water via turbines or motion of immersed body part)	

thus making conduction the form of energy transfer by which cryotherapy works.

The magnitude of the temperature change and secondary biophysical alterations will depend on several factors (Box 2-1).

The following equation summarizes the rate of heat transfer by conduction:

$$D = \text{Area} \times k \times (T_1 - T_2) \,/\, \text{thickness of tissue}$$

where D is the rate of heat loss (calories/second), *area* is the amount of body surface area cooled or heated (cm²), k is the thermal conductivity of tissues (calories/second/cm² °C/cm²) (Table 2-2), and T_1 and T_2 are the temperatures of the warm and cool surfaces (°C).

The greater the temperature gradient between the skin and the cooling source, the greater the resulting tissue temperature change may be. For example, following a 15-minute immersion of the forearm in a water bath of 1°C (34°F), subcutaneous tissue temperature dropped by 24°C (43°F).[6] With the same duration and

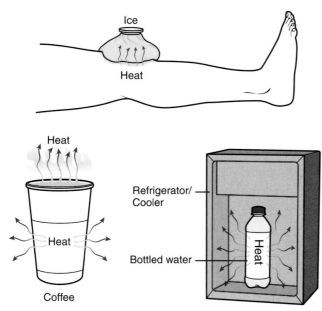

Fig 2•1 Heat abstraction. All cooling occurs via heat leaving one material and going in to another. Cold is never added to something to reduce its temperature.

Box 2•1	Factors Influencing Response to Cold Therapy

- Temperature difference between cold object and soft tissue
- Time of exposure
- Thermal conductivity of area being cooled
- Type and size of cooling agent
- Total body surface area cooled
- Activity level (increased activity→increased circulation→faster re-warming)
- Ability of cooling agent to maintain its temperature

Note that conversion of a *change* in temperature differs from conversion of absolute temperature

Table 2•2 Thermal Conductivities $(cal/s)/(cm^2 \times °C/cm)$		
Material/ Tissue	**Thermal Conductivity (k)**	
Silver	1.01	▲ Good Conductor
Aluminum	0.50	
Titanium	0.016	
Ice	0.005	
Water at 20°C (69°F)	0.0014	
Bone	0.0011	
Muscle	0.0011	▼ Poor Conductor
Fat	0.0005	
Air at 0°C (32°F)	0.000057	

area of immersion at 17°C (63°F), the decrease in temperature in the subcutaneous tissue was only 6°C (11°F).[7] See Box 2-2 for temperature conversion from Celsius to Fahrenheit and from Fahrenheit to Celsius. Table 2-3 provides some common temperature conversion values to add perspective.

Thermal conductivity (see Table 2-2) is a measure of the efficiency of a material or tissue to conduct heat. For example, metals are better heat conductors than are nonmetals. Tissues with high water content, such as muscle, have better thermal conductivity than do adipose tissues. Adipose acts as an insulator, providing resistance to heat transfer (gain or loss), and muscle usually underlies varying depths of adipose tissue. Therefore, the presence of adipose tissue can affect the rate of intramuscular cooling and rewarming.[8–10] While it took only 10 minutes to produce a 7°C

Box 2•2 **Temperature Conversion**
F = Fahrenheit temperature
C = Celsius temperature
$F = (9/5 \times C) + 32$
$C = 5/9\,(F - 32)$
Δ in C temperature = Δ in F temperature $\times$ 0.556
Δ in F temperature = Δ in C temperature/0.556

(12.5°F) temperature decrease in muscle underlying 1 cm (0.4 in.) of adipose tissue, it took 60 minutes to achieve the same temperature decrease in the presence of 3 to 4 cm (1.2 to 1.6 in.) of adipose tissue.[11]

KEY POINT! Thermal conductivity should be considered when cooling areas that have cutaneous or subcutaneous metal present, such as with body piercings, shrapnel, or joint replacements, and over scars that have altered circulatory response.

In addition to consideration of thermal conductivity, it is important to understand the effects of cold on blood flow to an injured area and why a cooled area can take such a long time to return to the precooled temperature. In fact, it can take a cooled area longer than a heated area to return to resting values. Arterial blood coming from the body core is warmer than the venous blood returning from the periphery. Arteries and veins course through the body in juxtaposition to each other. Normally, as warm blood flows toward the periphery, it passes by the cooler blood in veins that lie right next to the arteries. There is a countercurrent heat exchange between the warmer arterial blood and the cooler venous blood.

After an area is heated, arteriole vasodilation allows cooler blood to rush into the area and carry away the heat. Cold causes the opposite effect—a vasoconstriction of arterioles—resulting in a decrease in the amount of warm blood flowing into the area. Thus, countercurrent heat exchange is reduced, and the area may not rewarm very rapidly (Fig. 2-2). For example, when ice packs were applied around a dog's knee for 1 hour, it took more than 60 minutes after removing the cold source before tissue temperature returned to resting values.[12] When hot packs were applied for the same duration, temperatures rose and peaked within 15 minutes and then began to decline. The elevated temperature from hot-pack application caused a vasodilation, allowing cooler blood to flow into the area, dissipating heat. As long as the heat being added was greater than that

Table 2•3 **Values for Temperature Conversion***											
°C	−18	0	5	10	15	20	25	30	35	37	40
°F	0	32	41	50	59	69	77	86	95	98.6	104

*Some values are rounded off to the nearest whole integer.

Vasodilated artery carrying very warm blood after heating

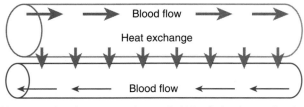

Vasoconstricted artery carrying cooled blood after ice application

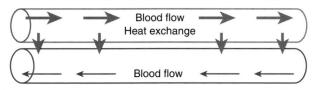

Fig 2•2 Heat exchange between an artery and a vein with (A) a vasodilated artery carrying very warm blood following a period of heating and (B) a vasoconstricted artery carrying cooler blood following a period of ice application.

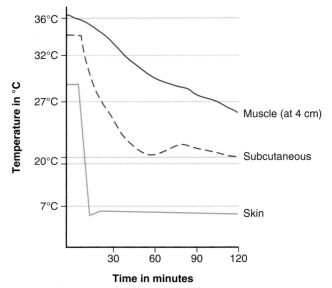

Fig 2•3 Temperature changes during ice pack application to the calf. *(Adapted from Bierman W, Friedlander M. The penetrative effect of cold. Arch Phys Ther. 1940;21:585.)*

being carried away, the temperature remained elevated. After the heat source was removed, heat was rapidly lost by convection and radiation. Clinically this implies that any examination or intervention that challenges a patient's muscle force generation should be avoided for a longer period of time following the application of cold versus an application of heat for a similar duration.

In another study, intramuscular temperature of the gastrocnemius muscle remained lowered for at least 3 hours following 20 minutes of cold baths at 10°C (50°F), for at least 4 hours following a 30-minute cold bath at the same temperature,[13] and for at least 1.75 hours following 20 minutes of ice packs.[14] The patient's level of activity can also influence the return of temperature to precooling levels. If exercise is performed following cooling, this will increase blood flow to the area, resulting in a faster rate of rewarming.[15]

Cryotherapy is used to lower the temperature of soft tissues, including subcutaneous tissue, muscle, and joints, for pain and edema control. Since cold modalities can lower temperatures in these tissues, the time of exposure and the presence of dressings or bandages are factors to be considered. The greater the target tissue depth, the longer it takes for the cold application to lower the temperature (Fig. 2-3).

Changes in skin temperature will occur very rapidly (typically within a minute) upon exposure to cold. Subcutaneous tissue and muscle temperature can also

be reduced by topical cold application, but additional time is required to allow for conduction of energy. Muscle temperature at a depth of 4 cm (1.6 in.) can be lowered by an average of 1.2°C (2.2°F) within 5 minutes when cooled with an agent at 10°C (50°F).[10] However, it can take as long as 30 minutes to lower muscle temperature at a depth of 4 cm by 3.5°C (6.3°F) using ice packs.[16]

KEY POINT! Lowering skin-surface temperature to 13.6°C (56.5°F) is sufficient to produce local analgesia;[17,18] a temperature of 10°C (50°F) can produce a 33% reduction in nerve conduction velocity.[19]

It is important to keep in mind that many of the studies done on tissue temperature change involved subjects who did not have an injury or pathology.[11,20] Tissue response to cold in the presence of new epithelialization, granulation, or capillary budding, as well as scar formation or impaired circulation can only be estimated. One study demonstrated that 1 hour of cooling with an ice-water/compression device following arthroscopic knee surgery led to an intra-articular temperature that was 7°C (12.6°F) lower than that of a control group that had no cooling.[21] Compared to presurgical, baseline intra-articular temperatures, the control group had a mean 5°C (9°F) increase while the cooled group had a mean decrease of 2°C (3.6°F). This tells us that, at a minimum, adding a cold modality after surgery can prevent a rise in intra-articular temperature, which often leads to increased swelling and pain.

Patient comfort should always be considered, regardless of treatment technique selected. Warren and associates[22] demonstrated greater intra-articular temperature reductions at 60 and 90 minutes of ice-bag application to the knee (12.8°C [23°F] and 15.2°C [27°F], respectively) compared to a commercial cold-compression device (7.1°C [13°F] and 9.7°C [17.5° F]). However, the ice-bag application was more painful than the cold-compression device. Similarly, when a continuous-flow cold device was compared to two intermittent-flow devices (one manually circulated and one automatically circulated), the continuous-flow unit was able to produce lower skin surface temperatures but was more painful than the intermittent-flow devices.[23]

The form in which cold therapy is applied (e.g., ice packs, ice massage, cold-water baths, or continuous-flow cold devices) can contribute to the degree of cooling. The magnitude of temperature change will be greater when ice packs are used, compared with cold-water baths or frozen gel packs. Greater internal energy is required to melt the ice, which occurs as the solid bonding forces of the ice molecules are broken apart. Energy is first used to change the ice to water before raising the surrounding temperature.[5] Four common cryotherapeutic agents were compared during a 20-minute application to the gastrocnemius muscle. Skin surface temperatures were lowered by 19.6°C (35°F) with crushed ice, 17°C (30.6°F) with ice-water immersion, 14.6°C (26°F) with frozen peas, and 13°C (23.5°F) with a cold gel pack.[24] In another study, ice massage was compared to cubed-ice bags during a 15-minute application. The ice massage reduced the intramuscular temperature by 4.3°C (7.7°F) while the ice bag reduced the temperature by 2.3°C (4.1°F).[25]

KEY POINT! Although ice massage may be able to cool a muscle at a faster rate compared to an ice bag, a prolonged ice massage may not be feasible, as it may take several ice-cup applications to cool the same area an ice bag can cover. Sustaining pressure and motion on an ice cup for more than 10 minutes may be very fatiguing, and an extended ice bag application may be more appropriate.

Convection

Heat abstraction by convection occurs when there is direct contact between the skin and moving fluid particles. The principal method of using convection in cryotherapy is a cold whirlpool; water moves over skin via turbines that circulate the water, or the patient moves the body part within the water. Heat abstraction occurs at a faster rate with convection versus conduction given the same medium (water) at the same initial temperature. This is because new (cooler) molecules are continually introduced to the skin surface when movement is occurring; when no motion occurs, molecules remain in contact with the skin surface and are warmed via conduction. Thus, when a body part is immersed in stationary cold water, the molecules in contact with the skin begin to warm and form a shield around the immersed limb. In addition, the specific heat of water is several thousands times that of air, and heat loss is 25 times greater in water versus air at a given temperature.[26]

Despite the ability of cold whirlpools to effectively cool body areas, they are usually practical for only distal extremities (e.g., elbow, wrist, or ankle) and can be uncomfortable. Cold whirlpools are not recommended in the acute phase of healing, as this puts the limb in a dependent position, encouraging edema in the distal extremity. However, in later stages of healing, when edema formation is less of a concern, cold whirlpools may be used to reduce pain prior to performing exercises that improve range of motion (ROM) and activities that increase weight-bearing tolerance. Additional information about interventions using whirlpools can be found in Chapter 5.

KEY POINT! The rate of heat loss through convection is evident to most people after spending time in a swimming pool, in a lake, or in the ocean. Immersion and movement in a cold pool, about 25.5°C (78°F), causes much faster heat loss than time spent in the same air temperature.

Evaporation

Vapocoolant sprays are used for temporary pain relief prior to stretching muscles with active trigger points or muscles with local spasm. These sprays use evaporation as a means of energy transfer. Vapocoolant sprays, such as Spray and Stretch and Instant Ice (both a blend of 1,1,1,3,3-pentafluoropropane and 1,1,1,2-tetrafluoroethane), are nonflammable, liquid, aerosol skin refrigerants that are bottled under pressure and are emitted in fine sprays (Spray and Stretch requires a physician's prescription while Instant Ice does not; Fig. 2-4). Both are nonozone depleting, as opposed to former types of vapocoolant sprays that contained fluoromethane. As the liquid leaves the pressurized canister, it begins to evaporate. When this transition occurs, the steam cools and, upon contact with the skin, extracts heat. The vapocoolant spray feels colder than room-temperature water sprayed on the skin, because, like alcohol, it evaporates more quickly than water. This cold sensation serves as a counterirritant stimulus to the thermal afferents that overlie the target muscle, causing a reflexive reduction in motor neuron activity and allowing stretch to occur more easily.[27] The spray is applied with only a few sweeps across the skin. The temperature of the spray upon skin contact is −9°C to −20°C (48°F to 68°F), depending upon the distance of the nozzle to the skin.[28]

Although skin temperature can drop to about 15°C (59°F) for a few seconds, changes in subcutaneous tissue and muscle temperatures are negligible.[29] Although few studies have been published examining the effects of vapocoolant spray, two studies demonstrated that

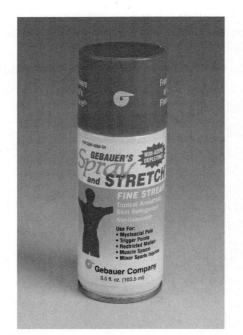

Fig 2•4 Vapocoolant spray. Gebauer's Spray and Stretch. *(Courtesy Gebauer Company, Cleveland, OH.)*

using it on the posterior aspect of the thigh could improve passive and active ROM of the hip with the knee extended. These ROM improvements, however, were relatively small (less than 2°).[30,31] A well-designed study using this technique to reduce pain from trigger points is warranted.

Biophysical Principles of Tissue Cooling

Many of the clinical uses of cold are predicated on the physiological changes resulting from reducing tissue temperature. Cold is used in the management of acute trauma because

1. the resulting arteriolar vasoconstriction reduces bleeding;
2. the decrease in metabolism and vasoactive agents (e.g., histamine and kinins) reduces inflammation and outward fluid filtration; and
3. the pain threshold is elevated.

A reduction in skeletal muscle spasm can be postulated as an interplay of factors, including a decrease in pain and a decrease in sensitivity of muscle-spindle afferent fibers to discharge. Muscle performance may be temporarily enhanced following short-duration cold, although this effect may reverse following cold applied for longer durations. Pain, and perhaps joint inflammation in certain inflammatory rheumatic diseases, can be decreased. However, there may also be an increase in joint stiffness secondary to the effect of cold, which increases tissue viscosity and decreases tissue elasticity. When tissue viscosity is increased and elasticity is decreased, the resistance to motion increases.

KEY POINT! Performing muscle-strength assessment after different durations of cold may lead to inaccurate findings: After a cold application of less than 5 minutes, a muscle may produce more force than when in its noncooled state,[32] while a longer cold application may reduce a muscle's ability to generate force compared to its noncooled state.[33]

Hemodynamic Effects

When cold is applied, the immediate response is vasoconstriction of the cutaneous blood vessels and reduction in blood flow. The amount of blood flow to an area is inversely proportional to the resistance factors that impede flow. Vessel diameter is the most significant factor relating to blood flow. Any influence that causes vascular smooth muscle to contract will reduce vessel diameter (vasoconstriction). Conversely, when smooth muscle tone decreases, as happens with heating, vessel diameter increases (vasodilation).

Exposure to cold for a short time (15 minutes or less) generally results in vasoconstriction of arterioles and venules. The mechanism of action causing vasoconstriction involves a number of factors, including the direct action of cold on smooth muscle,[34] a reduction in vasodilating neurotransmitters,[35] and a reflex cutaneous vasoconstriction. The viscosity of blood determines, in part, resistance to blood flow. If viscosity increases, so does resistance to blood flow. The increase in blood viscosity resulting from cold exposure contributes to the decrease in blood flow. Figure 2-5 summarizes the effects of cold on microcirculation.

Blood flow to the skin is primarily under neural control and plays an important role in thermoregulation. Vasoconstriction of cutaneous vessels occurs as part of the heat-retention mechanisms of the body.[36] When skin temperature is lowered, cold thermal sensors (free nerve endings) in the skin are stimulated, causing a reflex excitation of sympathetic adrenergic fibers. Increased activity of these fibers causes vasoconstriction. This reflex vasoconstriction can also result in a generalized cutaneous vasoconstriction that, to a lesser extent, may also occur in the contralateral extremity.[37,38] The decrease in cutaneous blood flow is greatest in the area that is directly cooled. For example, cutaneous blood flow in a hand cooled in ice water changed

from a resting value of 16 mL/100 mL per minute down to 2 mL/100 mL per minute (Fig. 2-6).[37]

As cooled blood returns to the general circulation, it stimulates the heat conservation area in the preoptic region of the anterior hypothalamus. Stimulation of this area will result in further reflex cutaneous vasoconstriction. If a large area of the body is cooled, shivering will occur as a heat-retaining mechanism.

Decreases in joint blood flow have also been demonstrated following cold application.[39] Ice packs at 0°C (32°F) applied to knee joints of dogs for 10 minutes resulted in a 56% average decrease in resting intra-articular blood flow. The flow returned to precooled values approximately 25 minutes after the cold was removed.

When tissue temperatures are reduced below 10°C (50°F) for a period of time, a cold-induced vasodilation may follow the initial period of vasoconstriction. This was first discovered in 1930, when Lewis[40] found that when fingers were immersed in an ice bath, skin temperature decreased dramatically during the first 15 minutes, then cyclically increased (due to vasodilation) and decreased (due to vasoconstriction). When skin temperature fell below 10°C, a neurotransmitter—termed "substance H," which is similar in action to histamine—was hypothesized to be released, resulting in arteriolar vasodilation. As warm blood came into the area and elevated skin temperature above 10°C, the ice bath was again effective in causing a vasoconstriction. This response occurs predominantly in apical areas

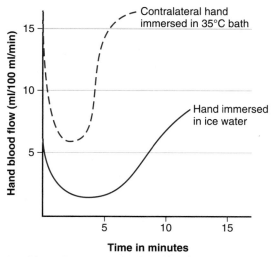

Fig 2•6 Blood flow to the hands following ice water immersion of one hand. *(Adapted from Folkow B, et al. Studies on the reaction of the cutaneous vessels to cold exposure. Acta Physiol Scand. 1963;58:342.)*

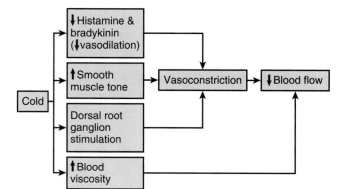

Fig 2•5 Effects of cold stimulus on local blood flow.

where arteriovenous (AV) anastomoses are located in the skin.[40,41]

Recently, the occurrence of cold-induced vasodilation has been both reproduced and challenged. Immersion of the middle finger for 30 minutes in water at 4°C (39°F) produced a rapid drop in finger pad and nail bed blood flow and temperature, followed by an increase in both measures (that remained well below pre-immersion values) and then a cycling of small increases and decreases (Fig. 2-7).[42] The response appears to be stronger in the fingers than in the toes for cold water immersion[43] and does not acclimate with repeated cold immersions.[44] One of the conclusions from Lewis's original work was that cold-induced vasodilation resulted in an increase in temperature, at times up to a sixfold increase, which led clinicians to use cold as a means to increase blood flow. This theory has since been discounted, however, as the sixfold increase was measured from the lowest immersion skin temperature of 2°C to the highest of 12°C (35.6°F to 53.6°F), while the preimmersion skin temperature was 31°C (88°F).[45] Therefore, while relatively small oscillations in blood flow and temperature do seem to occur in response to immersion in water less than 10°C (50°F), the overriding clinical effect is a dramatic reduction in both of these values during the time of immersion.

Posttraumatic Edema and Inflammation

For the first 24 to 48 hours following injury, cold is usually the modality of choice for the following reasons:

1. Fluid filtration into the interstitial tissue may be reduced with cold, owing to vasoconstriction and prevention of dramatic increases in microvascular permeability.[46]
2. Inflammation and pain may be reduced.
3. Local metabolism is decreased, leading to a reduction in cellular energy demands and, thus, a decrease in secondary hypoxic tissue injury.[45]

The choice of cold has largely been based on empirical evidence. The duration and temperature of the cold exposure can have significant effects on tissue swelling. Some laboratory animal studies are discussed in this section; clinical reports will be presented subsequently under "Clinical Indications for Cold Therapy."

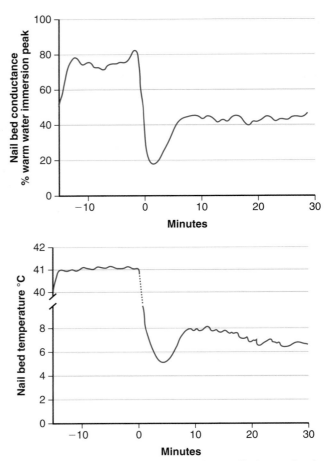

Fig 2•7 The effects of cold-induced vasodilation on (top) blood flow and (bottom) temperature of the nail bed during 30 minutes of immersion in 4°C (30°F) water. Blood flow was measured as a percent of maximal blood flow during warm-water immersion. Note the fluctuations (vasodilation and vasoconstriction) in blood flow and temperature that never approach preimmersion values. *(Adapted with permission from O'Brien C. Reproducibility of the cold-induced vasodilation response. J Appl Physiol. 2005;98:1334.)*

In most experiments using animal models, trauma was induced through some type of crushing force, resulting in soft-tissue damage or fracture. Cold was then applied for varying lengths of time. A summary of findings from studies that measured postinjury edema formation following the use of cold can be found in Table 2-4.[47–49] Figures 2-8 and 2-9 provide the reader with a graphic representation of some of these findings. These studies have generally shown a decrease or minimization of swelling if less-intense cold was used or if intense cold was applied for several hours or less. Prolonged intense cold may result in increased edema formation.[47,49–51] The increase in edema is likely due to reperfusion of superficial vessels damaged by

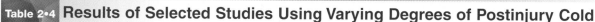

Table 2•4 **Results of Selected Studies Using Varying Degrees of Postinjury Cold**

Author	Injury Type	Type of Cold Application	Length of Intervention	Temperature/ Other Variables	Results	Clinical Relevance
Matsen et al[47]	Tibial fracture (rabbits)	Cold water bags	24 hours cold	5°C–15°C (41°F–59°F)	↑ edema vs. controls	Exposure to intense cold for a prolonged period of time immediately postinjury may result in greater edema formation compared with no cold, cold for a shorter period of time, or less-intense cold.
			24 hours cold	20°C–25°C (68°F–77°F)	No difference from controls	
			6 hours cold	10°C (50°F)	No difference from controls	
			24 hours	Room temperature water (controls)	—	
Dolan et al[48] (Fig. 2-8)	Fractured limb (rats)	Cold water immersion (with or without high-volt electrical stimulation)	3 hours cold	12.8°C (55°F)	↓ edema vs. controls	Application of cold immediately postinjury can reduce swelling compared to no treatment.
			3 hours electrical stimulation		↓ edema vs. controls	
			1 hour cold, then 2 hours electrical stimulation	12.8°C (55°F)	↓ edema vs. controls	
			No treatment (controls)		—	
McMaster & Liddle[49] (Fig. 2-9)	Fractured limb (rabbits)	Cold water immersion	1 hour	30°C (86°F)	5% ↑ edema	Postinjury application of intense cold, as well as cycling of cold, may lead to greater edema formation.
			1 hour	20°C (68°F)	12% ↑ edema	
			1 hour in/1 hour out/1 hour in	30°C (86°F)	11% ↑ edema	
			1 hour in/1 hour out/1 hour in	20°C (68°F)	14% ↑ edema	

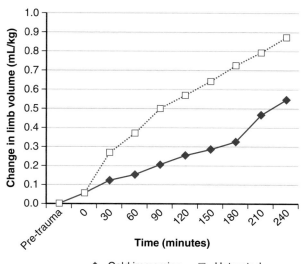

Fig 2•8 Changes in volume following trauma in treated (immersion in 12.8°C [55°F]) versus untreated limbs. *(Adapted with permission from Dolan MG, et al. Effects of cool-water immersion and high-voltage electric stimulation for 3 continuous hours on acute edema in rats. J Athl Train. 2003;38:327.)*

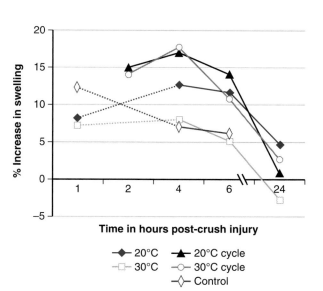

Fig 2•9 The effects of cold immersion on postcrush injury swelling in rabbits. Cycling consisted of 1-hour immersion/1 hour no immersion/1 hour immersion. Dashed lines indicate areas of missing data points. *(Adapted from McMaster WC, Liddle S. Cryotherapy influence on post-traumatic limb edema. Clin Orthop Rel Res. 1980;150:283.)*

cold-induced ischemia, which has also been shown to occur in noninjured tissues.[52]

While the presence of edema is of concern in rehabilitation, it is also important to consider how cryotherapy can affect changes in inflammatory exudates. Farry and Prentice[52] used cold to treat experimentally induced radiocarpal ligament sprains in pigs. Crushed ice packs were applied for 20 minutes, followed by a 1-hour rest period, followed by another 20 minutes of cold—a protocol similar to typical postinjury methods used by laypersons. Although the cold produced an increase in subcutaneous swelling, there was histological evidence of decreased inflammation. Only one of the 20 treated limbs had signs of a pronounced inflammatory response (i.e., numerous polymorphonuclear leukocytes, such as polymorphs, plasma cells, lymphocytes, and fibrinous exudate). All others had either no inflammatory cells or minimal to moderate amounts of polymorphs and lymphocytes.

Alterations in microcirculation in response to cryotherapy were studied by Schaser and associates.[35] Continuous cooling at 10°C (50°F) for 6 hours was compared to no cooling immediately following a closed soft tissue injury to rats. Measurements taken 24 hours postinjury showed that the rats who received the cold treatment demonstrated increased capillary density; narrowed venules with a corresponding increase in erythrocyte velocity; a reduction in adhering leukocytes, macrophages, and neutrophilic granulocytes; and a decrease in intramuscular pressure compared to the control group. Constant cooling for prolonged periods of time, as performed in this study, mimics the use of continuous cooling units that are becoming more prevalent in hospital and clinical settings.

Similar results were found by Lee and colleagues[53] when the effects of 10 minutes of intense cooling (3°C; 37.4°F), moderate cooling (27°C; 80.6°F), and room-temperature control (37°C; 98.6°F) on microcirculatory factors were studied in rats immediately following a crush injury. Both the intense and moderate cooling produced a reduction in venule diameter and in leukocyte adhesions, with the intense cooling producing the more dramatic responses. The intense cooling group showed a significant reduction in erythrocyte velocity whereas the moderate cooling group showed a significant increase in erythrocyte velocity.

The combined results of these two studies[35,53] suggest that immediate cooling of injured tissue can reduce secondary tissue damage by decreasing capillary dysfunction, decreasing venule diameter, and reducing the accumulation of leukocytes. The reduction of intramuscular pressure may also reduce the risk for compartment syndrome.

KEY POINT! Cold reduces the overall metabolism and oxygen demand of living tissues. When an adult tooth is knocked loose or if an extremity is accidentally amputated, emergency instructions include placing the tooth or lost body part in a container with ice (however, the ice cannot touch the vascular tissues). Cooling allows for longer survival of these tissues while they are separated from their natural blood supply because of the decrease in metabolism and oxygen requirements.

In summary, although postinjury cold application has not been shown to eliminate edema formation, moderate cooling for several hours or less may limit the extent of postinjury swelling. Intense cold, cycled cold, or cold applied for long periods of time may lead to greater edema formation. However, the positive factors of immediate cold application—including a lowered oxygen demand and metabolism,[45,54] reduced leukocyte and macrophage adherence, and decreased intramuscular pressure—outweigh the negative presence of increased edema, especially considering that edema can be better managed with the addition of compression and elevation.

Peripheral Nerve Effects

Cold can alter the conduction velocity and synaptic activity of peripheral nerves (Box 2-3). If the temperature of a nerve is decreased, there will be a corresponding decrease in sensory and motor conduction velocities, or even a failure of the nerve to conduct impulses. Synaptic transmissions can also be impeded or blocked. These

Box 2•3	**Effects of Cold on Peripheral Nerves**

- Increases threshold for depolarization
- Slows nerve conduction velocity
- Extreme cold can block nerve conduction

factors, in turn, can raise pain tolerance and pain threshold. The quantity of the change elicited depends on the duration and the degree of the temperature alteration.

Isolated cat nerves of various diameters and degrees of myelination were found to have different thresholds or sensitivities to cold stimuli.[55] In the saphenous nerve (afferent), reductions in nerve conduction velocity were observed first in small-diameter myelinated fibers. The fibers least sensitive to cold were small-diameter unmyelinated fibers. Cooling to 12°C (53.6°F) blocked conduction in A fibers, while considerably lower temperatures were required to block C-fiber conduction. Further examination showed that conduction in smaller-diameter A fibers (A-delta fibers) was affected first, while conduction in nerves with the largest diameter (A-alpha fibers) was affected last. When the motor fibers of the sciatic nerve were isolated and cooled, conduction was eliminated in the gamma fibers before the alpha fibers.

Cold can also decrease nerve conduction velocity in humans. When ice packs were applied over the ulnar nerve for 5 minutes, motor conduction velocity decreased by 6% followed by a return to precooling conduction within 15 minutes after ice removal.[56] In a similar study, ice packs were applied over the ulnar nerve for a longer period of time (20 minutes) with a resulting 29.4% decrease in motor conduction velocity. Thirty minutes after the ice packs were removed, the conduction velocity was still 8.3% lower than precooled values.[57] These studies indicate that longer applications of cold can progressively decrease motor nerve conduction velocity, and the longer the cold is applied, the longer it takes the nerve to return to precooled conduction velocity.

Ice pack application to the tibial nerve also resulted in decreased motor conduction velocity. Algafly and colleagues[19] cooled the tibial nerve of healthy subjects to 15°C (59°F) and then to 10°C (50°F) before rewarming back to 15°C. There were significant decreases in conduction velocities at both temperatures compared to the contralateral tibial nerve, which served as a control. At 15°C, motor conduction velocity had decreased by 17%, and at 10°C the decrease was 33% (Fig. 2-10, top). Pain tolerance and pain threshold were also measured in this study. Both significantly increased at 15°C and 10°C compared to the control site. Again, findings

at 10°C significantly differed from 15°C (Fig. 2-10, bottom). Results of this study indicate that application of cold to temperatures between 15°C and 10°C is effective in slowing motor nerve conduction as well as increasing the sensory stimulus needed to perceive pain.

KEY POINT! Although the effects of decreased or blocked nerve conduction velocity in sensory (afferent) nerves is desired for assistance with pain reduction, sensory nerves cannot selectively be cooled, and reduced motor ability should be considered if your patient will engage in activity after the application of cold.

Cryotherapy has resulted in cases of neurapraxia and case of axonotmesis in young athletes.[58] In each case, ice packs were applied either over a major nerve branch that was superficially located (i.e., over the peroneal

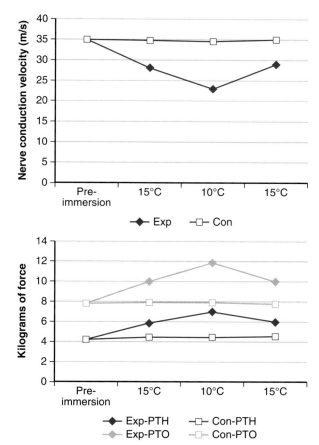

Fig 2•10 Changes in (top) nerve conduction velocity and (bottom) pain threshold (PTH) and pain tolerance (PTO) at skin temperatures of 15°C (59°F) and 10°C (50°F) compared to controls with no cooling. *Exp* = Experimental; *Con* = Control. *(Adapted with permission from Algafly AA, George KP. The effect of cryotherapy on nerve conduction velocity, pain threshold and pain tolerance. Br J Sports Med. 2007;41:366.)*

nerve at the lateral border of the knee) or around the thigh for up to 2 hours (in the case of axonotmesis). On two occasions, 1 hour of cryotherapy around the knee of a patient following a hamstring strain was reported to cause axonotmesis of the peroneal nerve.[59]

Muscle Performance Effects

Thermal agents can affect the ability of a muscle to generate tension. The effects of cold applied prior to muscle contraction or functional activities, and cold applied after muscle fatigue, have been examined and are discussed in this section.

Isometric force generation of the quadriceps was measured before and after 5 minutes of ice massage to the entire anterior thigh of healthy subjects.[32] After icing, the subjects demonstrated a 2 kg (4.4 lb) increase in isometric force generation compared to precooling values. Because muscle temperature was not expected to be lowered with such a short period of ice massage over the large muscle mass, the increase in force generation may have resulted from increased quadriceps blood flow via sympathetic nerve activity changes, as well as heightened psychological motivation to perform better posttest. Another explanation for the observed increase could have been the effect of short-duration cold on motor nerve excitability.[60] Facilitation of a single motor unit was seen after 1 to 2 minutes of icing over the biceps brachii muscle of healthy human subjects.[61]

When the duration of cold exposure is lengthened, muscle temperature will decrease. Following cold immersion of healthy legs for 30 minutes at 10°C to 12°C (50°F to 53.6°F), Oliver and associates[33] found that muscle temperature and plantarflexion strength decreased. This decrease could have been the result of reduced muscle blood flow at these lowered temperatures or the result of an increase in the viscous properties of the muscle. At 45 minutes postimmersion, plantarflexion strength began to increase over pretreatment values and continued to do so for the next 3 hours (Fig. 2-11).

While findings from these studies may be helpful in understanding the effects of cold on muscle force generation, the ability of individuals to perform functional activities following cold application is more clinically relevant. Fischer and colleagues[62] applied ice bags for 3 minutes and 10 minutes to the hamstrings of subjects' dominant leg. The 3-minute cooling had no

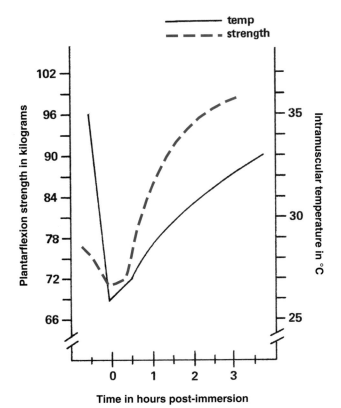

Fig 2•11 Plantarflexion strength and intramuscular temperature measurements postcold immersion at 10°C (50°F). *(Adapted from Oliver RA, et al. Isometric muscle contraction response during recovery from reduced intramuscular temperature. Arch Phys Med Rehabil. 1979;60:126.)*

effect on subjects' shuttle run time, vertical jump distance, or a co-contraction test that involved a timed, resisted lateral stepping activity. The 10-minute cooling, however, resulted in decreased vertical jump distance and slower shuttle run and co-contraction test times. These changes were also seen 20 minutes postcooling.

A similar study was conducted by Patterson and associates,[63] who immersed both lower legs of male and female subjects for 20 minutes in a 10°C (50°F) cold whirlpool. Pre- and posttesting consisted of a vertical jump, a 40-yard dash, and an agility test. Posttesting occurred at 5-minute intervals, beginning 2 minutes after cooling and ending 32 minutes after cooling. Vertical jump height was significantly decreased at all posttesting intervals, and the 40-yard dash and agility test times were both significantly slower for at least several posttest intervals. No measure returned to precooling levels by the end of the 32-minute posttest period.

The results of these studies are clinically important, in that some form of cold is often applied prior to exercise to reduce pain. Because muscle performance is negatively affected with cooling for 10 minutes or longer, caution should be taken if strenuous exercise or athletic activities are to be performed following muscular cooling.

KEY POINT! Because cold can alter muscle force generation, strength assessments on patients during initial and follow-up examinations should either be performed prior to or several hours after a cold modality has been used.

Cryotherapy may affect proprioception by altering the somatosensory input necessary for reflex integration of neuromuscular control. Therefore, the ability to safely and efficiently perform functional activities can be hindered by lack of joint position sense. Wassinger and colleagues[64] measured active joint position replication, path of joint motion replication, and throwing accuracy before and after a 20-minute ice bag application to subjects' dominant shoulders. While active joint position replication was not affected following the cold application, which supported findings of previous studies,[65,66] both the path of joint replication and throwing accuracy were significantly decreased.

In another study, medial-lateral postural sway increased significantly following 20 minutes of ice-water immersion (4°C; 39°F) of recently sprained ankles.[67] Medial-lateral sway was greater in involved versus uninvolved legs prior to immersion, and this difference increased following immersion. In the affected leg, significant pre- to postimmersion differences were found immediately after immersion and continued to be significantly different up to 20 minutes after the ankle was removed from the cold. Surenkok and associates[68] found similar results when measuring balance after a 30-minute cold gel pack application to the knee. Single-leg balance was significantly decreased immediately following removal of the gel pack. However, 5 minutes after the cold was removed, balance returned to and then surpassed normal levels.

Although the aforementioned studies indicate that proprioception may be hindered for short periods of time following cryotherapy, Berg and colleagues[69] found that application of an ice pack to the lateral ankle for 20 minutes did not alter peroneal reaction time when a sudden inversion force was introduced. Peroneal reaction time and peroneal muscle activity did not differ between cold and control sessions at 0, 15, and 30 minutes postcold application. This study used

healthy volunteers, so it is not known if individuals with acute or chronic ankle instability would demonstrate similar results.

The type of cold used in the previous studies varied, so it is difficult to compare findings. When ice bags or cold packs are used, cooling is relatively local and structures that are not cooled likely remain unaffected. In addition, as will be discussed in a later section in this chapter, the degree to which ice bags and cold gel packs reduce tissue temperature differs. When limbs are immersed in cold water, more tissues are affected, which may lead to more widespread changes in nerve conduction, force production, and joint position sense. Some studies suggest that proprioception is reduced immediately following application of cold; therefore, patients should be educated to use caution when ambulating or exercising immediately following cold application to the lower extremities. This is particularly important when treating a patient who may have an underlying balance deficit.

KEY POINT! Any examination or intervention that challenges balance, proprioception, accuracy, or agility should be avoided for a period of time following the application of a cold modality due to the reduction in somatosensory input that these tasks require.

Neuromuscular Effects

Conditions that result from central nervous system dysfunction, such as multiple sclerosis, cerebral palsy, and cerebrovascular accident, typically limit a person's ability to perform functional activities due to the presence of spasticity, muscle weakness, and inefficient movement patterns that lead to early fatigue. Spasticity often limits a person's ability to carry out purposeful movements at the variable speeds required to perform activities of daily living. Spasticity is associated with an increased resistance to passive stretch, increased deep-tendon reflexes, and clonus. Many therapeutic interventions are used to reduce spasticity, including positioning, modalities, and pharmacological interventions.

In some patients with spasticity, cold application can temporarily decrease the amplitude of deep-tendon reflexes (DTR)[70] and the frequency of clonus,[71–73] which may improve the patient's ability to participate in therapy programs. Cold facilitates alpha-motoneuron activity and decreases gamma-motoneuron firing. In order for spasticity to be reduced, the reduction in gamma activity should be proportionally greater than the increase in alpha activity. Spasticity reduction with cold may occur through at least two mechanisms:

1. A reflex decrease in gamma-motoneuron activity through stimulation of cutaneous afferents[71]
2. A decrease in afferent spindle discharge by direct cooling of the muscle[72,73]

Although the mechanisms responsible for the changes seen have not been fully elucidated, animal and human studies have been designed to clarify and provide a rationale for these observed responses. Some earlier studies are referenced for the interested reader but will not be elaborated on in this chapter.[70,72–77]

Knutsson[78] found that all patients with spasticity who were treated with 15 to 20 minutes of cold demonstrated a decrease in the frequency, duration, and threshold of clonus. Two-thirds also demonstrated a decrease in resistance to passive motion and an increase in active ROM. A short-duration application has also shown effectiveness in reducing spasticity of the masseter muscle in patients with cerebral palsy.[79] Significant increases in interincisal distance were found following a 1-minute icing procedure, which indirectly implies muscle relaxation.

Cooling vests have been studied for patients who may benefit from cooling on a more global level. One study examined the effects of a cooling garment on timed walking tests, spasticity, balance, and dexterity in individuals with multiple sclerosis.[80] Subjects who wore a cooled vest (stored in a freezer at $-20°C/-4°F$) for 45 minutes prior to performing the tests showed significant improvements in the timed walking tests and in several balance measures compared to those who wore a room-temperature vest. Subjectively, wearing the cooled vest led to less fatigue, spasticity, weakness, and balance and gait difficulties, and these improvements were reported to last 2 to 8 hours after the vest was removed. In a similar study,[81] individuals with myasthenia gravis demonstrated improvements in muscle strength, respiratory measures, and fatigue after wearing a cooling vest.

KEY POINT! If additional studies are able to demonstrate consistent benefits from cooling vests for managing spasticity, these devices may become just as common and available as ice packs or cold packs.

Grahn and colleagues[82] studied the effects of cooling one hand on exercise tolerance in 12 individuals with heat-sensitive multiple sclerosis. When one hand was cooled with a heat-extraction device, described as a curved metal device maintained at 18°C to 22°C (64.4°F to 71.6°F) on which the subjects rested one hand, treadmill walking tolerance increased from 33 minutes to 44 minutes.

These studies indicate that local or regional cooling may be beneficial to individuals with certain neurological conditions. The presence of spasticity, which can impede normal movement patterns, may be temporarily reduced, and this may encourage increased use of the affected limb during functional activities. Also, if cooling can improve endurance, strength, and walking efficiency, individuals may be encouraged to increase overall activity and may feel more confident participating in recreational and social activities. However, it should be noted that many individuals with spasticity report a worsening of symptoms when they become cold! Therefore, the use of cold is not appropriate for all individuals with a neurological condition.

Clinical Indications for Cold Therapy

Most clinicians will agree that in the acute phase (24 to 48 hours) following trauma, cold should be the modality of choice and should be administered as soon as possible following injury. Even though cold may be uncomfortable for the patient during the first few minutes, pain will ultimately be reduced, and edema, inflammation, and muscle spasm will most likely be lessened (Box 2-4).

Beyond the acute phase of injury, heat may be the agent of choice for intervention. But in many cases, cold has been a successful part of a therapeutic regimen to facilitate muscle contractions, reduce joint pain caused by arthritis, and lessen muscle spasm.

Box 2•4	Primary Goals With Use of Cold Therapy

- Limit edema formation
- Reduce pain
- Facilitate muscle relaxation
- Limit secondary hypoxic tissue injury

Acute Musculoskeletal Trauma

The most common applications of cryotherapy are for acute musculoskeletal trauma or postsurgical swelling and pain. One of the earliest clinical reports supporting cold therapy for edema control and pain management appeared in 1946.[83] A comparison was made between two groups of patients who had undergone a variety of orthopedic surgical procedures. One group (n = 479) had no cooling, while the other (n = 345) had ice bags over their soft casts for a 48-hour period, replaced every 4 hours. The group treated with ice packs required fewer swelling-related splitting of casts (5.31%) compared with the non-iced group (41.3%). The ice-treated group also had less inflammation, as evidenced by a lower white blood cell count and fewer fevers over 38.3°C (101°F). No subject in the iced group had apparent hematomas or hemarthrosis, compared with 16 of those in the group receiving no ice. Also, fewer narcotics were taken by those who were treated with ice, indicating that their pain was less. Reduction of analgesic intake following cold application also has been reported by others.[84,85]

Although intuition might lead us to believe that cold rather than heat during the early phases postinjury would lead to a faster recovery, this comparison was not reported until 1982 by Hocutt and associates.[86] Patients with severe ankle sprain were placed in one of three groups: (1) superficial heating one to three times per day for 15 minutes, plus elastic bandaging, initiated early after injury; (2) cold whirlpool one to three times per day at 7°C to 10°C (40°F to 50°F) or ice packs for 15 to 20 minutes, plus elastic bandaging, initiated early after injury; or (3) cold treatment initiated 36 hours after injury. Treatment was continued for a minimum of 3 days among all patients. The patients treated with early cold (within the first 36 hours) returned to full activity (running and jumping without pain) an average of 8 days before those treated with heat or delayed cold. Therefore, the time at which cryotherapy is initiated following trauma can be expected to influence the time course for functional outcome.

Compression and Elevation

Cold (ice) is most often used in conjunction with rest, compression, and elevation in managing acute trauma, represented by the acronym RICE: rest, ice, compression, and elevation. Several acronyms have been developed since the original RICE, including PRICE (P = "protection"; Table 2-5)[87] and RICES (S = "stabilization").[45] These added components have the common theme of preventing further injury by avoiding harmful activity or undue stresses and by using braces, wraps, or casts for support. Regardless of the acronym used, the goals of cold therapy are to reduce swelling and inflammation, prevent further injury, and return to functional activities as soon as possible.

In many circumstances, edema may be lessened with immediate application of cold, but results are inconsistent when cold is intense or applied for long durations. In addition, the use of cold does not appear to be

---

Table 2•5 **PRICE (Protection, Rest, Ice, Compression, and Elevation and Stabilization)**

Intervention	Technique	Rationale
Protection	• Avoid activity that may cause additional harm • Splints or braces for immobilization or relative immobilization	• Prevention of further injury or harmful stresses on inflamed tissues • Avoid unwanted motion of injured area
Rest	• Immobilization, limited weight bearing • Limited-range active motion	• Limit irritation of inflamed tissues • Provides opportunity to ice, compress, and elevate
Ice	• Ice packs • Ice baths • Controlled-cold devices	• Reduce bleeding • Control pain • Reduce microvascular permeability • Reduce metabolism to limit secondary hypoxic injury • Limit edema
Compression	• Light compressive bandages • Cold compression devices	• Limit edema • Maintain gains in edema reduction
Elevation	• Extremity positioned above heart level	• Reduce hydrostatic pressure to limit edema formation
Stabilization	• Use of splints, braces, wraps, or casts	• Provide support to allow surrounding musculature to relax • Prevent unwanted or unexpected motion

effective in reducing edema once it has already formed, so it is imperative to apply cold as soon as possible following injury.[45] None of the animal studies reported earlier incorporated the use of compression or elevation. Compression can help prevent and reduce edema by increasing external pressure on tissues, which limits fluid loss from vessels. In addition, compression increases the rate and degree of cooling compared to cold without compression[88,89] (Fig. 2-12). Elevation takes advantage of gravitational forces and decreases hydrostatic pressure of capillaries. When this pressure is reduced, less fluid is forced out of vessels, limiting edema formation.

Two groups of researchers investigated cold and compression for the postoperative management of patients following total knee arthroplasty (TKA).[90,91] Levy and Marmar[91] measured pain relief, swelling, blood loss, and ROM in 80 patients who underwent unilateral or bilateral TKA. The patients received either compression alone or combined cold and compression, provided by a commercially manufactured inflatable cuff filled with ice water. Those patients who received cold plus compression had less pain, less swelling, and a lesser degree of blood loss, while demonstrating a greater increase in ROM.

Healy and associates[90] compared types of cold compressive dressings applied to 105 knees after TKA. A commercially available cuff, consisting of an inflatable bladder filled with ice water, was used for one group of subjects; the control group was treated with elastic bandage wraps and ice packs. Knee ROM, swelling, narcotic requirements, and wound drainage were measured. There were no significant differences between the groups for any of the variables. Both studies[90,91] advocated the use of cold-compressive dressings for the postoperative treatment of TKA, but the type of cold-compressive dressing did not appear to make any significant difference.

Adding compression to cold therapy can also improve microcirculation and tissue oxygenation.[54] When a series of three 10-minute sessions of cryotherapy plus compression at the ankle was compared to the same protocol with cryotherapy alone, superficial and deep capillary blood flow was greater in the combined group during the recovery phases (between the 10-minute applications). Tendon oxygenation was also greater in the combined group during the recovery phases. Postcapillary venous filling pressures were decreased in both groups during the treatment and the recovery phases.

KEY POINT! Although prolonged elevation of an extremity is difficult to achieve while maintaining function, continual compression can often be provided in the form of braces, wraps, or cold-compression devices. This can help to counteract the increases in hydrostatic pressures and reduced venous return that occur when an extremity is in the dependent position.

The duration of cold and the extent of the resultant temperature drop are important factors to consider regarding effects on soft tissues. To lessen risk of thermal damage or an increase in limb volume during acute or postoperative phases from excessive cold exposure, the nature of the cold treatment must be taken into consideration. Less intense cold applied for durations of 20 to 30 minutes several times a day, in conjunction with elevation and compression, appears to be a logical choice.

Cold Application Over Casts and Bandages

The presence of casts or bandages should not preclude the use of cold for edema or pain control, although the time to reach a minimum skin temperature is longer than when applied directly to the skin. Okcu and

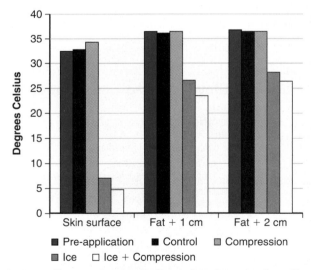

Fig 2•12 Temperature reductions at various depths with ice alone, compression alone, ice plus compression, and no treatment. *(Adapted with permission from Merrick MA, et al. The effects of ice and compression wraps on intramuscular temperature at various depths. J Athl Train. 1993;28:241.)*

Yercan[92] compared skin surface temperatures under two types of bandages and two types of casts in both injured (acute Grade III inversion ankle sprain) and uninjured individuals. Ice bags were applied over the casts or bandages. In all cases, skin surface temperature increased slightly immediately following application of the dressing or cast, but then dropped 7.3°C to 16.2°C (13°F to 29°F) below baseline. In both the injured and uninjured groups, the greatest temperature changes were reached with cooling over a plaster cast (average change 15°C; 27°F), and the smallest change was seen with the use of a Robert Jones bandage (alternating layers of cotton padding and gauze); the average change was 7.4°C (13.3°F). The time to reach the minimum recorded temperature was also shortest with the plaster cast (average 29 minutes) and longest with the Robert Jones bandage (average 47 minutes).

In a study by Ibrahim and colleagues,[93] the type of dressing was also shown to affect cooling. Cold was applied to the knees of healthy volunteers with a continuous cooling unit over no dressing, over a thin adhesive dressing (Tegaderm), and over a dressing of wool and crepe. The authors found that the wool and crepe dressing prevented the skin from reaching an effective cooling temperature of less than 20°C (68°F), whereas the skin temperatures with Tegaderm and no dressing both reached a temperature of 13°C (55.4°F). Similar results were found by Shibuya and associates,[23] where effective cooling was achieved with a continuous cooling unit placed over standard postsurgical dressings with and without one layer of Robert Jones bandaging; effective cooling was not achieved when two layers of the bandaging were used. Table 2-6 demonstrates the progression of most to least effective cooling over various dressing and casting materials based on several studies.[23,92–94]

KEY POINT! While studies have shown that cooling can occur when cold is applied over casts, it should be noted that it takes longer to achieve the same temperature under a fiberglass cast than it does under a plaster cast, and the presence of postsurgical dressings may prevent adequate cooling.

One of the underlying reasons for using cold after an acute musculoskeletal injury is to allow a more rapid return to function. However, few studies have looked at the effects of cryotherapy in conjunction with exercise or in relation to resumption of functional activities. Two systematic reviews point to the need for well-controlled studies in these areas.[95,96]

Pain and Muscle Spasm

As sequela to trauma, muscle spasm and pain often limit mobility and function. Many therapeutic techniques, including thermal agents, electrical stimulation, and manual therapy, are used with the common goals of reducing pain and muscle spasm, thus facilitating a more expedient recovery to normal function. In addition, many of these interventions may be used in lieu of pain medication. Patients can be easily instructed in the use of cold packs or ice massage at home for control of pain and muscle spasm.

Cooling the skin can elevate an individual's pain threshold[19,97] and reduce pain.[98] One theory for this process is that cold acts as a counterirritant,[99] and stimulation of thermal receptors in the skin (A-delta nerve fibers) may override pain signals from C fibers. Another theory involves a decrease in afferent input via reduced nerve conduction velocity.[19] Following acute injury or inflammation, severe pain can limit motion and ultimately lead to joint stiffness in the absence of intervention. Therapeutic interventions are aimed at reducing pain and inflammation and maintaining or increasing ROM.

Cryokinetics (cold plus exercise) was a technique popularized in the 1960s by Hayden[3] and Grant.[2] Hayden wrote about a group of 1,000 military patients who sustained sprains, strains, and contusions during training. Ice massage or ice-water immersion was used to provide analgesia before ROM exercises. All but

Table 2•6	Cooling Under Casts and Bandages	
Thin adhesive dressings		↑ Better Cooling
Plaster casts		
Fiberglass casts		
Standard elastic bandages		
Robert Jones dressing (layered padding* and elastic bandages)		↓ Poorer Cooling

*Typically a blend of cotton, crepe, rayon, or wool

three of the patients returned to active duty within 2 days, and most required only one physical therapy treatment. In Grant's study,[2] of the 7,000 patients with musculoskeletal injury from an army school, 90% had no more than three formal treatments with ice massage. Both Grant[2] and Hayden[3] cite that ice massage and exercise have the additional advantage of allowing patients to be more easily instructed in self-treatment. The goal behind cryokinetics is that the patient be able to perform pain-free, graded, progressive exercise following a period of tissue cooling (via cold immersion, ice massage, or ice bags).[45] However, exercise must not be performed to the extent that reinjury or increased inflammation occurs.

Cold in combination with static stretch or hold-relax techniques ("cryostretch") has been recommended for reducing muscle spasm or decreasing exercise-induced muscle soreness, thus increasing ROM. Cold is applied over the painful muscle using ice massage, ice packs, or cold packs. Either during or immediately following the cold application, the stretch is performed with the idea of returning the muscle to its normal resting length. Knight[45] suggests that when cold is used in conjunction with stretching, the area first be cooled until numbness is achieved, followed by cycles of passive stretch or hold-relax technique (a proprioceptive neuromuscular facilitation [PNF] technique).[100] This cycle of numbing and stretching is then repeated several times following periods of renumbing.

Delayed-Onset Muscle Soreness

Despite the positive effects of cold on pain and spasm, there is little research to support its use in reducing delayed-onset muscle soreness (DOMS). Prentice[101] induced muscle soreness in normal subjects through fatiguing concentric and eccentric contraction of the hamstrings. The following day, electromyographic (EMG) activity of the exercised muscle was increased from the pre-exercise measurement. EMG activity was measured as an indicator of muscle pain and spasm.[102] Following 20 minutes of cold packs and either static stretch or PNF slow-reversal-hold stretch to the hamstrings, EMG activity was reduced, suggesting a decrease in muscle soreness and spasm. These techniques were compared with an untreated control group and two groups that were given hot packs and static

stretch or PNF. Those who received cold had less measured EMG activity. Other studies have shown no significant benefit for using cold, either with ice-water immersion,[103,104] ice massage,[105] or contrast bath,[106] to reduce DOMS.

Myofascial Pain Syndrome

Myofascial pain syndrome is defined as "the sensory, motor, and autonomic symptoms caused by myofascial trigger points."[27] There are often accompanying ROM deficits in the area of the myofascial trigger point or area of referred pain. A trigger point in muscle may result from muscular strain or postural imbalance and may be associated with sensitized nerves, increased metabolism, and decreased circulation. Trigger points also are thought to be present in skin, ligaments, and fascia.

The pioneering work in trigger point localization and therapy was done by Janet Travell, MD.[29] According to Travell, active points are associated with a decrease in ROM and moderate to severe pain that is relatively constant. Latent trigger points may also lead to restricted ROM, but pain is present only on palpation. Both active and latent trigger points can be located by digital pressure. Trigger points can be treated using a variety of techniques, including spray and stretch, ice sweeps, ice massage, sustained deep pressure, ultrasound, electrical stimulation, and low-power laser.[107,108] Common areas of trigger points are around the cervical spine, shoulder girdle, lower back, and pelvis.[107] Trauma, poor body mechanics, and faulty posture are likely contributing forces.

A recent literature review highlights the need for well-controlled clinical studies regarding effective interventions for trigger points and myofascial pain syndrome.[108] It seems that the choice of treatment is largely based upon empiricism.[109] Interestingly, in spite of claims that vapocoolant spray and stretch techniques are widely used,[31] very few studies exist supporting its benefit in treating myofascial trigger points. A depiction of a spray and stretch treatment for a trigger point in the upper trapezius is shown in Figure 2-13A, and the spray and stretch technique is outlined in Case Study 2-4.

Ice massage has shown promise in reducing pain threshold sensitivity of trigger points.[110] When

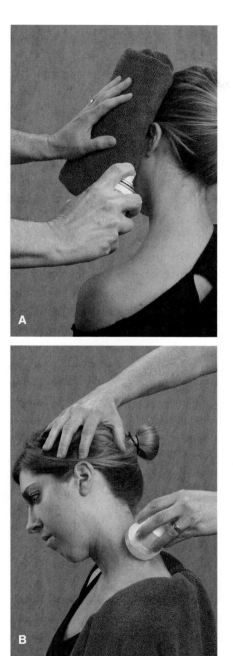

Fig 2•13 Options for myofascial trigger point treatment: (A) vapocoolant spray (and stretch) procedure for the upper trapezius; (B) ice cup plus stretch procedure for the levator scapula.

compared to sham ultrasound, 15 minutes of ice massage produced a significant decrease in trigger point pressure threshold and overall pain levels. Ice massage has also been shown to reduce pain pressure sensitivity of trigger points when compared to a menthol-based analgesic balm or placebo.[111] A technique for using ice massage and stretch for a trigger point in the

levator scapula is shown in Figure 2-13B. Ice is applied in a small area over the levator scapula trigger point in circular motions for 5 to 7 minutes. The duration of the ice application should be sufficient to produce analgesia and allow for deep-pressure massage over the trigger point and stretching of the neck muscles. Clinical trials comparing this technique to others in the management of trigger points would be beneficial.

Guidelines for Cryotherapy

Cold can be administered by a variety of methods. Those discussed in this section include ice packs, flexible frozen gel packs, ice massage, cold baths or whirlpools, vapocoolant sprays, and manual and mechanical controlled-cold and cold-compression units. The choice of which agent to use depends on accessibility, body part to be treated, whether simultaneous compression and elevation are required, and size of the area to be cooled. For example, the shoulder may be most effectively cooled using a cold pack wrapped around the joint (Fig. 2-14A), whereas the foot and ankle may be best covered by a cold immersion bath (Fig. 2-14B).

When considering cryotherapy, the practitioner must be familiar with the patient's medical status and how long it has been since the injury occurred. (Precautions for cryotherapy are discussed in a later section.) Before initiating treatment, a small area of skin should be tested for hypersensitivity.[112] If hypersensitivity is apparent, this should be documented and the cold discontinued. Signs of hypersensitivity include hives and wheals, the latter of which are raised, red, sometimes irregularly shaped areas that often burn or itch and can remain for 24 to 48 hours following exposure to cold (Fig. 2-15).

Following cryotherapy in any form, patients should avoid stresses for an hour or two that could potentially reinjure or aggravate the injury for which they were treated. The analgesia produced by the cold could mask exercise-induced pain, giving patients a false sense of security. Lowering of joint temperature can increase stiffness,[113] thereby decreasing reaction time and velocity of motion.[114] This, in combination with analgesia, may predispose patients to further injury.

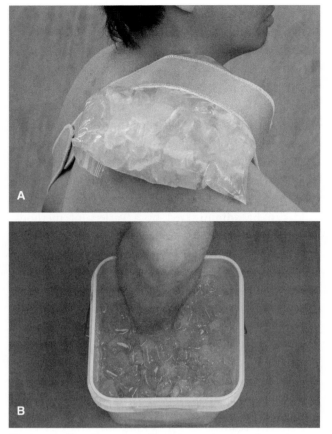

Fig 2•14 Cryotherapy options for various body regions: (A) ice bag for the shoulder (compression is added with sequential wrapping of the shoulder); (B) cold-bath immersion for the ankle (use of a toe cap will make immersion more comfortable yet allow cooling of the entire ankle).

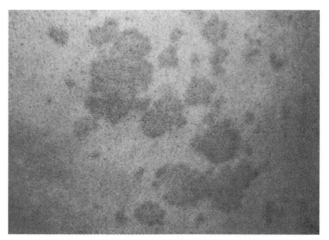

Fig 2•15 Example of wheals induced by exposure to cold.

When cold is applied to the skin, the area will become red. This occurs for two reasons. First, oxygen does not dissociate as freely from hemoglobin at lowered temperatures; therefore, the blood passing through the venous system is highly oxygenated, giving a red color to the skin. Second, after a 10- to 15-minute period of cooling, or upon removal of the cold stimulus, a reactive hyperemia may occur, bringing a greater amount of blood to the area.

Patients should be instructed about what to expect with application of a cold modality. When cold is to be applied for longer than several minutes, patients should be informed that they may initially feel intense cold, followed by a burning sensation, then aching, and finally numbness. Streator and associates[115] found that providing patients with information about the sensations they would likely experience resulted in a lower level of reported pain than when no information was provided.

The temperature of the cooling agent may influence the level of discomfort the patient can expect. Galvan and colleagues[116] found that pain ratings during immersion in ice water at 1°C (34°F) were 43% higher than immersion in 10°C (50°F) and 70% higher than immersion in 15°C (59°F) water. The authors also found that pain ratings across days and at the same temperature decreased, meaning that individuals somewhat adapted to the cold sensations. This may also be valuable information for patients, especially those who are reluctant to use cold after an initial uncomfortable experience.

KEY POINT! Informing patients that they will likely experience uncomfortable sensations (cold, burning, aching) before numbness with cold application and that these sensations often decrease in intensity with repeated applications may be beneficial in putting patients at ease and gaining their trust.

Generally speaking, conductive cooling is administered for 20 to 30 minutes, with longer time periods recommended for areas covered by significant adipose tissue.[8] Intermittent cold applications (e.g., 20 minutes on, followed by two cycles of 10 minutes off and 10 minutes on) are more effective in reducing tissue temperature, blood flow,[87,117] and pain with activity[118] than just one 20-minute application. This cycling of cold, rather than repeated prolonged use of cold packs or other cooling agents, is suggested to avoid or reduce the occurrence of any adverse responses to nerve or to blood vessels. In addition, if a patient remains inactive over several hours, repeated applications of cold for 30 minutes every 2 hours may produce a progressive cooling effect.[119]

Planned activity before, during, or immediately after cryotherapy should be considered in conjunction with the goals of using this modality. Cardiovascular exercise performed immediately prior to ice bag application will allow a more rapid cooling of muscular tissue due to increased blood flow that aids in the removal of heat from the cooled area.[120] When the goal is to achieve cooling at the level of muscular tissue, patients should refrain from activity while the cold modality is applied. Bender and colleagues[121] demonstrated that, despite evidence of skin surface cooling, no intramuscular cooling occurred while subjects walked on a treadmill with an ice pack secured to the calf (Fig. 2-16).

Based on this finding, wrapping an ice pack over a target area and then allowing the patient to carry on with functional activities will likely not provide the desired therapeutic effect. Finally, if the goal of cryotherapy is to reduce deep tissue temperature for 30 minutes to several hours, activity should be avoided after the cold application. Exercise following removal of ice packs from the gastrocnemius muscle increased subjects' intramuscular temperature to precooling levels

within 10 minutes, while the intramuscular temperature of the subjects who remained at rest continued to decline in this same 10-minute period.[15]

Selecting a Cooling Agent

When selecting a cooling agent, the clinician should consider which body area, and how much of the body surface, is to be cooled. For small areas (such as over a tendon, bursa, or small muscle belly), ice massage may effectively produce the cooling desired. If a distal extremity is to be cooled, as mentioned previously, a cool bath will most efficiently cover all surfaces. If there is concern about edema in distal extremities, a cold-compressive device may be most appropriate.

When cooling around a joint (such as the knee, elbow, or shoulder) or a larger muscle mass (such as lumbar or cervical paravertebral muscles), an ice pack secured with an elastic bandage or weighted to provide compression may be the best choice. Comparisons of various types of cooling agents will be presented in a later section, with most studies showing that ice or ice plus water in a plastic bag applied directly to the skin provides superior cooling compared to commercial gel packs or frozen peas, and any agent that requires toweling will be less effective than one that does not.[14,24,122]

Sometimes the decision of whether to use heat or cold for pain control is not always clear. Cold is always the appropriate choice in the acute phase of injury, while muscle spasms may respond to both heat (muscle relaxation) and cold (interruption of the pain/reflexive guarding cycle). The benefits of cold or heat with chronic inflammatory conditions are varied and may be patient-dependent. In this case, a trial of either heat or cold is within reason.

Contraindications and Precautions for Cryotherapy

Contraindications

Cryotherapy should not be used when treating patients who have specific cold-sensitivity symptoms. These conditions include, but are not limited to, cold urticaria, cryoglobulinemia, Raynaud's phenomenon,

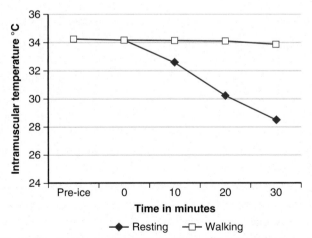

Fig 2•16 Intramuscular temperature of the gastrocnemius at rest and while walking on a treadmill with an ice bag secured to the calf. *(Adapted with permission from Bender AL, et al. Local ice-bag application and triceps surae muscle temperature during treadmill walking. J Athl Train. 2005;40:271.)*

and paroxysmal cold hemoglobinuria.[123] Cold urticaria can include both local and systemic reactions. In response to local cold application, patients develop wheals characterized by erythematous, raised borders, and blanched centers. Mast cell degranulation causes histamine to be released into the area, markedly increasing capillary permeability and leading to redness, swelling, and wheal formation. In severe cases, patients develop generalized swelling involving mucous membranes and viscera. Systemic reactions include flushing of the face, a sharp drop in blood pressure, increased heart rate, and syncope.[124]

Cryoglobulinemia is a disorder characterized by the presence of cryoglobulins, abnormal blood proteins that precipitate and form a gel when exposed to low temperatures (e.g., below body temperature). This precipitation of cryoglobulins results in the aggregation of serum proteins, which can lead to ischemia or gangrene. Cryoglobulinemia is associated with multiple myeloma; certain types of viral and bacterial infections, including hepatitis C; chronic liver disease; systemic lupus erythematosus (SLE); and other rheumatic diseases.[125]

Raynaud's phenomenon is a vasospastic disorder and can be either idiopathic or associated with other disorders, such as systemic scleroderma, SLE, thoracic outlet syndrome, and trauma. Smoking and caffeine can also worsen the frequency and intensity of the symptoms. Cycles of pallor, cyanosis, rubor, and normal color of the digits may be accompanied by numbness, tingling, or burning. Attacks are precipitated by exposure to cold or by emotional stress.[126]

Paroxysmal cold hemoglobinuria can occur following local or general exposure to cold. Hemoglobin, which is normally found within red blood cells, is released from lysed red cells and appears in the urine.

Cold should not be applied over areas of nerve regeneration or compromised circulation. For patients with peripheral vascular disease that affects arterial circulation, the vasoconstrictive effects of cold could potentially compromise an already nutritionally deprived area (Table 2-7).

Precautions

Because cold can cause a transient increase in systolic and diastolic blood pressures,[127,128] careful monitoring should take place when cryotherapy is used with hypertensive patients. Blood pressure should be monitored

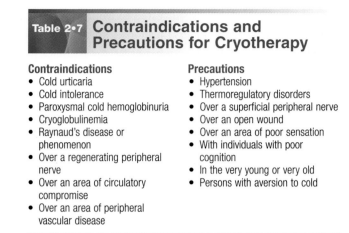

Table 2•7 Contraindications and Precautions for Cryotherapy

Contraindications	Precautions
• Cold urticaria	• Hypertension
• Cold intolerance	• Thermoregulatory disorders
• Paroxysmal cold hemoglobinuria	• Over a superficial peripheral nerve
• Cryoglobulinemia	• Over an open wound
• Raynaud's disease or phenomenon	• Over an area of poor sensation
• Over a regenerating peripheral nerve	• With individuals with poor cognition
• Over an area of circulatory compromise	• In the very young or very old
• Over an area of peripheral vascular disease	• Persons with aversion to cold

prior to and throughout treatment. Discontinue treatment if blood pressure rises.

Cold should be applied cautiously for individuals with hypersensitivity to cold, impaired circulation, and thermoregulatory disorders.[129] If, after careful consideration, cryotherapy is the treatment of choice for these patients, it is necessary to closely monitor the patient's response to treatment and make any adjustments to the treatment parameters. Decreasing the duration and adjusting the intensity of the cold application may produce the desired effects without eliciting adverse reactions.

Because cold temperatures may impede wound healing, precaution must be taken when aplying cold in the area of a wound. Lundgren and associates[130] demonstrated a 20% reduction in wound tensile strength in rabbits kept at environmental temperatures of 12°C (53.6°F) compared with those kept at 20°C (68°F). Only innervated animals showed this impaired healing response, suggesting a reflex cutaneous vasoconstriction (and thus a reduction in blood flow) with cold application. Until demonstrated otherwise, it is probably prudent to avoid vigorous cold application directly over a wound during the initial 2- to 3-week period of healing.

As mentioned earlier, prolonged cold application, from 1 to more than 2 hours, over an area containing a superficial peripheral nerve (e.g., around the medial epicondyle of the elbow or fibular head) can lead to neurapraxia or axonotmesis.[58,59] If cold is to be applied in an area of a superficial nerve, a small pad should be used between the cold source and the nerve for protection.

A survey of athletic trainers conducted by Nadler and colleagues[131] found that the most common complications from cryotherapy were from allergic reaction. Other complications were much less frequent and included intolerance/pain, burns, frostbite, and skin rash.

In addition to certain physiological factors contraindicating the use of cryotherapy, the patient's psychological response to this form of treatment should be taken into account. Some people have an aversion to cold and thus will not tolerate cryotherapy. This consideration is particularly important if cold is being used to decrease pain and promote skeletal-muscle relaxation.

Methods of Providing Cryotherapy

There are a variety of methods that can be used to provide effective cryotherapy. The following section describes the most common clinical applications of cold, all of which can be used by patients at home with proper instruction. A case study is presented for each type of cold modality to give the reader a clinical perspective. Table 2-8 provides information about the materials needed and the cost of different modes of therapeutic cold.

Cold Packs

Cold packs can be inexpensively purchased or easily made. They are typically composed of ice, ice plus water, water plus alcohol, gel, or chemicals (Fig. 2-17). The use of toweling over the skin is recommended for any agent that has the ability to reach temperatures below −1°C (30°F) because of the danger of skin damage. Any use of toweling, however, will decrease the effectiveness of the cooling agent.[132] When toweling is required, damp towels are superior to dry towels in facilitating energy transfer for thermal conduction.[45] If the towel is wet with room-temperature or lukewarm water, the initial contact with the skin will be more comfortable for the patient.

Crushed or cubed ice is typically placed in a plastic bag to create an ice pack. Ice is the most effective type of cold because it must undergo a phase change from solid to liquid, which causes greater heat extraction than when no phase change is required. Also, the temperature of the ice pack upon contact with the skin is typically just under 0°C (32°F), and this is safe to apply directly to the skin. Water can also be added to the ice in the bag. Dykstra and colleagues[14] found that this method reduced skin and intramuscular temperature to a greater extent than did cubed or crushed ice with no water (Fig. 2-18).

Table 2•8 Materials Needed and Average Cost of Typical Cryotherapy Agents		
Method	**Materials Required**	**Average Cost**
Frozen peas	• Purchased bag of peas, frozen for several hours • Thin wetted or dry towel for skin protection	$1–$3
Homemade ice bag	• Medium to large plastic bag (doubled for protection against leaking) • Ice cubes or crushed ice • Tap water (optional)	<$1
Homemade cold pack (with alcohol)	• Medium to large plastic bag (doubled for protection against leaking) • 1 cup isopropyl alcohol • 2–4 cups tap water • Thin wetted or dry towel for skin protection • Place in freezer several hours prior to use	$1–$3
Ice/cold bath	• Bucket or basin large enough to immerse the limb • Tap water • Ice cubes	$4–$10
Commercial cold packs (gel)	• Purchased gel pack • Thin wetted or dry towel for skin protection	$7–$50
Cold-compression units	• Appropriate sleeve for area to be cooled • Insulated cooler with hose	$60–$150
Continuous-cold compression units	• Appropriate sleeve for area to be cooled • Insulated motorized cooler with hose	$140–$280
Controlled cold-compression units	• Appropriate sleeve for area to be cooled • Insulated motorized cooler and compression pump with hose	$2,400–$2,700

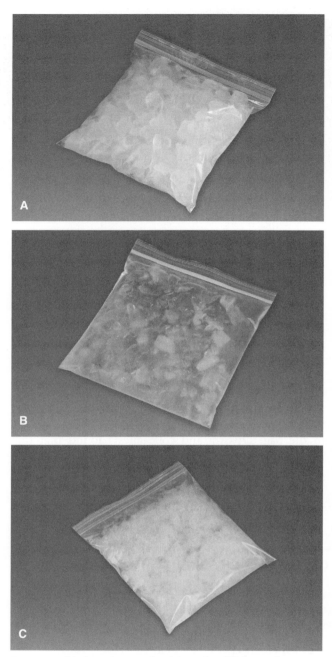

Fig 2•17 Various types of cold packs: (A) ice cubes; (B) ice cubes plus water; (C) crushed ice.

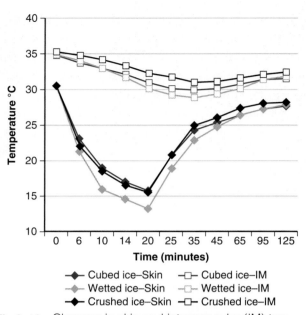

Fig 2•18 Changes in skin and intramuscular (IM) temperature with three different forms of ice pack during 20 minutes of application to the calf. *(Adapted with permission from Dykstra JH, et al. Comparisons of cubed ice, crushed ice, and wetted ice on intramuscular and surface temperature changes. J Athl Train. 2009;44:136.)*

A common recommendation for home cold packs is the use of bags of frozen vegetables (peas tend to be preferred because they are small, round, and conform well to body parts). While frozen peas may be a convenient, reusable, and low-cost alternative to ice packs, two studies have shown that frozen peas are not as effective in reducing skin-surface temperatures compared to ice packs or a mixture of water and alcohol.[24,122] Kennet and associates[24] also showed that the temperature of a bag of frozen peas taken from a freezer (−10°C; 14°F) was too cold for direct application to the skin and would require a layer of toweling. This toweling limits cooling by creating a barrier between the skin and the cold agent.

Commercial gel packs usually contain a silica gel and are available in a variety of sizes and shapes to contour the area to be treated (Fig. 2-19A). The flexible gel packs stored in a standard freezer will typically reach a temperature of −17°C (−1°F), which could cause frostbite if applied directly to the skin. Therefore, a layer of damp toweling is required. Gel packs are not as effective at cooling skin or intramuscular tissues when compared to ice packs or ice water packs.[24,122] This is because the gel does not go through a phase change, and therefore less energy is required for heat transfer. In addition, the requirement of toweling may also reduce the cooling effectiveness of this modality.

A mixture of water and isopropyl alcohol (2:1 to 4:1 ratio) can also be used as a homemade cold pack (Fig. 2-19B). The alcohol acts as antifreeze, which prevents the water from forming a solid and allows the pack to remain pliable, similar to the commercial gel packs. This mixture should be stored in the freezer for several hours prior to application. Because the

CASE STUDY 2•1 **ICE PACK**

A 42-year-old male is referred with a diagnosis of acute low back pain. Upon examination, he demonstrates pain and spasm in the right lumbar paraspinals. Hypertonicity of the musculature is observable and palpable, and the patient is limited in forward flexion, left lateral flexion, and right rotation as a result of pain and tightness.

CLINICAL DECISION-MAKING

1. Does the patient have a dysfunction, limitation, or problem that can be improved with the use of cryotherapy?
   Answer: Yes; muscle spasm and pain can be reduced with cryotherapy, allowing for performance of muscle stretching.

2. Is the patient appropriate for cryotherapy (i.e., do any of the general precautions or contraindications to cryotherapy apply to the patient, or are there any specific considerations regarding application of cryotherapy to this patient)?
   Answer: The patient should be asked about the presence of any contraindications or precautions for the use of cold. A small nearby area of skin should be tested with the cold modality to determine if hypersensitivity (wheals, hives) is present.

3. What are the specific goals to be achieved with the use of cryotherapy?
   Answer: Reduction of muscle spasm and pain to allow for stretching of tight musculature.

4. What specific form of cryotherapy would be appropriate for the patient?
   Answer: Ice packs are most appropriate because of the surface area to be treated and the desire to cool tissues at the muscular level. Commercial cold gel packs are also appropriate (but not as effective).

5. What specific parameters of cryotherapy are appropriate for the patient?
   Answer:
   Type of ice pack: Plastic bag filled with crushed ice, cubed ice, or ice with water. Commercial gel packs

are less effective but also appropriate (will use identical application technique except requires a layer of toweling between the cold pack and the patient's skin to prevent frostbite).
   Duration: Twenty minutes or until the area is numb (additional time is required if there is significant adipose tissue overlying the target tissue). If muscle stretching is to be performed, this can be done at the end of the 20-minute period, and then re-icing should occur for 5 to 10 minutes after the stretching period (this cycle can be repeated several times).

6. What are the appropriate and safe application procedures for ice packs?
   Answer:
   Instruct the patient: Inform the patient of the expected sensations of cold, burning, aching, and then numbness (analgesia).
   Preinspection: Inspect the area to be treated for skin compromise, and assess for intact sensation over the area to be treated.
   Equipment needed: Bag of ice; towels
   Patient position: Prone or sitting. If sitting, a wrap will be necessary to secure the ice pack to the affected area (this will also add a compressive force).
   Procedure: Place the ice pack directly on the patient's skin over the target area. A small weight can be placed on top of the ice pack to add a compressive force, which will allow for more effective cooling.
   Postinspection: Remove the ice pack and inspect the patient's skin. Redness will be present and may remain for 20 minutes or longer, depending on the patient's activity level or exercises performed. If stretching or light resistance is to be performed, it should be initiated as soon as possible after the ice pack is removed (a second or third application of cold may be necessary to renumb the area through an exercise session).

alcohol/water mixture can reach temperatures colder than ice, a thin layer of damp toweling should be placed between the skin and the pack. This type of cold pack has been shown to cool as effectively as a crushed ice pack over a 20-minute period (to a temperature of 10°C; 50°F).[122]

There are some cold packs that are chemically activated by squeezing or hitting them against a hard surface. These packs are usually marketed for first aid and designed for one-time use only. The chemical reaction inside some of the packs is at an alkaline pH and can cause skin burns if the package splits open

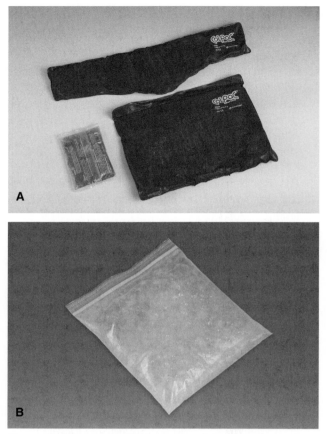

Fig 2•19 Examples of (A) commercial gel packs and (B) a homemade cold pack using a mixture of tap water and isopropyl alcohol (3 parts water to 1 part alcohol).

and the contents spill out. Therefore, these packs are not recommended for general use.

As mentioned in the "Acute Musculoskeletal Trauma" section, compression and elevation are often used to control edema and improve the cooling ability of the cold modality. Ice bags are usually the most readily available form of cold when acute injuries occur, and elastic bandages can provide excellent compression over the cold packs on most body regions.

Ice Massage

Ice massage is usually done over a small area (i.e., over a muscle belly, tendon, or bursa) or over trigger points before deep pressure release or massage. The technique is simple and can be taught to patients who can reliably follow directions for home use.

Water is frozen in paper or Styrofoam cups to make it easier for the practitioner to handle the ice. Just prior to use, the top of the cup is peeled back to expose the ice. Further peeling can occur as the ice melts. As an alternative, ice "lollipops" can be made by putting a wooden tongue depressor in the cup with the water (Fig. 2-20). The ice pop can be taken out of the cup and held by the tongue depressor for application. A 10 cm × 15 cm area (4 in. × 6 in.) can be covered in 5 to 10 minutes.[133] The ice is slowly rubbed over the skin using small overlapping circles or strokes.

KEY POINT! Styrofoam cups are often used for ice cups, as they allow for more comfortable handling of the cup due to the insulating properties of this material (i.e., the hand holding the ice cup will not become cold). However, Styrofoam is not biodegradable and therefore is not environmentally friendly. Wrapping a small washcloth around the base of the ice cup will prevent the hand from becoming too cold and is an environmentally friendly remedy to the handling problem.

During ice massage, the patient will probably experience the four common sensations of intense cold, burning, aching, then analgesia. However, the stages of burning and aching should each pass rapidly within about 1 to 2 minutes. A prolonged phase of aching or burning may result if the area covered is too large or if a hypersensitive response is imminent (see "Contraindications and Precautions for Cryotherapy"). Skin temperature will usually not drop below 15°C (59°F) when the ice is continually moved over the skin; therefore, the risk of damaging tissue and producing frostbite is minimal.

Vapocoolant Spray

Vapocoolant sprays are used to treat trigger points and to induce relaxation of tight muscles prior to stretching (the physiological basis is described in the "Evaporation" section). When treating trigger points, the patient is positioned comfortably and the muscle containing the trigger point is placed on passive stretch. Spraying is done in unidirectional sweeps along the muscle over the trigger point areas and over the areas of referred pain, while maintaining and gently increasing the passive stretch. The vapocoolant canister is held 12 to 18 inches away from the skin during spray applications. When using the spray to increase muscle length

CASE STUDY 2•2 PRICE

A 17-year-old male is referred with a diagnosis of acute Grade II right lateral ankle sprain that occurred 12 hours prior. Upon examination, he demonstrates notable effusion throughout the right ankle (lateral greater than medial), decreased ankle AROM (active range of motion) in all directions, and pain that increases with active or passive ankle motion and weight bearing.

CLINICAL DECISION-MAKING

1. Does the patient have a dysfunction, limitation, or problem that can be improved with the use of cryotherapy?
   Answer: Yes; pain can be reduced with cryotherapy, allowing for performance of range of motion within the patient's tolerance.

2. Is the patient appropriate for cryotherapy (i.e., do any of the general precautions or contraindications to cryotherapy apply to the patient, or are there any specific considerations regarding application of cryotherapy to this patient)?
   Answer: The patient should be asked about the presence of any contraindications or precautions for the use of cold. A small nearby area of skin should be tested with the cold modality to determine if hypersensitivity (wheals, hives) is present.

3. What are the specific goals to be achieved with the use of cryotherapy (specifically RICE)?
   Answer: The use of ice will reduce pain, allowing for initiation of gentle ROM exercises and at least partial weight bearing. Rest from typical or stressful activity will allow healing to proceed. Compression will help control effusion and edema and will increase the ice's cooling ability. Elevation will reduce joint effusion and edema.

4. What specific form of cryotherapy would be appropriate for the patient?
   Answer: Ice packs are most appropriate because these will conform well to the area.

5. What specific parameters of cryotherapy are appropriate for the patient?
   Answer:
   Type of ice pack: Plastic bag filled with crushed ice, cubed ice, or ice with water.

Type of compression: Elastic bandages (4 in. to 6 in. wide)
Duration: Twenty minutes or until the area is numb. If ROM exercises or weight bearing is to be performed, this can be done at the end of the 20-minute period, and then re-icing (with compression and elevation) may occur for 5 to 10 minutes following the stretching period (this cycle can be repeated several times).

6. What are the proper application procedures for RICE?
   Answer:
   Instruct the patient: Inform the patient of the expected sensations of cold, burning, aching, and then numbness (analgesia).
   Preinspection: Inspect the area to be treated for skin compromise and assess for intact sensation over the area to be treated.
   Equipment needed: Bag of ice or ice plus water; elastic bandage long enough to fully cover the ice bag and ankle; stack of towels or other materials to elevate the patient's leg.
   Patient position: Supine.
   Procedure: Place the ice pack directly on the patient's skin over the target area. Begin wrapping the elastic bandage around the ice pack and ankle and continue in a distal to proximal direction, stretching the elastic bandage to approximately 75% of its capacity.[45] Elevate the patient's lower extremity to a level above the heart and ensure that the leg is fully supported.
   Postinspection: Remove the elastic bandage and ice pack and inspect the patient's skin. Redness will be present and may remain for 20 minutes or longer, depending on the patient's activity level or exercises performed. If ROM or weight bearing is to be performed, it should be initiated as soon as possible after the ice pack is removed (a second or third application of cooling, compression, and elevation may be necessary to renumb the area and reduce any accumulated fluid caused by dependent positioning).

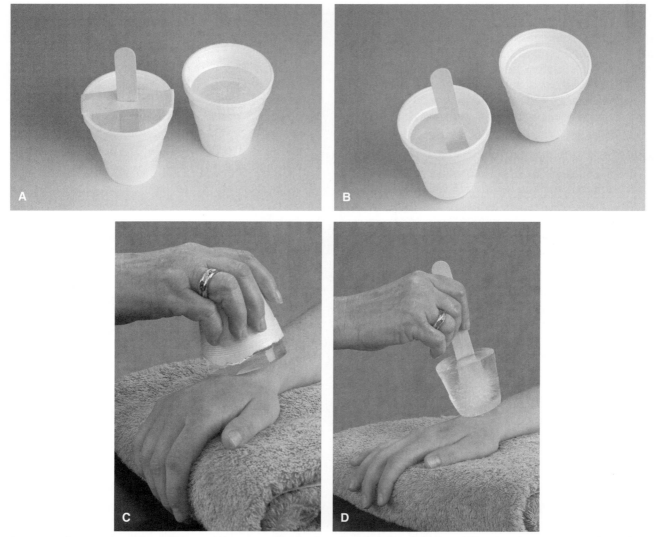

Fig 2•20 Ice cups and ice lollipops. (A) preparation for freezing; (B) after freezing; (C) using the ice cup on the wrist; (D) using the ice lollipop on the wrist.

without identified trigger points, the muscle is sprayed along its length from the proximal to the distal attachments. Repeated treatments during the same session are done only after the skin has been rewarmed to avoid frosting the skin.

Manual and Electric Cold Compression Units

Cold compression devices (Fig. 2-21) allow for manual circulation of cold water through a cuff that is applied over an extremity. A variety of sizes and shapes of cuffs and sleeves are available to conform to any joint or extremity. To fill or recirculate cold water into the cuff, the insulated ice-water-filled container is connected to the cuff by a hose and then elevated, allowing gravity to pull water into the cuff. Manual recirculation is recommended every 1 to 2 hours to maintain the cooling effect. However, specific temperature monitoring and adjustment are not possible with these units. Compression is achieved by pressure exerted from the filled cuff that is wrapped around the joint or extremity and secured with Velcro. One study demonstrated that the Aircast Cryo/Cuff device was capable of maintaining a skin surface temperature between 20.4°C and 28°C (68.7°F and 82.4°F) when applied over a standard postsurgical dressing. It should be noted that the authors recirculated the cold water in the sleeve every 15 minutes, versus every hour as recommended by the manufacturer.[23]

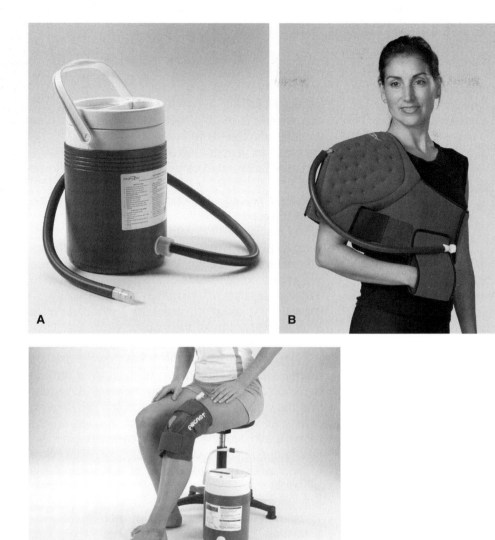

Fig 2•21 Cold compression units. (A) DonJoy ArcticFlow and (B) shoulder cuff; (C) Aircast Cryo/Cuff. *(Courtesy DJO Inc., Vista, CA.)*

Continuous-cold compression units (Fig. 2-22) are similar to the devices described previously, except they use an electric pump to circulate cold water at intervals or rates that can be set by the user, depending on the level of cooling desired. Water temperatures can be adjusted from 0°C to 40°C (32°F to 104°F), and the set temperature is maintained as long as the unit is on. Three studies[134–136] have investigated the differences in postoperative outcomes comparing continuous-cold units and traditional icing protocols. Although outcome variables differed between each study, pain, edema, range of motion, and medication use were improved to a greater extent in patients who used continuous-cold versus ice packs.

Because cooling temperatures can be set to levels that are unsafe for prolonged skin exposure,[23] patient education about appropriate temperature settings is imperative. Khajavi and colleagues[137] describe a case of severe compartment syndrome that resulted from improper use of a continuous-cold unit set at 0.5°C (33°F) and used continuously for 5 days following an arthroscopic procedure of the knee.

Controlled-cold compression units add the effect of adjustable levels of compression (typically 5 mm Hg to 75 mm Hg) at variable intervals. Thus, these units allow the treated area to receive a constant cold temperature along with intermittent periods of

CASE STUDY 2•3 **ICE MASSAGE**

A 28-year-old female is referred with a diagnosis of right lateral epicondylitis that began after she spent 9 hours painting fence posts 2 days ago. Upon examination, there is exquisite tenderness in the area surrounding the right lateral epicondyle, pain and limitations with right wrist extension, and intense pulling in the right proximal forearm with passive wrist flexion.

CLINICAL DECISION-MAKING

1. Does the patient have a dysfunction, limitation, or problem that can be improved with the use of cryotherapy?
   Answer: Yes; cryotherapy can be effective in reducing pain and inflammation.

2. Is the patient appropriate for cryotherapy (i.e., do any of the general precautions or contraindications to cryotherapy apply to the patient, or are there any specific considerations regarding application of cryotherapy to this patient)?
   Answer: The patient should be asked about the presence of any contraindications or precautions for the use of cold. A small nearby area of skin should be tested with the cold modality to determine if hypersensitivity (wheals, hives) is present.

3. What are the specific goals to be achieved with the use of cryotherapy?
   Answer: Reduce pain and allow the patient to perform ROM and stretching with less discomfort.

4. What specific form of cryotherapy would be appropriate for the patient?
   Answer: Ice massage (ice packs are also appropriate but would take longer and would not isolate the area as well).

5. What specific parameters of ice massage would be appropriate for the patient?
   Answer: Rubbing the ice directly on the skin over the affected area for 5 to 7 minutes or until analgesia (numbness) is achieved.

6. What are the proper application procedures for ice massage?
   Answer:
   Instruct the patient: Inform the patient of the expected sensations of cold, burning, aching, and then numbness in the treated area.
   Preinspection: Inspect the area for skin compromise and assess for intact sensation over the area to be treated.
   Equipment needed: Ice cup or ice popsicle; three small towels.
   Patient position: Sitting with the right arm in a comfortable position that allows easy access to the affected area. Once the patient is positioned, place two towels on either side of the proximal forearm to catch water drips.
   Procedure: If using the ice cup method, remove enough of the top of the cup to expose at least 1 inch of ice. Make sure to leave enough of the cup to hold on to (one of the small towels can be wrapped around the bottom of the cup to provide insulation for the hand holding the cup). After rubbing the ice briefly to make the top smooth (melting off any ice spurs or ridges), place the ice on the patient's skin over the affected area and begin moving the cup in small, slow circles. Continue for 5 to 7 minutes or until numbness is achieved. If the patient is to perform any stretching or ROM exercise, she should do so immediately after the ice massage. Renumbing may be required after several minutes of exercise, but the time required to achieve numbness again should be less than the first application. This cycle of numbing and exercise may be repeated several times.
   Postinspection: Remove the ice cup and discard. Dry the skin and inspect for any adverse effects. Redness will be present and may remain for 20 minutes or longer, depending on the patient's activity level or exercises performed.

compression. These units are most commonly found in sports medicine facilities and can cost several thousand dollars.

Cold Baths

When cooling the distal extremities, immersion of those parts in a cold bath is most practical (unless simultaneous elevation is desired, particularly in the presence of edema). This approach ensures circumferential contact of the cooling agent. Water temperatures for immersion vary from 10°C to 18°C (50°F to 64.4°F). The lower the temperature range, the shorter the duration of immersion required for cooling. In a previously mentioned study,[116] it was found that pain ratings were significantly higher during immersion in 1°C (34°F) and 10°C (50°F) temperatures

CASE STUDY 2•4 **VAPOCOOLANT SPRAY**

A 56-year-old female is referred with a diagnosis of headaches and right neck pain. Upon examination, several active myofascial trigger points are found in the right upper trapezius that, upon compression, reproduce the patient's lateral neck pain and headaches. She also reports tightness and discomfort with cervical flexion and left lateral flexion.

CLINICAL DECISION-MAKING

1. Does the patient have a dysfunction, limitation, or problem that can be improved with the use of cryotherapy?

   Answer: Yes; active myofascial trigger points may be treated with vapocoolant spray to reflexively inhibit the agonist muscle, followed by a stretch that is intended to normalize the affected muscle's length.

2. Is the patient appropriate for cryotherapy (i.e., do any of the general precautions or contraindications to cryotherapy apply to the patient, or are there any specific considerations regarding application of cryotherapy to this patient)?

   Answer: The patient should be asked about the presence of any contraindications or precautions for the use of cold. A small nearby area of skin should be tested with the vapocoolant spray to determine if hypersensitivity (wheals, hives) is present.

3. What are the specific goals to be achieved with the use of cryotherapy?

   Answer: Reflexive inhibition of active myofascial trigger points.

4. What specific form of cryotherapy would be appropriate for the patient?

   Answer: Vapocoolant spray.

5. What specific parameters of vapocoolant spray would be appropriate for the patient?

   Answer: Three to five slow (10 cm/sec; 4 in./sec), unidirectional sweeps of the spray in the direction of the pain pattern, avoiding direct overlap of each spray.[107]

6. What are the proper application procedures for vapocoolant spray (and stretch)?

   Answer:

   Instruct the patient: Inform the patient of the expected sensations of cold in the area to be sprayed.

   Preinspection: Inspect the area to be treated for skin compromise and assess for intact sensation over the area to be treated.

   Equipment needed: Vapocoolant spray; small towel to protect the patient's eyes.

   Patient position: Sitting with the right arm holding the edge of a chair and the right upper trapezius on slight stretch (cervical flexion, left lateral flexion, right rotation). Because the patient's head is rotated toward the spray, a small towel should be held over her eyes for protection from the spray.

   Procedure: Place the patient's right upper trapezius on a slight stretch (cervical flexion, left lateral flexion, right rotation), which should be maintained throughout the procedure, taking up any slack as the muscle relaxes. Begin spraying in the direction of the patient's pain pattern with the canister approximately 30 cm (12 in.) away from, and at a 30° angle to, the skin. The first sweep should go directly over the primary myofascial trigger point, and the remaining two to four sweeps should be along the referral pattern, in the same direction as the first sweep but not directly over it. Once the sweeps are completed, apply additional but gentle stretches to the upper trapezius, holding 20 to 30 seconds before the patient returns to normal alignment.

   Postinspection: The patient's skin may be slightly red over the treated area. Observe for any abnormal skin reaction to the spray. Because the spray evaporates quickly, there is little, if any, rewarming time required.

versus immersion in 15°C (59°F) water. However, pain ratings improved during both the 1°C and 10°C after the first several minutes of immersion, and average ratings never exceeded 4.5 on a 0 to 10 scale (0 = no pain, 10 = very, very strong pain) for any immersion temperature. As discussed in the "Convection" section, movement of the water particles over the skin, either with water turbulence or with movement of the body part, will increase the speed of cooling. A basin of water or a small whirlpool filled with water and crushed ice can be used (see Fig. 2-14B). The use of a toe cap will reduce the pain sensation in the toes, which tend to be the most painful during immersion.[138] Cold bath immersions can be used by patients at home with proper instruction.

CASE STUDY 2•5   COLD COMPRESSION DEVICE

A 32-year-old female is referred with a diagnosis of acute left knee sprain with suspicion of a torn anterior cruciate ligament. Upon examination, she demonstrates global knee pain and notable effusion. The patient's AROM is limited to 10° to 85°, and she ambulates with bilateral axillary crutches at 50% weight bearing on the left.

CLINICAL DECISION-MAKING

1. Does the patient have a dysfunction, limitation, or problem that can be improved with the use of cryotherapy?
   Answer: Yes; pain can be reduced with cryotherapy, allowing the patient to perform range of motion within her tolerance.

2. Is the patient appropriate for cryotherapy (i.e., do any of the general precautions or contraindications to cryotherapy apply to the patient, or are there any specific considerations regarding application of cryotherapy to this patient)?
   Answer: The patient should be asked about the presence of any contraindications or precautions for the use of cold. A small nearby area of skin should be tested with the cold modality to determine if hypersensitivity (wheals, hives) is present.

3. What are the specific goals to be achieved with the use of cryotherapy (specifically PRICE)?
   Answer: The use of cold will reduce pain, allowing for performance of ROM exercises and increased weight bearing. Compression will help control effusion and will increase the cooling ability of the ice water. Elevation may also be used to help with reduction of effusion.

4. What specific form of cryotherapy would be appropriate for the patient?
   Answer: A commercial cold-compression unit.

5. What specific parameters of cryotherapy are appropriate for the patient?
   Answer:
   Type of cold: Ice water in the cold-compression unit's container that is manually circulated through a wraparound cuff by raising and lowering the container.
   Duration: 20 to 30 minutes (with elevation to maximize effusion reduction) or until the area is numb

and swelling has reduced; if ROM exercises are to be performed, they can be done at the end of the initial period. This cycle of cooling/compression and exercise can be continued several times (cooling/compression time can be reduced after the first cycle unless more than 30 minutes have passed since the cold was removed).

6. What are the proper application procedures for a cold-compression device?
   Answer:
   Instruct the patient: Inform the patient of the expected sensations of cold, burning, aching, and then numbness (analgesia).
   Preinspection: Inspect the area to be treated for skin compromise and assess for intact sensation over the area to be treated.
   Equipment needed: Cold-compression device, ice, water; if elevation is necessary, use a stack of towels or other material to elevate the patient's leg.
   Patient position: Supine.
   Procedure: Fill the insulated cold-compression container with ice and then water to the levels indicated on the device. Place the cuff directly on the patient's skin surrounding the knee and secure with the Velcro on the cuff. Position the patient (supporting the leg in elevation as desired). Attach the hose from the container to the cuff, and fill the cuff with ice water according to the manufacturer's instructions. Once the cuff is full, release the hose. If continual cooling is desired, recirculate the water in the cuff after 15 minutes.
   Postinspection: Remove the cuff from the patient's knee and inspect the skin. Redness will be present and may remain for 20 minutes or longer, depending on the patient's activity level or exercises performed. If exercise is to be performed, it should be initiated as soon as possible after the cold-compression device is removed (a second or third application of cold-compression and elevation may be necessary to renumb the area and reduce any accumulated fluid caused by dependent positioning or exercise).

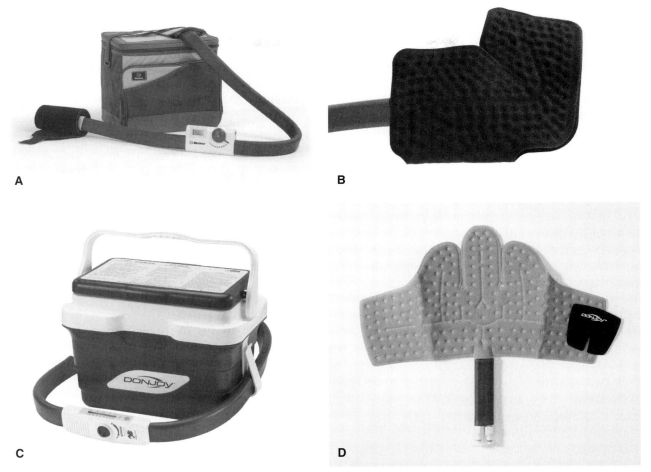

Fig 2•22   Controlled-cold compression units. (A) Bledsoe Cold Control and (B) shoulder wrap; (C) DonJoy IceMan and (D) ankle wrap. *(Courtesy Bledsoe Brace Systems, Grand Prairie, TX; and DJO Inc., Vista, CA.)*

Cold Gel

There are commercially available gels or creams that give the *perceived* sensation of cold. Most of these gels have chemicals such as ethanol and menthol as the active cold-forming agents. These creams or gels are applied to the skin overlying the area of injury and pain. One study demonstrated a decrease in pain and a decrease in perceived disability of higher magnitudes when cold gel was compared with placebo gel for soft-tissue injuries of the hand, knee, leg, or ankle.[139] The gel was applied on the skin four times daily for 2 weeks. Another study demonstrated a significant reduction in low back pain ratings in a group of patients who received chiropractic adjustments that included Biofreeze application versus adjustments

alone.[140] The appeal of these gels is their ease of application, ease of portability, and lack of need for refrigeration. However, actual cooling of the skin or subcutaneous tissues does not occur.

Assessment of Effectiveness and Expected Outcomes

As with any therapeutic technique, the decision to use cold modalities in a therapy program should be based on the treatment's goals. The goals of cold application are determined by the patient and the practitioner after examinations, including the history of the present problem and subjective and objective measures of impairments and current functional

CASE STUDY 2•6   COLD IMMERSION

The 17-year-old patient from Case Study 2-2 is now 10 days postinjury. His swelling is significantly reduced, although still present with prolonged standing. He is having difficulty performing some resistive and weight-bearing exercises without pain. Upon examination, he demonstrates 25% active ROM limitations in all ankle motions, mild to moderate pain with resistance in the directions of eversion and dorsiflexion, and difficulty completing a normal gait cycle (diminished passive ankle dorsiflexion in the terminal stance phase). The anterior and posterior talofibular ligaments, the calcaneofibular ligament, and the peroneal tendons are tender upon palpation.

CLINICAL DECISION-MAKING

1. Does the patient have a dysfunction, limitation, or problem that can be improved with the use of cryotherapy?
   Answer: Yes; pain can be reduced with cryotherapy, allowing for performance of ROM, resistive exercise, and increased weight-bearing tolerance to complete a normal gait cycle.

2. Is the patient appropriate for cryotherapy (i.e., do any of the general precautions or contraindications to cryotherapy apply to the patient, or are there any specific considerations regarding application of cryotherapy to this patient)?
   Answer: Because the patient has received cryotherapy in the form of ice packs during the acute phase of his injury, he should be safe for other forms of cryotherapy.

3. What are the specific goals to be achieved with the use of cryotherapy?
   Answer: The use of cold-bath immersion will reduce pain, allowing for performance of active ROM, light to moderate resistive exercises, and walking with a normalized gait pattern.

4. What specific form of cryotherapy would be appropriate for the patient?
   Answer: Cold-bath immersion will allow for more uniform cooling of the affected ligaments and tendons.

5. What specific parameters of cryotherapy are appropriate for the patient?
   Answer:
   Type of immersion: Basin filled with lukewarm to cool water and ice cubes.
   Duration: 20 minutes or until the area is numb.

6. What are the proper application procedures for cold immersion?
   Answer: Instruct the patient: Inform the patient of the expected sensations of cold, burning, aching, and then numbness (analgesia).
   Preinspection: Inspect the area to be treated for skin compromise and assess for intact sensation over the area to be treated.
   Equipment needed: Basin deep enough to allow water coverage of the patient's distal tibia; enough water to fill the basin to the stated level; ice cubes.
   Patient position: Sitting in a chair so the feet touch the floor.
   Procedure: Fill the basin with water and ice cubes to the required level. Placing a neoprene toe cap over the patient's forefoot will provide some insulation to the forefoot and will decrease the patient's discomfort.[138] Instruct the patient to immerse the ankle into the basin and ensure that the malleoli are below the water surface. The area will cool more effectively if the patient moves the limb within the water (convection). Once the area is numb, the patient may then remove the limb from the water, dry the area, and perform the desired exercises (ROM, resistance, gait). When the numbness has worn off or when the patient begins to feel discomfort, reimmersion can occur for 5 to 10 minutes until numbness has again been achieved. This cycle of numbing and exercise can be repeated several times.
   Postinspection: The immersed area will be red for 20 minutes or more following the cooling period. Observe the skin for any adverse reactions to cold.

status. The following outcome measures can be used in assessing effectiveness with cold:

- Edema—girth measures, volumetrics
- Pain—quantification via pain scales or questionnaires
- Range of motion—goniometric measures
- Functional movements—observation of gait quality or ease of active ROM
- Muscle guarding—reflected in joint ROM and muscle flexibility measures

Of course, the decision of which of these measures to use will depend on the body limitation being addressed by the treatment.

Documentation

Accurate recording of the treatment parameters, changes in patient response to treatment during and between sessions, and any modifications of the goals or treatment program should be documented. Specific parameters for cold applications include the type of cold agent, treatment duration, site of application, patient position, and use of concurrent compression or elevation. Further descriptions of changes in skin temperature or appearance, quality of edema, and sensation are also documented. Clinical notes include periodic reassessments of the patient's overall functional level, especially in relation to the impairments directly affected by intervention.

Documentation Tips

- Type of cold agent
- Treatment duration
- Site of cold application
- Position of patient for cold application
- Use of concurrent compression or elevation
- Change in skin appearance
- Patient response (i.e., change in pain, edema, ROM)
- Adverse responses

☐ REFERENCES

1. Licht S. *History of Therapeutic Heat and Cold.* 3rd ed. Baltimore: Williams & Wilkins; 1982.
2. Grant A. Massage with ice (cryokinetics) in the treatment of painful conditions of the musculoskeletal system. *Arch Phys Med Rehabil.* 1964;45:233–238.
3. Hayden C. Cryokinetics in an early treatment program. *J Am Phys Ther Assoc.* 1964;44(11):990–993.
4. Levine M, Kabat H, Knott M, Voss D. Relaxation of spasticity by physiological techniques. *Arch Phys Med Rehabil.* 1954;35:214–223.
5. Nave C, Nave B. *Physics for the Health Sciences.* 2nd ed. Philadelphia: WB Saunders; 1980.
6. Clarke R, Hellon R, Lind A. Vascular reactions of the human forearm to cold. *Clin Sci.* 1958;17(1):165–179.
7. Abramson D. Physiologic basis for the use of physical agents in peripheral vascular disorders. *Arch Phys Med Rehabil.* 1965;46:216–244.
8. Lehmann J, DeLateru B. *Cryotherapy.* Baltimore: Williams & Wilkins; 1990.
9. Lowdon B, Moore R. Determinants and nature of intramuscular temperature changes during cold therapy. *Am J Phys Med.* 1975;54(5):223–233.
10. Wolf S, Basmajian J. Intramuscular temperature changes deep to localized cutaneous cold stimulation. *Phys Ther.* 1973;53(12):1284–1288.
11. Otte J, Merrick M, Ingersoll C, Cordova M. Subcutaneous adipose tissue thickness alters cooling time during cryotherapy. *Arch Phys Med Rehabil.* 2002;83:1501–1505.
12. Wakim K, Porter A, Krusen K. Influence of physical agents of certain drugs on intra-articular temperature. *Arch Phys Med.* 1951;32:714–721.
13. Johnson D, Moore S, Moore J, Oliver R. Effect of cold submersion on intramuscular temperature of the gastrocnemius muscle. *Phys Ther.* 1979;59(10):1238–1242.
14. Dykstra J, Hill H, Miller M, Cheatham C, Michael T, Baker R. Comparisons of cubed ice, crushed ice, and wetted ice on intramuscular and surface temperature changes. *J Athl Train.* 2009;44(2):136–141.
15. Myrer J, Measom G, Fellingham G. Exercise after cryotherapy greatly enhances intramuscular rewarming. *J Athl Train.* 2000;35(4):412–416.
16. Bierman W, Friedlander M. The penetrative effect of cold. *Arch Phys Ther.* 1940;21:585–593.
17. Bugaj R. The cooling, analgesic, and rewarming, effects of ice massage on localized skin. *Phys Ther.* 1975;55:11–19.
18. Jutte L, Merrick M, Ingersoll C, Edwards J. The relationship between intramuscular temperature, skin temperature, and adipose thickness during cryotherapy and rewarming. *Arch Phys Med Rehabil.* 2001;82(6):845–850.
19. Algafly A, George K. The effect of cryotherapy on nerve conduction velocity, pain threshold, and pain tolerance. *Br J Sports Med.* 2007;41:365–369.
20. Enwemeka C, Allen C, Avila P, Bina J, Konrade J, Munns S. Soft tissue thermodynamics before, during, and after cold pack therapy. *Med Sci Sports Exerc.* 2002;34(1):45–50.
21. Martin S, Spindler K, Tarter J, Detwiler K, Petersen H. Cryotherapy: an effective modality for decreasing intra-articular temperature after knee arthroscopy. *Am J Sports Med.* 2001;29(3):288–291.
22. Warren T, McCarty E, Richardson A, Michener R, Spindler KP. Intra-articular knee temperature changes: ice versus cryotherapy device. *Am J Sports Med.* 2004;32(2):441–445.
23. Shibuya N, Schinke T, Canales M, Yu G. Effect of cryotherapy devices in the postoperative setting. *J Am Podiatr Med Assoc.* 2007;97(6):439–446.
24. Kennet J, Hardaker N, Hobbs S, Selfe J. Cooling efficiency of 4 common cryotherapeutic agents. *J Athl Train.* 2007;42(3):343–348.
25. Zemke J, Andersen J, Guion W, McMillan J, Joyner A. Intramuscular temperature responses in the human leg to two forms of cryotherapy: ice massage and ice bag. *J Orthop Sports Phys Ther.* 1998;27(4):301–307.
26. Eldlich R. Bioengineering principles of hydrotherapy. *J Burn Care Rehabil.* 1987;8:579–584.
27. Simons D, Travell J, Simons L. *Travel & Simons' Myofascial Pain and Dysfunction: The Trigger Point Manual.* Vol 1. Baltimore: Lippincott, Williams, & Wilkins; 1999.
28. Gebauer C. *Gebauer's Spray and Stretch: Topical Aerosol Skin Refrigerant.* Cleveland, OH; 2006.
29. Travell J, Simons D. *Myofascial Pain and Dysfunction: The Trigger Point Manual.* Baltimore: Williams & Wilkins; 1983.

30. Halkovich L, Personius W, Clamann H, Newton R. Effect of fluori-methane spray on passive hip flexion. *Phys Ther.* 1981;61(2):185–189.

31. Kostopoulos D, Rizopoulos K. Effect of topical aerosol skin refrigerant (Spray and Stretch technique) on passive and active stretching. *J Body Mov Ther.* 2008;12:96–104.

32. McGown H. Effects of cold application on maximal isometric contraction. *Phys Ther.* 1967;47:185–192.

33. Oliver R, Johnson D, Wheelhouse W, Griffin PP. Isometric muscle contraction response during recovery from reduced intramuscular temperature. *Arch Phys Med Rehabil.* 1979;60:126–129.

34. Perkins J, Li M, Nicholas C, Lassen W, Gertler P. Cooling and contraction of smooth muscle. *Am J Physiol.* 1950;163:14–26.

35. Schaser K, Disch A, Stover J, Lauffer A, Bail H, Mittlmeier T. Prolonged superficial local cryotherapy attenuates microcirculatory impairment, regional inflammation, and muscle necrosis after closed soft tissue injury in rats. *Am J Sports Med.* 2007;35(1):93–102.

36. Guyton A, Hall J. *Textbook of Medical Physiology.* 10 ed. Philadelphia: WB Saunders; 2000.

37. Folkow B, Fox R, Krog J, Odelram H, Thoren O. Studies on the reaction of the cutaneous vessels to cold exposure. *Acta Physiol Scand.* 1963;58:342–354.

38. Isii Y, Matsukawa K, Tsuchimochi H, Nakamoto T. Ice-water hand immersion causes a reflex decrease in skin temperature in the contralateral hand. *J Physiol Sci.* 2007;57(4):241–248.

39. Cobbold A, Lewis O. Blood flow to the knee joint of the dog: effect of heating, cooling and adrenaline. *J Physiol.* 1956;132:379–383.

40. Lewis T. Observations upon the reactions of the vessels of the human skin to cold. *Heart.* 1930;15:177–208.

41. Fox R, Wyatt H. Cold-induced vasodilation in various areas of the body surface in man. *J Physiol.* 1962;162:289–297.

42. O'Brien C. Reproducibility of the cold-induced vasodilation response. *J Appl Physiol.* 2005;98:1334–1340.

43. Van der Struijs N, Van Es E, Raymann RJ, Daanen H. Finger and toe temperatures on exposure to cold water and cold air. *Aviat Space Environ Med.* 2008;79(10):941–946.

44. Mekjavic I, Dobnikar U, Kounalakis S, Musizza B, Cheung S. The trainability and contralateral response of cold-induced vasodilation in the fingers following repeated cold exposure. *Eur J Appl Physiol.* 2008;104:193–199.

45. Knight K, Draper D. *Cryotherapy Beyond Immediate Care.* Baltimore: Lippincott, Williams & Wilkins; 2008.

46. Deal D, Tipton J, Rosencrance E, Curl W, Smith T. Ice reduces edema. *J Bone Joint Surg.* 2002;84(9):1573–1578.

47. Matsen F, Questad K, Matsen A. The effect of local cooling on post fracture swelling. *Clin Orthop Relat Res.* 1975;109:201–206.

48. Dolan M, Mychaskiw A, Mattacola C, Mendel F. Effects of cool-water immersion and high-voltage electric stimulation for 3 continuous hours on acute edema formation in rats. *J Athl Train.* 2003;38(4):325–329.

49. McMaster W, Liddle S. Cryotherapy influence on post-traumatic limb edema. *Clin Orthop Relat Res.* 1980;150:283–287.

50. Jezdinsky J, Marek J, Ochonsky P. Effects of local cold and heat therapy on traumatic oedema of the rat hind paw: I: Effects of cooling on the course of traumatic oedema. *Acta Universitatis Palackianea Olomucensis Facultatis Medicae.* 1973;66:185–199.

51. Marek J, Jezdinsky J, Ochonsky P. Effects of local cold and heat therapy on traumatic oedema of the rat hind paw: II: Effects of cooling on the course of traumatic oedema. *Acta Universitatis Palackianea Olomucensis Facultatis Medicae.* 1973;66:203–228.

52. Farry P, Prentice N, Hunter A, Wakelin C. Ice treatment of injured ligaments: an experimental model. *N Z Med J.* 1980;91:12–14.

53. Lee H, Natsui H, Akimoto T, Yanagi K, Ohshima N, Kono I. Effects of cryotherapy after contusion using real-time intravital microscopy. *Med Sci Sports Exerc.* 2005;37(7):1093–1098.

54. Knobloch K, Grasemann R, Spies M, Vogt P. Midportion achilles tendon microcirculation after intermittent combined cryotherapy and compression compared with cryotherapy alone. *Am J Phys Med.* 2008;36(11):2128–2138.

55. Douglas W, Malcolm J. The effect of localized cooling on conduction in cat nerves. *J Physiol.* 1955;130:53–71.

56. Zankel H. Effect of physical agents on motor conduction velocity of the ulnar nerve. *Arch Phys Med Rehabil.* 1966;47:787–792.

57. Lee J, Warren M, Mason S. Effects of ice on nerve conduction velocity. *Physiotherapy.* 1978;64:2–6.

58. Drez D, Faust D, Evans J. Cryotherapy and nerve palsy. *Am J Sports Med.* 1981;9(4):256–257.

59. Collins K, Storey M, Peterson K. Peroneal nerve palsy after cryotherapy. *Phys Sportsmed.* 1986;14(5):105–108.

60. Knutsson E, Mattsson E. Effects of local cooling on monosynaptic reflexes in man. *Scand J Rehabil Med.* 1969;52:166–168.

61. Clendenin M, Szumski A. Influence of cutaneous ice application on single motor units in human. *Phys Ther.* 1971;51(2):166–175.

62. Fischer J, Van Lunen B, Branch J, Prione J. Functional performance following an ice bag application to the hamstrings. *J Strength Cond Res.* 2009;23(1):44–50.

63. Patterson S, Udermann B, Doberstein S, Reineke D. The effects of cold whirlpool on power, speed, agility, and range of motion. *J Sports Sci Med.* 2008;7:387–394.

64. Wassinger C, Myers J, Gatti J, Conley K, Lephart S. Proprioception and throwing accuracy in the dominant shoulder after cryotherapy. *J Athl Train.* 2007;42(1):84–89.

65. Dover G, Powers M. Cryotherapy does not impair shoulder joint position sense. *Arch Phys Med Rehabil.* 2004;85:1241–1246.

66. Ozmun J, Thieme H, Ingersoll C, Knight K. Cooling does affect knee proprioception. *J Athl Train.* 1996;31:8–11.

67. Kernozek T, Greany J, Anderson D, Van Heel D, Youngdahl R, Benesh B. The effect of immersion cryotherapy on medial-lateral postural sway variability in individuals with a lateral ankle sprain. *Physiother Res Int.* 2008;13(2):107–118.

68. Surenkok O, Aytar A, Tuzun E, Akman M. Cryotherapy impairs knee joint position sense and balance. *Isokinet Exerc Sci.* 2008;16:69–73.

69. Berg C, Hart J, Palmieri-Smith R, Cross K, Ingersoll C. Cryotherapy does not affect peroneal reaction following sudden inversion. *J Sport Rehabil.* 2007;16:285–294.

70. Mecomber S, Herman R. Effects of local hypothermia on reflex and voluntary activity. *Phys Ther.* 1971;51(3):271–282.

71. Hartvikksen K. Ice therapy in spasticity. *Acta Neurol Scan.* 1962;38(3):79–83.

72. Miglietta O. Electromyographic characteristics of clonus and influence of cold. *Arch Phys Med Rehabil.* 1964;45:502–503.

73. Miglietta O. Action of cold on spasticity. *Am J Phys Med.* 1973;52:198–205.

74. Eldred E, Lindsley D, Buchwald J. The effect of cooling on mammalian muscle spindles. *Exp Neurol.* 1960;2:144–157.

75. Newton M, Lehmkuhl D. Muscle spindle response to body heating and localized muscle cooling: implications for relief of spasticity. *J Am Phys Ther Assoc.* 1965;45(2):91–105.

76. Urbscheit N, Johnson R, Bishop B. Effects of cooling on the ankle jerk and H-response in hemiplegic patients. *Phys Ther.* 1971;51(9):983–988.

77. Wolf S, Letbetter W. Effect of skin cooling on spontaneous EMG activity in triceps surae of the decerebrate cat. *Brain Res.* 1975;91:151–155.

78. Knutsson E. Topical cryotherapy in spasticity. *Scand J Rehabil Med.* 1970;2:159–162.

79. dos Santos M, de Oliveira L. Use of cryotherapy to enhance mouth opening in patients with cerebral palsy. *Spec Care Dentist.* 2004;24(2):232–234.

80. Nilsagard Y, Denison E, Gunnarsson L. Evaluation of a single session with cooling garment for persons with multiple sclerosis—a randomized trial. *Disabil Rehabil Assist Technol.* 2006;1(4):225–233.

81. Mermier C, Schneider S, Gurney A, Weingart H, Wilmerding M. Preliminary results: effects of whole-body cooling in patients with myasthenia gravis. *Med Sci Sports Exerc.* 2006;38(1):13–20.

82. Grahn D, Murray J, Heller H. Cooling via one hand improves physical performance in heat sensitive individuals with multiple sclerosis: a preliminary study. *BMC Neurol.* 2008;8(14).

83. Schaubel H. Local use of ice after orthopedic procedures. *Am J Surg.* 1946;72:711–714.

84. Lessard L, Scudds R, Amendola A, Vaz M. The efficacy of cryotherapy following arthroscopic knee surgery. *J Orthop Sports Phys Ther.* 1997;26(1):14–22.

85. Ohkoshi Y, Ohkoshi M, Nagasaki S. The effect of cryotherapy on intra-articular temperature and postoperative care after anterior cruciate ligament reconstruction. *Am J Sports Med.* 1999;27(3):357–362.

86. Hocutt J, Jaffee R, Rylander C, Beebe J. Cryotherapy in ankle sprains. *Am J Sports Med.* 1982;10(5):316–319.

87. Bleakley C, O'Connor S, Tully M, Rocke L, MacAuley D, McDonough S. The PRICE study (Protection Rest Ice Compression Elevation): design of a randomised controlled trial comparing standard versus cryokinetic ice applications in the management of acute ankle sprain. *BMC Musculoskelet Disord.* 2007;8:125.

88. Janwantanakul P. Cold pack/skin interface temperature during ice treatment with various levels of compression. *Physiotherapy.* 2006;92(4):254–259.

89. Merrick M, Knight K, Ingersoll C, Potteiger J. The effects of ice and compression wraps on intramuscular temperatures at various depths. *J Athl Train.* 1993;28(3):236–245.

90. Healy W, Seidman J, Pfeiffer B, Brown P. Cold compressive dressing after total knee arthroplasty. *Clin Orthop Relat Res.* 1994;299:143–146.

91. Levy A, Marmar E. The role of cold compression dressings in the postoperative treatment of total knee arthroplasty. *Clin Orthop Relat Res.* 1993;297:174–178.

92. Okcu G, Yercan H. Is it possible to decrease skin temperature with ice packs under casts and bandages? *Arch Orthop Trauma Surg.* 2006;126:668–673.

93. Ibrahim T, Ong S, Saint Clair Taylor G. The effects of different dressings on the skin temperature of the knee during cryotherapy. *Knee.* 2005;12(1):21–23.

94. Kaempffe F. Skin surface temperature reduction after cryotherapy to a casted extremity. *J Orthop Sports Phys Ther.* 1989;10:448–450.

95. Bleakley C, McConough S, MacAuley D. The use of ice in the treatment of acute soft-tissue injury: a systematic review of randomized controlled trials. *Am J Phys Med.* 2004;32(1):251–261.

96. Hubbard T, Aronson S, Denegar C. Does cryotherapy hasten return to participation? A systematic review. *J Athl Train.* 2004;39(1):88–94.

97. Benson T, Copp E. The effects of therapeutic forms of heat and ice on the pain threshold of normal shoulder. *Rheumatol Rehabil.* 1974;13:101–104.

98. Chapman C. Can the use of physical modalities for pain control be rationalized by the research evidence? *Can J Physiol Pharmacol.* 1991;69:704–712.

99. Gammon G, Starr I. Studies on the relief of pain by counterirritation. *J Clin Invest.* 1941;2:13–20.

100. Kisner C, Colby L. *Stretching for Impaired Mobility.* 5th ed. Philadelphia: FA Davis; 2007.

101. Prentice W. An electromyographic analysis of the effectiveness of heat or cold and stretching for inducing relaxation in injured muscle. *J Orthop Sports Phys Ther.* 1982;3(3):133–140.

102. Cobb C, DeVries H, Urban R, Luekens C, Bagg R. Electrical activity in muscle pain. *Am J Phys Med.* 1975;54(2):80–87.

103. Bailey D, Erith S, Griffin P, et al. Influence of cold-water immersion on indices of muscle damage following prolonged intermittent shuttle running. *J Sports Sci.* 2007;25(11):1163–1170.

104. Sellwood K, Brukner P, Williams D, Nicol A, Hinman R. Ice-water immersion and delayed-onset muscle soreness: a randomised controlled trial. *Br J Sports Med.* 2007;41:392–397.

105. Gaze H, van Someren K. The efficacy of ice massage in the treatment of exercise-induced muscle damage. *Scand J Med Sci Sports.* 2005;15(6):416–422.

106. Vaile J, Gill N, Blazevich A. The effect of contrast water therapy on symptoms of delayed onset muscle soreness. *J Strength Cond Res.* 2007;21(3):697–702.

107. Daniels J, Ishmael T, Wesley R. Managing myofascial pain syndrome. *Phys Sportsmed.* 2003;31(10):39–45.

108. Dommerholt J. Myofascial pain syndrome—trigger points. *J Musculoskelet Pain.* 2009;17(2):202–209.

109. Hou C, Tsai L, Cheng K, Chung K. Immediate effects of various physical therapeutic modalities on cervical myofascial pain and trigger-point sensitivity. *Arch Phys Med Rehabil.* 2002;83:1406–1414.

110. Huddleston L, Walusz H, McLeod M, Evans T, Ragan B. Ice massage decreases trigger point sensitivity and pain. The National Athletic Trainers' Association Annual Meeting and Clinical Symposia. Indianapolis, IN: The National Athletic Trainers' Association; 2005.

111. Walusz H, McLeod M, Huddleston L, Evans J, Ragan B. Ice massage alters sensory discrimination when compared to menthol-based analgesic balm and placebo. The National Athletic Trainers' Association Annual Meeting and Clinical Symposia. Indianapolis, IN; 2005.

112. Olson J, Stravino V. A review of cryotherapy. *Phys Ther.* 1972;52(8):840–853.

113. Wright V, Johns R. Physical factors concerned with the stiffness of normal and diseased joints. *Bull Johns Hopkins Hosp.* 1960;106:215–231.

114. Fox R. Local cooling in man. *Br Med Bull.* 1961;17:14–18.

115. Streator S, Ingersoll C, Knight K. Sensory information can decrease cold-induced pain perception. *J Athl Train.* 1995;30(4):293–296.

116. Galvan H, Tritsch A, Tandy R, Rubley M. Pain perception during repeated ice-bath immersion of the ankle at varied temperatures. *J Sport Rehabil.* 2006;15:105–115.

117. Karunakara R, Lephart S, Pincivero D. Changes in forearm blood flow during single and intermittent cold application. *J Orthop Sports Phys Ther.* 1999;29(3):177–180.

118. Bleakley C, McDonough S, MacAuley D. Cryotherapy for acute ankle sprains: a randomised controlled study of two different icing protocols. *Br J Sports Med.* 2006;40:700–705.

119. Palmer J, Knight K. Ankle and thigh skin surface temperature changes with repeated ice pack application. *J Athl Train.* 1996;31(4):319–323.

120. Long B, Cordova M, Brucker J, Demchak T, Stone M. Exercise and quadriceps muscle cooling time. *J Athl Train.* 2005;40(4):260–263.

121. Bender A, Kramer E, Brucker J, Demchak T, Cordova M, Stone M. Local ice-bag application and triceps surae muscle temperature during treadmill walking. *J Athl Train.* 2005;40(4):271–275.

122. Kanlayanaphotporn R, Janwantanakul P. Comparison of skin surface temperature during the application of various cryotherapy modalities. *Arch Phys Med Rehabil.* 2005;86: 1411–1415.

123. Ritzmann S, Levin W. Cryotherapies: a review. *Arch Intern Med.* 1961;107:186–204.

124. Wanderer A. Cold urticaria syndromes: historical background, diagnostic classification, clinical and laboratory characteristics, pathogenesis, and management. *J Allergy Clin Immunol.* 1990;85(6):965–981.

125. Schumacher H. *Cryoglobulinemia.* 9th ed. Atlanta: Arthritis Foundation; 1988.

126. Porter RS, Kaplan JL, Homeier BP. The Merck Manual of Patient Symptoms: A Concise, Practical Guide to Etiology, Evaluation, and Treatment. Whitehouse Station, NJ: Merck Research Laboratories; 2008.

127. Boyer J, Fraser J, Doyle A. The haemodynamic effects of cold immersion. *Clin Sci.* 1980;19:539–550.

128. Claus-Walker J, Halstead L, Carter R, Campes R. Physiological responses to cold stress in healthy subjects and in subjects with cervical cord injuries. *Arch Phys Med Rehabil.* 1974;55:485–490.

129. Harchelroad F. Acute thermoregulatory disorders. *Clin Geriatr Med.* 1993;9(3):621–639.

130. Lundgren C, Muren A, Zederfeldt B. Effect of cold vasoconstriction on wound healing in the rabbit. *Acta Chir Scand.* 1959;118:1–4.

131. Nadler S, Prybicien M, Malanga G, Sicher D. Complications from therapeutic modalities: results of a national survey of athletic trainers. *Arch Phys Med Rehabil.* 2003;84:849–853.

132. Janwantanakul P. Different rate of cooling time and magnitude of cooling temperature during ice bag treatment with and without damp towel wrap. *Phys Ther Sport.* 2004;5(3):156–161.

133. Waylonis G. The physiologic effect of ice massage. *Arch Phys Med Rehabil.* 1967;48(1):37–42.

134. Barber F. A comparison of crushed ice and continuous flow cold therapy. *Am J Knee Surg.* 2000;13:97–102.

135. Hochberg J. A randomized perspective study to assess the efficacy of two cold-therapy treatments following carpal tunnel release. *J Hand Ther.* 2001;14:208–215.

136. Woolf S, Barfield W, Merrill K, McBryde A. Comparison of a continuous temperature-controlled cryotherapy device to a simple icing regimen following outpatient knee arthroscopy. *J Knee Surg.* 2008;21:15–19.

137. Khajavi K, Pavelko T, Mishra A. Compartment syndrome arising from use of an electronic cooling pad. *Am J Sports Med.* 2004;32(6):1538–1541.

138. Misasi S, Morin G, Kemler D, Olmstead P, Pryzgocki K. The effect of a toe cap and bias on perceived pain during cold water immersion. *J Athl Train.* 1995;30:49–52.

139. Airaksinen O, Kyrklund N, Latvala K, Kouri J, Gronblad M, Kolari P. Efficacy of cold gel for soft tissue injuries: a prospective randomized double-blinded trial. *Am J Sports Med.* 2003;31(5):680–684.

140. Zhan J, Enix D, Snyder B, Giggey K, Tepe R. Effects of Biofreeze and chiropractic adjustments on acute low back pain: a pilot study. *J Chiropr Med.* 2008;7(2):59–65.

chapter 3

Therapeutic Heat

Sandy Rennie, PT, PhD | Susan L. Michlovitz, PT, PhD, CHT

The use of therapeutic heat (thermotherapy) in the treatment of various conditions has been around for thousands of years. Understanding the physiological and biomechanical principles of therapeutic heat is one of the elements to successful treatment of the patient. The clinician must be well versed with the various conditions for which these modalities are used and aware of the contraindications to using therapeutic heat. This text provides clinicians with the tools necessary to have a safe and effective outcome with their patients.

Warmth is associated with tranquility and relaxation. Heating of injured tissue has been used for centuries for relieving pain and reducing muscle spasms. In physical therapy, locally applied heating modalities are used to promote relaxation, provide pain relief, increase blood flow, facilitate tissue healing, decrease muscle spasm, and prepare stiff joints and tight muscles for exercise.[1–23] Several studies[24–28] have examined the frequency of use of thermal agents as interventions in physical therapy treatments. These studies, which are from Australia,[24,25] Canada,[26,27] and England,[28] indicated that the percentage of daily use of therapeutic heating agents, such as hot packs and paraffin wax, ranged from 36.5% to 95% in various practice settings.

The physiological effects of elevating tissue temperature are included in the rationale for selecting these modalities as part of a therapy paradigm. Elevating collagen tissue temperature, for example, can alter viscoelastic properties, thus enhancing the effects of passive stretch for increasing range of motion.[10–12,15–17,29,30]

Many thermal modalities are available for tissue heating (Box 3-1). Some heating modalities primarily cause an increase in skin and superficial subcutaneous tissue temperature. Thermotherapy modalities, such as moist heat packs, paraffin wax, and fluidized therapy (Fluidotherapy), are used to:

1. Heat superficial joints, such as the hand, which has little soft tissue covering
2. Cause a heating effect in deeper structures, such as muscle, through reflex mechanisms
3. Heat soft tissue (muscle, tendon, superficial joint capsule) in order to increase its extensibility

If the goal of intervention is to increase the temperature of deeper tissues, such as the knee joint capsule or the muscle belly of the quadriceps muscle, then another heating modality is logically selected.

Heating modalities, including continuous shortwave diathermy and continuous-wave ultrasound, can increase tissue temperature at depths ranging from 3 to 5 cm without overheating the skin and subcutaneous tissues. Therapeutic ultrasound is discussed in Chapter 4, and shortwave diathermy is covered in Chapter 6.

Biophysical Effects of Temperature Elevation

Many sequelae can occur as a result of an increase in temperature of body tissues. The occurrence and magnitude of these physiological changes are dependent upon several factors,[31] including:

1. Extent of the temperature rise
2. Rate at which energy is being added to the tissue
3. Volume of tissue exposed
4. Composition of the absorbing tissue
5. Capacity of the tissue to dissipate heat (largely a factor of blood supply)

Box 3·1	**Thermal Modality Options**

To increase tissue temperature within 1 to 3 cm depth:
- Moist heat packs (e.g., hot packs)
- Paraffin wax bath
- Fluidotherapy
- Warm whirlpool
- Microwavable gel packs
- Air-activated heat wraps
- Electric heating pads

To increase tissue temperature within 1 to 5 cm depth:
- Continuous ultrasound
- Continuous shortwave diathermy

To meet therapeutic levels of vigorous heating, study results[1,10] indicate that tissue temperature must be elevated to between 40°C and 45°C (104°F and 113°F). Within these temperatures, hyperemia, which is indicative of increased blood flow, will occur. Above this range, there is potential for tissue damage. Below 40°C (104°F), heating is considered to be only mild.[1,10,13,14,28] Behavioral regulation, or how the body responds, and subjective responses associated with surface temperatures are illustrated in Table 3-1.

KEY POINT! Tissue temperature should be elevated to 40°C to 45°C for a therapeutic effect.

The rate of temperature rise in response to the addition of thermal energy can influence physiological responses. Temperature elevation increases local blood flow,[2,3,10,13,14,32–38] thus cooler blood comes into the area and acts to remove some of the heat produced. If the rate of temperature increase is very slow, the amount of heat added could be balanced out by the convective effect of cooler blood, so therapeutically effective heating levels may not be obtained. On the other hand, if temperature rises faster than excess heat can be dissipated, heat may build up to a point that stimulates pain receptors and may also cause tissue damage. The goal of heating is to achieve a therapeutic level of temperature elevation without causing adverse responses.

Physiological alterations can occur at the site of local temperature rise and in areas remote from the area of heat absorption. Usually, the larger the tissue volume affected by the addition of thermal energy, the greater the likelihood for reflex, or consensual, changes in other areas and for systematic alterations. An increase in forearm temperature as a result of hot pack application could be expected to cause an increase in local blood flow, with minimal or no alterations in overall peripheral vascular resistance. On the other hand, immersing a person in a water bath of 40°C (104°F) could result in systemic changes, such as a decrease in mean blood pressure, an increase in heart rate, and an increase in pulmonary minute ventilation.[1]

Several physiological responses to temperature elevation are important to understand when considering a heating modality for therapeutic purposes. The most relevant changes to address include alterations in

Table 3•1	**Behavioral Regulation and Subjective Responses Associated with Surface Temperatures**	

Temperature (°C)	Body and Environmental Temperatures	Subjective Feeling Associated With Surface Temperatures
60		
55		
50		Tissue damage, burning pain
45		Very hot
40	Normal range of resting	Hot
35	temperature of body 36.3°C–37.3°C	
30		Warm
25		Neutral
20	Region of thermal environmental comfort	Cool
15		Cold
10		Very cold
5	Behavioral regulation	
0		

metabolic activity, hemodynamic function, neural response, skeletal muscle activity, and collagen tissue's physical properties. These changes, in part, serve as a foundation for the use of heat as an effective therapeutic modality. In addition, understanding the adverse reactions to the addition of thermal energy is imperative for administering a safe intervention.

Metabolic Reactions

Chemical reactions in cells of the body are influenced by temperature. Generally speaking, chemical activity in cells and metabolic rate will increase twofold to threefold for each 10°C (50°F) rise in temperature.[35,39] Therefore, energy expenditure will increase with increasing temperature. With even mild increases in tissue temperature, the oxygen-hemoglobin dissociation curve shifts to the right, making more oxygen available for tissue repair.[6] However, as temperature rises past a certain point, usually 45°C to 50°C (113°F to 122°F), human tissues will burn because the metabolic activity required to repair tissue is not capable of keeping up with thermally induced protein denaturation.

KEY POINT! Metabolic reactions to heat include the following:

- Cell activity and metabolic rate increases two to three times for each 10°C temperature increase
- Increase in oxygen uptake by tissues.

An increase in chemical reaction rate can also have positive effects on human function. Oxygen uptake by tissues will increase.[32] Therefore, theoretically, more nutrients will be available to promote tissue healing.[5,6]

Vascular Effects

Increasing tissue temperature is usually associated with vasodilation and thus with an increase in blood flow to the area.[1,2,6,9,13,14,32–38,40,41] However, this general statement can be misleading. It is important to know which regions have increased blood flow. The control mechanisms are different for blood flow to different structures—for example, skin compared with skeletal muscle. Therefore, responses to temperature change will not always be the same; or if a response is in the same direction, it may not be of the same magnitude.

Skin blood flow has an important role both in nutrition and in the maintenance of constant core body temperature of 37°C (98.6°F), and it is primarily under the control of sympathetic adrenergic nerves.[42,43] Vasodilation of resistance vessels of the skin will occur as a means of losing heat through local or reflex mechanisms. The skin is unique in that it has specialized vessels, called arteriovenous (AV) anastomoses, which have an important role in heat loss.[43] These shunt vessels go from arterioles to venules to venous plexuses, thus bypassing the capillary bed. The blood flow through these anastomoses is under neural control. Activation occurs in response to reflex activation of temperature receptors or to stimulation of heat loss mechanisms triggered in part by the circulation of warmed blood through the preoptic region of the anterior hypothalamus. These AV shunt vessels are found in the hands (palms and fingertips), feet (toes and soles), and face (ears, nose, and lips).

As mentioned previously, blood flow changes in the skin can be caused by local[1,34,42,44] or reflex[41] mechanisms. Vasodilation of the heat-exposed skin can be proposed to occur as a result of three factors:

1. An axon reflex
2. Release of chemical mediators secondary to temperature elevation
3. Local spinal cord reflexes

Heat applied to the skin stimulates cutaneous thermoreceptors. These sensory afferents carry impulses to the spinal cord. Some of these afferent impulses are carried through branches antidromically toward skin blood vessels, and a vasoactive mediator is released. This results in vasodilation through an axon reflex (Fig. 3-1).

Heat produces a mild inflammatory reaction. Chemical mediators of inflammation, including histamine and prostaglandins, are released in the area and act on resistance vessels to cause vasodilation (Fig. 3-2). In addition, temperature elevation causes sweat secretion, and the enzyme kallikrein is released from sweat glands. This enzyme acts on a globulin, kininogen, to release bradykinin.[45] Vasodilation of resistance vessels (i.e., small arteries and arterioles) and an increase in

capillary and postcapillary venule permeability occur because of the action of these chemical mediators on smooth-muscle tone and endothelial cell contractility, respectively. Because of an increase in capillary hydrostatic pressure and permeability, outward fluid filtration from vascular to extravascular space is favored. Therefore, heat within the therapeutic range can potentially increase interstitial fluid and cause mild inflammation.

A local spinal cord reflex is elicited through heat-activated cutaneous afferent stimulation. This reflex results in a decrease in postganglionic sympathetic adrenergic nerve activity to the smooth muscles of blood vessels.[46] A schematic of the reflex is diagrammed in Figure 3-3.

Vasodilatory effects of this reflex response are not limited to the area heated; rather, there will be a consensual (reflex) response in areas remote from the application site. When one area of the body (e.g., the lower back) is heated, increases in skin blood flow occur in distal extremities of the body that are not directly heated.[47–49] This principle of reflex vasodilation is considered to be safe to use with patients who have peripheral vascular disease (PVD).[47] For example, cutaneous blood flow to the feet could be increased by applying heat to the lower back.

KEY POINT! Consensual heating to improve circulation in persons with PVD is not a usual rationale for using heat in clinical practice. In this instance, physiological response does not equate with clinical utility.

Skeletal muscle blood flow is primarily under metabolic regulation and demonstrates the greatest response

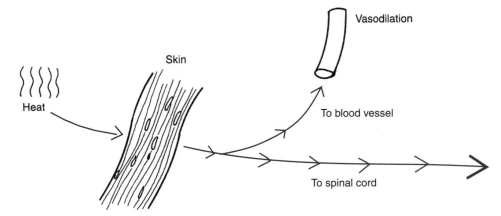

Fig 3•1 Schematic diagram of an axon reflex.

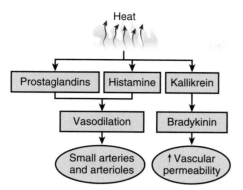

Fig 3•2 Metabolic effects of heat.

to increases or decreases in levels of exercise. When heating modalities are given, minimal change in skeletal muscle blood flow is expected. This notion is supported by two reports on heat lamp (infrared) application. Crockford and Hellon[33] measured venous oxygen content following 20- to 30-minute exposures of the forearm. Superficial venous oxygen content increased, but there was no change in muscle blood flow. Wyper and McNiven[50] reported no change in muscle blood flow following heat (infrared heat lamp) treatment. Similarly, Robertson et al.[15] found that the lesser effect of superficial heat compared to deep heat in examining tissue extensibility suggests the contribution of any skin response or any reflex vasodilation from heating the skin is minimal. Draper and Hopkins[8] measured intramuscular (vastus medialis oblique) and intracapsular (suprapatellar pouch) temperatures of 11 healthy human subjects following 2 hours of application of an air-activated heat wrap for continuous low-level heat therapy. They found significant differences in skin, intramuscular, and intracapsular temperatures compared to control subjects.

Heat is often used before exercise. Both heat and exercise can increase blood flow. Greenberg[36] compared moist heat packs alone, exercise alone, and moist heat packs plus exercise. Heat was applied for 20 minutes. Exercise consisted of squeezing a rubber ball once per second for 1 minute. The increase in blood flow from exercise was greater than with heat; however, the effects of moist heat packs plus exercise were additive and greater than either modality used alone.

Kauranen and Vanharanta[51] compared the effects of hot and cold packs on motor performance of normal hands. The forearm, from elbow to fingers, was placed between two hot packs for 20 minutes on three successive days, and functional testing followed each heat treatment. The same procedure occurred the next week with cold packs, except the application was for 15 minutes. Reaction time, movement speed, tapping speed, and coordination for upper extremity motor control were measured. Results demonstrated that cold decreased all fine motor tasks. Heat decreased simple reaction time; however, finger-tapping speed was increased. The authors suggest that patients completing fine motor tasks may find it more difficult if cold is applied prior to activity, compared to heat.[51]

Mayer et al.[20] examined the use of continuous low-level heat wrap therapy and exercise in treatment of low back pain. Four treatment groups (heat wrap alone, heat wrap plus exercise, exercise alone, and back pain booklet) were examined daily for 5 days. The heat-plus-exercise group had the heat wrap applied for 1 hour before commencing the directional preference-based exercise program. Results indicated that the combination of low-level heat wrap therapy and directional preference-based exercise during the treatment of low

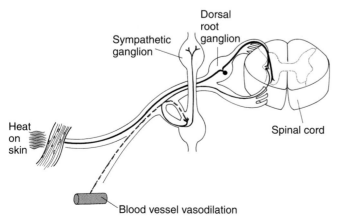

Fig 3•3 Heat applied to the skin leads to vasodilation. The change in activity of postganglionic sympathetic adrenergic fibers secondary to local heating is diagrammed.

back pain significantly improved functional outcomes and pain relief compared with the control groups for either intervention alone.[20] Johnson and Park[52] found that the onset of vigorous exercise led to cutaneous vasoconstriction, which is the body's method of shunting blood to the muscles. This means that during vigorous exercise, the patient's skin may feel cool because the blood is being shunted to the skeletal muscles. In general, cold application appears to limit or decrease functional ability, whereas heat may improve or augment physical performance or ability.

Neuromuscular Effects

Heat is used therapeutically to provide analgesia[6,9,13,41,42,53,54] and to assist in the resolution of pain and muscle-guarding spasms.[1,9,55–57] Although the mechanisms of action are not totally understood, the underlying basis for use is heat's ability to elevate pain threshold,[41,58] alter nerve conduction velocity,[59–62] and change muscle spindle firing rates.[6,9,13,56,63] The increased firing rate of thermoreceptors in cutaneous tissue may block input from the primary nociceptive afferents to the dorsal horn (the "thermal gate theory").[6,9,13,56] Figure 3-4 provides an interesting depiction of the mechanisms of pain relief brought about by heat. In addition, temperature elevation of skeletal muscle can temporarily change the muscle's ability to build tension and sustain prolonged activity.[64,65]

Raising subcutaneous tissue temperature using a variety of heating modalities has been demonstrated to alter sensory nerve conduction velocity.[60–62] The most pronounced changes appear to occur during the first 1.5°C to 2°C (2.7°F to 3.6°F) temperature increase.[60] However, the relevance of these findings to therapeutic use is not readily apparent. Heating over the area of a peripheral nerve can elevate the pain threshold. Fifteen minutes of high-intensity heat lamp (infrared radiation) was administered over the medial aspect of the elbow—that is, over the ulnar nerve. Pain threshold measurements distal to the site of application, over the tip of the little finger, revealed analgesia.[58] Direct heating over the area where pain was measured also produced analgesia. Kelly et al.[62] found that fluidized therapy (Fluidotherapy) decreased sensory nerve latency of the superficial radial nerve after 20 minutes of application, suggesting analgesic effects at the site of

application and at sites distal to the application. The clinical correlate is that heat can be a useful adjunct to reduce pain before performing stretching exercises, joint mobilization techniques, or active exercise.[1–3,5–7,11,12,16,17,30,42,66–68] Following proper education, including written instructions, heat can easily be used on a home basis prior to exercise.

Nadler et al.[69] and Davis et al.[70] suggested that some of the benefits of topical heat therapy may be mediated directly in the brain. Functional brain imaging has shown central effects of non-noxious warming of the skin with increased activity of the thalamus and posterior insula of the brain, supporting the beneficial psychosomatic effects of heat.

Muscle-guarding spasms can result from the overuse of a muscle during exercise or from activation of a protective mechanism that guards against moving painful joints. Pain can be the event triggering a reflex, tonic muscle contraction, thus beginning the pain-spasm-pain cycle.[1,5,6,13,14,71,72] The muscle spindle afferents that alter their rate of firing, primarily in response to tonic or static stretch, are the type II afferents. Elevating muscle temperature to about 42°C (107.6°F) will decrease the firing rate of the type II afferents and will increase the firing of the type Ib fibers from Golgi tendon organs (GTOs).[1,6,13,14,63] Therefore, with decreased firing of the type II afferents and increased GTO activity, we could predict a decreased firing of the alpha motoneuron, and thus a reduction of tonic extrafusal fiber activity.

Heating modalities, such as moist heat packs, are not likely to elevate muscle temperature to the degree necessary to alter type II or type Ib activity. Therefore, another mechanism must be postulated to account for the reduction in muscle spasm when the skin overlying the muscle is heated. Heating the skin has been demonstrated to produce a decrease in gamma (γ) efferent activity and sensory nerve action potential latencies.[35,62] With a decrease in γ activity, the stretch on the muscle spindle would be less, thus reducing afferent firing from the spindle. This indirect method ultimately results in decreased alpha (α) motoneuron firing, and thus less muscle spasm. Another theory for the mechanism reducing muscle tension comes from Kettenmann et al.[72] These authors used objective electroencephalogram (EEG) measurements in patients who had acute

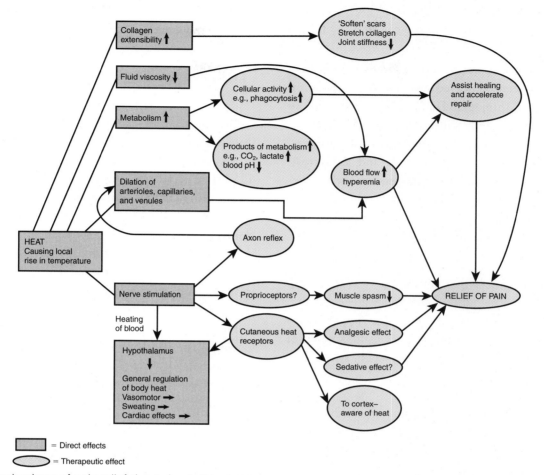

Fig 3•4 Mechanisms of pain relief due to heat. *(Adapted with permission from Wells PW, Frampton V, Bowsher D. Pain Management in Physical Therapy. 2nd ed. Oxford, Butterworth-Heinemann; 1994:154.)*

low back pain and found acute therapeutic relaxation after wearing a back heat wrap for a minimum of 4 hours. The authors believe this reduction of pain and muscle tension was due to a decrease in nociceptive information load.

Heating modalities have also been used to help prevent or decrease the effects of delayed-onset muscle soreness (DOMS) after exercise[23,55] Sumida et al.[55] found the pain of eccentric-induced DOMS was reduced 30 minutes after applying hot packs to the skin overlying the painful muscle compared to cold pack and control groups. The authors suggested that the visual analogue scale (VAS) pain rating decreased because heat is soothing and produces feelings of comfort. Using a prevention group, a treatment group, and control groups, Mayer et al.[23] examined the use of a wearable heat wrap to the low back region after

eccentric exercise induced DOMS. For the prevention group, they found that 4 hours of wearing the heat wrap before exercise decreased pain intensity, disability, and self-reported physical function by 47%, 52%, and 45% respectively. In the treatment group, pain relief was 138% greater at 24 hours postexercise compared to the cold pack group. Mayer et al.[23] suggested that the most plausible explanations for the efficacy of heat wraps in preventing and decreasing low back DOMS are a combination of the heat wrap's thermal effect on muscle tissue, the analgesic properties of topical heat, and the fact that subjects can remain active while wearing the heat wrap.

Elevating muscle temperature can also alter strength and endurance. In a study of normal volunteers, Chastain[64] used a deep-heating modality (continuous shortwave diathermy) over the quadriceps. During the first 30 minutes after terminating the heat, isometric strength was decreased, followed by an increase for the next 2 hours of measurement.

Strength and endurance decreases following heating have also been reported in other studies on humans.[65,73] Immediately after immersion in whirlpools whose temperatures ranged from 40°C to 43°C (104°F to 109.4°F), quadriceps strength and endurance were reduced.[73] Edwards and associates[65] found similar results following immersion of the lower extremity in a water bath of 44°C (111.2°F) for 45 minutes. The muscle temperature after the 45-minute immersion had reached a value of 38.6°C (101.3°F) from a normal mean of 35.1°C (95.2°F).

KEY POINT! The practitioner should be aware of the changes in muscle performance following heat (and cold) application, particularly when planning strengthening programs or performing valid assessments of performance such as manual muscle testing.

Connective Tissue Effects

Temperature elevation, in combination with a sustained stretch, can alter the viscoelastic properties of connective tissues.[8,10–12,14–17,35,74–77] The viscous properties of connective tissue permit a residual elongation after stretch is applied, then released. This is referred to as *plastic deformation*, or *elongation*.[78] An elastic structure will stretch under tension but will return to its original length when the load is removed. The elastic properties of connective tissue result in recoverable deformation.[77-79]

KEY POINT! The effects of heat on connective tissue include

- increased elasticity
- decreased viscosity
- decreased joint stiffness
- increased muscle flexibility

Connective tissue will progressively shorten, and joint contractures will develop following injury if full-range-of-motion exercises are not performed.[80] Adhesions, or the loss of ability of tissue layers to glide past one another, will also develop. Lacerations and crush and burn injuries result in scar tissue and often limit mobility.

Heat and stretch of connective tissue will result in plastic elongation.[77,78,81,82] Two factors must be considered in determining effective intervention strategies:

1. Temperature elevation—site, time, and amount
2. Stretch—duration, amount, and velocity

Greater residual length changes will occur when a stretch is applied during the time the tissue temperature is elevated at therapeutic levels (between 40°C and 45°C [104°F and 113°F]).[11,12,15,16,29] For in vivo experiments on rat tail tendon, temperature was elevated in a water bath of 45°C (113°F) for 10 minutes; then elongation was performed and maintained until cooling to resting values occurred.[81] This was compared with stretch in a water bath of 25°C (77°F). Length increases were greater in the 45°C (113°F) bath, with less evidence of tissue damage.[82]

For patients with frozen shoulder, Leung and Cheing[11] compared 20-minute superficial (hot pack) and deep (shortwave diathermy) treatments prior to stretching exercises. They found a significant improvement in all groups in all outcome measures except for shoulder flexion range. The improvement in the shoulder score index (activities of daily living) and in the ROM was significantly better in the deep heating group than in the superficial heating group. Similarly, Knight et al.[77] compared the effects of superficial heat (hot packs for 15 minutes), deep heat (continuous ultrasound, 1.5 W/cm^2 for 7 minutes), and stretch alone (control) on the extensibility of the plantar flexors. They found heat prior to stretch increased both active ROM (AROM) and passive ROM (PROM) compared to the control group, and the deep heat group obtained the greatest increases in AROM and PROM.

Three techniques reportedly provide for permanent elongation of collagen tissue:

1. Constant load of enough magnitude to overcome tissue elasticity
2. Rapid stretch followed by a period of holding in that position
3. Constant rate of stretching using a slow, steady stretch[29,77,78,83]

Lower loads of longer duration result in less tissue damage[31,78,79,83] and greater increases in joint ROM.[31,78–80,82,84] Lentell and associates[31] demonstrated an increase in long-term improvement in shoulder flexibility when their subjects were treated with moist heat packs prior to low-load, prolonged stretch. Two groups (ice and stretch, and heat and stretch) showed an improvement in shoulder flexibility compared with controls. However, only the heat-and-stretch group showed significant gains in shoulder flexibility compared with those who received stretching alone.[30]

Joint stiffness is a common complaint among patients with rheumatoid arthritis and osteoarthritis (degenerative joint disease). Joint stiffness has the physical components of elasticity, viscosity, inertia, plasticity, and friction. Joint stiffness in normal subjects and in patients with rheumatoid arthritis is mainly attributable to the elastic properties of joint capsular structures.[7,85] Following immersion of the hands in a water bath of 43°C (109.4°F) for 10 minutes, there was a slight decrease in finger joint stiffness.[76] Heating of the hand to 45°C (113°F) with a heat lamp (infrared) resulted in a 20% reduction in metacarpophalangeal stiffness compared with heating to a temperature of 33°C (91.4°F).[77]

A controlled pilot study involving patients with rheumatoid arthritis was conducted to compare and assess the effects of ice versus heat on shoulder pain and limited mobility.[68] The heat-treated group showed a greater increase in shoulder abduction and flexion than the ice-treated group, although this difference was not statistically significant. In a systematic database search, Ayling and Marks[7] found paraffin wax applications were accompanied by significant improvements in rheumatoid arthritic hand function when followed by exercise. Similarly, Robinson et al.[22] concluded that patients with rheumatoid arthritis can use thermotherapy palliatively or as an adjunct therapy combined with exercises, and they found that wax baths were especially helpful in the treatment of arthritic hands. Clearly, heating can result in decreased joint stiffness and increased tissue extensibility, thus facilitating ease of motion and gains in ROM.

Physical Principles of Heat

Heat flow through matter (tissues) varies with the nature of the material (type of tissue) and is called *thermal conductivity*.[42] Changes in surface tissue temperature from heating modalities depend on the intensity of the heat applied, the time of heat exposure, and the thermal medium (product of thermal conductivity, density, and specific heat) for surface heat.[85] The greatest degree of temperature elevation with heating modalities occurs in the skin and the subcutaneous tissues within 0.5 to 2.0 cm from the skin surface.[86] In areas of adequate blood supply, temperature will increase to a maximum within 6 to 8 minutes of exposure.[32,36,58] Muscle temperature at depths of 1 to 2 cm will increase to a lesser degree and will require a longer duration of exposure (15 to 30 minutes) to reach peak values.[32,40,58, 86] At a depth of 3 cm and using clinically tolerable intensities, muscle temperature elevation will be about 1°C (1.8°F) or less.[14,16,32,86]

In joints of the hand and wrist or foot and ankle, with relatively little soft tissue covering, heating modalities can raise intra-articular temperatures.[3,88,89] In fact, a 20-minute exposure of the foot to dry heat fluidized therapy (Fluidotherapy) at 47.8°C (118°F) was shown to increase joint capsule temperature in the foot.[3] Even though there can be a reflex vasodilatory response on the unheated opposite extremity, no reflex temperature changes would be expected to occur.[89]

After the peak temperature is reached, there is a plateau effect, or a slight decrease in skin temperature, over the remainder of the heat exposure.[32,36,40,58] In contrast, a study by Kelly et al.[62] using fluidized therapy found that skin temperature remained significantly above pretreatment levels 20 minutes after completion of the treatment. Typical temperature responses of areas with intact circulation are given in Table 3-1.

Fat provides insulation against heat; it has a low thermal conductivity (see Table 3-1). Therefore, areas under adipose tissue are likely to be minimally affected by heating modalities. In order to elevate deep tissues to therapeutically desired levels without burning the skin and subcutaneous tissue, a heating modality such as continuous ultrasound or shortwave diathermy should be selected.

Heat Transfer

The primary methods of heat transfer for heating modalities are conduction, convection, and radiation.[1,31,86] *Conduction* is a method of heat transfer in which the kinetic motion of atoms and molecules of one object is passed on to another object. This kinetic motion, often described as "atoms jostling one another,"[42,86] is increased when one object is heated more than another and occurs more effectively if the objects are solids.[42,86] More details on principles of conduction are presented in Chapter 2.

Convection is the bulk movement of moving molecules, either in liquid or gaseous form, that transfers heat from one place to another.[42,86] The fluid movement can be pumped, such as blood within the body is pumped by the heart and warms all the parts to which it travels, or movement may occur because a heated liquid or gas, being less dense, floats upward.[42,86]

Radiation is the conversion of heat energy to electromagnetic radiation.[42,86] All objects at temperatures above absolute zero ($-273°C$) both emit and absorb radiant energy. Any heated object or element, such as an infrared heat lamp, gives off radiant heat. If an object or body part is brought close enough to the radiant energy source, heat will be absorbed. Radiant heat application using infrared lamps is rarely, if ever, used today in rehabilitation; therefore, it will not be discussed further.

Conductive Heat Modalities

Moist heat packs and paraffin wax baths are commonly used heating modalities for clinical use. For home use, many patients use electric heating pads, microwavable heat packs, air-activated heat wraps, and paraffin wax baths. These modalities transfer heat to the body via conduction, because they are in contact with the skin and are at a much higher temperature than the skin surface to which they are applied. Therefore, thermal energy is lost from the modality and gained by the tissues. The quantity of heat gained and the subsequent physiological responses to it are dependent upon several factors, including but not limited to:

1. thermal conductivity of the tissues
2. body volume exposed
3. time of exposure.

Moist Heat Packs or Hot Packs

Commercially available moist heat packs consist of canvas or nylon cases filled with a hydrophilic silicate or some other hydrophilic substance or sand (Fig. 3-5). Moist heat packs are stored in a thermostatically controlled cabinet in water that is at a temperature between

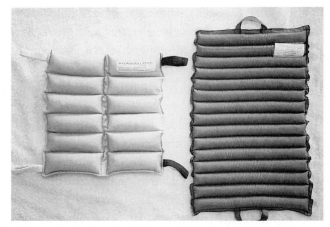

Fig 3•5 Two commercially available hot packs. These are heated in a thermostatically controlled unit.

70°C and 75°C (158°F and 167°F).[1,40,42,86] Moist heat packs come in a variety of shapes and sizes and should be chosen on the basis of the size and contour of the body part(s) to be treated.

The hot pack should completely cover the intervention area and should be secured in place (Figs. 3-6 and 3-7). The pack should not be secured so tightly that the patient cannot remove it if it becomes too hot. The pack should be covered with layers of terry-cloth toweling or commercial hot pack covers. While there appears to be no definitive number of layers of toweling for wrapping moist heat packs, the consensus is about six to eight layers, depending on towel thickness. Commercial hot pack covers often need another layer or two of toweling to ensure adequate insulation from the hot pack.

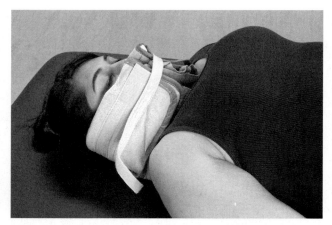

Fig 3•6 Hot pack application to the neck prior to exercise.

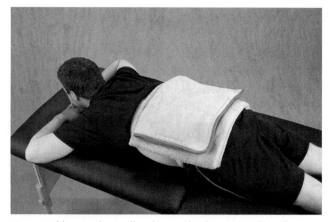

Fig 3•7 Hot pack application to the lower back before soft-tissue mobilization and exercise. Note that the patient is in the prone position. If indicated for patient comfort, a pillow may be added under the abdomen.

KEY POINT! The quality of the towels used with a heat pack should be considered. Because air acts as an insulator, newer, fluffier towels hold more air to insulate, thus retaining heat. Worn, thin towels will hold less heat and thus dissipate it sooner.

As with all forms of heating modalities, the patient should feel only a mild to moderate sensation of heat during application; the old adage "the hotter the better" could result in skin burns. A significant early change in skin color may suggest overheating. Fair-skinned individuals may turn bright pink-red[40] or blotchy red and white, while darker-skinned individuals may exhibit areas of darker and lighter color. Fyfe[40] suggests frequent monitoring of the patient until about the 9- to 10-minute mark after warmth is first perceived, when the maximum heating begins to dissipate. If the pack feels too hot to the patient or the therapist detects distinct skin color change, more toweling should be added, or the hot pack should be removed.

KEY POINT! The practitioner should monitor the patient during hot pack application. It is advisable to check under the hot pack after about 5 minutes to observe the skin color and the patient's subjective feelings about the amount of heat being perceived.

Patients should be advised not to lie with full body weight directly on top of moist heat packs, particularly when the intended intervention area is on the trunk. Body weight will squeeze water from the pack and may accelerate the rate of heat transfer. In addition, local

circulation could be reduced through compression of vessels, thus reducing circulatory convective cooling (dissipation of the heat). Both factors could cause overheating of the skin. Along this same line, the use of weights, such as sandbags, to hold the packs in position can potentially create hot spots in the patient's tissues.

If moist heat packs are to be used at home by caregivers or reliable patients, adequate instructions should be provided. There are a variety of methods of using moist heat at home by patients or caregivers, including commercial moist heat packs (hydrophilic silicate) and small water tanks for storage; sand packs, which can be heated either in water or in a microwave oven; and gel packs, which can also be heated in water or in a microwave oven. A common rubber hot-water bottle covered with moist toweling will also suffice.

All forms of moist heat packs should be inspected regularly for leaks and should be discarded if leaking occurs. When hydrophilic silicate moist heat packs become old and worn, they leak the pastelike material within them, and they should be discarded, as should gel packs that leak.

Clinically, moist heat packs are used mostly to help reduce pain and muscle spasm and to help improve tissue extensibility.[1,2,4–6,9,11,16,19,29,30,41,42,57,68,78,90] The moist heat from these packs rates quite highly among patients relative to their comfort, heating ability, and effectiveness.

Compared with other heating modalities, or other modalities used to treat pain, moist heat packs fare well, although not significantly better. Several studies[11,16,22,68,76,77] indicated that while the moist heat packs decreased pain and muscle spasm and improved ROM, they were not significantly better than other modalities. Williams and associates[68] found that moist heat packs did improve ROM at the shoulder more than did ice, although not significantly. Interestingly, however, most of the patients in the ice intervention group asked if they could be treated with heat instead of ice once the study was completed. Leung and Cheing[11] found that hot packs did increase shoulder function, ROM, and pain relief; however, the shortwave diathermy group fared better in all three measurements. Similarly, Minton[16] found both hot packs and ice packs improved straight-leg hip ROM following application to the hamstring muscles with no significant difference between them. However, the increase in

CASE STUDY 3•1   THERAPEUTIC HEAT FOR LOW BACK PAIN

Your patient is a 65-year-old female with chronic, intermittent low back pain (LBP) sustained 14 years ago during a low-speed motor vehicle accident where she sustained a compression fracture of a lumbar vertebra. The patient still complains of pain and stiffness most mornings and several days each month when pain lasts all day and limits her activity. Diagnostic imaging from 1 year ago shows moderate degenerative joint disease/osteoarthritis throughout the lumbar and lower thoracic spine without central canal or neuroforaminal stenosis. Examination reveals approximately 50% of expected lumbar motion in all directions when tested in standing, limited by "grabbing" pain in flexion and extension; negative neurological screen; pain and mild motion limitation with joint play testing of the lumbar vertebra; and pain with palpation of lumbar spinous processes and adjacent paraspinal muscles, which feel especially taut on the right side.

CLINICAL DECISION-MAKING

1. Does the patient have a dysfunction, limitation, or problem that can be improved with the use of therapeutic heat?

   Answer: The patient demonstrates decreased active ROM, decreased passive intervertebral joint play, and increased pain with palpation. Application of therapeutic heat is indicated for all of these and can be an effective and complementary adjuvant to the complete rehabilitation plan.

2. Is the patient appropriate for therapeutic heat? Do any of the general precautions or contraindications to therapeutic heat apply to the patient, or are there any specific considerations regarding the application of therapeutic heat to this patient?

   Answer: The patient's symptoms and history are appropriate for the use of therapeutic heat. Contraindications in this situation include treatment over areas of recent or potential hemorrhage, malignancy, acute inflammation, infection, poor thermal sensation, or where heat rubs have been recently applied.

3. What are the specific goals to be achieved with the use of therapeutic heat?

   Answer: Goals of treatment include decreasing pain, decreasing muscle spasm, increasing range of motion, increasing function without pain.

4. What specific aspects of therapeutic heat would be appropriate for this patient?

   Answer: Options for heating include moist heat pack, warm whirlpool, electric heating pad, and low-level continuous heat wrap. Moist heat pack is easy to use and may deliver heat to deeper tissues than electric heating pad. Heat wrap can deliver heat over a long duration and may allow a person to be more active during the treatment. Between 10 and 30 minutes for moist heat pack or electric heating pads, and up to 8 hours for heat wrap. Paraffin and Fluidotherapy are not practical options for treating the lumbar spine.

5. What are the proper application procedures for therapeutic heat?

   Answer: Any position with the spine unloaded and in a neutral position should be fine. Supine with hips/knees flexed is a good option for most people (comfortable, decreased stress on low back) but requires more frequent skin checks since the body weight can compress the vessels in the back that would otherwise dissipate excess heat; prone may put the patient's spine into too much extension, but this can be corrected with pillows under the abdomen. The size of the heating pack, pad, or wrap selected should be appropriate for the size of the area to be treated. A moist hot pack should be wrapped in a hot pack cover with several layers of additional toweling used to provide safe and adequate heating. More layers of pads or towels are needed if the patient is to lie atop the pack. Instruct the patient to contact you if the heat increases to an uncomfortable level. Return to check on the patient after 5 minutes. If the pack is too hot to the patient, or the therapist detects distinct changes in skin color, more toweling should be added or the hot pack should be removed. Following treatment, always inspect the skin.

ROM following hot pack application was deemed to be from the increased tissue temperature, the increased extensibility of collagen, and the relaxed psychological response of the subjects. It was felt that the cryotherapy increased ROM because of its inhibitory effect on muscle spasm and pain, yet these were all normal subjects with no known pathology.[16] (See Box 3-2 for advantages and disadvantages of using moist heat packs.)

Paraffin Wax

Paraffin wax has several physical characteristics that make it an efficient source of heat. First, it has a low melting point, around 54°C (129°F). This can be lowered further by adding more paraffin oil or mineral oil, so the wax remains molten at temperatures between about 45°C and 54°C (113°F and 129°F). This molten state allows for a more even distribution of the wax around the part to be treated (usually distal extremities). Second, paraffin has a low specific heat, which means that it does not feel as hot as water of the same temperature; therefore, there is much less risk of a burn. Third, it conducts heat more slowly than water at the same temperature, thus allowing the tissues to heat up more slowly, also decreasing the risk of a burn. This is particularly important when treating patients with sensitive skin or diminished skin sensation—for example, following burns.[66,91]

The paraffin mixture of a paraffin wax to oil (six or seven parts wax to one part oil) is commercially available and is melted and stored for use in thermostatically controlled stainless-steel or plastic containers. These wax baths come in a variety of sizes; the smaller ones are ideal for patient use at home (Fig. 3-8).

Paraffin is most commonly used for the distal extremities, including the fingers, hand, wrist, and perhaps elbow in the upper limb, and the toes, foot, and ankle in the lower limb. There are two principal techniques of application:

1. Dip and wrap
2. Dip and reimmerse

Dip-and-wrap is the more practical of the two options. For both methods, the extremity to be treated should be washed and dried and all jewelry removed from it. If a ring(s) cannot be removed, it should be covered with a piece of adhesive or surgical tape to prevent the wax from getting trapped in the ring crevices. When treating the hand and wrist, for example, the fingers should be slightly spread apart, the wrist relaxed, and the hand and wrist dipped into the wax to a few centimeters above the wrist joint. The hand is then removed from the wax and held above the bath until the wax has stopped dripping and becomes opaque; then the hand is dipped again (Fig. 3-9).

The patient should be reminded not to move the hand and fingers so as not to break the seal of the glove

---

Box 3•2	**Advantages and Disadvantages of Using Moist Heat Packs**

Advantages
1. Ease of preparation and application
2. Variety of shapes and sizes available
3. Moist, comfortable heat
4. Relatively inexpensive to purchase and replace (assuming a tank is already owned)

Disadvantages
1. No method of temperature control once applied to patient
2. Does not readily conform to all body parts
3. Sometimes awkward to secure in place on a patient
4. Does not retain heat for longer than about 20 minutes
5. A passive intervention; patient exercise cannot be performed simultaneously
6. May leak and then must be discarded (hydrophilic or gel packs)

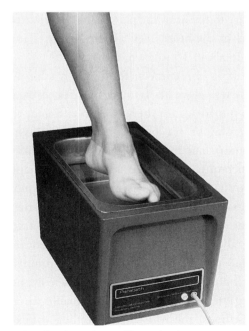

Fig 3•8 Application of paraffin to the foot. *(Courtesy of Talcott Laboratories, Houston, PA.)*

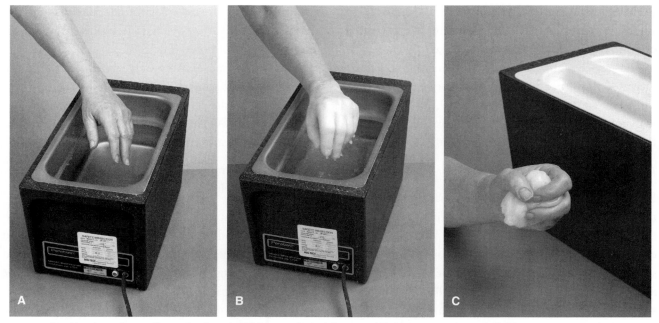

Fig 3•9 Application of paraffin to the hand. (A) Note relaxed fingers. (B) Note wax glove. (C) After wax removal, the patient can do light grip exercises before discarding wax.

being formed. This procedure is repeated about 8 to 10 times until a solid wax glove has formed around the fingers, hand, and wrist. The hand is then placed in a plastic bag and wrapped with a towel to help retain the heat. The end of the wrapped towel should be folded over to close the end of the extremity. Otherwise, the wrapped towel essentially makes a chimney and heat can escape. If there is a potential for edema to increase secondary to the heat, the part should be elevated above the level of the heart until the treatment time is over, usually in about 15 to 30 minutes.[86,92,93]

The dip-and-reimmerse technique is a bit different. After the wax glove has formed, the area covered by the glove is put back into the wax bath and kept there for the duration of the heat intervention (about 10 to 20 minutes). The most vigorous responses with respect to temperature elevation and blood flow changes will occur with the dip-and-reimmerse technique.[86,92–94] This technique is not well suited for most patients who are predisposed to edema or who cannot sit comfortably in the position required for intervention. This technique also precludes other patients from using the wax bath during that time period. If there are potential intervention areas that are not amenable to either of these methods, the wax can be applied with a paintbrush, using up to 10 coats of wax.

When using paraffin to improve skin pliability over healed burn areas, a temperature of 47°C (116.6°F) has been suggested.[66] Paraffin also lubricates and conditions the skin because of the mineral oil content.[95] This can be particularly useful when treating a scarred skin area. Using wax and stretching, Head and Helms[91] demonstrated a maintainable average increase in ROM of 7° to 10° in the joints of patients with burn scars. If wax is applied over a skin-grafted area, the graft should be stable and nonfragile, and the application should occur at least 10 days postgraft.[91] Intervention is daily for 2 to 3 weeks.

Paraffin baths are often used as part of an intervention program in patients with rheumatoid arthritis. Wax is applied during the nonflare phases to decrease pain and increase tissue extensibility. Dellhag and associates[96] found wax baths to be an effective intervention for this population. Although they found no significant therapeutic effects with wax bath interventions alone, there was a significant improvement in stiffness, ROM, and grip function when the wax intervention was followed by active exercise. In a Cochrane Review, Robinson et al.[22] suggested that paraffin wax baths combined with exercises can provide beneficial short-term effects for rheumatoid arthritic hands.

Paraffin baths have been used in patients with systemic sclerosis (scleroderma). Sandqvist et al.[97] found that after 1 month of daily treatment, paraffin hand baths significantly improved finger flexion and extension, thumb abduction, wrist flexion, and perceived stiffness and skin elasticity over the baseline values of the nontreated (control) hand.

Relative to other heat modalities, paraffin wax may not be significantly better at decreasing pain or increasing joint ROM. Hoyrup and Kjorvel[67] compared whirlpool and wax interventions for hand therapy. They measured hand volume, ROM, and level of pain immediately prior to and following 3 weeks of intervention. While all subjects showed significant improvements in ROM and decreased pain levels, no major differences were found between the modalities.

Paraffin should not be applied over open wounds because of the risk of burning the tissues. Patients with infected skin lesions should not use wax, as it may exacerbate the lesion. When contagious skin conditions or warts are present, prior to immersion in the wax bath, the area is covered with a bandage or some form of plastic skin film to prevent the wax bath from becoming contaminated. See Box 3-3 for advantages and disadvantages of paraffin wax.

Electric Heating Pads

A method of applying a low-level heat over a long time (e.g., hours) has been available for years in the form of electric heating pads. The disadvantages of electric heating pads are the patient must be at the site of an electrical outlet, and some of these pads may heat up enough to produce superficial burns.

Electric heating pads primarily are used at home for temporary pain relief. They are usually square but also may be shaped like a cervical moist heat pack. The pads may have an adjustable intensity control, but they should not be used during sleep in case the pad is inadvertently left on. See Box 3-4 for advantages and disadvantages of electric heating pads.

Air-Activated, Wearable Heat Wraps

Commercially available wearable heat wraps are air activated and can be worn for up to 8 hours at a time. These heat wraps are made of cloth embedded with multiple disks made of iron powder, activated charcoal,

---

Box 3•3 Advantages and Disadvantages of Paraffin Wax

Advantages
1. Low specific heat allows for application at a higher temperature than water without the risk of a burn.
2. Low thermal conductivity allows for heating of tissues to occur more slowly, thus reducing the risk of overheating the tissues.
3. Molten state allows for even distribution of heat to areas like fingers and toes.
4. First dip traps air and moisture to create more even heat distribution.
5. Oils used in the wax add moisture to the skin.
6. Wax remains malleable after removal, allowing for use as an exercise tool.
7. Paraffin provides a comfortable, moist heat.
8. Replacing the wax is relatively inexpensive (assuming bath is already owned).

Disadvantages
1. Paraffin wax is effective only for distal extremities in terms of ease of application.
2. The most effective method of application is the bath, which limits accessibility for other body parts to be treated effectively.
3. There is no method of temperature control once applied.
4. The heating lasts only about 20 minutes.
5. It is a passive intervention; patient exercise cannot be performed simultaneously.

Box 3•4 Advantages and Disadvantages of Electric Heating Pads

Advantages
1. Readily available for purchase at a reasonable cost for long-term use
2. A convenient method of at-home heat application to be used prior to exercise
3. Provides a comfortable, dry heat sensation

Disadvantages
1. Can cause skin and subcutaneous tissue burns if patient inadvertently falls asleep with the pad turned on
2. Patient must be near an electrical outlet during use
3. A passive intervention; patient exercise cannot be performed simultaneously

---

sodium chloride, and water. The disks are spaced throughout the cloth's application surface; when the wrap is removed from its sealed pouch and exposed to oxygen, the disks oxidize, producing an exothermic reaction, thus producing heat.[14] These wearable heat wraps maintain a temperature of about 40°C (104°F), elevate tissue temperature, and can be worn during activities of daily living, work, and sleep. The wraps are available in different sizes and shapes to accommodate body size and contour (Fig. 3-10).

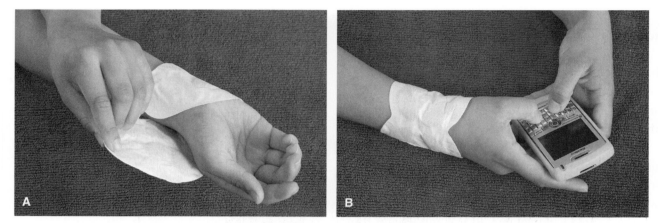

Fig 3•10 Air-activated heat wrap. (A) Wrap being applied to the wrist. (B) Using the hand with wrap in place.

Improved trunk flexibility, reduced pain, and less muscle stiffness in patients with lower back pain were reported by Nadler et al.[98] in a trial of continuous low-level heat (e.g., 8 hours of continuous wear) using air-activated heat wraps (Fig. 3-11). This study showed that the effects were greater with the heat wrap than with oral placebo medication.[98] Another study showed similar effects when the heat wrap therapy was compared with ibuprofen and acetaminophen.[99] This study was performed on patients with acute lower back pain; therefore, it is unlikely that loss of motion was due to adaptive shortening of connective tissue. The positive results could be attributed in part to pain reduction and perhaps a reduction in muscle-guarding spasms.[99] These heat wraps have also been effective in low pain control when used during sleep.[100]

Kettenmann et al.[72] examined the impact of low-level heat wrap therapy on acute low back pain by taking objective electroencephalogram measures in addition to other psychophysical measurements. They found the heat wrap group had reduced low back pain, a better night's sleep, a decreased number of daytime naps, and everyday situations being less stressful compared to the control group. Mayer and colleagues[20] found the combination of low-level heat wrap and directional preference-based exercise during the treatment of acute low back pain significantly improved functional outcomes compared with either intervention alone or with the control group. Patients with wrist pain due to sprains/strains and arthritis had relief with a wrist wrap as compared with placebo medication.[101] Another study by Mayer and associates[23]

found low-level heat wrap therapy was of significant benefit in the prevention and the early phase treatment of delayed-onset muscle soreness of the low back. These studies showed that the relief low-level, air-activated heat wraps provided is based on the length of application, which varied from 4 to 8 hours, compared to the 15- to 30-minute application of hot packs or paraffin wax.[23] See Box 3-5 for advantages and disadvantages of air-activated, wearable heat wraps.

Convective Heating: Fluidotherapy (Fluidized Therapy)

Fluidotherapy is a dry-heat modality that transfers heat energy by forced convection. Borrell and coworkers[3] suggest that for heating, it is irrelevant whether the modality is providing wet or dry heat, provided that the skin temperature is raised to the same temperature by both modalities. The Fluidotherapy system uses air-fluidized solids as the heat transfer medium. Warm air is uniformly circulated through the bottom of a bed of finely divided cellulose particles (finely ground corn cob, dubbed "cellex") in a container. The solid particles become suspended when the stream of air is forced through them, making the fluidized bed demonstrate properties similar to those of liquids.[3] The viscosity of the air-fluidized system is low, allowing a patient to submerge body parts into the fluidized bed and suspend these parts similarly to a fluid bath, thus permitting exercise with relative ease.[102,103] The heat transfer characteristics within the fluidized bed and to parts submerged in it are similar to those of a mildly agitated liquid.[102] The combination of air flowing around the

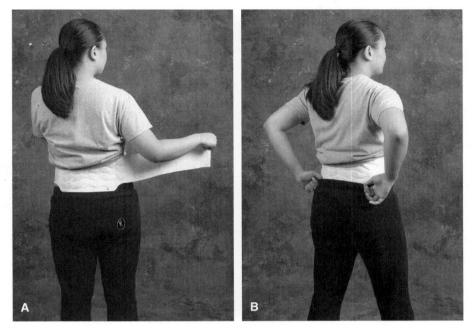

Fig 3•11 (A) Air-activated heat wrap being applied to lower back. (B) Patient can wear wrap under clothing.

high surface area of the finely divided particles and the bulk movement of solids produces high heat fluxes and uniform temperatures throughout, thus providing a strong massaging action, sensory stimulation, and levitation.[103]

Fluidotherapy units come in a variety of sizes and are best used for treating the distal extremities. For joints and distal body parts, the patient places the body part through the entrance sleeve of the Fluidotherapy unit (Fig. 3-12). The sleeve is then secured to keep the cellulose particles from escaping. As the air stream is blown in, the particles become suspended and the treated body part feels as though it is immersed in a moving liquid bath, such as a whirlpool.

Both temperature and the amount of particle agitation can be varied. Temperature ranges are typically between 38.8°C to 47.8°C (102°F to 118°F). The lower ranges are recommended for patients who have a greater predisposition for edema formation or who are in beginning programs for desensitization, as they may not be able to tolerate higher temperatures. Agitation can be controlled for patient comfort. In addition,

Box 3•5	Advantages and Disadvantages of Air-Activated Heat Wraps

Advantages
1. Dry heat prevents clothing from getting wet.
2. Wraps provide a comfortable and low-profile heat source.
3. Wraps can be worn during activity and sleep.
4. Patients can easily be instructed in safe application.
5. Wraps are relatively inexpensive for short-term use.
6. Active exercises may be performed during wear.
7. When used as directed, wraps do not heat up to more than 40°C.

Disadvantages
1. Wraps can be used only one time.
2. If needed for extended periods of time, the expense must be considered.

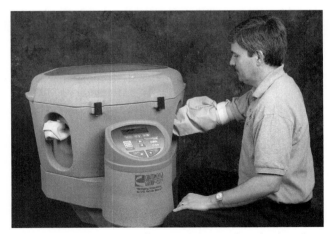

Fig 3•12 Fluidotherapy (fluidized therapy) to the hand and wrist.

varying degrees of agitation can be used in a program of desensitization for hypersensitive areas.

Patients can perform exercises while the affected body part(s) is within the cabinet. This is particularly effective for the distal extremities, such as the wrist, hand, fingers, ankle, foot, and toes. If heat and stretch is desired, dynamic splinting can be used during the time of heat intervention to provide a gentle stretch, or stretching techniques can be used immediately following immersion in Fluidotherapy.

If there is an open wound on a body part that needs to be treated, the wound can be protected by a plastic barrier or bag to prevent any fine cellulose particles from becoming embedded in the wound and to minimize the risk of cross-contamination.

The effects of Fluidotherapy on nerve conduction velocity and skin temperature in normal subjects was examined by Kelly and colleagues.[62] They found that Fluidotherapy (heat plus tactile stimulation) significantly elevated superficial skin temperature compared to tactile stimulation alone and no treatment (control group). In addition, they found a concomitant decrease in distal sensory latency of the superficial radial nerve action potential as the skin temperature increased. The authors suggest that the higher skin temperatures obtained with Fluidotherapy may be of benefit clinically when the aim of treatment is to increase soft tissue extensibility or reduce joint stiffness with active or passive movements.[62]

The effectiveness of Fluidotherapy as a heating modality was compared with paraffin wax and hydrotherapy by in vivo temperature measurements.[3] Joint capsule and muscle temperatures in the hands and feet were measured at various depths. Fluidotherapy produced the greatest increase in tissue temperatures in all areas. The authors' conclusion was that Fluidotherapy delivered more heat than paraffin wax or hydrotherapy because higher temperatures can be tolerated in a dry environment.[3] However, this conclusion is questionable, because paraffin wax in particular allows tissues to be immersed in a bath with an operating temperature of 45°C to 54°C (113°F to 129°F), compared with the Fluidotherapy range of 39°C to 48°C (102.2°F to 118.4°F).

Alcorn and coworkers[104] used Fluidotherapy and exercise in the management of patients with sickle cell anemia. They demonstrated a marked reduction in the length of hospitalization (compared with the length of hospitalization by the same patients during previous episodes); a major reduction in the dosage of analgesics previously administered; and a marked improvement in spine, trunk, and extremity ROM and gait. See Box 3-6 for advantages and disadvantages of Fluidotherapy.

Clinical Application: Principles and Indications

Heating modalities are used in therapeutic programs to assist in the reduction of pain and stiffness, to alleviate muscle spasm, to increase ROM, and to improve tissue healing by increasing blood flow and nutrients to an area. When heat is applied to the trunk, shoulders, hips, or knees, it is usually considered a mild heat. The site of dysfunction is often well below the surface, and the heat will produce desired responses through reflex mechanisms by stimulation of cutaneous afferents. Mild heating usually elevates temperature at the site of pathology to less than 40°C (104°F) and may be thought of as having a soothing, counterirritant effect.[29]

When a higher temperature—for example, between 40°C and 45°C (104°F and 113°F)—is desired at the involved structure, the appropriate modality for the intervention must be chosen. Paraffin, for example, may be a vigorous heater of the finger joints but only a mild heater of the shoulder. The principles of mild versus vigorous heating are summarized in Table 3-2.

Box 3•6 Advantages and Disadvantages of Fluidotherapy

Advantages
1. Convenient and easy to administer
2. Temperature of application can be controlled.
3. Agitation of dry particles can be controlled for comfort.
4. Variety of unit sizes allows for most body areas to be treated.
5. Allows for some active exercise to be carried out during intervention
6. Provides a dry, comfortable heat
7. Can be used for desensitization of hypersensitive hands/fingers or feet/toes

Disadvantages
1. Relatively expensive modality to purchase
2. Some patients are intolerant to the enclosed container (claustrophobic feeling).
3. Some patients are intolerant to the dry materials used.

CASE STUDY 3•2 THERAPEUTIC HEAT TO IMPROVE RANGE OF MOTION ▰

Your patient is a 38-year-old construction worker who had his right hand crushed under a heavy weight at work 3 months ago. He suffered fractures to his second, third, and fourth proximal phalanges and to his second and third metacarpals, and he dislocated the metacarpal-phalangeal joint of his thumb. His hand was immobilized in a splint for 6 weeks. He is unable to return to work due to the significant loss of function of his right hand. Your examination reveals decreased ROM of flexion, extension, and opposition of the thumb; decreased ROM of flexion and extension of the second, third, and fourth metacarpal-phalangeal joints; weakness of the hand intrinsic muscles; and pain with closing his hand and grasping objects.

CLINICAL DECISION-MAKING

1. Does the patient have a dysfunction, limitation, or problem that can be improved with the use of therapeutic heat?

   Answer: The patient has significant dysfunction and limitations, including decreased ROM, strength, and pain that presently keep the patient from returning to work. Therapeutic heat can be used as part of the rehabilitation plan to allow the patient to complete ROM and hand-strengthening exercises that will lead to further functional retraining.

2. Is the patient appropriate for therapeutic heat? Do any of the general precautions or contraindications to therapeutic heat apply to the patient, or are there any specific considerations regarding the application of therapeutic heat to this patient?

   Answer: The patient's dysfunctions and limitations are appropriate for use of therapeutic heat. Contraindications in this situation include treatment over areas of recent or potential hemorrhage, malignancy, acute inflammation, infection, poor thermal sensation, peripheral vascular compromise, or where heat rubs have been recently applied.

3. What are the specific goals to be achieved with the use of therapeutic heat?

   Answer: The primary goals are to decrease pain and to increase extensibility of soft tissue in order to gain more range of motion in the restricted joints. Job-specific functional goals will be incorporated as appropriate.

4. What specific aspects of therapeutic heat would be appropriate for this patient?

   Answer: Options for heating for this case include warm whirlpool, paraffin wax bath, and Fluidotherapy. Whirlpool and Fluidotherapy would allow for the patient to perform active exercises during treatment; paraffin wax is a passive treatment. Moist heat packs or low-level heat wrap therapy would not work very well with the hand, wrist, and fingers because of their flat surface.

5. What are the proper application procedures for therapeutic heat?

   Answer: Several therapeutic heating agents may be used for this patient, including warm whirlpool (38°C; 100°F) for 15 to 20 minutes, Fluidotherapy (40°C; 104°F) for 15 to 20 minutes, and paraffin wax using the dip-and-wrap method for 20 minutes. Because restoring hand mobility is a primary interest, warm whirlpool and Fluidotherapy are preferred because active ROM activities can be performed while the heat is applied. If restrictions from scarring are present, paraffin wax may assist in softening and mobilizing the restricted scar.

Table 3•2 **Comparison of Mild and Vigorous Heating[1]**

	Mild	**Vigorous**
Temperature elevation site of pathology	Low	High
Degree of temperature increase	Warmth—up to 40°C comfortable sensation of warmth	Near tolerance levels up to 45°C
Rate of rise of temperature	Slow	Rapid
Clinical examples	To cervical area for reducing muscle spasm upper trapezius	Fluidotherapy at 45°C to the hand to increase tissue extensibility before ROM exercises

Intervention time with all heating modalities usually ranges from 15 to 30 minutes. This duration will allow time for maximal tolerable increases in tissue temperature and blood flow. However, with certain heat modalities, such as air-activated heat wraps, a much longer time of application is used. (See the previous section on air-activated heat wraps.)

Despite the widespread clinical use of heating modalities, there are very few well-designed clinical studies that address the efficacy of these modalities in a therapeutic regimen. The remainder of this chapter will discuss safety issues and application techniques based on purported physiological rationales and the clinical experience of the authors. Details regarding specific studies related to the use of thermotherapy for pain control, reduction of muscle-guarding spasm, and increasing ROM are discussed in Chapter 13.

Contraindications and Precautions to Thermotherapy

Before using heat in therapeutic intervention, the therapist should determine the status of the patient's circulation and his or her sensitivity to temperature and pain. The skin overlying the intervention area should be tested for thermal sensation using hot and cold water in test tubes or with other hot and cold objects, such as spoons. Pain sensation can be determined by using the pinprick versus the blunt test. This information is necessary because determining the safe level of heat requires that the patient be able to perceive when the pain threshold has been reached. Response of thermal receptors in the skin is illustrated in Figure 3-13.

The following is a list of contraindications to the use of heating modalities:

- Application over areas with a lack of intact thermal sensation (risk of burn if patient cannot distinguish between hot and cold)
- Application over areas of vascular insufficiency or vascular disease (risk of burn if circulation is inadequate to dissipate heat in tissues)
- Application over areas of recent hemorrhage or potential hemorrhage (heat will increase bleeding)
- Application over areas of known malignancy (while the exact nature of what may happen

when superficial heat is applied over a known malignancy is unknown, heat may increase activation and movement of malignant cells)
- Application over areas of acute inflammation (heat will aggravate and potentially increase inflammatory response)
- Application over infected areas where infection may spread or where cross-contamination may occur (heat may cause infection to spread to other areas)
- Application over areas where liniments or heat rubs have recently been applied (heat will increase risk of burn because vessels are already dilated from the presence of liniment; the vessels cannot dilate further to dissipate more heat)
- Application in any situation deemed unreliable by the physical therapist (unreliable situations, such as language difficulties, put patients at risk because they may not understand the therapist's instructions)

Clinical Decision-Making

The decision to use a thermal modality as part of a total intervention program should be based on a combination of factors, including the patient's diagnosis and medical status and the objective findings of the physical therapy examination. It is not until this information is gathered that the intervention goals are established. The plan of intervention to obtain these goals can include a thermal modality when indicated. It should be noted that, in most situations, it is only appropriate to apply one type of heating modality. To include two, such as paraffin and whirlpool to the hand in one session, would most likely be redundant. In certain situations, combining two electrophysical agents may be complementary to the treatment goals, such as the use of transcutaneous electrical stimulation (TENS) with a hot pack for the treatment of pain.[90] Intervention is executed and follow-up completed. The procedures for clinical decision-making and carrying out the intervention are outlined in Box 3-7.

Heat Versus Cold

There are clinical situations when either heat or cold may be selected to meet intervention objectives or when

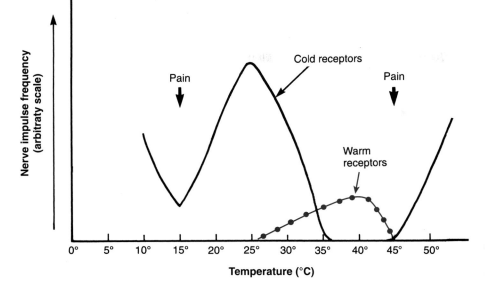

Fig 3•13 Responses of thermal receptors in the skin. *(Adapted with permission from Low J, Reed A. Electrotherapy Explained: Principles and Practices. Oxford, Butterworth Heinemann; 1990:177.)*

one is clearly preferred over the other. Often the choice between heat and cold is empirical, but before the decision is made, certain factors should be considered:

1. Stage of injury or disease
2. Area of body treated
3. Medical status
4. Patient preference, which may be determined by cold or heat hypersensitivity
5. Decision to use thermal modalities as part of a home program

Cold is the preferred modality during the acute stages of inflammation; heat at this stage may further aggravate inflammation. In patients who can tolerate cryotherapy, this may be chosen for reducing muscle spasm (see Chapter 2). Cold can also reduce pain around joints before ROM exercises and may be easier for the patient to apply at home. On the other hand, heat may be better tolerated psychologically by persons with pain or muscle spasm, resulting in increased patient compliance with intervention programs. Temperature elevation will decrease joint stiffness and increase connective tissue extensibility, so if either of these is the intervention goal, heat is the modality of choice. In addition, heat to distal extremities seems to be tolerated better than cold. The advantages and disadvantages of using heat or cold are briefly outlined in Figure 3-14.

Box 3•7	**Procedure for Clinical Decision-Making and Execution of Intervention With a Thermal Modality**

1. Assess patient.
2. Establish intervention goals based on results of patient assessment and consultation.
3. Select intervention plan, including thermal modality when applicable, to meet these goals.
4. Choose thermal modality.
5. Select position for intervention.
6. Apply thermal modality (followed by exercise or other appropriate techniques).
7. Reassess and determine if intervention should continue or be modified or discontinued.
8. Establish a home program (which can include a thermal modality).

HEAT vs. COLD

Heat	
Advantages: ↓ Pain ↑ Tissue extensibility ↓ Stiffness	*Disadvantages:* May cause ↑ swelling

Cold	
Advantages: May prevent further swelling ↓ pain	*Disadvantages:* ↑ stiffness ↓ tissue extensibility

Fig 3•14 Intervention choice: heat versus cold.

Factors to Consider for Therapeutic Heat Techniques

The decision of which heat modality to select primarily depends on the location of the involved structure, the pathophysiology, and the degree of temperature elevation desired (Fig. 3-15). Generally speaking, deep heat is usually selected during the remodeling phase of an injury or a disease when tissue contractures persist or when heat is required deep into a joint.

When treating a patient with pain, muscle spasm, or both, the patient's position must be carefully selected and should be the most comfortable possible, particularly considering that the patient may need to remain in that position for up to 30 minutes. If muscle spasm is present, the muscle(s) should not be in a position of "undue stretch" until some pain relief has occurred. If the patient has joint pain, the joint should be positioned in an open-packed position, with the ligaments and joint capsule in a slackened position; this will lessen the intra-articular pressure[105] and the stress on joint structures.

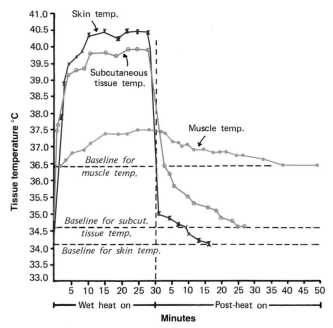

Fig 3•15 Curves representing changes in skin, subcutaneous tissue, and muscle temperatures obtained during and after 30 minutes of wet heat topically applied to the forearm. *(Adapted with permission from Abramson, et al. Changes in blood flow, oxygen uptake and tissue temperatures produced by the topical application of wet heat. Arch Phys Med Rehabil. 1961;42:305.)*

As has been previously described,[31,77] the use of heat combined with low-load prolonged stretch may be amenable to elongating tissues secondary to contracture, as heat increases extensibility of collagen tissue.

Wet Versus Dry Heat

Many patients say they have heard that moist heat is more penetrating, and thus more effective, than dry heat. Few clinical studies that examine the efficacy of one versus the other in obtaining functional intervention goals are available. Cosgray et al.[106] compared hamstring length treated with moist hot packs and with the Pneumatherm, a device that delivers pulsed, dry hot air to the skin at temperatures of approximately 49°C (120°F). They found that the dry heat produced greater increases in hamstring length than moist heat or controls. It has been determined that dry heat can elevate surface temperatures to a greater degree but that moist heat can elevate temperature to a slightly deeper level.[107]

Home Application of Therapeutic Heat Modalities

In most cases, it is desirable to provide a patient with an at-home means for pain control and for reducing stiffness before exercise. Gel packs, sand packs, and bead packs are commercially available and can be heated in either a water container or a microwave oven for short-duration heat applications (e.g., up to 20 or 30 minutes). Both paraffin wax baths and Fluidotherapy units are available in home-use sizes, which are generally for the hands, wrists, and feet. Electric heating pads also provide relief and are available in various sizes. A rubber hot water bottle filled with hot tap water and covered with a moist towel will also provide mild, comfortable heat. Adequate, clear, and concise instructions should be written down for the home patient, including the intervention time, method, frequency of application, and any special instructions and precautions to prevent inadvertent burns from excess heat.

Safety of Heat Application

The adverse responses that can occur with heat application primarily include the chance of increasing swelling, in the case of acute edema, and the chance of causing superficial tissue burns. Barillo et al.[108] reviewed 4,510 records of patients admitted to one burn center between January 1978 and July 1997. Eleven admissions were due to burns caused by therapeutic application of heat.

Assessment of Effectiveness and Expected Outcomes

The use of heat in a therapy program is based on the goals of the treatment. The goals are determined by the patient and the therapist after a thorough evaluation of the patient, including the history of the present problem and subjective and objective measures of impairments and current functional status. The following outcomes and measures can be used for assessing effectiveness with heat:

- Pain—quantification via scales (see Chapter 13)
- Range of motion—goniometric measures
- Muscle guarding—reflected in joint ROM and muscle flexibility measures

Of course, the decision as to which of these measures to use will depend on the impairment being assessed.

Documentation

The astute clinician realizes the importance of documenting the specifics of intervention techniques and patient response to therapeutic intervention. Information included in the intervention record is outlined in the Documentation Tips that follow. Without such information, it is often difficult to replicate techniques and to adjust the plan of care as needed. A copy of home instructions should be kept with the patient's file.

Documentation Tips

- Thermal modality used
- Method of application, including duration
- Body area treated
- Patient position for intervention
- Special precautions or application concerns

REFERENCES

1. Lehmann JF, deLateur BJ. Therapeutic heat. In: Lehmann JF, ed. *Therapeutic Heat and Cold.* 4th ed. Baltimore: Williams & Wilkins; 1990.
2. Baker RJ, Bell GW. The effect of therapeutic modalities on blood flow in the human calf. *J Orthop Sports Phys Ther.* 1991;13:23.
3. Borrell RM, Parker R, Henley EJ, et al. Comparison of in vivo temperatures produced by hydrotherapy, paraffin wax treatment, and Fluidotherapy. *Phys Ther.* 1980;60:1273–1276.
4. Levi SJ, Maihafer GC. Traditional approaches to pain. In: Echternach J, ed. *Pain.* New York: Churchill Livingstone; 1987.
5. Halvorsen, GA. Therapeutic heat and cold for athletic injuries. *Phys Sports Med.* 1990;18:87.
6. Allen RJ. Physical agents used in the management of chronic pain by physical therapists. *Phys Med Rehabil Clin North Am.* 2006;17:315–345.
7. Ayling J, Marks R. Efficacy of paraffin wax baths for rheumatoid arthritic hands. *Physiotherapy.* 2000;86(4):190–201.
8. Draper DO, Hopkins JT. Increased intramuscular and intracapsular temperature via ThermaCare® knee wrap application. *Med Sci Monit.* 2008;14(6):7–11.
9. Fedorczyk J. The role of physical agents in modulating pain. *J Hand Ther.* 1997;10:110–121.
10. Hardy M, Woodall W. Therapeutic effects of heat, cold and stretch on connective tissue. *J Hand Ther.* 1998;11:148–156.
11. Leung MSF, Cheing GLY. Effects of deep and superficial heating in the management of frozen shoulder. *J Rehabil Med.* 2008;40:145–150.
12. Lin YH. Effects of thermal therapy in improving the passive range of knee motion: comparison of cold and superficial heat applications. *Clin Rehabil.* 2003;17(6):618–623.
13. Nadler SF, Steiner DJ, Erasala GN, Hengehold DA, Abeln SB, Weingand KW. Continuous low-level heatwrap therapy for treating acute nonspecific low back pain. *Arch Phys Med Rehabil.* 2003;84:329–334.
14. Trowbridge CA, Draper DO, Freland JB, Jutte LS, Eggett DL. Paraspinal musculature and skin temperature changes: comparing the ThermaCare HeatWrap, the Johnson & Johnson Back Plaster, and the ABC Warme-Pflaster. *J Orthop Sports Phys Ther.* 2004;34:549–558.
15. Robertson VJ, Ward AR, Jung P. The effect of heat on tissue extensibility: a comparison of deep and superficial heating. *Arch Phys Med Rehabil.* 2005;86:819–825.
16. Minton J. A comparison of thermotherapy and cryotherapy in enhancing supine, extended-leg, hip flexion. *J Athl Train.* 1993;28(2):172–176.
17. Brodowicz GR, Welsh R, Wallis J. Comparison of stretching with ice, stretching with heat, or stretching alone on hamstring flexibility. *J Athl Train.* 1996;31(4):324–327.
18. Chou R, Huffman LH. Nonpharmacologic therapies for acute and chronic low back pain: a review of the evidence for an American Pain Society/American College of Physicians Clinical Practice Guideline. *Ann Intern Med.* 2007;147:492–504.
19. French SD, Cameron M, Walker BF, Reggars JW, Esterman AJ. A Cochrane review of superficial heat or cold for low back pain. *Spine.* 2006;31(9):998–1006.
20. Mayer JM, Ralph L, Look M, et al. Treating acute low back pain with continuous low-level heat wrap therapy and/or exercise: a randomized controlled trial. *Spine J.* 2005;5:395–403.
21. Rakel B, Barr JO. Physical modalities in chronic pain management. *Nurs Clin North Am.* 2003;38:477–494.
22. Robinson V, Brosseau L, Casimiro L, et al. Thermotherapy for treating rheumatoid arthritis. Cochrane Database of Systematic Reviews, Issue 2. Art. No.:CD002826. DOI: 10. 1002/14651858.CD002826; 2002
23. Mayer JM, Mooney V, Matheson LN, et al. Continuous low-level heat wrap therapy for the prevention and early phase treatment of delayed-onset muscle soreness of the low back: a randomized controlled trial. *Arch Phys Med Rehabil.* 2006;87:1310–1317.

24. Robertson VJ, Spurritt D. Electrophysical agents: implications of their availability and use in undergraduate clinical placements. *Physiotherapy*. 1998;84(7):335–344.

25. Chipchase LS, Williams MT, Robertson VJ. A national study of the availability and use of electrophysical agents by Australian physiotherapists. *Physiother Theory Pract*. 2009;25(4):279–296.

26. Lindsay DM, Dearness J, McGinley CC. Electrotherapy usage trends in private physiotherapy practice in Alberta. *Physiother Can*. 1995;47(1):30–34.

27. Nussbaum EL, Burke S, Johnstone L, Laliffe G, Robitaille E, Yoshida K. Use of electrophysical agents: findings and implications of a survey of practice in Metro Toronto. *Physiother Can*. 2007;59(2):118–131.

28. Pope GD, Mockett SP, Wright JP. A survey of electrotherapeutic modalities: ownership and use in the NHS in England. *Physiotherapy*. 1995;81(2):82–91.

29. Kitchen S. Thermal effects. In: Watson T, ed. *Electrotherapy: Evidence-Based Practice*. 12th ed. Edinburgh: Churchill Livingstone Elsevier; 2008.

30. Warren G. The use of heat and cold in the treatment of common musculoskeletal disorders. In: Hertling D, Kessler RM, eds. *Management of Common Musculoskeletal Disorders*. 2nd ed. Philadelphia: Harper & Row; 1989.

31. Lentell G, Hetherington T, Eagan J, Morgan M. The use of thermal agents to influence the effectiveness of a low-load prolonged stretch. *J Orthop Sports Phys Ther*. 1992;16:200–207.

32. Abramson DI, Mitchell RE, Tuck S, et al. Changes in blood flow, oxygen uptake and tissue temperatures produced by the topical application of wet heat. *Arch Phys Med Rehabil*. 1961;42:305.

33. Crockford GW, Hellon RF. Vascular responses in human skin to infra-red radiation. *J Physiol*. 1959;149:424.

34. Crockford GW, Hellon RF, Parkhouse J. Thermal vasomotor response in human skin mediated by local mechanisms. *J Physiol*. 1962;161:10.

35. Erasala GN, Rubin JM, Tuthill TA, et al. The effect of topical heat treatment on trapezius muscle blood flow using power Doppler ultrasound. In: Proceedings, Annual Conference and Exposition of the American Physical Therapy Association; June 20–24, 2001.

36. Greenberg RS. The effects of hot packs and exercise on local blood flow. *Phys Ther*. 1972;52:273.

37. Krusen EM, et al. Effects of hot packs on peripheral circulation. *Arch Phys Med*. 1950;31:145.

38. Reid RW, Foley JM, Prior BM, et al. Mild topical heat increases popliteal blood flow as measured by MRI. *Med Sci Sports Exerc*. 1999;31(5):S208.

39. Hardy JD, Bard P. Body temperature regulation. In: Mountcastle VB, ed. *Medical Physiology*. Vol. 2. 14th ed. St Louis: Mosby; 1979.

40. Fyfe M. Skin temperature, colour, and warmth felt, in hydrocollator pack applications to the lumbar region. *Aust J Physiol*. 1982;28:12.

41. Wadsworth H, Chanmugam APP. *Electrophysical Agents in Physiotherapy*. 2nd ed. Marrickville, NSW, Australia: Science Press; 1988.

42. Low J, Reed A. *Electrotherapy Explained: Principles and Practice*. Oxford, UK: Butterworth-Heinemann; 1990.

43. Berne R, Levy MN. *Cardiovascular Physiology*. 3rd ed. St Louis: Mosby; 1993.

44. Fox HH, Hilton SM. Bradykinin formation in human skin as a factor in heat vasodilation. *J Physiol*. 1958;142:219.

45. Milnor WR. Autonomic and peripheral control mechanisms. In: Mountcastle VB, ed. *Medical Physiology*. Vol. 2. 14th ed. St Louis: Mosby; 1979.

46. Guyton AC, Hall JE. *Textbook of Medical Physiology*. 10th ed. Philadelphia: Saunders; 2000.

47. Abramson DI, Bell Y, Tuck S, et al. Changes in blood flow. O_2 uptake and tissue temperatures produced by therapeutic physical agents. III. Effect of indirect or reflex vasodilation. *Am J Phys Med*. 1961;404:5.

48. Abramson DI, Tuck S, Chu LS, et al. Indirect vasodilation in thermotherapy. *Arch Phys Med Rehabil*. 1965;46:412.

49. Wessman MS, Kottke FJ. The effect of indirect heating on peripheral blood flow, pulse rate, blood pressure and temperature. *Arch Phys Med Rehabil*. 1967;48:567.

50. Wyper DJ, McNiven DR. Effects of some physiotherapeutic agents on skeletal muscle blood flow. *Physiotherapy*. 1976;62:83.

51. Kauranen K, Vanharanta H. Effects of hot and cold packs on motor performance of normal hands. *Physiotherapy*. 1997;83:340–344.

52. Johnson JM, Park MK. Effect of heat stress on cutaneous vascular responses to the initiation of exercise. *J Appl Physiol*. 1982;53:744.

53. Kanui TI. Thermal inhibition of nociceptor-driven spinal cord nerves in rats. *Pain*. 1985;21:231.

54. Barbour LA, McGuire DB, Kirchott KT. Non-analgesic methods of pain control used by cancer outpatients. *Oncol Nurs Forum*. 1986;13:56.

55. Sumida KD, Greenberg MB, Hill JM. Hot gel packs and reduction of delayed-onset muscle soreness 30 minutes after treatment. *J Sport Rehabil*. 2003;12:221–228.

56. Kaul MP, Herring SA. Superficial heat and cold—how to maximize the benefits. *Phys Sportsmed*. 1994;22:65–74.

57. Forster N, Palastanga A. *Clayton's Electrotherapy: Theory and Practice*. 9th ed. London: Balliere-Tindall; 1985.

58. Lehmann JD, Brunner GD, Stow RW. Pain threshold measurements after therapeutic application of ultrasound, microwaves and infrared. *Arch Phys Med Rehabil*. 1958;39:560.

59. Abramson DI, Chu LS, Tuck S, et al. Effect of tissue temperatures and blood flow on motor nerve conduction velocity. *JAMA*. 1966;198:1082.

60. Currier DP, Kramer JF. Sensory nerve conduction: heating effects of ultrasound and infrared. *Physiother Can*. 1982;34:241.

61. Halle JS, Scoville CR, Greathouse DG. Ultrasound's effect on the conduction latency of the superficial radial nerve in man. *Phys Ther*. 1981;61:345.

62. Kelly R, Beehn C, Hansford A, Westphal KA, Hale JS, Greathouse DG. Effect of Fluidotherapy® on superficial radial nerve conduction and skin temperature. *J Orthop Sports Phys Ther*. 2005;35:16–23.

63. Mense S. Effects of temperature on the discharges of muscle spindles and tendon organs. *Pflugers Arch*. 1978;374:159.

64. Chastain PB. The effect of deep heat on isometric strength. *Phys Ther*. 1978;58:543.

65. Edwards HT, Harris RC, Hutman E, et al. Effect of temperature on muscle energy metabolism and endurance during successive isometric contractions, sustained to fatigue, of the quadriceps muscle in man. *J Physiol*. 1972;220:335–352.

66. Burns S, Conin T. The use of paraffin wax in the intervention of burns. *Physiother Can*. 1987;39:258.

67. Hoyrup G, Kjorvel L. Comparison of whirlpool and wax interventions for hand therapy. *Physiother Can*. 1986;38:79.

68. Williams J, Harvey J, Tannenbaum H. Use of heat versus ice for the rheumatoid arthritic shoulder: a pilot study. *Physiother Can*. 1986;38:8.

69. Nadler SF, Weingand K, Kruse RJ. The physiologic basis and clinical application of cryotherapy and thermotherapy for the pain practitioner. *Pain Physician*. 2004;7:395–399.

70. Davis KD, Kwan CL, Crawley AP, Mikulis DJ. Functional MRI study of thalamic and cortical activations evoked by cutaneous heat, cold, and tactile stimuli. *J Neurophysiol.* 1998;80:1533–1546.

71. DeVries H. Quantitative electromyographic investigation of the spasms theory of muscle pain. *Am J Phys Med.* 1966;45:119.

72. Kettenmann B, Wille C, Lurie-Luke E, Walter D, Kobal G. Impact of continuous low level heatwrap therapy in acute low back pain patients: subjective and objective measurements. *Clin J Pain.* 2007;23(8):663–668.

73. Wickstrom R, Polk C. Effect of whirlpool on the strength endurance of the quadriceps muscle in trained male adolescents. *Am J Phys Med.* 1961;40:91.

74. LeBan MM. Collagen tissue: implications of its response to stress in vitro. *Arch Phys Med Rehabil.* 1962;43:461.

75. Wright V, Johns RJ. Quantitative and qualitative analysis of joint stiffness in normal subjects and in patients with connective tissue diseases. *Ann Rheum Dis.* 1961;20:36.

76. Backlund L, Tiselius P. Objective measurements of joint stiffness in rheumatoid arthritis. *Acta Rheum Scand.* 1967;13:275.

77. Knight CA, Rutledge CR, Cox ME, et al. Effect of superficial heat, deep heat and active exercise warm-up in the extensibility of the plantar flexors. *Phys Ther.* 2001;81(6):1206–1214.

78. Reid DC. *Sports Injury Assessment and Rehabilitation.* New York: Churchill Livingstone; 1992.

79. Sapega AA, Quedecfeld TC, Moyer RA, Butler RA. Biophysical factors in range-of-motion exercise. *Phys Sports Med.* 1981;9:57.

80. Kottke FJ, Pauley DL, Ptak RA. The rationale for prolonged stretching for correction of shortening of connective tissue. *Arch Phys Med Rehabil.* 1966;47:345.

81. Lehmann JF. Effect of therapeutic temperatures on tendon extensibility. *Arch Phys Med Rehabil.* 1970;51:481.

82. Warren GC, Lehmann JF, Koblanski JN. Heat and stretch procedures: an evaluation using rat tail tendon. *Arch Phys Med Rehabil.* 1976;57:122.

83. Akai M, Oda H, Shirasaki Y, Tateishi T. Electrical stimulation of ligament healing: an experimental study of patellar ligament of rabbits. *Clin Orthop.* 1988;235:298.

84. Light KE, Nuzik S, Personius W, Barstrom A. Low-load prolonged stretch vs. high-load brief stretch in treating knee contractures. *Phys Ther.* 1984;64:330.

85. Wright V, Johns RJ. Physical factors concerned with the stiffness of normal and diseased joints. *Bull Johns Hopkins Hosp.* 1960;106:215.

86. Robertson V, Ward A, Low J, Reed A. *Electrotherapy Explained: Principles and Practice.* 4th ed. Edinburgh: Butterworth Heinemann Elsevier; 2006.

87. Whyte HM, Reader SR. Effectiveness of different forms of heating. *Ann Rheum Dis.* 1951;10:449.

88. Mainardi CL, Walter JM, Spiegel PK, et al. Rheumatoid arthritis: failure of daily heat therapy to affect its progression. *Arch Phys Med Rehabil.* 1979;60:390.

89. Wakim KG, Porter AN, Krusen KH. Influence of physical agents and of certain drugs on intra-articular temperature. *Arch Phys Med Rehabil.* 1951;32:714.

90. Cetin N, Aytar A, Atalay A, Akman MN. Comparing hot pack, short-wave diathermy, ultrasound, and TENS on isokinetic strength, pain, and functional status of women with osteoarthritic knees. *Am J Phys Med Rehabil.* 2008;87:443–451.

91. Head MD, Helms PA. Paraffin and sustained stretching in the treatment of burn contractures. *Burns.* 1977;4:136.

92. Fox J, Sharp T. *Practical Electrotherapy: A Guide to Safe Application.* Edinburgh: Churchill Livingstone Elsevier; 2007.

93. Belanger A-Y. *Therapeutic Electrophysical Agents: Evidence Behind Practice.* 2nd ed. Philadelphia: Lippincott Williams Wilkins; 2010.

94. Abramson DI, et al. Effect of paraffin bath and hot fomentation on local tissue temperature. *Arch Phys Med Rehabil.* 1965;45:87.

95. Stimson CW, Rose GB, Nelson PA. Paraffin bath as thermotherapy: an evaluation. *Arch Phys Med Rehabil.* 1958;39:219.

96. Dellhag B, Wollersjö I, Bjelle A. Effect of hand exercise and wax bath treatment in rheumatoid arthritis patients. *Arthritis Care Res.* 1992;5:87.

97. Sandqvist G, Akesson A, Eklund M. Evaluation of paraffin bath treatment in patients with systemic sclerosis. *Disabil Rehabil.* 2004;26(16):981–987.

98. Nadler SF, Steiner DJ, Erasala GN, et al. Continuous low-level heatwrap therapy for treating acute nonspecific low back pain. *Arch Phys Med Rehabil.* 2003;84(3):329–334.

99. Nadler SF, Steiner DJ, Erasala GN, et al. Continuous low-level heat wrap therapy provides more efficacy that ibuprofen and acetaminophen for acute low back pain. *Spine.* 2002;27(10): 1012–1017.

100. Nadler SF, Steiner DJ, Petty SR, et al. Overnight use of continuous low-level heat wrap therapy for relief of low back pain. *Arch Phys Med Rehabil.* 2003;84:335–342.

101. Michlovitz S, Hun L, Erasala GN, et al. Continuous low level heat wrap is effective for wrist pain. *Arch Phys Med Rehabil.* 2004;85(9):1409–1416.

102. Henley EJ. Fluidotherapy®. *Crit Rev Phys Rehabil Med.*1991;3:151.

103. Borrell RM, Henley EJ, Ho P, Hubbell MK. Fluidotherapy®: evaluation of a new heat agent. *Arch Phys Med Rehabil.* 1977;58:69.

104. Alcorn R, Bowser B, Henley EJ, Holloway V. Fluidotherapy® and exercise in the management of sickle cell anemia. *Phys Ther.* 1984;64:1520.

105. Eyring EJ, Murray WR. The effect of joint position on the pressure of intra-articular effusion. *J Bone Joint Surg.* 1964; 46-A(6):1235.

106. Cosgray NS, Lawrance SE, Mestrich JD, Martin SE, Whalen RL. Effect of heat modalities on hamstring length: a comparison of Pneumatherm, moist heat pack, and a control. *J Orthop Sports Phys Ther.* 2004;34:377–384.

107. Abramson DI, Tuck S, Lee SW, et al. Comparison of wet and dry heat in raising temperature of tissue. *Arch Phys Med Rehabil.* 1967;48:654.

108. Barillo DJ, Coffey EC, Shirani KZ, Goodwin CW. Burns caused by medical therapy. *J Burn Care Rehabil.* 2000;21(3):269–273.

chapter 4

Therapeutic Ultrasound

Susan L. Michlovitz, PT, PhD, CHT | Karen J. Sparrow, PT, PhD

Ultrasound (US) is a therapeutic modality commonly used for improving connective tissue extensibility, including managing scar tissue, promoting pain relief in musculoskeletal injuries, and enhancing tissue healing and remodeling in the care of tendinopathies. There is clear evidence from well-designed animal studies that ultrasound (US) has many positive effects on connective tissue characteristics, pain and tissue inflammation, and healing. The same concordance has not been reported in the clinical literature in effectiveness studies using human subjects, albeit there is moderate evidence for some techniques and clinical indications. This chapter will discuss the physical principles of ultrasound (e.g., acoustical energy, the transmission and absorption of ultrasound in soft tissues, common clinical uses of ultrasound, and safety issues in application). We need well-designed clinical trials using ultrasound to determine characteristics of those patients who could benefit from this treatment and to determine dosages that would positively affect alterations of body function, such as loss of ROM and pain.

Physical Principles

The Nature of Acoustic Energy

Ultrasound is a form of acoustic, or sound, energy. Sound waves are mechanical pressure waves. Unlike transmission of electromagnetic energy—such as that delivered by diathermy, in which individual particles such as photons or electrons may travel unhindered through a vacuum—transmission of acoustic energy requires a medium such as a coupling gel when treating human tissues.

KEY POINT! Because US energy requires a medium for transmission, the ultrasound applicator is "coupled" to the skin surface via a layer of water-soluble gel.

Sound waves travel by mechanically deforming or vibrating molecules. A vibrating molecule "bumps" into an adjacent molecule, transfers energy, and thus sets the adjacent molecule in motion. This chain reaction continues to propagate throughout a material until the energy is dissipated (i.e., absorbed by tissues). Molecules that are close together collide more quickly than widely dispersed molecules. This means that sound energy travels faster through denser connective tissues, such as tendon and bone. Nonetheless, energy is more quickly dissipated, overcoming the greater resistance to molecular vibration in denser materials.

The number of oscillations a molecule undergoes during 1 second defines the frequency of a sound wave and is measured in hertz (Hz): 1 Hz = 1 cycle/second; 1 MHz = 1 million cycles/second. Audible sound ranges between 16 and 20,000 Hz. Sound energy at frequencies greater than 20,000 Hz is defined as *ultrasound.*

Generally, low-frequency sound waves diverge in all directions as they leave the energy source, like light from an open flame. At higher frequencies, waves are more collimated, diverging less as they leave the energy

source, like light leaving a flashlight. The frequencies used for therapeutic ultrasound devices produce a well-collimated cylindrical beam.

KEY POINT! Due to the collimated beam of US, the energy can be delivered to a well-delineated and focused area. US is not appropriately used over large surface areas like the low back. It is an inefficient way of heating the paraspinal musculature because of the small area of the transducer and because of the only moderate capabilities of muscle to absorb US. (Note: Continuous shortwave diathermy is a much better choice to heat larger areas and will be discussed in Chapter 6.)

Production of Ultrasound Waves

Sound waves travel in a sinusoidal pattern as they travel through a medium. A positive pressure phase, where molecules adjacent to the energy source are compressed together, is followed by a negative pressure phase, where molecules in the same region disperse. As the wave propagates, additional molecules undergo compression and dispersion. Areas of compression or increased molecular density are referred to as *condensations,* and the areas of decreased molecular density are referred to as *rarefactions* (Fig. 4-1).

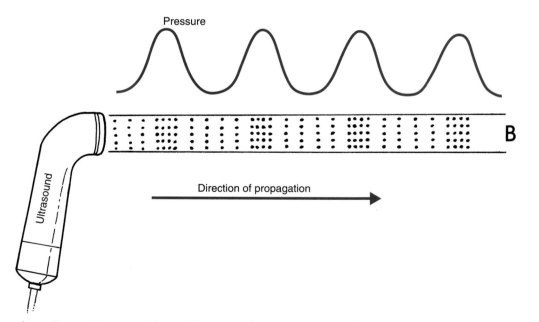

Fig 4•1 Diagram of a collimated ultrasound beam (B) coming from an ultrasound (US) applicator. The associated pressure wave is diagrammed; areas of increased molecular concentration (:::) are condensations. Areas of decreased molecular concentrations are rarefactions (::).

In ultrasound, the pressure waves are generated by oscillations of a piezoelectric crystal induced by passing voltage from a high-frequency alternating current across its face. Piezoelectricity is a property of many naturally occurring and synthetic crystals and refers to the phenomenon in which the crystal generates an electric voltage when mechanically compressed. If the crystal is expanded rather than compressed, a voltage of the opposite polarity is produced. Similarly, applying voltage to the crystal can induce it to compress or expand. Changes in polarity of the applied voltage result in expansion of a compressed crystal, and vice versa. This is known as the *reverse piezoelectric effect* (Fig. 4-2).

Repeated cycles of compression and expansion of the crystal produce the ultrasound pressure wave, with the frequency of the wave determined by the frequency of the imposed alternating electrical current across the crystal. *Wavelength* is defined as the distance between two successive peaks in the pressure wave. Wavelength is inversely related to frequency and is represented by the equation

$$\text{Velocity} = \text{Frequency} \times \text{Wavelength}$$

Characteristics of the Ultrasound Wave

Frequency: 1 or 3 MHz

Ultrasound is characterized by its frequency, mode, and intensity. Most modern therapeutic ultrasound machines in clinical use are dual-frequency units, allowing the operator to select a frequency of either 1 MHz or 3 (or 3.3) MHz. At higher frequencies, more frequent molecular oscillations occur, and increased work is required for sound waves to overcome molecular friction. Theoretically, this means that more energy is absorbed in superficial tissues and less is available for transmission to deeper tissues. Generally, 3 MHz is selected when the target tissue is within 1 to 2 cm from the body surface, and 1 MHz is used when the target tissue is greater than 2 cm beneath the skin.

Mode: Continuous Wave or Pulsed

Ultrasound waves may be delivered in two modes: in an uninterrupted stream or in periodic intervals in which energy is flowing for a brief duration (in milliseconds, or msec) and then no energy is flowing (in msec).

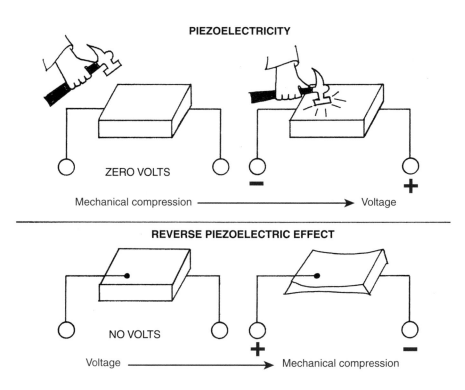

PIEZOELECTRICITY

ZERO VOLTS

Mechanical compression ⟶ Voltage

REVERSE PIEZOELECTRIC EFFECT

NO VOLTS

Voltage ⟶ Mechanical compression

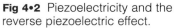

Fig 4•2 Piezoelectricity and the reverse piezoelectric effect.

When the flow of ultrasound is delivered as an uninterrupted stream, it is referred to as *continuous wave mode,* and when delivered with periodic interruptions, it is referred to as *pulsed mode* (Fig. 4-3). Pulsed-mode ultrasound is further characterized by its duty cycle, which is the fraction of time during a single pulse period that the ultrasound beam is present, usually expressed as a percentage. It is calculated using the following equation:

Duty cycle = duration of pulse (time on)/pulse period
(time on + time off)

KEY POINT! Continuous-wave US is often associated with its use for heating effects. Pulsed US at 20% is used for nonthermal effects, and pulsed US at 50% will most likely produce very mild heating effects. But with 50% duty cycle, the peak of the US energy can have a positive mechanical effect on movement of ions across cell membranes.

Most therapeutic ultrasound machines allow the user to select from a range of duty cycles between 5%

and 50%, but most studies on effects of US on tissues have used duty cycles of 20% or 50%.

Intensity: Watts/cm²

The strength of the ultrasound wave is determined by the quantity of energy, or acoustic power, produced by an ultrasound transducer and is measured in watts (W). Power emitted is not uniform across the surface of the ultrasound transducer. The outer edge of the piezoelectric crystal is cemented to the undersurface of a metal end plate; consequently, less vibration occurs along the periphery relative to the central portion of the crystal. In addition, waves emitted from different points across the surface of the crystal interfere with one another. This means that some regions of the ultrasound beam will be more intense than others as it exits the transducer (Fig. 4-4).

The effective radiating area (ERA) of a transducer is a measure of the actual cross-sectional area of the ultrasound beam as it exits the metal end plate and is expressed in square centimeters (cm²). It is determined by the size and vibrational properties of the

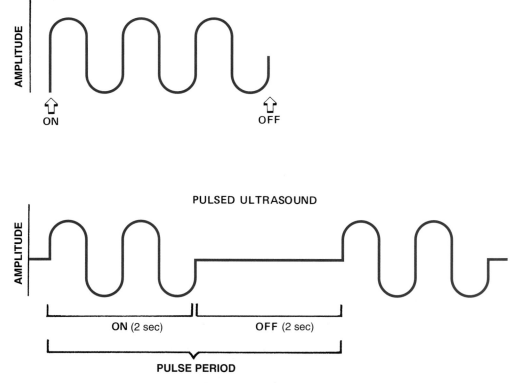

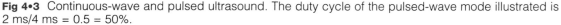

Fig 4•3 Continuous-wave and pulsed ultrasound. The duty cycle of the pulsed-wave mode illustrated is 2 ms/4 ms = 0.5 = 50%.

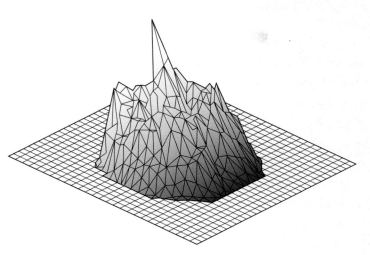

Fig 4•4 Hydrophone graphic of an ultrasound beam.

piezoelectric crystal and is always smaller than the cross-sectional area of the metal end plate. Figure 4-5 shows two transducers of different cross-sectional areas. Accordingly, the ERA of each differs and is smaller than the cross-sectional area.

The term *spatial peak intensity* (I_{SP}) refers to the acoustic power of the ultrasound beam at its highest point (Fig. 4-6). This peak typically occurs somewhere within the central third of the ERA. Spatial average intensity (I_{SA}), however, is a measure of the average acoustic power across the ERA and is expressed in watts per square centimeter (W/cm²). This measure is commonly referred to clinically as *intensity* and is labeled as such on output meters of ultrasound units. The beam-non-uniformity ratio (BNR) of a transducer is the ratio between its spatial peak intensity and its spatial average intensity. Smaller ratios correspond to a more uniform ultrasound beam. The BNR is

determined by the quality of the crystal and the construction of the transducer. Ultrasound units with lower BNRs are typically more expensive to manufacture and to purchase. Generally, ratios that are less than or equal to 6:1 are considered acceptable for clinical use. In the United States, the Food and Drug Administration (FDA) requires that the manufacturer indicate the BNR on the ultrasound unit. This is often labeled on the coaxial cable of the US applicator.[1]

In pulsed-mode ultrasound, intensity must be further qualified because the duty cycle impacts the total quantity of energy generated. The term *spatial average temporal peak intensity* (I_{SATP}) refers to the spatial average intensity of the ultrasound beam between

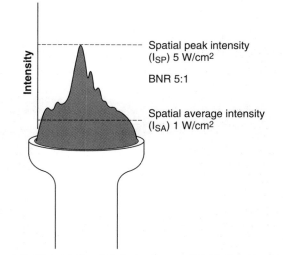

Fig 4•6 The relationship between spatial peak intensity (I_{SP}), beam nonuniformity ratio (BNR), and spatial average intensity (I_{SA}). When the BNR is 5:1, the spatial peak intensity for the ultrasound beam is five times its spatial average intensity.

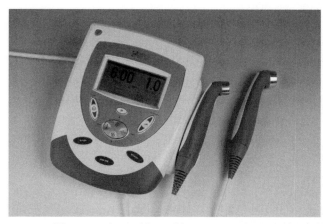

Fig 4•5 Ultrasound machine with two transducers of different cross-sectional areas.

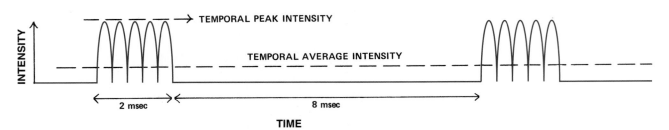

Fig 4•7 A typical pulsing pattern. The total pulse period is 10 msec. The pulse duration on time is 2 msec; pulse off time is 8 msec. The duty cycle is 0.20 (20%).

interruptions during pulsed ultrasound (Fig. 4-7). In and of itself, this measure has limited usefulness, because it does not quantify the degree to which the energy output is decreased when factoring in the duty cycle. Conversely, spatial average temporal average intensity (I_{SATA}) does account for the impact of the duty cycle. It is calculated by multiplying I_{SATP} by the duty cycle:

$$I_{SATA} = I_{SATP} \times \text{duty cycle}$$

For example, pulsed ultrasound delivered at 2.0 W/cm² using a 20% duty cycle is documented as I_{SATA} = 0.4 W/cm². In physical therapy practice, particularly in the United States, use of the term I_{SATA} is infrequent. Instead, intensity is typically described by its spatial average and the duty cycle is noted. The advantage of using I_{SATA} is that it allows for easy comparison of energy outputs between continuous and pulsed-mode treatments. For example, assuming that the duration of treatment is the same, continuous ultrasound at I_{SA} = 0.5 W/cm² generates the same net energy output as pulsed ultrasound at 1.0 W/cm² using a 50% duty cycle (I_{SATA} = 0.5 W/cm²). But, perhaps some of the effects of pulsed ultrasound are related to the peak intensity of the pulse.

Ultrasound Interaction With Biological Tissues

Propagation of Ultrasound Waves in Tissue

In gases and liquids, molecular vibration occurs only in longitudinal waves, parallel to the direction of energy flow. In solids, however, molecular vibration also occurs in transverse waves, perpendicular to the direction of energy flow. This is due to the strong three-dimensional intermolecular bonds present in solid media. With the exception of compact bone, biological tissues behave acoustically as liquids. In bone, ultrasound travels in longitudinal and transverse waves, but in other biological tissues, ultrasound travels exclusively in longitudinal waves.

Like electromagnetic energy, acoustic energy can be transmitted, absorbed, reflected, and refracted. What happens to the energy is determined by the specific properties of the materials in its path and the angle from which the energy strikes them. These concepts dictate how ultrasound interacts with biological tissue. *Acoustic impedance* refers to a material's ability to transmit sound and is related to the molecular density and structure of the material. If acoustic impedance is low, transmission is high and the material absorbs little sound. If acoustic impedance is high, the material absorbs more of the energy and less is available for transmission. For example, blood and other body fluids have low impedance, and bone has the highest impedance of all biological tissues.

When acoustic energy travels through a homogeneous medium, it does so in a straight line. Reflection and refraction occur when energy is transmitted between materials with different impedances. The magnitude of the difference between materials at the boundary determines how much reflection and refraction occur (Fig. 4-8). For example, as ultrasound travels from subcutaneous tissue to muscle, some of the energy is reflected back into subcutaneous tissue. When ultrasound travels from muscle to bone, however, a greater percentage of energy is reflected because of the more drastic change in impedance at the interface between the muscle and bone. When a wave strikes a boundary that is directly perpendicular to its path, the angle of reflection is directly back toward its source. When a wave strikes a boundary at an angle, however,

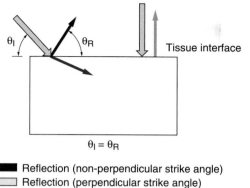

■ Reflection (non-perpendicular strike angle)
☐ Reflection (perpendicular strike angle)
■ Refraction

Fig 4•8 Reflection and refraction. θ_I = incident angle; θ_R = reflected angle.

the angle of reflection is equal to and opposite the strike angle. When a reflected wave travels back through its original path, it is possible that it will interact with sound waves traveling away from the energy source in the exact opposite direction. If both waves are in phase with each other, the energies from both are added together, creating an area of more intense energy in the tissue. This is known as a *standing wave* (Fig. 4-9). The potential for creating standing waves is minimized when the ultrasound transducer is moved during treatment, not held stationary. Waves are also bent as they pass from one medium to another in proportion to the difference in acoustic impedance. This is known as *refraction* and it is minimized when waves strike directly perpendicular to a boundary between tissues of varying collagen densities.

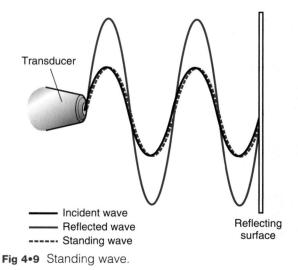

Fig 4•9 Standing wave.

—— Incident wave
—— Reflected wave
----- Standing wave

Reflecting surface

Factors Influencing Energy Absorption

As ultrasound waves travel through a tissue, all or part of the energy may be absorbed, changing into the kinetic energy of molecular vibration. Energy not reflected, refracted, or absorbed is transmitted through the tissue until it encounters a change in tissue density. At the boundary and in the next tissue layer, energy may be reflected, refracted, absorbed, or transmitted again. Each time some of the energy is absorbed, reflected, or refracted, less energy is available to transmit through subsequent interfaces and into deeper tissues. *Attenuation* is a measure of the decrease in sound energy as the sound wave travels, either by absorption, reflection, or refraction. Table 4-1 lists the attenuation of a 1 MHz ultrasound beam in several biological tissues. Generally, denser tissues with high protein content, especially collagen, are the most effective absorbers of ultrasound energy.

In therapeutic ultrasound, the amount of energy absorbed by the target tissue is dependent on several factors. As discussed previously, ultrasound frequency is one factor that determines depth of penetration. The generalization that 3 MHz should be used for treating superficial tissues and 1 MHz should be used for deeper tissues is perhaps an oversimplified guideline. Several studies, which will be discussed in subsequent sections, have demonstrated therapeutic effects in superficial tissues using 1 MHz. In addition, a thermal imaging study of fresh pig cadaver tissue demonstrated no difference in the tissue depth of thermal changes during ultrasound at different frequencies.[2] Temperature increases in tissue result not only from molecular friction in the region of maximal ultrasound absorption,

Table 4•1	Attenuation of a 1 MHz Ultrasound Beam	
Tissue	**Attenuation (%/cm)**
Blood	3
Fat	13
Muscle	24
Blood vessel	32
Skin	39
Tendon	59
Cartilage	68
Bone	96

but also from conductive heating of adjacent tissues distant from the frequency predicted region of maximal absorption. Also, because not all effects of ultrasound are thermal in nature, energy traveling through tissue, even with little absorption, may cause therapeutic changes.

Intensity of the ultrasound wave is another factor that influences depth of penetration. Since energy is attenuated as the sound wave travels toward the target tissue, either at interfaces or in more superficial tissues, it is logical that the net energy arriving at the target tissue will be greater if the initial intensity of the wave is higher. Logically, the number and nature of interfaces through which the ultrasound beam must pass, as well as the tissue composition of the intervening layers, affects the net amount of energy that reaches the target tissue. Finally, the proportion of arriving energy actually absorbed by the target tissue will depend on its particular tissue composition.

Of course, all of the preceding factors affecting energy absorption at the target tissue assume that the ultrasound wave passes into the patient's body in the first place. Ultrasound cannot effectively travel through air. At an interface between the metal faceplate of an ultrasound transducer and air, essentially all of the energy is reflected back toward the transducer. A medium that effectively transmits ultrasound and is without pockets or bubbles of air is necessary (see the "Application Techniques" section). The ultrasound beam must also be directed exactly over the target tissue and perpendicular to the surface of the skin. If the angle of the ultrasound beam is greater than 15° relative to perpendicular, the beam is refracted and runs parallel to the skin rather than into it (Fig. 4-10).

Effects of Ultrasound as a Basis for Therapeutic Use

Thermal and Mechanical Effects

When tissues absorb ultrasound and kinetic energy increases, friction between the molecules results in heat production. Depending on the intensity and length of time ultrasound is applied and the physical properties of the tissue, an increase in tissue temperature may occur. As described in Chapter 3, increasing tissue temperature is associated with potentially desirable physiological changes, such as decreased muscle guarding, decreased pain perception, increased tissue extensibility, and increased blood flow. Because ultrasound is categorized as a "deep heating modality," these same physiological changes are usually considered to be effects, albeit indirect ones, of ultrasound treatment as well. However, it is critical to realize that in order for ultrasound to produce these effects, specific tissue temperature increases must occur. Lehman[3] and Lehman and colleagues[4,5] reported that a tissue temperature elevation of 1°C (1.8°F) increases metabolic rate. Elevations in the range of 2°C (3.6°F) to 3°C (5.4°F) reduce muscle spasm and pain and increase blood flow, and temperature increases of 4°C (7.2°F) or greater are necessary to boost collagen extensibility and inhibit sympathetic activity.

However, apart from production of frictional heat, therapeutic ultrasound is also hypothesized to cause other mechanical effects in tissue. Ions present within and around cells, as well as intracellular and extracellular fluids in tissue exposed to ultrasound energy, are subjected to small-magnitude movements. This flux is referred to as *microstreaming* and has been implicated in altering cell membrane permeability and cellular

Fig 4•10 Schematic diagram showing reflection and refraction of ultrasound at a muscle-bone interface. (A) A wave arriving perpendicular to the boundary. (B) A wave arriving at an angle of 35° from the perpendicular. *(Adapted with permission from Behrens/Michlovitz. Physical Agents. 2nd ed. Philadelphia: FA Davis; 2006: 62.)*

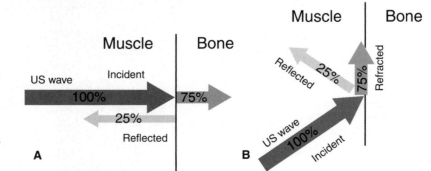

activity found with ultrasound application at therapeutic intensities.[6,7] Small gas bubbles that may be present in body fluids exposed to ultrasound are subject to compression during condensations and to expansion during rarefactions. This pulsation of gas bubbles is called *cavitation* and may contribute to diffusional changes across the cell membrane and thus to altered cellular function.[8] At high ultrasound intensities, a violent collapse or implosion of gas bubbles resulting in tissue destruction may occur. This is referred to as *unstable cavitation* and is very unlikely during ultrasound at therapeutic intensities.[9]

KEY POINT! The nonthermal effects of ultrasound are produced by both continuous and pulsed modes, but generally speaking, pulsed US is used for these mechanical effects, including stable cavitation and acoustic streaming.

Muscular Effects

Draper and colleagues[10] described the heating effects of therapeutic ultrasound at various intensities on uninjured triceps surae muscle in 24 college students. Results are summarized in Table 4-2. Muscle temperature was measured at depths of 0.8 and 1.6 cm beneath the skin during 3 MHz ultrasound and at 2.5 and 5 cm beneath the skin during 1 MHz ultrasound. Temperatures did not differ between the two muscle

Table 4•2	**Mean Muscle Temperature Increase (°C) During Ultrasound Treatment of Human Triceps Surae at Either 1 or 3 MHz**[10]			
	Intensity (W/cm²)		Time (min)		
		2.5	5.0	7.5	10
1 MHz	0.5	*	*	*	0.5
	1.0	*	1.0	1.25	1.75
	1.5	1.0	1.75	2.5	3.5
	2.0	1.25	2.25	3.25	4.0
3 MHz	0.5	0.75	1.5	2.0	3.0
	1.0	2.5	3.5	5.0	5.75
	1.5	2.75	5.0	**	**
	2.0	4.0	**	**	**

*Temperature increase < 0.5°
**Treatment terminated due to subject discomfort
Adapted from Draper et al.[10]

depths measured during treatment at either frequency. The treatment area was twice the effective radiating area (ERA) of the sound head. The rate and magnitude of muscle heating depended not only on treatment intensity and duration, but also on frequency. On average, superficial muscle temperature increased 4°C (7.2°F) over baseline within 2.5 minutes when treated at 2.0 W/cm² delivered at 3 MHz, but the same temperature increase in deeper muscle tissue required 10 minutes to achieve when delivered at 2.0 W/cm² at 1 MHz. When ultrasound was delivered at 0.5 W/cm² and 1 MHz, the temperature increase never reached 1°C (1.8°F), even after 10 minutes of treatment. However, at 3 MHz, the same treatment intensity resulted in an increase of 3°C (5.4°F) over a 10-minute treatment.

KEY POINT! The implication is that much longer treatment times with higher intensities are required to achieve vigorous muscle heating when the target tissue is deep and 1 MHz is used than when more superficially located muscle tissue is treated using 3 MHz.

To date, it appears that no published studies have examined the duration of temperature elevation in human muscle following ultrasound treatment.

Connective Tissue (Tendon/Ligament) Effects

US is used to increase tissue extensibility and alter scar. Relative to muscle, it appears that larger temperature increases may be achieved at faster rates when a dense connective tissue such as tendon is treated with ultrasound. Thus, US would be an appropriate choice for this goal. One reason that tendon heats faster and more intensely than muscle during ultrasound is because of its higher collagen content,[11] but another likely reason is its relative avascularity. In well-vascularized tissues such as muscle, a homeostatic cooling mechanism of vasodilation and increased local blood flow is initiated in response to increasing tissue temperature. This response is diminished when fewer blood vessels are present, such as in tendon and ligament.

Chan and colleagues[12] described the heating effects of 3 MHz ultrasound applied at 1.0 W/cm² for 4 minutes over uninjured patellar tendons in 16 college students. When the treatment area was two times the effective radiating area of the sound head (2 × ERA), the average temperature increase within the tendon was 8°C (14.4°F) immediately following treatment, and temperature did not return to baseline until 20 minutes post-treatment. When the treatment area was 4 × ERA, the temperature increase immediately following treatment was approximately 5°C (9°F), and temperature returned to baseline within 15 minutes. Since temperature increases of 4°C (7.2°F) (or greater are thought to be necessary to improve connective tissue extensibility, it stands to reason that therapeutic stretching should take place in a treatment session within the "window of opportunity." In this study, at 2 × ERA, temperature increases greater than 4°C (7.2°F) were reached halfway through the 4-minute treatment and were maintained for 4 additional minutes following cessation of treatment. While treatment using 4 × ERA was also able to produce a temperature increase greater than 4°C (7.2°F), it took more than 3 minutes to achieve and was only maintained for 2 minutes after treatment, meaning that the therapeutic window for stretching was decreased 50%.

KEY POINT! If the intent of ultrasound treatment is to maximize the effect of therapeutic stretching, these results suggest that stretching should immediately follow ultrasound treatment or begin concurrently with it and continue for at least 4 minutes afterward.

Effects on Joint Pain

Ultrasound has been commonly used to reduce joint stiffness and pain in patients with arthritis. Studies for pain control are discussed in Chapter 13, but one new study is worthy of mention.[12a] Continuous ultrasound applied at 1 MHz frequency, 1.0 W/cm² power for 5 minutes was capable of reducing pain in the knees of patients with osteoarthritis. In this randomized, controlled study, ultrasound was compared to sham ultrasound and found to have superior effects.

Hemodynamic Effects

The theoretical construct that explains ultrasound's potential ability to increase blood flow is straight forward. As ultrasound energy is absorbed by tissue, temperature elevation occurs. In response to an increase in temperature in healthy tissue, local blood flow to the area increases to dissipate heat and restore temperature homeostasis. The actual evidence in the literature regarding blood flow and ultrasound is not as simple. Early studies examining the effects of ultrasound on blood flow employed widely varying and often incompletely described treatment parameters, models, and measurement methodologies. Not surprisingly, findings were confusing, with some groups reporting changes and others not. More recently, Robinson and Buono[13] studied the effects of 1 MHz continuous-wave ultrasound at 1.5 W/cm² for 5 minutes on cutaneous and muscular blood flow in the forearm in 20 healthy adults. They reported no significant differences between treated arms and control arms immediately following treatment. The treatment area was 16 to 25 times the ERA. In contrast, increased blood flow was demonstrated in the popliteal artery during and after 1 MHz continuous-wave ultrasound over the triceps surae at either 1.0 or 1.5 W/cm² in 20 healthy adults.[14] The treatment area was two times the ERA. Changes were statistically similar, and no further blood flow increases occurred with treatment times greater than 5 minutes. Ultrasound at 3 MHz was not effective at increasing blood flow. The primary difference between the treatments in the Robinson and Buono study and the study by Fabrizio et al.[14] at 1 MHz was the size of the treatment area. Based on Draper's work,[10] it can be hypothesized that Fabrizio and colleagues obtained a muscle temperature increase of approximately 1.75°C (31.8°F) during the 5-minute treatment at 1.5 W/cm² and approximately 1°C (1.8°F) during the 5-minute treatment at 1.0 W/cm². Given the extremely large treatment area used by Robinson and Buono,[13] it is unlikely that any change in muscle temperature occurred. Unfortunately, no single study has directly correlated temperature increase and blood flow response during ultrasound.

Nonthermal effects produced by US may also be involved in hemodynamic responses during treatment. Lota[15] found increased superficial blood flow in the foot during application of ultrasound over the lumbar paraspinal region in humans. He hypothesized that the increase was due to reflexive vasodilation secondary to a stimulative effect on lumbar sympathetic ganglia. Fabrizio et al.[14] hypothesized that changes in cell membrane permeability during ultrasound may stimulate local histamine release and changes in vascular tone.

CASE STUDY 4•1 ULTRASOUND TO REDUCE PAIN FROM CALCIFIC TENDINITIS

Mr. Swaggle, a 57-year-old male carpenter, has right shoulder pain that rates 8/10 with elevation and a 4/10 at rest. His pain interrupts his sleep. He has been diagnosed with calcific tendinitis of the supraspinatus.

CLINICAL DECISION-MAKING

1. Does the patient have a problem that can be improved with the use of ultrasound?
   Answer: Yes, ultrasound can be used to reduce pain and accelerate resorption of calcium deposits.

2. Is the patient appropriate for application of ultrasound (i.e., do any of the general precautions or contraindications to ultrasound apply), or are there any specific considerations regarding application of ultrasound to this patient?
   Answer: No

3. What are the specific goals to be achieved with the use of ultrasound?

Answer: Reduce pain during shoulder elevation to 3/10 in 2 to 3 weeks and 1/10 at rest.

4. What specific parameters of ultrasound would be appropriate for the patient?
   Answer: pulsed 20 to 50% duty cycle, 1.0 MHz, 1.5 W/cm^2 for a total of 10 minutes to the supraspinatus tendon and immediately surrounding tissues. Use a moving applicator with direct coupling.

5. What are the proper (i.e., effective and safe) application procedures related to this case example?
   Answer: Prescreen sensation and circulation. Monitor patient response. He should feel either a mild sensation or no warmth in the shoulder. The arm should be positioned in extension and internal rotation to expose the tendon from under the acromion process of the scapula.

CASE STUDY 4•2 ULTRASOUND TO REDUCE PAIN AND INCREASE TISSUE EXTENSIBILITY

Mrs. Smith, a 75-year-old female with osteoarthritis and diabetes, has right knee pain that rates 5 out of 10 upon walking a block. Her pain has worsened over the past 2 weeks.

CLINICAL DECISION-MAKING

1. Does the patient have a problem that can be improved with the use of ultrasound?
   Answer: Yes, ultrasound can be used to reduce pain and joint stiffness.

2. Is the patient appropriate for application of ultrasound (i.e., do any of the general precautions or contraindications to ultrasound apply), or are there any specific considerations regarding application of ultrasound to this patient?
   Answer: In a woman this age with diabetes, we would be concerned about her peripheral circulation and peripheral sensation. You screen for distal pulses and for sensation to the foot and leg. Both

appear to be intact. The foot is not cold or cool to the touch and there are no sores on her feet.

3. What are the specific goals to be achieved with the use of ultrasound?
   Answer: Reduce pain during walking to a 2 out of 10 within 2 to 3 weeks.

4. What specific parameters of ultrasound would be appropriate for the patient?
   Answer: CW, 1.0 MHz, 1.0 to 1.5 W/cm^2 for a total of 10 to 15 minutes around the medial and lateral knee. Use a moving applicator with direct coupling.

5. What are the proper (i.e., effective and safe) application procedures related to this case example?
   Answer: Prescreen sensation and circulation. Monitor patient response. She should feel either a mild sensation or warmth in the knee.

When the treatment objective is to increase blood flow—whether to increase supply of nutrients to an area, to facilitate tissue repair, or to wash away the nociceptive sensitizing by-products of the inflammatory process—ultrasound parameters should be selected carefully. Based on the evidence, the treatment area should be limited to 2 × ERA and the frequency should be 1 MHz. Intensity and time parameters should likely be chosen to ensure muscle heating of at least 1°C (1.8°F).

Even though maximal blood flow elevation may occur within 5 minutes, longer treatment times may be indicated to maintain blood flow elevation. Blood flow appears to return to baseline levels within 1 minute after treatment ends.[14]

Effects of US on Nerve

Motor nerve conduction velocities (MNCV) have been demonstrated to increase, decrease, or remain unchanged when exposed to ultrasound, depending upon the treatment parameters and the particular investigation. Zankel[16] found that ultrasound over the volar forearm at 1 MHz and 1.0 W/cm^2 for 5 minutes was not sufficient to alter ulnar MNCV, but when intensity was increased to 2.0 W/cm^2 or treatment time was increased to 10 minutes, MNCV decreased. In contrast, Farmer[17] found that ultrasound delivered at 1.0 to 2.0 W/cm^2 over the ulnar nerve decreased MNCV, but at higher intensity, MNCV increased.

Sensory nerve conduction velocities (SNCV) appear to increase with thermal doses of ultrasound. Currier et al.[18] reported increased conduction in the lateral cutaneous branch of the radial nerve following ultrasound at 1 MHz, 1.5 W/cm^2 for 5 minutes. In a similar study, Halle and colleagues[19] also found increased superficial radial SNCV with ultrasound treatment at 1 MHz, 1.0 W/cm^2 between 5 and 20 minutes. In both studies, increases in subcutaneous tissue temperature were noted. It is unclear whether the changes in nerve conduction velocity seen with ultrasound are solely due to increased tissue temperature or whether additional mechanisms are at play.

KEY POINT! ▶ The relationship between nerve conduction velocity changes and pain perception is unknown.

Lehmann et al.[20] found an elevated pain threshold following 0.8 MHz ultrasound at 1.5 W/cm^2. It is important to realize that pain perception may be altered not only by direct effects of ultrasound on neurological tissue, but also by associated vascular and thermal changes in the treated region.

Posttraumatic Effects: Inflammation and Tissue Repair

The rationale for using ultrasound during recovery from injury is outlined in Table 4-3.

In Vitro Research

Several in vitro studies have demonstrated that ultrasound has a stimulative effect on cells active during acute inflammation and tissue repair. Harvey and colleagues[21] found that 3 MHz ultrasound treatment at intensities of 0.5 to 2.0 W/cm^2 was associated with increased protein synthesis by cultured human fibroblasts. In a study of cultured fibroblasts from neonatal rats in a simulated injury model, Ramirez and colleagues[22] concluded that 1 MHz ultrasound at 0.4 W/cm^2 stimulated collagen synthesis and cellular proliferation. Macrophages, the dominant cell type present in wounds by about the fourth or fifth day following injury, secrete factors that stimulate fibroblast proliferation.[23] Young and Dyson[24] discovered that cultured macrophages treated with ultrasound at frequencies of either 0.75 or 3 MHz at 0.5 W/cm^2 had a mitogenic effect on fibroblast proliferation. In a study by Mortimer and Dyson,[25] calcium uptake, typically reflective of cellular activity, increased in cultured fibroblasts after a 5-minute exposure to ultrasound using a 20% duty cycle, 1 MHz, at intensities of 0.5 to 1.0 W/cm^2.

Wound Healing

Young and Dyson[26] examined the effects of 0.1 W/cm^2 intensity ultrasound applied for either 5 or 7 consecutive days at 0.75 or 3 MHz to surgically induced skin wounds in a rat model. At 5 days post-injury, rats treated with ultrasound had more new blood vessel formation, as measured by microfocal x-ray techniques, in the region of the granulated tissue than did sham-treated controls. However, by day 7, there was no longer a significant difference. In another animal study, done by Byl and colleagues,[27] Yucatan pigs' wounds were sonicated using a 20% duty cycle, 1 MHz frequency at an intensity of 0.5 W/cm^2 for 3 days and then at 1.5 W/cm^2 for 2 days. After 7 days total healing time, sonicated wounds demonstrated significant differences when compared to sham-treated controls. The treated wounds were smaller, and they had increased breaking strength, collagen deposition, and mast cell degranulation. In a follow-up study, the same group found that the lower dose (0.5 W/cm^2) was more effective than the higher dose (1.5 W/cm^2) at enhancing collagen deposition and breaking strength when applied daily for either 5 or 10 total treatments.[28]

The majority of human trials studying the effects of ultrasound on wound healing have been limited to patients with chronic venous or pressure ulcers. A systematic review of randomized controlled trials of therapeutic ultrasound for treatment of pressure sores through 1999 found no apparent benefit.[29] A 1998 meta-analysis of ultrasound therapy for chronic leg ulceration found a modest effect on healing rate after 4 or 8 weeks of treatment in comparison to control, but there was no significant difference in number of healed ulcers.[30] Casual observation might suggest that the data from human trials conflicts with the generally positive evidence from animal research on ultrasound and wound healing. However, it is important to realize that the surgically induced skin wounds treated in the animal studies are not the same as chronic skin ulcerations. The former represents traumatic injury of previously normal tissue, where the predictable cascade of acute inflammation followed by tissue repair is expected. Chronic venous stasis and pressure ulcerations represent the end stage of progressive tissue breakdown resulting from prolonged local ischemia. Since the inflammatory response is largely vascularly mediated, healing is impaired. In a human study where the nature of the wounds more closely approximated those used in the animal model studies, ultrasound treatment was found to be effective. The scientific logic behind the use of US for healing indolent wounds has been demonstrated best in controlled situations with laboratory animals. It is not apparent that this success has been consistent in humans with open wounds and delayed healing such as pressure ulcers.[31]

Muscle Healing and Contusions

The effects of low-intensity therapeutic ultrasound treatment on healing of acute muscle injury have been studied in animal models. This has also been used for recovery in humans following injury (Table 4-3). Rantanen and colleagues[32] examined the effects of pulsed ultrasound on myoregeneration following contusion with transverse rupture of the rat gastrocnemius. Beginning 3 days after injury, limbs in the treatment group received ultrasound at 3 MHz, 20% duty cycle, 1.5 W/cm^2 (I_{SATA} = 0.3 W/cm^2) for 6 minutes, for 2 consecutive days followed by 1 day off. At 10 days post-injury, a significant increase in the proliferation of

Table 4•3	Rationale for Use of Ultrasound During Healing From Injury

Inflammatory Phase	• US can stimulate release of growth factors
	  – In vitro and animal model work (Level 5 evidence)
	• Angiogenesis promoted by pulsed US
	  – Animal model work (Level 5 evidence)
	• Reduce inflammation by transcutaneous transmission of drug?
	  – Phonophoresis (weak to no evidence)

Proliferative Phase	• Angiogenesis promoted by pulsed US
	  – Animal model work (Level 5 evidence)
	• Fibroplasia promoted by pulsed US
	  – Animal model work (Level 5 evidence)

Remodeling Phase
Improve connective tissue extensibility
	• Use US in CW mode to elevate tissue temperature
	• Effects on scar
	  – Common use
	  – Need evidence

the myogenic precursor satellite cells and fibroblasts was demonstrated in muscles treated with ultrasound in comparison to controls, but no difference was seen in actual myotube production. The authors concluded that there was no overall morphological benefit of ultrasound treatment.

Later work by Markert et al.[33] examined a low dose of continuous wave (CW) US at 0.1 W/cm^2 for 5 minutes per day in a rat gastrocnemius contusion model. Exercise was also included, with both being delivered separately or together in various iterations. Using their experimental protocol, the investigators could not find any muscle fiber regeneration attributed to either US or exercise or both in combination. It is unclear if ultrasound would be an effective treatment to enhance recovery after muscle contusion. Certainly a well-controlled clinical trial could be warranted. Pre- and posttesting could be done using imaging ultrasound.

Peripheral Nerve Healing

Preliminary evidence suggests that low-intensity ultrasound may help facilitate healing of peripheral nerve injuries. In the rat model, Crisci and Ferreira[34] found an increased quantity of regenerating nerve fibers, increased myelinization, increased diameter of nerve fibers, and increased Schwann cell activity following transection of the sciatic nerve and treatment with pulsed ultrasound, in comparison to sham-treated controls. The treatment parameters were 1.5 MHz,

I_{SATA}=16 mW/cm^2, 20 minutes daily for 12 days. Mourad and colleagues[35] examined the effect of pulsed ultrasound treatment in rats following crush injury to the sciatic nerve. Ultrasound was delivered at 2.25 MHz, I_{SATA} = 0.25 W/cm^2, for 1 minute, three times weekly for 30 days. In comparison to controls, treated rats showed a statistically significant acceleration of foot function recovery.

Tendon and Ligament Healing

Several studies have examined the effects of ultrasound on tendon injuries in animal models. When CW ultrasound at 1.5 W/cm^2 (frequency not reported) was administered for 3 minutes every other day following surgically induced partial ruptures of Achilles tendons in rats, tensile strength was noted to be significantly greater than controls for tendons treated for 3 weeks but not those treated for 2 weeks.[36] Treated tendons displayed more densely aggregated collagen fibrils with more parallel orientation. Another study using the same injury model and ultrasound intensity found significantly greater breaking strength in treated rat tendons following partial rupture, compared to controls at 5, 9, 15, and 21 days post-injury.[37]

In contrast to these two studies, Turner and colleagues[38] found no change in the mechanical strength of transected and repaired chicken tendons treated with ultrasound beginning 1 week after surgery and continuing for 5 weeks, relative to sham-treated sutured tendons. The parameters used in this study were 3 MHz, 25% duty cycle, 1.0 W/cm^2 for 4 minutes, three times weekly. When comparing this study to the other two, it's worth noting the lack of treatment during the first postoperative week.

Enwemeka[39,40] led two investigations that examined the effects of continuous underwater 1 MHz ultrasound, 5 minutes daily, for the first 10 days post-injury on the healing of ruptured rabbit Achilles tendons. The first study used an intensity of 1.0 W/cm^2 and the second used 0.5 W/cm^2. Both studies demonstrated better resistance to tensile loading and higher energy absorption in tendons treated with ultrasound relative to sham-treated controls, but a treatment intensity of 0.5 W/cm^2 was more effective than 1.0 W/cm^2. More recently, Saini et al.[41] confirmed the positive results observed with 10 days of 1 MHz ultrasound at 0.5 W/cm^2 following Achilles tendon rupture in dogs.

They found that dogs treated with ultrasound resumed normal gait earlier, and the treated tendons showed histological evidence of more advanced healing relative to controls, even as long as 40 days after injury.

Only one published study to date has examined the effects of ultrasound on ligament healing in an animal model. Takakura and colleagues[42] found superior biomechanical properties in healing rat medial collateral ligament transections 12 days post-injury, following daily treatments with 1.5 MHz pulsed ultrasound, I_{SATA} = 30 mW/cm^2, for 20 minutes. In spite of the largely positive results seen in animal model research on ultrasound and tendon and ligament healing, a systematic review of placebo-controlled human trials on ultrasound for treatment of acute lateral ankle sprains did not support its use.[43] In addition, a recent randomized placebo-controlled human trial of adding thermal ultrasound (1 MHz continuous, I_{SATA} = 1.5 W/cm^2, for 10 minutes, for 15 days) to a multi-modal physical therapy regimen in patients with shoulder soft tissue disorders also found no significant effect.[43a] In this study, the patients' duration of symptoms prior to treatment was at least 4 weeks and averaged 8 months. However, it should be noted that human studies of low-intensity ultrasound therapy using treatment parameters similar to those found to be beneficial in animal models of tendon and ligament healing are absent in the literature. Clinical studies are certainly warranted on patients to facilitate tendon healing not only following tendon repair but also in tendinopathies where tendons have gone through a process of angiofibroblastic hyperplasia.

Fracture Healing and Articular Cartilage Repair

Over the past decade, the use of low-intensity pulsed ultrasound has emerged as an effective treatment for facilitation of fracture healing. Many of the animal and human studies demonstrating effects have used the same ultrasound treatment parameters: 20% duty cycle, 1.5 MHz, I_{SATA} = 30 mW/cm^2, for 20 minutes daily. Typically, specific ultrasound units designed to deliver only these fixed parameters were used in the studies. Known as the Sonic Accelerated Fracture Healing System (SAFHS), these units are commercially available (e.g., EXOGEN Ultrasound Bone Healing System, Smith & Nephew), in the United States (Fig. 4-11).

Using these parameters, Pilla et al.[44] found that surgically induced fibula fractures in rabbits treated with

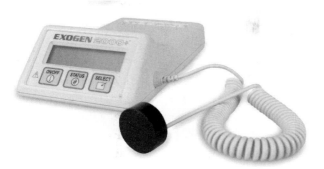

Fig 4•11 Exogen 2000. *(Reprinted with permission from Smith & Nephew Orthopaedics, Memphis, Tennessee.)*

ultrasound demonstrated accelerated healing by a factor of 1.4 to 1.6 in comparison to contralateral sham-treated fractures. Also with SAFHS, Azuma and colleagues[45] found that the torsional strength of healing rat femur fractures treated with ultrasound was superior to the strength of contralateral sham-treated controls, even with no differences in bone mineral content or fracture callus area between groups. Wang and associates[46] also found a beneficial treatment effect using the same fracture model and a very similar treatment regimen.

In a double-blind, randomized, placebo-controlled trial of patients with tibial shaft fractures, Heckman and colleagues[47] found a 38% reduction in healing time with SAFHS. In another, similarly designed study, Kristiansen et al.[48] found a 38% reduction in healing times of distal radius fractures with SAFHS. In both studies, fractures were closed and minimally displaced, and treatment with ultrasound commenced within the first week following injury.

A third trial that was a randomized, double-blind, placebo-controlled study on patients with scaphoid fractures confirmed the results of the first two. Mayr et al.[49] found that treatment with SAFHS accelerated healing time by 31% relative to controls. In addition to facilitation of fresh-fracture healing, pulsed low-intensity ultrasound with SAFHS parameters or very similar ones has been demonstrated to facilitate bone healing in patients with chronic nonunion fractures who failed previous treatments[50,51] and to accelerate bony fusion following spinal arthrodesis in rabbits.[52,53] Recent work suggests that beneficial effects on bone healing may be possible with even lower doses and less frequent applications. Heybeli and colleagues[54] demonstrated that healing rat femur fractures exposed to a diagnostic ultrasound device (7.5 MHz, I_{SATA} = 11.8 mW/cm²) for 10-minute sessions once every 5 days were measurably superior to controls with as few as three or eight treatments. Although research to date has been limited to experimental animal models, it also appears that low-intensity pulsed ultrasound similar to SAFHS has the potential to stimulate articular cartilage repair in induced arthritis.[55,56]

It is noteworthy that none of the previously referenced studies used conventional clinical ultrasound units. It is possible, yet unestablished, that similar results could be obtained with conventional units as used in physical therapy practice. An example of how the SAFHS parameters could be approximated with a conventional therapeutic ultrasound unit is illustrated in Table 4-4.

With the exception of facilitation of bone healing, most of the evidence supporting the use of ultrasound for posttraumatic inflammation and tissue repair has been limited to animal models. In the absence of clinical trials, in practice, it is prudent to approximate those treatment regimens that resulted in therapeutic benefit on similar tissues in animal models. There is a clear

Table 4•4 Comparison of SAFHS and the Most Similar Parameter Selections Available on a Conventional Therapeutic Ultrasound Unit

Parameter	SAFHS (EXOGEN 2000)	Conventional Unit (Omnisound 3000C)
Frequency	1.5 MHz	1.0 MHz
BNR	3:1	2.9:1
Duty cycle	20%	20%
I_{SA}	0.16 W/cm²	0.15 W/cm²
I_{SATA}	30 mW/cm²	30 mW/cm²
ERA	3.88 cm²	5.0 cm²
Treatment time	20 min	20 min

Adapted from technical specifications of EXOGEN 2000 (Smith-Nephew, Memphis, TN) and Omnisound 3000C (Accelerated Care Plus, Sparks, NV).

trend suggesting that low intensities are most likely to be effective and that treatment should begin as soon as possible after injury. However, it is unclear whether use of continuous or pulsed mode is a variable that determines treatment effect. Studies have demonstrated successful treatment effects using both modes.

A recent systematic review concluded that the evidence to date to support this technique for fracture healing is weak.[57] More well-designed clinical trials are warranted.

Instrumentation for Delivering Therapeutic Ultrasound

The basic components of therapeutic ultrasound units are the console, coaxial cable, and transducer. The console houses a transformer that raises incoming voltage from the power source, which is usually house current (60 Hz at 110 volts). A battery may power smaller, portable units. An oscillator circuit within the console modifies the incoming frequency to the designated level for ultrasound. A coaxial cable transfers the electrical energy from the console to the transducer. The transducer houses a piezoelectric crystal, where the high-frequency electrical energy is converted to ultrasound energy, as previously described. The wafer-thin (2 to 3 mm) crystal is typically made of ceramic and is cemented to the undersurface of the transducer's metal faceplate. The outer surface of the faceplate is in contact with the patient. A wand or applicator handle is attached to the transducer. Transducers are available in a variety of sizes for different applications, but the most frequently used are 5 cm² and 10 cm². A typical ultrasound unit is depicted in Figure 4-12.

The controls for operating the US equipment are typically found on the console and often may involve a series of sequential steps using LED-activated buttons. A power switch (e.g. on/off) and treatment timer in minutes are always included. The intensity control allows the user gradual, incremental adjustment. Most output meters are calibrated to read in watts per square centimeter (W/cm²) (spatial average intensity), but some read in watts (acoustic power) or allow the user to choose either. A frequency control is usually present that allows the user to select from at least two choices. Frequencies of 1 MHz and 3 MHz are standard. Most contemporary US units include various duty cycle

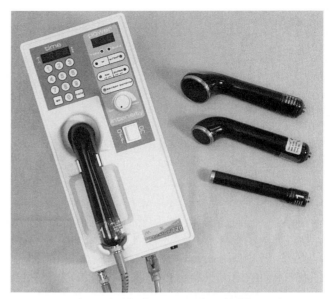

Fig 4•12 A typical ultrasound unit. Note the varying sizes of the transducers.

options for pulsed ultrasound. Many units have a pause button that allows the user to temporarily interrupt treatment while retaining treatment settings. Some newer units include contact monitors and thermistors that trigger an automatic shutoff in case of inadequate coupling or transducer overheating. Figures 4-13 and 4-14 picture

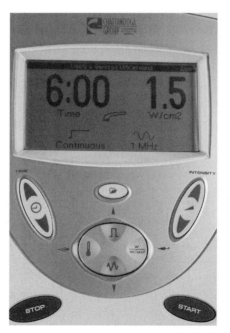

Fig 4•13 Demonstrates the dosage used to heat over a knee joint.

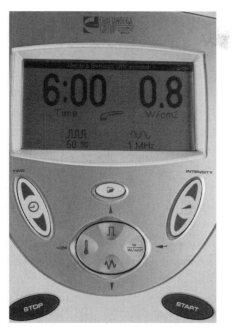

Fig 4•14 Demonstrates the dosage used to treat tendinopathy at the wrist.

the panel of one ultrasound machine with setup for pulsed and CW ultrasound. Figure 4-13 is set up to demonstrate the dosage used to heat over a knee joint, and Figure 4-14 is set up to deliver ultrasound to the wrist. Note the differences in frequency and intensity for both.

Application Considerations

Indications

With appropriate parameter selections, therapeutic ultrasound may be an effective means of temporarily increasing tissue temperature or blood flow over a small treatment area (Box 4-1). Low-intensity ultrasound

---

may be indicated to facilitate healing. Dosage guidelines are included in Box 4-2.

Contraindications

Sometimes, increasing tissue temperature, blood flow, metabolic activity, or cell proliferation in an area is undesirable or perhaps even dangerous. Therapeutic ultrasound is contraindicated in such instances (Box 4-3).

Ultrasound waves may interfere with the electrical circuitry of cardiac pacemakers. Treatment with therapeutic ultrasound should be limited to areas remote from the pacemaker, such as the distal aspects of the extremities. Positioning should ensure that the ultrasound waves are directed away from the patient's trunk. Specific effects of therapeutic ultrasound on the fetus are unknown. Diagnostic obstetrical ultrasound, generally considered to be without fetal risk, typically employs very low intensities, ranging between 0.1 and 60 mW/cm^2.[58]

There is no clear consensus regarding the safety of therapeutic ultrasound over epiphyseal plates in children. Historically, it was considered contraindicated based on animal research demonstrating retardation of growth and damage to the epiphyseal plate following

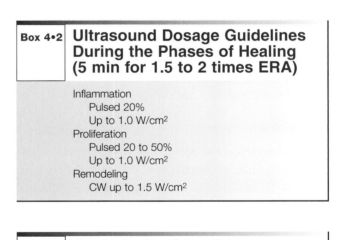

Box 4•2 | **Ultrasound Dosage Guidelines During the Phases of Healing (5 min for 1.5 to 2 times ERA)**

Inflammation
    Pulsed 20%
    Up to 1.0 W/cm^2
Proliferation
    Pulsed 20 to 50%
    Up to 1.0 W/cm^2
Remodeling
    CW up to 1.5 W/cm^2

Box 4•1 | **Indications for Therapeutic Ultrasound**

As a deep-heating modality:
• Joint contracture and scar tissue
• Pain and muscle spasm
• Subacute or chronic soft tissue inflammation (when increased tissue temperature or blood flow is desired)
To facilitate healing:
• Acute injury or inflammation of soft tissue
• Acute injury or inflammation of peripheral nerve
• Open wounds
• Fracture (using specialized equipment)

Box 4•3 | **Contraindications for Therapeutic Ultrasound**

• In the region of a cardiac pacemaker
• During pregnancy; over pelvic, abdominal, or lumbar regions
• Eyes and testes
• In a region of active bleeding or infection
• In a region of a tumor/malignancy
• In the region of a deep vein thrombosis or thrombophlebitis
• Over the heart, stellate, or cervical ganglia
• Over epiphyseal plates of growing bones

high-intensity ultrasound delivered using a stationary transducer.[59,60] More recently, some texts have reported that at clinically applicable intensities, ultrasound over open epiphyseal plates should be safe and is no longer considered a contraindication[61,62] but rather may be used with caution.[63,64]

However, experiments using animal explant models of growing bone have demonstrated that ultrasound stimulates endochondral ossification. Daily 20-minute pulsed ultrasound treatments at very low intensity (I_{SATA} = 0.03 W/cm^2) for 7 days resulted in significant increases in the length of metatarsal diaphyses relative to untreated controls[65] and increases in matrix production by chondrocytes in the epiphyseal region.[66] In contrast, Ogurtan and colleagues[67] recently reported that 5-minute daily pulsed ultrasound treatments at either I_{SATA} = 0.5 or 0.2 W/cm^2 for up to 20 days had no significant effect on the growth rate of the radius and ulna in immature rabbits. However, these results must be interpreted with caution, because each group consisted of only five rabbits, and variability within each data set suggests that statistical power was likely quite low. Because of the potential for damage to the growth plate with intense thermal ultrasound and for increased stimulation of bone formation even with very minimal ultrasound exposure, it is this author's opinion that in the absence of compelling data to suggest otherwise, application of therapeutic ultrasound at any intensity over epiphyseal regions in skeletally immature patients is contraindicated (see Box 4-3).

Precautions

When considering the application of therapeutic ultrasound, particularly thermal doses, it is important to consider several factors to ensure safety. As with any thermal modality, the patient's ability to accurately perceive and communicate about changes in pain and temperature perception is a major safeguard against injury. For this reason, the therapist must be very cautious when applying ultrasound over areas with sensory deficits and on patients who are unable to clearly communicate. The circulatory status and vascularity of tissue in the treated region must also be considered. If local circulation is impaired by peripheral vascular disease, or if the tissue has little inherent vascularity, excessive temperature elevation may occur because heat generated during

ultrasound cannot be adequately dissipated. Although treatment over areas with plastic or metal implants, such as those used in fracture fixation, joint repair, and replacement, is not contraindicated, caution is warranted. Plastic materials used in joint replacement components and as bone cement are highly absorptive of ultrasound waves.[68] In theory, this means that any heating effects of ultrasound on tissues in the vicinity of a plastic implant may be intensified by conduction of heat from the implant. Because metals largely reflect ultrasound, the potential for creating standing waves in the tissue between the transducer and a metal implant is increased. Proper ultrasound application technique minimizes risk of excessive heating, but in no case should ultrasound treatment be uncomfortable. When pain is reported during treatment, therapists should respond rapidly by decreasing ultrasound intensity.

Application Techniques

Keep the Applicator Moving!

A moving sound applicator technique is preferred for administering therapeutic ultrasound. Because of beam nonuniformity with a high spatial peak intensity in the center of the beam, the distribution of energy beneath a stationary applicator is uneven. Some small areas underlying the transducer may receive a disproportionately high percentage of the emitted energy, and other areas may receive very little. The potential for creating standing waves in regions of reflected ultrasound also increases if the transducer is stationary. When ultrasound is delivered in continuous mode at sufficient intensity, focal areas of painful, intense heat (often referred to as "hot spots") can occur and potentially cause tissue damage. In contrast, when the applicator is moved slowly in a smooth, rhythmical pattern over the treatment area, a more even spatial distribution of energy occurs. Either longitudinal stroking or overlapping circular movements can be used. The US applicator can also be moved more rapidly without losing any therapeutic effects; the key is to maintain good contact with the coupling gel on the skin surface.

Logically, as the size of the treatment area increases, the effective dosage delivered to any one region decreases, as does the potential for any therapeutic heating. As a general rule, the total treatment area should be 1.5 to 2 times the ERA of the transducer.

Application of very low-intensity pulsed ultrasound to facilitate fracture healing typically employs a stationary applicator positioned directly over the fracture site. Most units designed for such use incorporate fixed parameters to ensure patient safety and can fine-tune US energy better than most units available for traditional rehabilitation uses.

Direct Contact Coupling Is Preferred

Ultrasound waves do not travel effectively through air; therefore, a coupling medium must be used to transmit ultrasound energy between the transducer and the patient's body. When the surface of the treatment area is relatively flat and is at least as large as the transducer face, the simplest and most convenient method of ultrasound application is direct contact. Typically, a thin layer of highly transmissive water-soluble gel is spread on the area to be treated, and the transducer is applied in direct contact with the gel-covered skin. The purpose of the coupling gel is to eliminate as much air as possible between the transducer and the skin, thereby maximizing the amount of ultrasound energy entering the patient's body.

KEY POINT! Adequate coupling is needed because complete reflection of ultrasound waves will occur at an interface between the transducer's metal faceplate and any air pockets or bubbles present in the gel.

From a therapeutic standpoint, energy emitted from areas of the transducer not in contact with the body is wasted, but the reflected energy may cause overheating and damage to the transducer itself. Therefore, therapists should choose an appropriately sized transducer. Treatment in the region of small bony prominences (e.g., lateral malleolus of the ankle or medial epicondyle of the elbow) and small, irregular surfaces like the fingers and toes necessitate a smaller transducer (Figs. 4-15 through 4-19). Commercially available, water-soluble ultrasound gel is by far the most common coupling agent used for direct-contact ultrasound application, but water-soluble lotions specifically designed for ultrasound application are also available. Although less frequently used, now that many commercially prepared ultrasound gels and lotions are readily available at reasonable cost, mineral oil may

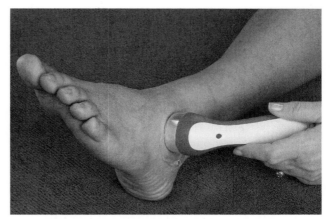

Fig 4•15 The sound head should be proportionate to the surface area that is to be treated. The large sound head in this image exceeds the surface area and will result in poor transmission of ultrasound energy.

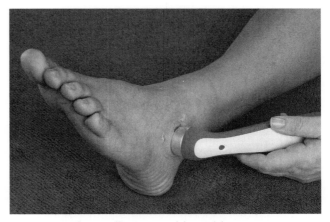

Fig 4•16 A smaller sound head is more appropriate for the lateral ankle, thus improving transmission of ultrasound energy.

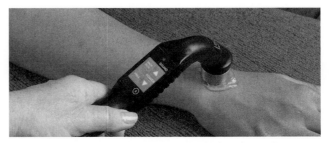

Fig 4•17 Ultrasound over dorsal wrist prior to mobilization to increase wrist flexion.

also serve as a direct coupling agent. Its transmissivity is similar to that of commercially prepared ultrasound gel.[69] Single-application packages of sterile ultrasound gel are commercially available for use in treating over open wounds or surgical incisions.

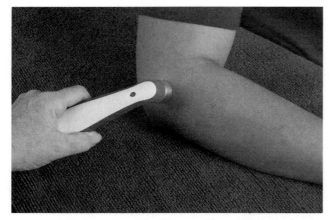

Fig 4•18 Ultrasound with small applicator over lateral epicondyle.

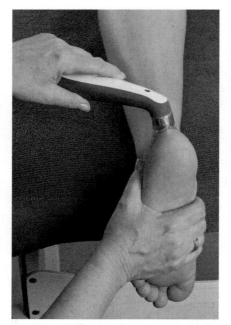

Fig 4•19 Ultrasound over Achilles tendon using a small sound head.

Indirect Coupling Methods Are Overrated

With the advent of smaller transducers, there is less concern about effectively coupling US to the skin surface. But sometimes, direct-contact ultrasound application may not be the favored choice. If pressure from moving the transducer on the skin causes pain or if an appropriately sized transducer is unavailable for treating an irregularly shaped or small surface, an indirect application method, where the transducer does not directly contact the skin, must be used.

In the water-immersion method, the part to be treated, typically the hand or foot, is submerged in a basin of water and the transducer is moved over the treatment area from a distance of about 1 to 2 cm away. Plastic basins are recommended over metal ones to minimize reflection. Air bubbles often accumulate on the transducer's faceplate and on the patient's skin during underwater ultrasound application, decreasing transmission if they are not quickly wiped away by the operator during treatment. Two studies have compared tissue temperature change with ultrasound treatments of equal intensity delivered with either an underwater or topical aqueous gel technique.[70,71] Both found that temperature increases were 40% to 60% lower using the underwater technique. Using an in vitro pig tissue model, Klucinec and colleagues[72] found that ultrasound delivered underwater transmitted only about 32% as much energy as when delivered using direct contact with gel. These findings suggest that treatment intensity should be substantially increased when using an underwater delivery technique to approximate the same tissue temperature increases expected from use of a direct-contact method. Likewise, when clinicians use a direct-contact method hoping to achieve the same therapeutic effects demonstrated in experimental studies that employed underwater treatments, treatment intensity must be substantially decreased.

Other indirect methods employed for ultrasound application include use of gel or water-filled bladders or aqueous gel pads. Although rarely used today, a cushionlike offset, made with either a tied latex glove filled with gel or water or a gel-filled condom covering the transducer, has been used as an alternative method for treating highly sensitive areas or areas with irregular contours. More recently, disposable aqueous gel pads designed specifically for ultrasound application have become commercially available and are increasingly used clinically as an alternative to either water immersion or bladder methods. The clear, flexible water-based pads are 2 cm thick and 9 cm in diameter. The pad is used as an offset between the skin and the transducer, either as the sole coupling agent or in combination with a thin layer of gel on either side of the pad.

In addition to water immersion, Klucinec and colleagues[72] examined ultrasound transmission through pig skin using bladder methods or a gel pad in comparison to transmission using direct-contact application with gel. Latex gloves filled with either tap water or gel transmitted only 66% and 50% as much energy, respectively. A gel-filled condom transmitted even less energy. Transmission measured using the gel pad and a thin layer of gel added on either side of the pad was superior to transmission using the gel alone. Merrick and colleagues[73] found similar levels of muscle heating in human volunteers using either direct-contact application with gel or indirect application with gel pads, suggesting they are equivalent coupling methods. With the exception of gel pads, indirect methods of ultrasound application appear to be significantly less efficient means of transmitting acoustic energy, relative to direct contact using gel. In addition, treatment involving indirect methods is generally more difficult to set up and administer. Gel pads, while effective, add expense. The availability of small transducers that can be efficiently coupled to skin via coupling gel may negate the need for gel pads in most instances.

KEY POINT! When the contour of the treatment area and availability of appropriately sized transducers allow, direct contact is the preferred method of ultrasound application.

When an indirect application method is indicated, gel pads appear to be the best option. If other indirect methods are used, clinicians must recognize that transmission is decreased and must alter parameter selections accordingly.

Assessment of Intervention Outcomes

Measurement and Expected Outcomes

Pain assessment is often a useful measure of treatment effectiveness with therapeutic ultrasound. Changes in resting or baseline pain levels may be evaluated during treatment, immediately after treatment, or from one treatment session to the next. Likewise, tenderness to palpation and level of discomfort with a particular movement or resisted test may be appropriate measures, depending on the patient's condition. For example, decreased pain during or immediately following treatment may be reported when a thermal dose of ultrasound is applied over a painful trigger point. On the other hand, with a more chronic condition, reported pain levels with resisted testing of the plantar flexor muscles, for instance, may be expected to gradually decrease over several treatment sessions when low-intensity ultrasound is used for treating an Achilles tendinopathy. If ultrasound is used to increase soft tissue extensibility during or immediately prior to stretching, then obviously range-of-motion measurements are indicated. With ultrasound, like most other physical therapy interventions, the ultimate measure of treatment effectiveness is seeing an improvement in patient function.

Documentation of Ultrasound Treatment

Treatment with therapeutic ultrasound should be thoroughly documented in the patient record. In addition to ultrasound parameters, the specific treatment area, patient position, application technique, transducer size, and when the ultrasound was sequenced within the treatment session should be included. Any adverse reactions during treatment should be noted as well as the clinician's response. For example, "The patient reported an increase in anterior knee pain approximately 4 minutes into treatment. The knee was repositioned to approximately 60°, and the patient tolerated the rest of treatment without any discomfort."

Documentation Tips

Treatment area
- Patient position
- Frequency
- Mode

Intensity
- Duty cycle (%)
- Treatment duration
- Application technique
- Transducer size
- Sequence within treatment session
- Other
  - Example:
  - 1 MHz, 100% duty cycle, 2.0 W/cm^2, 2 cm^2 sound head, 10 min

Phonophoresis: Is It a Viable Option?

The term *phonophoresis* refers to the use of ultrasound to enhance delivery medication through the skin.

Historically, in physical therapy the most common application has been to treat musculoskeletal inflammatory conditions. A steroidal anti-inflammatory medication (e.g., hydrocortisone or dexamethasone) compounded into ultrasound gel or a commercially prepared lotion containing nonsteroidal anti-inflammatory agents such as methyl salicylate is used as the coupling medium. Ultrasound is theorized to enhance transdermal diffusion of medications through such mechanisms as dilating points of entry (e.g., hair follicles, sweat glands), increasing local circulation, increasing kinetic energy of local cells and the medication itself, and increasing cell membrane permeability.[74] To date, however, the evidence demonstrating efficacy and effectiveness of phonophoresis for treating musculoskeletal inflammatory conditions is weak at best.

The use of phonophoresis in physical therapy has been perpetuated based largely on the results of two studies. In 1967, Griffin and colleagues[75] published results of a double-blind human study comparing hydrocortisone phonophoresis to ultrasound, using the same treatment parameters in patients with arthritis of various joints. They found that the combination of ultrasound and steroid was more effective at reducing pain than ultrasound alone. In an older study, Kleinhort and Wood[76] compared phonophoresis with either 1% or 10% hydrocortisone preparations in patients with a variety of musculoskeletal inflammatory conditions. Patients treated with 10% hydrocortisone phonophoresis had more pain relief than patients treated with the lower concentration. Neither study included a nonsonicated control group.

Cameron and Monroe[77] studied the relative transmission of ultrasound through common media used for phonophoresis and found that hydrocortisone-impregnated gels and most salicylate preparations effectively blocked transmission of ultrasound waves. Lidex gel (containing the corticosteroid fluocinonide), Thera-Gesic cream (containing menthol and methyl salicylate), and betamethasone 0.05% in ultrasound gel were found to be good transmitters, allowing at least 80% transmission. The implication of this study is that patients who demonstrated a therapeutic effect from hydrocortisone phonophoresis in the previous two studies likely benefited not from the hydrocortisone itself, but rather from less ultrasound energy exposure at the target tissue, since the hydrocortisone largely blocked transmission of sound waves.

Studies have also examined motility of medications, either directly or indirectly, following phonophoresis. Benson et al.[78] found no differences relative to sham treatment in the amount of benzydamine hydrochloride (a topical nonsteroidal anti-inflammatory) left in gel, following either continuous or 50% duty cycle pulsed phonophoresis at a variety of frequencies. Using an experimental animal model in which hydrocortisone penetration was indirectly assessed by measuring collagen deposition in subcutaneous tissue, Byl and colleagues[79] found no difference between hydrocortisone rubbed on the skin and phonophoresis using the same concentration of hydrocortisone.

Interestingly, in the same study, dexamethasone was found to decrease collagen deposition in subcutaneous tissue when applied with phonophoresis but not when rubbed on the skin. This study may suggest that it is possible to increase tissue delivery of dexamethasone with phonophoresis. One small clinical trial lends limited support to this hypothesis. In a human study of patients with myofascial trigger points, phonophoresis with dexamethasone and lidocaine was compared to sham phonophoresis using the same drugs and ultrasound using the same parameters.[80] Because separate groups treated with only dexamethasone phonophoresis or lidocaine phonophoresis were not included, the relative contribution of each agent is unclear.

In summary, there is a paucity of evidence supporting the use of phonophoresis for musculoskeletal inflammatory conditions. Most of the topical agents and medications historically used for phonophoresis by physical therapists do not effectively transmit ultrasound. Of those agents demonstrated to be effective transmitters, no published studies have demonstrated enhanced penetration through the skin with phonophoresis or, more importantly, added therapeutic benefit. More research in this area, particularly exploring the use of dexamethasone, is indicated. However, at present, there is inadequate evidence to support the use of phonophoresis as an effective physical therapy treatment modality.

REFERENCES

1. Ferguson BH. *A Practitioner's Guide to Ultrasonic Therapy Equipment Standard.* Rockville, MD: U.S. Department of Health and Human Services, Public Health Service, Food and Drug Administration; 1985.
2. Demmink JH, Helders PJM, Hobaek H, Enwemeka C. The variation of heating depth with therapeutic ultrasound frequency in physiotherapy. *Ultrasound Med Biol.* 2003;29:13–118.
3. Lehmann JF. *Therapeutic Heat and Cold.* 4th ed. Baltimore: Williams and Wilkins; 1990.
4. Lehmann JF, DeLateur BJ, Stonebridge JB, Warren G. Therapeutic temperature distribution produced by ultrasound as modified by dosage and volume of tissue exposed. *Arch Phys Med Rehabil.* 1967;48:662–666.
5. Lehmann JF, DeLateur BJ, Warren G, Stonebridge JB. Heating produced by ultrasound in bone and soft tissue. *Arch Phys Med Rehabil.* 1967;48:397–401.
6. Lota MJ, Darling RC. Change in permeability of the red blood cell membrane in a homogenous ultrasonic field. *Arch Phys Med Rehabil.* 1955;36:282.
7. Harvey W, Dyson M, Pond JB, Grahame R. The stimulation of protein synthesis in human fibroblasts by therapeutic ultrasound. *Rheumatol Rehabil.* 1975;14:237.
8. Lehmann JF, Guy AW. Ultrasound therapy. In: Reid J, Sikov MR, eds. *Interaction of Ultrasound and Biological Tissues.* DHEW Pub. FDA 73–8008, Session 3:8; 1971:141–152.
9. Williams AR. *Ultrasound Biological Effects and Potential Hazard.* New York: Academic Press; 1983.
10. Draper DO, Castel JC, Castel D. Rate of temperature increase in human muscle during 1 MHz and 3 MHz continuous ultrasound. *J Orthop Sports Phys Ther.* 1995;22:142–150.
11. Goss SA, Dunn F. Ultrasonic propagation properties of collagen. *Phys Med Biol.* 1980;25:827–837.
12. Chan AK, Myrer WM, Measom GJ, Draper DO. Temperature change in human patellar tendon in response to therapeutic ultrasound. *J Athl Train.* 1998;33:130–135.
12a. Ozgenel L, Aytekin E, Durmuşoglu G. A double-blind trial of clinical effects of therapeutic ultrasound in knee osteoarthritis. Ultrasound Med Biol. 2009;35(1):44–49.
13. Robinson SE, Buono MJ. Effect of continuous-wave ultrasound on blood flow in skeletal muscle. *Phys Ther.* 1995;75:145–149.
14. Fabrizio PA, Schmidt JA, Clemente FR, et al. Acute effects of therapeutic ultrasound delivered at varying parameters on the blood flow velocity in a muscular distribution artery. *J Orthop Sports Phys Ther.* 1996;24:294–302.
15. Lota M. Electronic plethysmographic and tissue temperature studies of effect of ultrasound on blood flow. *Arch Phys Med Rehabil.* 1965;44:315–322.
16. Zankel HT. Effect of physical agents on motor nerve conduction velocity of the ulnar nerve. *Arch Phys Med Rehabil.* 1966;47:787–792.
17. Farmer W. Effect of intensity of ultrasound on conduction velocity of motor axons. *Phys Ther.* 1968;48:1233–1237.
18. Currier DP, Greathouse D, Swift T. Sensory conduction: effect of ultrasound. *Arch Phys Med Rehabil.* 1978;59:181–185.
19. Halle JS, Scoville CR, Greathouse D. Ultrasound's effect on conduction latency of the superficial radial nerve in man. *Phys Ther.* 1981;61:345–350.
20. Lehmann JF, Bruner GD, Stow RW. Pain threshold measurements after therapeutic application of ultrasound, microwaves and infrared. *Arch Phys Med Rehabil.* 1958;39:560.
21. Harvey W, Dyson M, Pond JB, Grahame R. The stimulation of protein synthesis in human fibroblasts by therapeutic ultrasound. *Rheumatol Rehabil.* 1975;14:237.
22. Ramirez A, Schwane JA, McFarland C, Starcher B. The effect of ultrasound on collagen synthesis and fibroblast proliferation in vitro. *Med Sci Sports Exerc.* 1997;29:326–332.
23. Wharton W, Gillespie GY, Russell SW, Pledger WJ. Mitogenic activity elaborated by macrophage-like cell lines acts as competence factors for BALB/c 3T3 cells. *J Cell Physiol.* 1982;110:93–100.
24. Young SR, Dyson M. Macrophage responsiveness to therapeutic ultrasound. *Ultrasound Med Biol.* 1990;16:809–816.
25. Mortimer AJ, Dyson M. The effect of therapeutic ultrasound on calcium uptake in fibroblasts. *Ultrasound Med Biol.* 1980;16:261–269.
26. Young SR, Dyson M. The effect of therapeutic ultrasound on angiogenesis. *Ultrasound Med Biol.* 1990;16:261–269.
27. Byl N, McKenzie AL, West JM, et al. Low-dose ultrasound effects on wound healing: a controlled study on Yucatan pigs. *Arch Phys Med Rehabil.* 1992;73:656–664.
28. Byl N, McKenzie AL, Wong T, et al. Incisional wound healing: a controlled study of low and high dose ultrasound. *J Orthop Sports Phys Ther.* 1993;18:619–628.
29. Flemming K, Cullum N. Therapeutic ultrasound for pressure sores. Cochrane Database Syst Rev, 4, CD001275; 2000.
30. Johannsen F, Gam AN, Karlsmark T. Ultrasound therapy in chronic leg ulceration: a meta-analysis. *Wound Repair Regen.* 1998;6:121–126.
31. Baba-Akbari Sari A, Flemming K, Cullum NA, Wollina U. Therapeutic ultrasound for pressure ulcers. Cochrane Database Syst Rev. 2006 Jul 19;3:CD001275.
32. Rantanen J, Thorsson O, Wollmer P, et al. Effects of therapeutic ultrasound on the regeneration of skeletal myofibers after experimental injury. *Am J Sports Med.* 1999;27:54–59.
33. Markert CD, Maerrick MA, Kirby TE, Devor ST. Nonthermal ultrasound and exercise in skeletal muscle regeneration. *Arch Phys Med Rehabil.* 2005;86:1304–1310.
34. Crisci AR, Ferreira AL. Low-intensity pulsed ultrasound accelerates the regeneration of the sciatic nerve after neurotomy in rats. *Ultrasound Med Biol.* 2002;28:1335–1341.
35. Mourad PD, Lazar DA, Curra FP, et al. Ultrasound accelerates functional recovery after peripheral nerve damage. *Neurosurgery.* 2001;48:1136–1140.
36. Frieder S, Weisberg J, Fleming B, Stanek A. A pilot study: the therapeutic effect of ultrasound following partial rupture of Achilles tendon in male rats. *J Orthop Sports Phys Ther.* 1988;10:39–46.
37. Jackson BA, Schwane JA, Starcher BC. The effect of ultrasound therapy on the repair of Achilles tendon injuries in rats. *Med Sci Sports Exerc.* 1991;23:171–176.
38. Turner SM, Powell ES, Ng CS. The effect of ultrasound on the healing of repaired cockerel tendon: is collagen cross-linking a factor? *J Hand Surg Br.* 1989;14:428–433.
39. Enwemeka CS. The effect of therapeutic ultrasound on tendon healing: a biomechanical study. *Am J Phys Med Rehabil.* 1989;6:283–287.
40. Enwemeka CS, Rodriguez O, Mendosa S. The biomechanical effects of low-intensity ultrasound on healing tendons. *Ultrasound Med Biol.* 1990;16:801–807.
41. Saini NS, Roy KS, Bansal PS, et al. A preliminary study on the effects of ultrasound therapy on the healing of surgically severed Achilles tendons in five dogs. *J Vet Med A Physiol Pathol Clin Med.* 2002;49:321–328.
42. Takakura Y, Matsui N, Yoshiya S, et al. Low-intensity pulsed ultrasound enhances early healing of medial collateral ligament injuries in rats. *J Ultrasound Med.* 2002;21:283–288.

43. Van der Windt DAWM, Van der Heijden GJMG, Van den Berg SGM, et al. Ultrasound therapy for acute ankle sprains. Cochrane Database Syst Rev. 1, CD001250; 2002.

43a. Gursel YK, Ulus Y, Bilgic A, et al. Adding ultrasound in the management of soft tissue disorders of the shoulder: a randomized placebo-controlled trial. *Phys Ther.* 2004;84: 336–343.

44. Pilla AA, Mont MA, Nasser PR, et al. Non-invasive low intensity pulsed ultrasound accelerates bone healing in the rabbit. *J Orthop Trauma.* 1990;4:246–253.

45. Azuma Y, Ito M, Harada Y, et al. Low-intensity pulsed ultrasound accelerates rat femoral fracture healing by acting on various cellular reactions in the fracture callus. *J Bone Miner Res.* 2001;16:671–680.

46. Wang S-J, Lewallen DG, Bolander ME, et al. Low intensity ultrasound treatment increases strength in a rat femoral fracture model. *J Orthop Res.* 1994;12:40–47.

47. Heckman JD, Ryaby JP, McCabe J, et al. Acceleration of tibial fracture-healing by non-invasive, low intensity pulsed ultrasound. *J Bone Joint Surg Am.* 1994;76:26–34.

48. Kristiansen TK, Ryaby JP, McCabe J, et al. Accelerated healing of distal radius fractures with the use of specific, low-intensity ultrasound. *J Bone Joint Surg Am.* 1997;79: 961–973.

49. Mayr E, Rudzki M, Borchardt B, et al. Does low intensity, pulsed ultrasound speed healing of scaphoid fractures? [German]. *Handchir Mikrochir Plast Chir.* 2000;32:115–122.

50. Nolte PA, van der Krans A, Patka P, et al. Low intensity pulsed ultrasound in the treatment of nonunions. *J Trauma.* 2001;51:693–702.

51. Mayr E, Frankel V, Ruter A. Ultrasound—an alternative healing method for nonunions. *Arch Orthop Trauma Surg.* 2000; 120:1–8.

52. Glazer PA, Heilmann MR, Lotz JC, Bradford DS. Use of ultrasound in spinal arthrodesis: a rabbit model. *Spine.* 1998;23:1142–1148.

53. Aynaci O, Onder C, Piskin A, Ozoran Y. The effect of ultrasound on the healing of muscle-pediculated bone graft in spinal fusion. *Spine.* 2002;27:1531–1535.

54. Heybeli N, Yesildag A, Oyar O, et al. Diagnostic ultrasound treatment increases the bone fracture-healing rate in an internally fixed rat femoral osteotomy model. *J Ultrasound Med.* 2002;21:1357–1363.

55. Huang MH, Ding HJ, Chai CY, et al. Effects of sonication on articular cartilage in experimental osteoarthritis. *J Rheumatol.* 1997;24:1978–1984.

56. Cook SD, Salkeld SL, Popich-Patron LS, et al. Improved cartilage repair after treatment with low-intensity pulsed ultrasound. *Clin Orthop.* 2001;391(Suppl):S231–S243.

57. Busse JW, Kaur J, Mollon B, Bhandari M, Tornetta P 3rd, Schünemann HJ, Guyatt GH. Low intensity pulsed ultrasonography for fractures: systematic review of randomised controlled trials. *BMJ.* 2009;338:b351. doi: 10.1136/bmj.b3558.

58. Diagnostic Ultrasound Imaging in Pregnancy. NIH Consensus Statement; 1984;5:1–16.

59. Bender LF, James JM, Herrick JR. Histologic studies following exposure of bone to ultrasound. *Arch Phys Med Rehabil.* 1954;35:555.

60. DeForest RE, Herrick JF, James JM. Effects of ultrasound on growing bone: an experimental study. *Arch Phys Med Rehabil.* 1953;34:21.

61. Nussbaum EL. Therapeutic ultrasound. In: Behrens BJ, Michlovitz SL, eds. *Physical Agents Theory and Practice for the Physical Therapist Assistant.* Philadelphia: FA Davis; 1996:105.

62. McDiarmid TM, Ziskin MC, Michlovitz SL. Therapeutic ultrasound. In: Michlovitz SL, ed. *Thermal Agents in Rehabilitation.* 3rd ed. Philadelphia: FA Davis; 1996:205.

63. Belanger A-Y. Acoustic radiation: ultrasound. In: Belanger A-Y, *Evidence-Based Guide to Therapeutic Physical Agents.* Philadelphia: Lippincott Williams & Wilkins; 2002: 249.

64. Starkey C. Ultrasound. In: *Therapeutic Modalities.* 2nd ed. Philadelphia: FA Davis; 1999: 298.

65. Nolte PA, Klein-Nulend J, Albers GH, et al. Low-intensity ultrasound stimulates endochondral ossification in vitro. *J Orthop Res.* 2001;19:301–307.

66. Zhang ZJ, Huckle J, Francomano CA, Spencer RG. The influence of pulsed low-intensity ultrasound on matrix production of chondrocytes at different stages of differentiation: an explant study. *Ultrasound Med Biol.* 2002;28:1547–1553.

67. Ogurtan Z, Celik I, Izci C, et al. Effect of experimental therapeutic ultrasound on the distal antebrachial growth plates in one-month-old rabbits. *Vet J.* 2002;164:280–287.

68. Krotenberg R, Ambrose L, Mosher R. Therapeutic ultrasound effect on high density polyethylene and polymethyl methacrylate. *Arch Phys Med Rehabil.* 1986;67:618.

69. Warren GC, Koblanski JN, Sifelmann R. Ultrasound coupling media: their relative transmissivity. *Arch Phys Med Rehabil.* 1976;57:218–222.

70. Forrest G, Rosen K. Ultrasound: effectiveness of treatments given under water. *Arch Phys Med Rehabil.* 1989;70:28–29.

71. Draper DO, Sunderland S, Kirkendall DT, Ricard M. A comparison of temperature rise in human calf muscles following applications of underwater and topical gel ultrasound. *J Orthop Sports Phys Ther.* 1993;17:247–251.

72. Klucinec B, Scheidler M, Denegar C, et al. Transmissivity of coupling agents used to deliver ultrasound through indirect methods. *J Orthop Sports Phys Ther.* 2000;30:263–269.

73. Merrick MA, Mihalyov MR, Roethemeiser JL, et al. A comparison of intramuscular temperature during ultrasound treatments with coupling gel or gel pads. *J Orthop Sports Phys Ther.* 2002;32:216–220.

74. Byl NN. The use of ultrasound as an enhancer for transcutaneous drug delivery: phonophoresis. *Phys Ther.* 1995;75: 539–553.

75. Griffin JE, Enternach JL, Price RE, Touchstone JC. Patients treated with ultrasonic driven hydrocortisone and with ultrasound alone. *Phys Ther.* 1967;47:594–601.

76. Kleinhort J, Wood F. Phonophoresis with 1% versus 10% hydrocortisone. *Phys Ther.* 1975;55:1320–1324.

77. Cameron MH, Monroe LG. Relative transmission of ultrasound by media customarily used for phonophoresis. *Phys Ther.* 1992;72:142–148.

78. Benson HA, McElnay JC, Harland R. Use of ultrasound to enhance percutaneous absorption of benzydamine. *Phys Ther.* 1989;69:113–118.

79. Byl NN, McKenzie A, Halliday B, et al. The effects of phonophoresis with corticosteroids: a controlled pilot study. *J Orthop Sports Phys Ther.* 1993;18:590–600.

80. Moll JM. A new approach to pain: lidocaine and Decadron with ultrasound. *USAF Med Serv Dig.* 1977;30:8–11.

chapter 5

Hydrotherapy
The Use of Water as a Therapeutic Agent

Elaine L. Bukowski, PT, DPT, (D) ABDA |
Thomas P. Nolan Jr., PT, DPT, OCS

ydrotherapy is a therapeutic intervention that uses water to facilitate physiological effects and enable patients to achieve therapy goals. Hydrotherapy usually takes place in a large pool or a stainless-steel tank known as a whirlpool. The properties of water provide treatment options that might otherwise be difficult or impossible to provide with land-based interventions. For example, in a pool, the patient can be placed in non-weight-bearing positions—supine, prone, or sitting—with the use of buoyant devices. Weight-bearing in a pool can be varied depending on the water's depth and the patient's position.

Hydrotherapy in a pool, often called "aquatic therapy," has wide therapeutic applications for interventions for pediatric, geriatric, cardiopulmonary, neurological, and orthopedic populations.[1–20] Aquatic therapy can be used to promote relaxation, improve circulation, restore mobility, strengthen muscles, provide gait training with less stress on weight-bearing joints, stimulate the vestibular system, facilitate sleep, increase one's capacity for stress, and improve psychological and emotional outlook.[8,9,21–26] The temperature and buoyancy of water, combined with decreased body weight and joint compression, and the psychological effects of participating in an enjoyable activity, can reduce pain and muscle spasms and increase range of motion.[1,2] A recent systematic review and meta-analysis on the effectiveness of aquatic exercise in relieving pain in adults with neurological or musculoskeletal problems concluded that further studies on specific aquatic exercise techniques

with robust methodological designs and detailed reporting of temperature, depth, and care setting are needed.[27]

Hydrotherapy is often combined with exercise for therapeutic effects. Slow, rhythmic movements combined with rotary-type motions may decrease spasticity of muscles. For example, a 38-year-old male with cerebral palsy attended aquatic therapy for gait dysfunction secondary to an adverse reaction to antianxiety medication. He performed slow, rhythmic, and rotary movements in the pool and had improvement in the tone in his lower extremities, which resulted in less spasticity and a more normal gait pattern. Aquatic therapy was chosen for this patient to increase endurance, improve static and dynamic posture, and increase independence in ambulation with a walker.[28]

CASE STUDY 5•1 SELECTING POOL THERAPY FOR A PATIENT WITH CEREBRAL PALSY

A 38-year-old male with cerebral palsy is referred for balance and gait training secondary to severe balance and endurance problems that were the result of a medication reaction used to treat anxiety. Prior to this, the patient ambulated independently, played sports, and was active in his community. Upon testing, the patient demonstrated decreased balance and endurance and inability to ambulate without a walker.

CLINICAL DECISION-MAKING

1. Does the patient have a dysfunction, limitation, or problem that can be improved with the use of pool therapy?
   Answer: Yes, pool therapy can be used to improve endurance, balance, and gait.

2. Is the patient appropriate for pool therapy? Do any of the general precautions or contraindications to pool therapy apply to the patient, or are there any specific considerations regarding the application of pool therapy to this patient?
   Answer: None of the precautions or contraindications applies to this patient. He is able to enter the pool using a ramp and handrails with the assistance of the practitioner. Pool therapy is an appropriate intervention for him.

3. What are the specific goals to be achieved with the use of pool therapy?
   Answer: Improved endurance and balance and decreased use of assistive device for ambulation.

4. What specific aspects of pool therapy would be appropriate for this patient?
   Answer: The force of buoyancy can be used to resist movement and improve endurance, and the slow, rhythmical movements combined with rotary-type motions promote improved tone in the lower extremities and a more normal gait. Seated bicycling, and ambulating back and forth and sideways in different water depths will also promote improved endurance and balance and a more normal gait.

5. What are the proper application procedures for pool therapy?
   Answer: Inform the patient of the purpose and procedure, including the schedule of pool therapy sessions and the need for appropriate swimwear. Assess the patient's previous swimming experiences and his expectations for the sessions.
   Pre-session: Determine the techniques to be used during the session (seated activities versus standing activities, depth of water to assist or challenge balance, types and speeds of movements to achieve goals of session).
   Pool session: Monitor vital signs to ensure patient safety. Use safest method for entry into pool. Proceed with activities chosen for session and modify as needed.
   Post-session: Assess balance and gait as patient exits pool, including trying a different method of exit from that used for entry. Assess balance and gait on land and monitor vital signs. Determine progression of next pool therapy session.

Hydrotherapy can facilitate exercises designed to strengthen muscles. Repetitive exercises in water and swimming strokes can improve coordination, and the warmth of the water can increase blood supply to the musculoskeletal tissues. Kicking exercises in water can stimulate venous return, and the hydrostatic pressure provided by deeper water can help move fluids upward, all of which can assist with improving circulation insufficiency.[29]

KEY POINT! Hydrostatic pressure is present against any body part immersed in water; the deeper the body part is immersed, the greater will be the pressure.

A 23-year-old male baseball player had surgery to repair a rotator cuff and glenoid labrum tear. Postoperatively, he was limited to 90° of shoulder flexion and abduction range of motion (ROM). Aquatic therapy was included as part of his rehabilitation program. The use of water provided buoyancy to assist, support, and resist shoulder exercises. Turbulence of the water and the speed of movement facilitated exercise to increase ROM and strength of the involved shoulder while maintaining ROM and strength of the elbow and wrist joints of the involved side.[16,30]

Hydrotherapy can facilitate exercise programs for patients who cannot tolerate exercise on land. A 64-year-old female received aquatic therapy for treatment of low back pain because she could not tolerate land-based exercises when she first started physical therapy. She was able to exercise her back musculature while moving her lower body in the water.[16] A 55-year-old female with restricted weight-bearing following total hip arthroplasty secondary to osteoarthritic

---

CASE STUDY 5•2   SELECTING POOL THERAPY FOR A PATIENT FOLLOWING SHOULDER SURGERY

A 23-year-old male is referred for increased ROM and strengthening of the right shoulder secondary to rotator cuff and labrum repair. Upon testing, the patient was limited to 90° of flexion and abduction of the shoulder and weakness of the rotator cuff muscles and the anterior and middle deltoid.

CLINICAL DECISION-MAKING

1. Does the patient have a dysfunction, limitation, or problem that can be improved with the use of pool therapy?
   Answer: Yes, pool therapy can be used to improve ROM and increase the strength of the rotator cuff and anterior and middle deltoid muscles.

2. Is the patient appropriate for pool therapy? Do any of the general precautions or contraindications to pool therapy apply to the patient, or are there any specific considerations regarding the application of pool therapy to this patient?
   Answer: None of the precautions or contraindications apply to this patient. The surgical site is healed, and there is no opening or drainage that would be of concern. Pool therapy is an appropriate intervention for him.

3. What are the specific goals to be achieved with the use of pool therapy?
   Answer: Increased ROM and increased strength of the rotator cuff and anterior and middle deltoid muscles.

4. What specific aspects of pool therapy would be appropriate for this patient?
   Answer: The force of buoyancy can be used to assist the motions of the involved muscles and to resist movement and improve strength of these muscles while maintaining ROM and strength of the elbow and wrist joints of the involved side.

5. What are the proper application procedures for pool therapy?
   Answer: Inform the patient of the purpose and procedure, including the schedule of pool therapy sessions and the need for appropriate swimwear. Assess the patient's previous swimming experiences and his expectations for the sessions.
   Pre-session: Determine the techniques to be used during the session (seated, standing, prone or supine activities; depth of water to assist motions or challenge muscle; types and speeds of movements to achieve goals of session).
   Pool session: Monitor vital signs to ensure patient safety. Use safest method for entry into pool. Proceed with activities chosen for session and modify as needed.
   Post-session: Assess ROM and strength of involved muscles. Determine progression of next pool therapy session.

changes experienced decreased body weight and joint compression during exercises in a pool; this resulted in improved ROM and increased strength of the involved musculature.[10,11,31,32] A systematic review and meta-analysis on the effectiveness and safety of aquatic exercise in the treatment of knee and hip osteoarthritis suggested the need for more studies of clearly defined patient groups with long-term outcomes.[20]

Patients who have inadequate orofacial control can benefit from hydrotherapy by working on lip closure and bubble blowing, provided there are no problems with their swallowing mechanisms. Holding one's breath in water, gradually increasing the time in the pool, and swimming can improve endurance or respiratory function for patients with pulmonary dysfunction.[33–36] Impairments and functional deficits, including inadequate sitting and standing balance and ambulatory dysfunction, can be addressed with pool therapy.[33,34]

Patients with balance deficits can benefit from aquatic therapy because hydrostatic pressure and buoyancy help to support the body. Balance in chest-deep water is easier, and practiced recovery from disturbed balance can facilitate head-righting and trunk control.

Aquatic therapy can facilitate a patient's arousal because of the changed environment when entering a pool. Splashing, kicking, and turbulence of water can also improve alertness. Patients with hypersensitivity disorders can benefit from aquatic therapy by gradually immersing one extremity at a time into the pool, and performing enjoyable activities in the pool can help decrease hypersensitivity. Aquatic therapy can also be beneficial for patients with cognitive impairments, including perceptual-spatial problems such as neglect of distance or depth, poor eye-hand coordination, poor concept of midline, decreased sequencing abilities, and poor socialization skills.[37] In addition, psychological

---

CASE STUDY 5•3 SELECTING POOL THERAPY FOR A PATIENT WITH LOW BACK PAIN

A 64-year-old female is referred for strengthening of the back musculature secondary to low back pain and inability to tolerate land-based exercises. Upon testing, the patient was able to walk limited distances and was unable to move the trunk freely during any activities.

CLINICAL DECISION-MAKING

1. Does the patient have a dysfunction, limitation, or problem that can be improved with the use of pool therapy?
   Answer: Yes, pool therapy can be used to decrease pain, improve ROM, and increase the strength of the trunk musculature.

2. Is the patient appropriate for pool therapy? Do any of the general precautions or contraindications to pool therapy apply to the patient, or are there any specific considerations regarding the application of pool therapy to this patient?
   Answer: None of the precautions or contraindications apply to this patient. Pool therapy is an appropriate intervention for her.

3. What are the specific goals to be achieved with the use of pool therapy?
   Answer: Decreased pain, increased ROM, increased strength of the trunk musculature, and increased endurance.

4. What specific aspects of pool therapy would be appropriate for this patient?
   Answer: The buoyancy can be used to support the body while the muscles can be worked. The buoyancy can assist the motions of the involved muscles and can resist movement and improve strength of these muscles while improving endurance.

5. What are the proper application procedures for pool therapy?
   Answer: Inform the patient of the purpose and procedure, including the schedule of pool therapy sessions and the need for appropriate swimwear. Assess the patient's previous swimming experiences and her expectations for the sessions.
   Pre-session: Determine the techniques to be used during the session (seated, standing, prone or supine activities; depth of water to assist motions or challenge muscle; types and speeds of movements to achieve goals of session).
   Pool session: Monitor vital signs to ensure patient safety. Use safest method for entry into pool. Proceed with activities chosen for session and modify as needed.
   Post-session: Assess ROM and strength of involved muscles and endurance for ambulation on dry land. Determine progression of next pool therapy session and eventual progression to land-based exercises.

impairments,[38,39] such as depression, lack of confidence, or decreased motivation, can be addressed with aquatic therapy. Athletes can also benefit from aquatic therapy because water becomes an isophysiological environment that requires similar functional physiology used in competitive sports. Sport-specific movement patterns can be performed in water, and their intensity can be increased over time, depending on the athletes' functional improvements on land.[25]

Whirlpools are used for treating a variety of musculoskeletal conditions (Box 5-1). Cold whirlpools are typically used to help control pain and swelling of acute sprains and strains. Warm whirlpools are often used to facilitate motion and exercise for subacute and chronic stages of sprains and strains. Stretching of contractures may be facilitated by the simultaneous or immediate application of a warm whirlpool. Whirlpools may be applied following orthopedic surgery (after the surgical skin wounds are fully healed) to help soften scar tissue, reduce pain, and promote restoration of motion. Healing bone fractures may benefit from whirlpool once clinical union has been achieved. The fluidity and pressure properties of whirlpools assist in removing dry, scaly skin after casts have been removed, and the thermal and buoyancy properties of a warm whirlpool assist in increasing mobility.[40]

Patients with osteoarthritis or rheumatoid arthritis may benefit from whirlpool. The water's buoyancy effects will help support the affected joints and help to decrease pain and increase mobility. The thermal effects of a warm whirlpool may help decrease the pain of arthritis.[41–45] The relaxing effect of warm-water whirlpools is well known. Anxious patients may benefit from partial or full immersion in a whirlpool to facilitate cooperation with rehabilitation procedures.[38] The patient may use earplugs or headphones to blunt the noise of the turbine; this promotes relaxation while in the whirlpool.

Box 5•1	**Musculoskeletal Conditions Treated by Whirlpool**

- Sprains and strains
- Contractures
- Postsurgical repair of joints and soft tissues
- Healing fractures of bones
- Osteoarthritis
- Rheumatoid arthritis

Historically, whirlpools have been used in the care of open wounds. Whirlpools provide a method of cleansing through the addition of a bactericidal agent or mechanically debriding a wound to remove surface necrotic material when the patient is unable to tolerate more selective forms of debridement. The mechanical effects of whirlpools may stimulate formation of granulation tissue and, in conjunction with the appropriate water temperature, may soften tissues and stimulate circulation in the affected area. The increase in local circulation may boost the amount of oxygen, antibodies, leukocytes, and nutrition supplied to the tissues and enhance the removal of metabolites. The amount of systemic medications, such as antibiotics, available to the wound area may also be increased by the improved circulation, which helps to diminish or prevent infection. Whirlpools may also create sedation and analgesia, which may aid in reducing pain caused by the open wound or surrounding tissues. Unfortunately, whirlpools can prolong or prevent wound closure and are contraindicated for ulcers due to venous insufficiency, edema, or lymphedema. Therefore, using a whirlpool to treat an open wound must be carefully considered based on the known advantages and disadvantages of this modality.

Physical Properties of Water

An appreciation of the unique properties of water, including an understanding of its static and dynamic properties as they apply to immersion and exercise, is important to appropriately and effectively use hydrotherapy for therapeutic interventions. This section will discuss the physical properties of water, including buoyancy, viscosity, hydrostatic pressure, hydrodynamics, thermodynamics, physiological effects, and mechanics.

Buoyancy

One of the most important properties of water is buoyancy. Archimedes' principle states that "the buoyant force on a body immersed in a fluid is equal to the weight of the fluid displaced by that object."[46] A body or body part immersed in water will experience this buoyant force, which in effect reduces the force of gravity on the body. Thus, exercise of the extremities can be assisted by the effect of buoyancy. A person standing in water up to the neck can raise an extremity with the assistance of buoyancy. Buoyancy can also resist movement. An extremity moved downward against the force of buoyancy will encounter resistance to movement (Fig. 5-1). Resistance exercises for strengthening can be performed against the force of buoyancy. For example, a patient recovering from a surgical repair to his rotator cuff can use the buoyant force to raise the extremity from the side of the body to 90° of flexion or abduction while standing in neck-deep water. When returning the extremity to the side, buoyancy will be used as a resistance.

When a body is immersed or partially immersed in water, it is subjected to two opposing forces: buoyancy and gravity. The body will remain balanced, and no movement will take place if these forces are equal and opposite of each other. When these forces are unequal and unaligned, as when part of the body is out of the water while part of the body remains in the water, then the body will tend to move or rotate. This rotary motion may cause instability when an individual is partially immersed in water. The buoyancy of an object in water depends on its density (mass per unit volume). Objects that are denser than water will have less buoyancy and will tend to sink. Objects that are less dense than water will experience more buoyancy and will tend to float. The specific gravity of an object is defined as the ratio of the object's density to the water's density

at 4°C (39.2°F). Specific gravity is a number without dimensions or units. The specific gravity of water is 1.0, whereas the specific gravity of the body with air in the lungs is 0.974[47] (Table 5-1). Objects with a specific gravity less than 1.0 will displace a proportional amount of water. Therefore, the body will displace about 90% of water when immersed, and about 2.6% will float. This enables a person lying supine in water to keep his or her face out of the water while the remainder of the body is immersed slightly below the surface (Fig. 5-2).

Buoyancy of the body will be affected by the amount of air in the lungs. Fully inflated lungs will increase buoyancy, and deflated lungs will decrease buoyancy. Buoyancy is also dependent upon body composition. Obese individuals will have increased buoyancy because fat tissue has a lower specific gravity. Individuals with increased bone density will experience less buoyancy than those with bones that are less dense.

Table 5•1	Specific Gravity of Water, Ice, and Human Tissues
Substance	**Specific Gravity**
Water	1.0
Ice	0.917
Average human body with air in lungs	0.97
Average human body without air in lungs	1.1
Subcutaneous fat	0.85
Bone (femur)	~1.85
Bone (vertebral body)	~0.47

From Hecox, et al.[47]

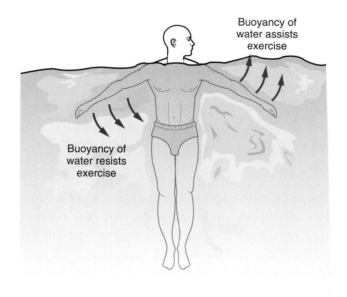

Fig 5•1 Exercising with buoyancy assists exercise; exercising against buoyancy resists exercise.

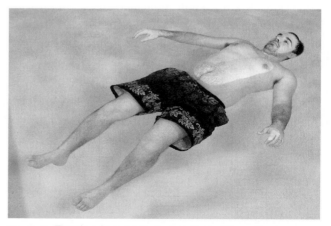

Fig 5•2 Floating in a pool demonstrates the effects of buoyancy.

Viscosity and Hydrostatic Pressure

Two properties of water that add to its therapeutic capabilities are *viscosity* and *hydrostatic pressure*. Viscosity is the internal friction present in liquids secondary to the cohesive forces between the molecules. When an arm or a leg is moved through water, the viscosity of the water will tend to resist this movement. The faster the limb is moved, the greater the resistance secondary to viscosity. Therefore, varying the speed of exercise will change the amount of resistance to exercise.

This principle can be applied to the patient with the rotator cuff problem described earlier and to many other patients. The viscosity of the water will act as resistance as the affected upper extremity is moved through the water: The faster the movement, the greater the resistance encountered. Therefore, the exercises performed in the pool can accomplish the goal of strengthening the shoulder musculature.

Hydrostatic pressure is the force that water exerts on the body or body part. This force impacts the body equally from all directions at a given depth of immersion. The amount of hydrostatic pressure will vary depending on the depth of immersion of the body part. A person standing in a pool of water up to his neck will have a greater amount of hydrostatic pressure against his feet than against his trunk or shoulders (Fig. 5-3).

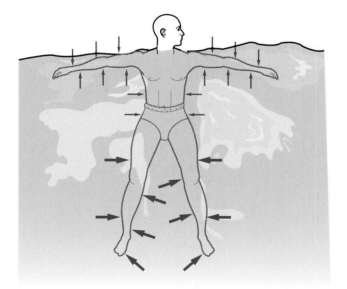

Fig 5•3 The amount of hydrostatic pressure against the body depends upon the depth of submersion of the body part. Smaller arrows represent lower hydrostatic pressure; larger arrows represent greater pressure.

Therefore, when a patient exercises near the water's surface, she will encounter less resistance than when exercising at a greater depth. This increased pressure may encourage venous return in a proximal direction from the lower extremities. Jamison[48,49] advocated this therapeutic effect of aquatic therapy, combined with the effect of viscosity, for increasing lymph flow and reducing edema in patients with lymphedema. However, the dependent position of the body part may cancel this effect. McCulloch and Boyd[50] found that the combination of heat and the dependent position of an extremity in a whirlpool have the potential to encourage lower extremity swelling.

Hydrodynamics

Water in motion has physical properties known as *hydrodynamics*. This includes the dynamics of two types of fluid flow. Streamline or laminar flow occurs when each particle of the fluid follows a smooth path without crossover of parts. Turbulent flow is the flow of fluids in erratic, small, whirlpool-like circles called *eddy currents* or *eddies*.[46] Turbulent water creates more resistance to movement. Movement of a body part in water at rest will encounter minimal turbulence, although the movement itself will create some turbulence. Movement against turbulent water will encounter more resistance as experienced when moving a body part in a whirlpool when the water is agitated.[47]

Thermodynamics: Heat Transfer

Physiological effects of hydrotherapy depend on the temperature of the water, the amount of the body immersed in the water, and whether the person receiving the treatment is at rest or moving. The water's temperature will affect the temperature of the tissues in the water. Heat will be transferred primarily by convection when the patient is moving in the water or when the water moves across the skin's surface. When the body and the water are at rest, some heat will be transferred by conduction. However, the layer of water immediately adjacent to the skin may act as a "sealer," which tends to inhibit conductive heat transfer. Agitation of the water in a whirlpool will limit this sealer effect.[47] The body will also lose heat by radiation and evaporation, depending on the amount of the body that is immersed and the environment's temperature and humidity.

Radiation is the exchange of electromagnetic energy between the warmer surface of the body and the cooler surrounding air, and evaporation is the loss of body fluids to the environment by sweating. These processes do not occur when the body surface is immersed in water. Care must be taken to expose a sufficient amount of body surface to the environment outside the hydrotherapy tank or pool to allow for radiational cooling and evaporation. The ability of the body to lose heat to help maintain a constant core temperature is limited when the hydrotherapy environment is too warm or too humid. The hydrotherapy environment must be kept at a comfortable temperature, usually an air temperature between 18.3°C and 26.7°C (65°F and 80°F) and a lower humidity (between 50% and 65%).[51,52]

Another property of water related to heat transfer is specific heat. The amount of heat required to change the temperature of a given material is proportional to the mass of the material and to the temperature change. This can be expressed in the following equation:

$$Q = mc\,\Delta T$$

where Q is the amount of heat, *m* is the mass of the material, *c* is the specific heat, and ΔT is the change in temperature.[46] Specific heat is a measure of the amount of energy (heat) stored in a material and the amount of energy required to heat the material. Water has one of the highest specific heats of all substances (1.00 kcal/kg·C° at 15°C).[46] This is evident in the difference in heat between water and paraffin. Paraffin is usually applied to the skin at a temperature between 45°C and 54°C (113°F and 129.1°F); water at these temperatures would likely feel too hot and may burn the skin.

Physiological Effects of Water

Hemodynamics

The hemodynamic effects of hydrotherapy include local changes in circulation and systemic effects on cardiac function. The water's temperature will either cause an increase in localized circulation secondary to vasodilation or a decrease in localized circulation secondary to vasoconstriction. Generally, warm water temperatures, about 35.5°C (95.9°F), will result in vasodilation, and cold water temperatures below 27°C (80.6°F)

will cause vasoconstriction. Table 5-2 summarizes the physiological effects of commonly used water temperatures for hydrotherapy.

Immersion of most of the body (with the head out of the water) or just the face will result in a set of cardiovascular effects known as the *dive reflex*.[53] These effects include bradycardia, peripheral vasoconstriction, and preferential shunting of blood to vital organs. However, these effects are dependent on the water's temperature. Immersion in warm or hot water increases heart rate, and immersion in water at body temperature has a neutral effect on heart rate.[54]

Immersion in water may affect blood pressure. Enhanced venous return secondary to a rise in central venous pressure with immersion increases cardiac volume, which causes an increase in right atrial pressure and increased cardiac output (assuming normal cardiac pump mechanics). However, the effect on blood pressure may be blunted secondary to the effects of the dive reflex, resulting in bradycardia.

KEY POINT! When exercising in water, monitoring heart rate may not be an accurate reflection of cardiovascular stress. Therefore, monitoring perceived exertion is preferred over monitoring of heart rate.

The effects on the cardiovascular system (sudden vasoconstriction, decrease in heart rate, and increase in heart volume from increased venous return) may not be

Table 5•2	Water Temperature Classification for Hydrotherapy
Very cold	33°F–55°F; 1°C–13°C
Cold	56°F–65°F; 14°C–18°C
Cool	66°F–80°F; 19°C–26°C
Tepid	81°F–92°F; 27°C–32°C
Neutral	93°F–96°F; 33°C–35°C
Warm	97°F–99°F; 36°C–37°C
Hot	100°F–104°F; 38°C–40°C
Very hot	105°F–110°F; 41°C–43°C
Expected Physiological Effect of Water Temperatures	
Very cold, cold, cool	Vasoconstriction, analgesia, possible anesthesia
Tepid and neutral	Likely no loss of body heat or change in core temperature or limb size (best temperature range for pool exercise)
Warm and hot	Vasodilation, analgesia, relaxation
Very hot	Same as warm and hot temperatures but may cause rapid fatigue and overheating

tolerated by some, particularly those with cardiovascular deficits. To limit the effects on the cardiovascular system, it is best to enter the water slowly, wetting the face and hands first, and avoid full-body immersions in cold water.[53]

Effects of Water on the Respiratory System

Immersing the body in water may affect the ability to breathe. Hydrostatic pressure against the chest will tend to inhibit lung expansion. Also, increased circulation to the center of the body during immersion will increase circulation in the chest cavity, further inhibiting lung expansion. Maximal oxygen uptake is lower during most forms of water exercise than during exercise on land.[53]

Effects of Water on Renal Function

Water immersion can affect renal function, resulting in increased urine output (diuresis), increased sodium excretion, and increased potassium excretion. These effects can be potentiated when the individual is immersed in cold water. Patients should empty their bladders prior to entering a therapeutic pool.

Effects of Water on the Neurological System

Effects of water immersion on the neurological system are primarily temperature dependent. The effects of cold and heat on the neurological system are discussed in Chapters 2 and 3. Warm water tends to be relaxing, whereas cold water tends to be invigorating or stimulating. Whether these effects are secondary to direct effects on the nervous system or are examples of psychological responses is debatable and requires further study.

Effects of Water on the Muscular System

Direct effects on the muscular system are probably secondary to temperature effects, such as increased muscular blood flow secondary to immersion of a muscle in warm water. Clinical use of hydrotherapy for relaxation of muscle spasm may in part be a result of increased blood flow by immersion in warm water. Agitation of the water, as in a whirlpool bath, may also help relax muscle spasms by increasing sensory stimulation of the water against the skin overlying the spastic muscle, resulting in analgesia that will help break the "pain/

spasm" cycle. Muscle strength may be increased with exercise in water, especially when exercising against turbulence. There is no evidence that muscles at rest will be strengthened by placing the limb in still or agitated water; however, the relaxing, stimulating, or analgesic effects of a whirlpool may be helpful preparation for an exercise program. For example, a patient with low back pain may benefit from the effects of whirlpool agitation against the back prior to starting an exercise program on land or in a pool.

Mechanical Effects of Water

The mechanical effects of water primarily occur during agitation in a whirlpool or with application of a forceful stream to the body such as with a wound-irrigation device. The force of the water can help débride loose necrotic tissue in a wound and cleanse the wound of dirt and other contaminants. Water has a softening effect on tissue, which may facilitate debridement of necrotic tissue. However, water applied to wounds may damage new granulation tissue, and prolonged soaking may cause maceration of intact skin.[55]

Aquatic (Pool) Therapy

Indications, Precautions, and Contraindications

Most patients will be able to participate in aquatic therapy; however, there are precautions that should be considered before proceeding with pool therapy. Patients who are fearful of water may experience increased symptoms, such as muscle guarding or improper technique during exercises. Some patients may be leery of losing their balance or sinking to the bottom. In instances like these, a gradual orientation to the water may be necessary, including using flotation devices or starting slowly in shallow water to build confidence.[25] Patients with neurological involvement, such as those with multiple sclerosis, may fatigue quickly when exercising in water greater than 33°C (91.4°F).[56–58] Patients with controlled epilepsy may need to be monitored for medication compliance prior to treatment and for responses during treatment. Anyone with cardiovascular problems, such as high or low blood pressure or a history of angina, heart disease, or compromised pump mechanics, will require close monitoring during treatment.[6,7,59] Meyer and Leblanc[60] reviewed selected publications on patients with left ventricular dysfunction or stable congestive heart failure. They made the following suggestions for rehabilitation and secondary prevention:

1. Temporary abnormal hemodynamic responses may be elicited by immersion up to the neck.
2. Water therapy is absolutely contraindicated in patients with decompensated congestive heart failure.
3. Feeling good in water does not equate with left ventricular toleration of increased volume loading caused by immersion.
4. If patients with previous severe myocardial infarctions or congestive heart failure can sleep supine, they may be able to tolerate bathing in a half-sitting position provided immersion does not exceed the xiphoid process.
5. Patients with Q-wave myocardial infarctions older than 6 weeks may exercise in a pool for orthopedic reasons provided that they do so in an upright position and immersion does exceed the xiphoid process.

An algorithm to support clinical decision-making for prescribing swimming to patients with left ventricular dysfunction or stable congestive heart failure can be found in the article by Meyer and Leblanc.[60]

Patients with open wounds may participate in pool therapy if the wound is covered and secured with a waterproof dressing. Patients with catheters, colostomies, intravenous lines, or other open lines may participate in pool therapy; however, they will require proper clamping and fixation. Similar precautions should be followed for patients who have G-tubes and suprapubic appliances. These patients should be observed for any adverse reactions to pool therapy. Patients with medically controlled seizure disorders or fear of water should be monitored for any adverse reactions to the treatment.

There are several factors that must be considered when deciding whether pool therapy is appropriate for a patient. Any situation that creates the potential for contamination of the water is considered a contraindication for aquatic therapy. Open wounds without occlusive dressings, incontinence of bowel or bladder,

skin infections, menstruation without internal protection, and patients with isolation precautions are included in this category of contraindications. A general rule to follow is patients should be free of bowel and bladder accidents for at least 5 days prior to pool therapy. Patients with a history of uncontrolled seizures during the last year, severe cardiac precautions, acute fever, upper respiratory infection, severe mental disorders, and severe pulmonary conditions, especially with vital capacity less than 1,500 milliliters, are considered poor candidates for aquatic therapy since these conditions may be exacerbated by water immersion. Patients with halo vests are not candidates for pool therapy, because the site of the halo pins' insertion into the skull is considered an open wound. See Table 5-3 for a complete list of contraindications for aquatic (pool) therapy.

Clinical Controversy

Patients with arthritis of the knees, hips, and spine are often prescribed aquatic therapy by their physicians. There are many benefits of exercise in a pool; however, do these benefits justify the cost of resources required for aquatic therapy? Can patients with arthritis benefit equally as well with therapeutic exercise programs in rehabilitation clinics ("land" therapy)? What is the optimal number of exercise sessions per week for aquatic therapy? And how many sessions of aquatic therapy are needed for improved patient function? When can patients be discharged from aquatic therapy programs to pool exercise programs that they can perform independently? Does the chronic nature of arthritis justify long-term aquatic therapy programs? These are some of the questions that practitioners must consider when initiating aquatic therapy programs for patients with arthritis.

Pools and Pool Area

Therapeutic pools vary in size and shape, depending on the patient populations served and the space allocations at a given facility. Traditional swimming pools, specially designed therapeutic pools, and self-contained exercise units can be used for aquatic therapy. Traditional swimming pools are at least 100 feet long and 25 feet wide, with a bottom that begins to slope at a depth of 3 to 4 feet and gradually increases to a depth of 8 to 10 feet. This type of pool can accommodate several groups of patients and the practitioners who are

Table 5•3 Aquatic (Pool) Therapy Precautions and Contraindications[92]

Precaution/Contraindication	Explanation
Aspiration risk	Follow precautions if patient has a history of aspiration.
Bowel or bladder incontinence	If this is uncontrolled, patient cannot enter pool because of danger of cross-contamination of other tissues and other people in the pool.
Tracheostomy	Contraindication because of respiratory concerns
Catheters	Patients with indwelling catheters require proper clamping and fixation.
Infectious diseases	Contraindication for aquatic therapy because of the danger of spreading infection to others in the pool.
Cardiovascular problems	Contraindicated in patients with decompensated congestive heart failure. Monitor vital signs of patients with other cardiovascular problems, such as uncontrolled blood pressure.
Cognitive impairments	Concerns with safety when entering and leaving pool. Must be monitored closely while in pool.
Uncontrolled seizures	Contraindication because of danger of having a seizure while in the pool.
Tetraplegia or high paraplegia	Difficulty with thermoregulation. Monitor patient and temperature of water and air to prevent heat prostration and hypothermia.
Respiratory compromise, vital capacity less than 1 L	Contraindication if immersion is likely to exacerbate symptoms
Open wounds	Must be covered with waterproof dressing to prevent infection and maceration of periwound tissue.
Fever	Exercise in the pool stresses the cardiopulmonary and immune system.
Dry skin or skin rashes or rash	Time in pool may exacerbate dryness.
Fear of water	May increase symptoms, such as muscle guarding or improper techniques during exercise
Fear of losing balance or sinking	Need to gradually orient with use of flotation devices in shallow water or starting in shallow water to build confidence
Neurological impairments	May fatigue quickly in water greater than 33°C (91.4°F).
Severe kidney disease during immersion	May be unable to adjust to fluid loss
Menstruation without internal protection	May contaminate pool

conducting the therapy session (Fig. 5-4). Smaller, self-contained exercise pools are designed for individual patient use (Fig. 5-5). These units do not allow for the practitioner to be in the pool with the patient; therefore, they are not appropriate for patients who have low functional levels and who require assistance in the pool.

Access to a traditional pool is by ramp, stairs, ladders, or mechanical overhead lift. Some specially designed pools have floors that have adjustable heights to permit easier access. Therapeutic pools have a built-in filtration and chlorination system. The room in which the pool is housed needs to be adequately ventilated to avoid condensation accumulating on walls, windows, and floors. Water on floors can cause slippery conditions that can lead to patient or practitioner slips

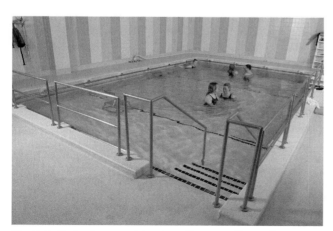

Fig 5•4 Patients exercising in a therapeutic pool.

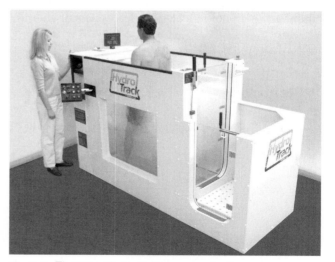

Fig 5•5 Therapeutic hydrotherapy unit. *(Photo courtesy of Ferno-Washington, Inc.)*

and falls. Immediate drying of wet floors with sponges or towels is a must. Use of nonslip floor mats or rubber or plastic grids around whirlpool tanks may help prevent slips and falls. Patients should wear sandals with nonskid soles or other similar footwear when walking on therapeutic pool aprons. Careful guarding of patients during transfers in and out of the pool will also help prevent falls. A private area for changing clothes, showering, and cooling down should be available to the patient following therapeutic exercise sessions.

Access to the smaller self-contained exercise pools is either via a door and steps located on one side of the unit or from a stair or two inside the unit. These units usually have their own filtration system and may include built-in exercise stations, varying water depths, and integrated treadmills. Some pools produce adjustable currents that increase exercise resistance and simulate wave action.

There are many types of equipment that can be used in pool therapy sessions. These include floats, resistive paddles, paddle boards, swim fins, flotation vests, parallel bars, treadmills, handrails, weighted stools and chairs, and weighted walkers. Examples of patients exercising with equipment can be seen in Figures 5-6 through 5-8. The type of equipment used during a particular session is based on the patient's current functional level and the goals for the aquatic therapy session.

Pool Care and Safety Precautions

Regular care and cleaning of therapeutic pools is essential to avoid the buildup of *Pseudomonas aeruginosa*,[61–63] a bacteria that causes folliculitis infections. Organic contaminants in a pool reduce the effectiveness of chlorine

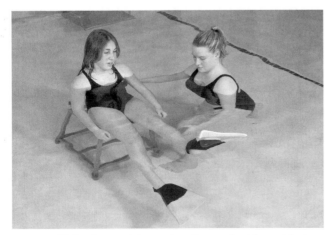

Fig 5•6 Patient exercising using fins on feet for added resistance in therapeutic pool.

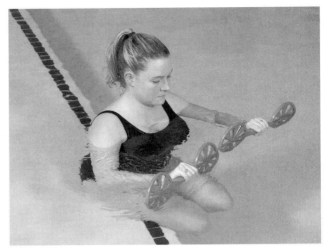

Fig 5•7 Patient exercising her upper extremities using paddles in therapeutic pool.

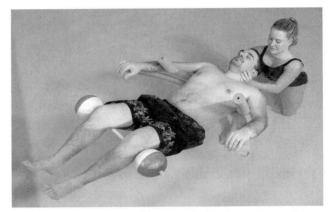

Fig 5•8 Therapist stretching cervical spine while patient uses foam noodles for buoyancy in therapeutic pool.

when used as a bactericidal agent. Frequent use of pools increases the total organic carbon as well as ammonia and organic nitrogen found in the pool. Regular care of therapeutic pools should include at least weekly cleaning and twice-daily chlorine and pH level tests. Walking surfaces leading up to and around the pool should be slip-resistant and kept free of barriers.

Safety rules and regulations and emergency procedures should be established. Rules and regulations should be posted and observed by both patients and staff. An obvious danger whenever a patient is immersed in water is drowning.

KEY POINT! Patients who are immersed in large whirlpools or therapeutic pools should be monitored continuously, especially if they have decreased mental function or drowsiness secondary to the effects of medication.

Children must always be closely supervised. Life preservers should be available for all therapeutic pools. At least one staff member who is CPR certified should be present at all times in case of an emergency.

Clinical Applications of Therapeutic Pools

Practitioners should meet with patients prior to exercise in a therapeutic pool to discuss the treatment schedule and the procedures to be used. The patient's previous swimming experiences should be addressed, including any fear of water and his or her expectations for the session. Other topics to be discussed with patients prior to entering a therapeutic pool include any bowel and bladder problems, use of any assistive or adaptive devices, type of clothing to be worn while in the pool and after leaving the pool, and medications.

KEY POINT! Practitioners should have a complete list of the patient's current medications and discuss with the patient any effect these medications may have while exercising in the pool. Medications that cause drowsiness or sedation, such as muscle relaxants, require close monitoring of the patient while he or she is in the pool.

The practitioner should be aware of the increased demand placed on the patient's cardiovascular and pulmonary systems. Core temperature can be increased by the water temperature, and muscular contraction places a greater demand on heat dissipation, the respiratory system, and the exposed integument. General considerations should include a maximum immersion time of 20 minutes for noncompromised cardiopulmonary patients and less time for elderly, hypertensive, or cardiopulmonary patients. It may be advisable to initiate treatment for 10 minutes and increase as tolerated.[64,65]

Vital signs must be monitored to ensure patient safety. Water temperatures vary, and therapeutic pool temperatures cannot be quickly adjusted. In general, water temperatures between 36°C and 37°C (96.8°F and 98.6°F) are considered high and between 30°C and 34.5°C (86°F and 94.1°F) are considered low. High temperatures may be recommended for patients with disease processes, such as rheumatoid arthritis (except in the acute stage), while low temperatures may be recommended for patients with spasticity or for those

whose immersion time may last 20 to 45 minutes. A patient's fatigue factor should be considered when choosing therapeutic pool temperatures.[58,59]

A complete review of specific types of exercises and exercise programs is beyond the scope of this text. For more information on aquatic exercise programs, see Box 5-2 for a list of references, and see Box 5-3 for websites related to aquatic therapy.

Box 5·2	**References for Aquatic Therapy Exercises**

Duffield MH, Skinner AT, Thompson AM. *Duffield's Exercise in Water*. Philadelphia: W.B. Saunders; 1983.

Kisner C, Cobly LA. *Therapeutic Exercise, Foundations and Techniques*. 5th ed. Philadelphia: F.A. Davis; 2007.

Koury JM. *Aquatic Therapy Programming—Guidelines for Orthopedic Rehabilitation*. Champaign, IL: Human Kinetics; 1996.

Lepore M, Gayle GW, Stevens FS. *Adapted Aquatics Programming—A Professional Guide*. 2nd ed. Champaign, IL: Human Kinetics; 2007.

Norm A, Bates H. *Aquatic Exercise Therapy*. Philadelphia: W. B. Saunders; 1996.

Norton CO, Jamison LJ. *A Team Approach to the Aquatic Continuum of Care*. St. Louis, MO: Elsevier Health Sciences; 2000.

Rosenstein, AA. *Water Exercises for Parkinson's: Maintaining Balance, Strength, Endurance, and Flexibility*. Rev ed. Enumclaw, WA: Idyll Arbor; 2008.

Sova, R. *Aquatics: The Complete Reference Guide for Aquatic Fitness Professionals*. Port Washington, WI: DSL; 2000.

Sova, R. *Essential Principles of Aquatic Therapy and Rehabilitation*. Port Washington, WI: DSL; 2003.

Vargas, LG. *Aquatic Therapy: Interventions and Applications*. Enumclaw, WA: Idyll Arbor; 2004.

Box 5·3	**Websites Related to Aquatic Therapy**

http://www.ncpad.org/exercise
This website is maintained by the National Center on Physical Activity and Disability, based at the University of Illinois. It has definitions of aquatic therapy techniques, a list of conditions in which aquatic therapy is useful, sample programs, sample techniques, program modifications, and more basic information.

http://www.aeawave.com
This website provides standards and guidelines for aquatic fitness programming from the Aquatic Exercise Association.

http://www.mayoclinic.com/health/aquatic-exercise/SM00055&slide=1
This website provides basic instruction on a few simple aquatic exercises through a short series of slides with accompanying information.

A Word About Hot Tubs and Jacuzzis

Hot tubs and Jacuzzis are popular in many health clubs and homes. These types of units are not intended for aquatic pool sessions because of their small size and high water temperature. Water temperatures are generally in the 38.9°C to 40.5°C (102°F to 104.9°F) range, which places a greater demand on the cardiovascular and pulmonary systems. Regular care and cleaning of hot tubs and Jacuzzis is required to avoid the buildup of *P. aeruginosa*.[61–63] The high temperatures and turbulence of the water in hot tubs and Jacuzzis increases the potential for the presence of pathogens. A good filtration and chlorination system, similar to those found in therapeutic pools, is an essential requirement for all hot tubs and Jacuzzis.

Whirlpools

Whirlpools are enclosed stainless-steel or acrylic tanks of various sizes that are used clinically to provide therapeutic effects. These tanks have an attached motor, called a *turbine,* that agitates the water in the tank to create the "whirlpool" effect. Smaller tanks can be portable and filled with a hose; larger tanks are nonportable and have attachments to faucets to provide water to the tank. Whirlpools are intended to be used as single-patient treatments and must be drained and cleaned after each use.

Types of Whirlpools

Whirlpools are available in various sizes to accommodate either a body part or full-body (with the face out of the water) immersion. Small whirlpools are designed to treat distal parts of the upper or lower extremities. They are often portable, with attached wheels for ease of movement (Fig. 5-9). Larger whirlpools can accommodate the entire upper or lower extremity or partial or full immersion of the body. Low-boy tanks have low walls that allow for ease of transfer in and out of the tank (Fig. 5-10). Patients in a low-boy are usually in a long-sitting position during treatment. High-boy tanks, sometimes referred to as *hip tanks,* require a chair or lift to transfer in and out of the tank (Fig. 5-11). Patients in a high-boy tank are usually sitting on a removable seat attached to rungs on the side of the tank, or they may sit on a high

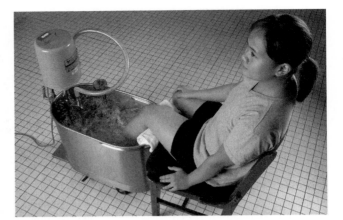

Fig 5•9 Small portable (ankle/foot/hand) whirlpool.

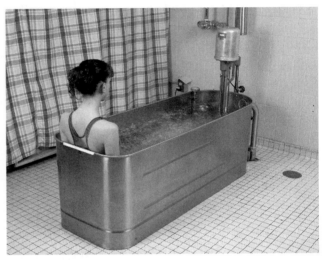

Fig 5•10 Low-boy whirlpool.

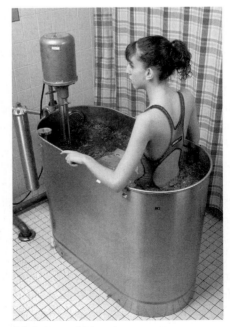

Fig 5•11 High-boy whirlpool.

chair outside the tank with their lower extremity dangling in the tank. Burn tanks are specially designed for treating patients with burns. They are usually larger than extremity tanks and require a lift for patient transfer into and out of the tank. Some of these tanks are designed without seams; this helps prevent infections by limiting sites in the tank that are more difficult to clean and disinfect.[54]

Hubbard tanks are large whirlpools designed for full-body (with the face out) immersion. The first Hubbard tank was designed in 1928 primarily for underwater exercise.[66] The wide top and bottom and narrow middle (Fig. 5-12) allows the patient to exercise the extremities and provides the practitioner access to the patient for assistance with exercise. Patients are typically lowered into the tank on a stretcher by an overhead hydraulic hoist. Hubbard tanks are used for patients who require full-body immersion and who are unable to stand or transfer safely into and out of whirlpools. These tanks usually have two whirlpool turbines that can be moved around the perimeter of the tank to direct and control the agitation pattern. Some tanks have a walking trough with parallel bars for gait training. A typical Hubbard tank holds over 400 gallons of water. The cost of the water, which in most cases must be heated, and the time and personnel required to fill, empty, and clean the Hubbard tank after each use causes this modality to be more expensive than other therapeutic alternatives. Some health-care facilities have removed their Hubbard tanks as a cost-cutting and space-saving measure.

Turbine

The turbine is the electrical motor pump that creates the agitation in a whirlpool (Fig. 5-13). A switch on the top of the turbine turns the motor on or off. Attached to the turbine are two or three tubular metal shafts. One of these tubes is the drive shaft, which contains an impeller housed in a casing at the bottom of the tube. The amount of water ejected at the base of the drive shaft determines the force of the ejected water. Adjusting the throttle near the top of the shaft can control the amount of water ejected. The other tube is called the *breather tube*. The amount of air mixing with the ejected water (aeration) at the base of the breather tube can be adjusted by turning the butterfly valve near the shaft's top. Agitation of the water in the whirlpool tank can be regulated by adjusting the force of the ejected water and the amount of aeration. The entire turbine assembly is usually mounted on a spring-loaded adjustable pole on the side of the whirlpool tank. This allows for height and side-to-side adjustments of the turbine, which enables the clinician to direct the ejected water toward or away from the body or body part in the whirlpool tank.

Near the bottom of the turbine's middle shaft, on the side, is a small hole. This hole must be under the surface of the water whenever the turbine motor is turned on. Care must also be taken to ensure that the turbine ejector at the bottom of the turbine shaft is not blocked by bandages, wound packing, or patient fingers or toes.

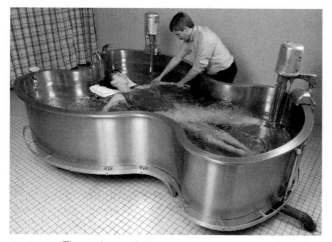

Fig 5•12 Therapist assisting patient as she exercises in Hubbard tank.

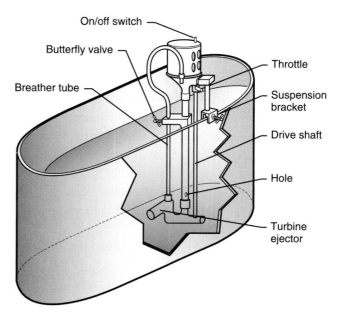

Fig 5•13 Turbine attached to a whirlpool.

Electrical Safety

Electrical safety is an essential concern for all hydrotherapy devices that have an attached turbine. Ground fault circuit interrupters (GFCIs) are required for all hydrotherapy outlets. The function of the GFCIs should be checked, and the condition of the turbine wire should be inspected for damage prior to performing any whirlpool treatments. The attachment of the turbine on the adjustable pole should also be inspected to be certain it is tightly secured. An unsecured turbine could come loose during position adjustments and fall into the whirlpool tank, potentially causing a fatal electrical shock. Patients should be instructed to *never* touch the turbine, including the on/off switch, when it is running.

Clinical Applications for Whirlpools

Preparatory Considerations

Before initiating a whirlpool treatment, the therapeutic objectives of the treatment should be determined. These may include (1) facilitation of exercise either for assistance or resistance, (2) promotion of muscle relaxation and pain relief, (3) mechanical debridement of wound surface exudates and necrotic tissue, and (4) stimulation of circulation for wound care. Next, the proper temperature should be selected, based on the patient's medical condition and treatment objectives. (Commonly used temperatures and their corresponding generic names are listed in Table 5-2.) In general, temperatures between 36.5°C to 40.5°C (98°F and 105°F) are reasonable when using heat, except in the presence of peripheral vascular disease, sensory loss, or full-body immersion. With peripheral vascular disease, the skin temperature of the extremity to be immersed can be a guideline to help determine water temperature and should not be greater than 1°F or 1°C above skin temperature. In the presence of cardiovascular or pulmonary disease, the temperature should not exceed 38°C (100°F).

The body part to be treated should be inspected for skin temperature, presence of edema, open lesions, color, muscle spasm, and sensation. The treatment procedure and safe operation of the whirlpool should be explained to the patient to reduce anxiety and promote safety. The patient should be positioned comfortably using padding or pillows as needed. The whirlpool may then be activated and the agitation force set initially at a minimal level and increased as needed. Be sure not to direct the agitation directly toward any body area that may cause tissue damage or increased pain. The patient should not be left unattended during the treatment session. Patients on a lift chair or stretcher should be secured by straps when immersed in whirlpools or secured by straps if sitting in an elevated chair during lower extremity treatment in an extremity tank.

Whirlpool Duration

The length of time for treatment in a whirlpool must be based on sound physiological judgment and on the treatment objectives. The duration of treatment also depends upon the pathologies being treated. When used strictly as a heating modality, the usual duration is 20 minutes, depending on the patient's medical condition. Borrell and colleagues[67] demonstrated that 20 minutes was a long enough time to increase skin, muscle, and joint capsule temperature in the hand and foot.

Abramson and associates[68] demonstrated that a 20-minute application of moist heat increased blood flow, and further exposure of up to 2 hours had no real effect on increasing the peak response obtained at the 20-minute mark. When using a whirlpool to débride and clean a wound, the duration will vary from 5 to 20 minutes, depending on the amount of necrotic tissue and patient tolerance. Niederhuber, Stribley, and Koepke[69] found that 20 minutes of agitation in a whirlpool was optimal for removing skin bacteria. A duration of 10 to 30 minutes is recommended for patients who are exercising in the whirlpool, depending on the patient's medical status.

Cleaning and Disinfecting Whirlpools

No chemical additives are necessary in whirlpool water when the skin is intact (use of chemical additives for open wounds is discussed later in this chapter). Whirlpool tanks must be drained, cleaned, and disinfected after each use. Practitioners should wear gloves and goggles to protect the hands and eyes when doing this. The inside surface of the tank, turbine tubes, and drains should first be manually scrubbed with a cleanser, then thoroughly rinsed with clean water. Next, a disinfectant should be applied to the inside of the tank and turbine tubes (following label-recommended dilutions) for no more than 10 minutes. The tank is then thoroughly rinsed and dried. Sterilization of whirlpool tanks is not practical or necessary.[70]

Lower Extremity Techniques

Lower extremity immersion or immersion to the midthoracic level can be achieved by using either a high-boy or low-boy whirlpool tank. The high-boy tank requires that the patient be able to flex the hip and knee. The length of this tub does not allow for full extension of the average adult's lower extremity and limits the amount of ROM exercise a person can perform while in the whirlpool. However, its depth allows a greater body surface area to be submerged safely and comfortably, including submersion up to the midthoracic region. The low-boy tank is not as deep but has greater length than the high-boy, and it affords the patient the ability to fully extend the lower extremities and perform full-motion exercises for the knees. When only the distal portion of the lower extremity has to be immersed, either a small extremity tank or a high-boy tank with the use of the whirlpool chair is the appropriate choice.

In summary, the high-boy and low-boy afford greater body-surface immersion than a small extremity tank, while the low-boy may allow for greater lower extremity extension than the high-boy. If a patient is unable to safely transfer into one of these tubs, the high-boy or low-boy can be fitted with a hydraulic chair lift or "Hoyer lift."

Upper Extremity Techniques

When treating the upper extremity, the patient should be seated comfortably next to the extremity tank, with a towel or other form of padding on the tank edge to avoid constricting the circulatory and lymphatic system (Fig. 5-14).

KEY POINT! Use of a whirlpool for treating the upper or lower extremity deserves special consideration because the dependent position of the extremity in the tank may promote edema, especially when higher temperatures are used.

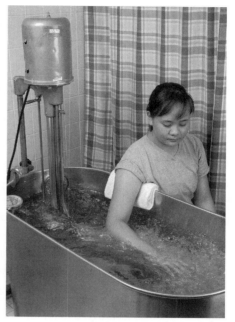

Fig 5•14 Whirlpool treatment to the hand and forearm. Caution should be used to avoid a totally dependent position of the hand. If possible, active ROM exercises should be performed during the treatment to encourage venous and lymphatic return, thus minimizing edema formation.

Magness and coworkers[71] studied the effect of whirlpool on volume in the upper extremity. They measured upper extremity volume in 20 normal male and female volunteers before and after the immersion of the same extremity for 20 minutes in a whirlpool bath at temperatures ranging from 33.5°C to 44.4°C (92.3°F to 111.9°F). In addition, 20 patients with various upper extremity disorders were treated by whirlpool in the same manner at temperatures ranging from 37.8°C to 40°C (100°F to 104°F) for 20 minutes. The results revealed a significant increase in volume for the normal subjects, which were directly related to increased water temperature. There was also a significant increase in volume of the patient's extremity, and the rise in volume was greater than in the normal subjects at the specific temperatures treated.

Hoyrup and Kjorvel[72] studied the effect of whirlpool and paraffin dips on hand volume, ROM, and pain in patients with traumatic hand injuries. The patients received whirlpool at 43°C (109.4°F) and paraffin dips at 50°C (122°F). One half of each group performed exercises; the other half did not. A significant reduction in pain and increase in motion were found. There was no significant change in hand volume during a 3-week period.

However, daily increases in volume were significant, and the changes were significantly greater in the whirlpool group. Therefore, these studies suggest exercising discrimination when choosing to use a whirlpool to treat upper extremity disorders in patients for whom edema is a primary concern.

Clinical Controversy

Using the whirlpool for acute sprains allows the practitioner to apply cold water to the entire circumference of a joint and allows for active ROM during the treatment. The goal is to decrease edema by the effects of cold and assist active movement of the joint to help maintain mobility. However, the dependent position of the extremity in the whirlpool tank inhibits venous return, which may limit edema reduction and possibly exacerbate edema in the joint. Therefore, practitioners must consider whether other cryotherapy modalities would be a better choice for acute sprains when the goal is to limit or decrease edema.

Full-Body Immersion

Large, full-body immersion tanks such as the Hubbard tank can be used for the following: (1) a patient with arthritis who is in an exacerbation phase and is unable to negotiate transfer into a smaller tank but who requires the use of heat and water to help with exercising, maintaining ROM, and providing pain relief; (2) a patient with paresis of the extremities who is actively able to move his or her extremities in the buoyancy of water but unable to do so without such assistance; (3) a patient with extensive burns; (4) an elderly or debilitated patient with an open wound on the buttocks, hip, or back. After a full-body immersion, whirlpool patients may experience some light-headedness, especially if the water was very warm. This may be avoided by having the patient rest in a lying or sitting position for 5 to 10 minutes before standing.

Contrast Bath

A contrast bath requires two whirlpool tubs or plastic basins (Fig. 5-15). One is filled with cold water at a tem-

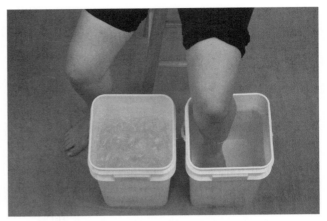

Fig 5•15 Contrast bath for ankle sprain. Tub on the right contains warm water; tub on the left contains cold water.

perature ranging from 13°C to 18°C (55°F to 65°F), and the other is filled with hot water at a temperature ranging from 38°C to 43°C (100°F to 110°F). The tubs or basins should be large enough to accommodate immersion of the extremity. A common technique is to first place the extremity into the hot water for 3 or 4 minutes, followed by immersing the extremity in the cold water for 1 or 2 minutes. This cycle continues for 20 to 30 minutes, with the last immersion in the hot water if the condition is chronic, cold water if the condition is subacute. The specific times for immersion can vary, although a hot-to-cold water ratio of 3:1 or 4:2 is typically used. The cycling of immersion of the limb in hot and cold water is thought to trigger a vascular pumping action caused by vasodilation (hot water) and vasoconstriction (cold water). Hypothetically, this will stimulate local circulation in the treated extremity and, to a lesser extent, increase circulation in the contralateral untreated extremity. However, any change in circulation that may occur is likely to be limited to superficial vasculature only.

Fiscus et al.[73] studied the effects of a 4:1 (hot:cold) contrast bath on circulation in the lower legs of 24 healthy men. Fluctuations in blood flow occurred during the 20-minute contrast bath; however, the authors believed that these changes were likely secondary to changes in cutaneous circulation and not intramuscular circulation. Several other studies failed to show significant changes in muscle temperature in subjects who received contrast baths.[74–76] A study by Cote and colleagues[77] found that contrast baths *increased* edema in postacute sprained ankles. The use of contrast bath for edema reduction is not supported by research and needs further study.

Contrast baths have been recommended for pain relief and desensitization. Kuligowski and associates[78] found decreased pain perception and improved elbow flexion following contrast baths after eccentric contractions of the elbow flexors. Vaile et al.[79] studied the effect of contrast baths on delayed-onset muscle soreness (DOMS). Subjects who received contrast baths following lower extremity exercise had a reduction in the physiological and functional deficits associated with DOMS, including improved recovery of isometric force and dynamic power and a reduction in localized edema. Hamlin[80] compared "contrast temperature water therapy" to active recovery in athletes. After running sprints, subjects were immersed in hip-height cold water for 1 minute, followed by 1 minute hot water showers for three cycles. Compared to the active postsprint recovery group, the contrast water therapy group had a substantial decrease in blood lactate concentration and heart rate.

KEY POINT! Contraindications and precautions for the use of contrast baths are based on the effects of heat, cold, and water. Patients who have any contraindications for the use of heat, cold, or water should not receive contrast baths.

Patients with small-vessel vascular disease secondary to diabetes, arteriosclerotic endarteritis, or Buerger's disease may not be able to tolerate the rapid change in temperatures used in contrast baths. Circulation in these patients must be monitored carefully. Contrast baths may be contraindicated for these patients depending on the severity of the disease.

Indications for Whirlpool Treatments

Musculoskeletal Conditions

Whirlpools have been used to treat musculoskeletal conditions such as sprains and strains. Cool or cold whirlpools are typically used to help control pain and swelling of acute sprains and strains, and warm or hot

whirlpools are often used to facilitate motion and exercise for subacute and chronic stages of sprains and strains. Range of motion of stiff or painful joints may be facilitated by whirlpool treatment. Stretching of soft tissue contractures may be aided by the simultaneous or immediate preapplication of a warm whirlpool. Whirlpools may be applied after orthopedic surgery (after the surgical skin wounds are fully healed) to help soften scar tissue, reduce pain, and promote restoration of motion. Patients with healing fractures may benefit from whirlpool once clinical union has been achieved. The fluidity and pressure properties of whirlpools assist in removing dry, scaly skin after casts have been removed, and the thermal and buoyancy properties of a warm whirlpool may assist in increasing joint and limb mobility.[40]

Patients with osteoarthritis or rheumatoid arthritis may benefit from whirlpool. The buoyancy effects of the water will decrease weight-bearing compression forces on the affected joints and can decrease joint pain and facilitate exercise. The thermal effects of a warm or hot whirlpool may help decrease the pain of arthritis.[41–45]

Circulatory Conditions

The use of whirlpools to reduce swelling of an extremity is controversial. The hydrostatic pressure of water and its effects on circulation and renal function may help to reduce postoperative peripheral edema.[81] The use of a cool or cold water whirlpool will cause vasoconstriction and reduce vascular permeability. This may also help to reduce edema. However, the dependent position of an extremity required for using a whirlpool may inhibit edema reduction. Although Dolan et al.[82] found that immersing the hind limbs of rats in the dependent position in cold water effectively curbed edema formation, McCulloch and Boyd[50] found that placing the lower extremities of humans in the dependent position in an empty whirlpool tank for 20 minutes increased limb volume. Warm or hot water is contraindicated, because heat will increase tissue temperature and intravascular pressure,[83] thereby increasing inflammation and peripheral arterial blood flow, which will likely increase edema.[71,72,84] The effect of a warm or hot whirlpool on blood flow was studied by Cohen and colleagues.[85] They reported

CASE STUDY 5•4   SELECTING PARAMETERS FOR WHIRLPOOL

Six weeks ago, a 72-year-old female with a history of osteoporosis fell while walking in her yard. She sustained a Colles' fracture of her right wrist. She had a closed reduction and cast application to the right forearm, wrist, and hand. The cast was removed 3 days ago, and today she has mild swelling of the wrist and significant loss of ROM. She has poor tolerance to passive stretching and joint mobilization of the wrist.

CLINICAL DECISION-MAKING

1. Does the patient have a dysfunction, limitation, or problem that can be improved with the use of hydrotherapy?
   Answer: Yes, loss of ROM secondary to stiffness, contracture, and pain of a joint or joints is an indication for using hydrotherapy to help decrease pain and facilitate active and passive ROM.

2. Is the patient appropriate for hydrotherapy (i.e., do any of the general precautions or contraindications to hydrotherapy apply), or are there any specific considerations regarding applying hydrotherapy to this patient?
   Answer: As long as this patient has intact sensation and can sit with her arm in a whirlpool, then she should be able to safely receive hydrotherapy treatment for her right lower arm. The mild edema in her wrist will need to be monitored, since any increase in edema following whirlpool will require discontinuation of this treatment.

3. What are the specific goals to be achieved with the use of hydrotherapy?
   Answer: Decreased pain in wrist; increased tolerance for passive ROM, stretching, and joint mobilization; and increased mobility of the wrist and forearm.

4. Do you have the specific type of hydrotherapy that is appropriate for this patient?
   Answer: A small whirlpool on a stand or pedestal would be best, or a high-boy tank, so the patient

can sit on a chair with her arm comfortably inside the tank (see Fig. 5-14).

5. What specific hydrotherapy parameters would be appropriate for this patient?
   Answer: To decrease pain and facilitate improved mobility of the wrist and forearm, the following parameters would be appropriate:
   Water temperature: warm (97°F–99°F; 36.1°C–37.2°C) or cool (66°F–80°F; 18.9°C–26.7°C) if edema is present in the hand or wrist.
   Agitation: Begin with a low setting, with the force directed at the wrist and forearm if tolerated; gradually increase agitation to maximally tolerated level.
   Duration: 15 minutes
   Frequency: At the beginning of each treatment session, either daily or every other day, until pain and stiffness are no longer limiting tolerance to stretching, joint mobilization, and exercise

6. What are the proper (i.e., effective and safe) application procedures for hydrotherapy related to this case example?
   Answer: Inform the patient of the purpose and procedure. Be sure to explain the anticipated sensation and effect of the whirlpool and have her immediately report any discomfort to the practitioner.
   Preinspection: Inspect the area to be treated for skin compromise and sensation. Measure the circumference of the wrist to determine amount of edema present.
   Patient position: Patient should be able to sit comfortably in a chair with her arm in the whirlpool tank and a towel for padding under her axilla.
   Postinspection: Remove the arm from the water, dry the skin with a towel, and inspect the skin for any signs of irritation or adverse effects. Measure the circumference of the wrist to determine if the treatment increased or decreased wrist edema.

---

a 21% increase in extremity blood flow after a 38.6°C (101.5°F) whirlpool and a 50% increase in extremity blood flow after a 42.5°C (108.5°F) whirlpool. There was no significant difference in extremity blood flow in extremities immersed in whirlpools without agitation and those immersed in whirlpools with agitation. Therefore, the effect on blood flow is more likely dependent upon the temperature of the water

rather than any mechanical effects of whirlpool agitation.

Psychological Conditions

The relaxing effects of warm water whirlpools are well known. Anxious patients may benefit from partial or full immersion in a whirlpool to facilitate cooperation with rehabilitation procedures.[38] Partial immersion in a cool or cold whirlpool may stimulate drowsy or stuporous patients to facilitate participation in rehabilitation.

Wound Care

In the past, whirlpools were commonly used to treat open wounds, such as burns and ulcers of the skin. Whirlpools provide a method of mechanically cleansing and debriding a wound to remove surface necrotic material in patients who cannot tolerate more selective techniques. In addition, the mechanical effects of a whirlpool may facilitate improved circulation to the wound and stimulate formation of granulation tissue. The increase in local circulation may raise the levels of oxygen, antibodies, leukocytes, and nutrition supplied to the tissues and may enhance the removal of metabolites. The amount of

systemic medications, such as antibiotics, available to the wound area may also be increased by the improved circulation, which helps to diminish or to prevent infection.

Whirlpools also create sedation and analgesia, which may aid in reducing pain caused by the open wound or surrounding tissues. However, the force of the water jet is difficult to calibrate and may damage new granulation tissue, inhibiting wound healing. Immersion of wounds in whirlpools may also cause maceration of wound tissue, promote edema of the dependent limb, and cause cross-contamination of other tissues.[86] These disadvantages of whirlpools and the development of pulsed lavage devices for wound irrigation has decreased the use of whirlpools for treating wounds. See Table 5-4 for a list of whirlpool precautions and contraindications.

Table 5•4 Whirlpool Precautions and Contraindications

Precaution/Contraindication	Explanation
Malignancies	Danger of metastasis due to increased blood flow with warm or hot water temperatures
Sensory impairments	Danger of burns if water is too hot
Hypersensitivity to cold	Cold urticaria may occur
Incontinent bladder or bowel	May contaminate water and cause infection, particularly if receiving whirlpool for an open wound
Pulmonary disease	Poor ability to resist hydrostatic pressures with full-body immersion; monitor patient for signs of respiratory distress.
Cardiac insufficiency	May have difficulty adapting to maintain thermal homeostasis; limit maximum immersion time to 10 minutes initially and monitor vital signs during treatment.
Unstable blood pressure	Blood pressure problem may be exacerbated with full immersion in hot or cold water.
Impaired circulation	Patients with peripheral vascular disease (diabetes, arteriosclerosis): danger of burns; do not place in water temperatures greater than 35°C (95°F).
Thrombophlebitic areas	Use of warm or hot water whirlpool is contraindicated because of the danger of dislodging the clot with enhanced circulation in the area.
Skin infection	May cause cross-contamination of the other body parts immersed in the water.
Skin ulcers caused by venous insufficiency, edema, or lymphedema	Contraindicated because whirlpool can prolong or prevent wound closure
Tissue flaps or recent skin grafts	May not tolerate the agitation or may not be able to compensate for extremes of heat or cold
Skin conditions such as atopic eczema, ichthyosis, and senile pruritus	May exacerbate condition due to removal of natural skin moisture
Post-op surgical incisions with dehiscence, sutures, or staples	Contraindicated because may cause dehiscence of incision or contamination resulting in infection
Edema	May increase edema if warm or hot water is used
Acute febrile episode	May exacerbate fever if warm or hot water is used
Acute inflammation	May aggravate inflammation if warm or hot water is used
Danger of hemorrhaging	May increase bleeding if warm or hot water is used
Thermal regulation impairment	Danger of thermal shock if fully immersed in warm or hot water because convection and sweating may be impaired
Rheumatic arthritis (RA)	Warm or hot water contraindicated in the acute stage
Multiple sclerosis	May increase fatigue and weakness in water temperatures above 31°C (88°F)
Uncontrolled epilepsy	Full-body immersion contraindicated because of increased risk of drowning during an attack
Confusion or impaired cognition	May not be able to report problems or discomfort
Fear of water	May refuse full-body immersion or induce panic
Alcohol or drug ingestion	Reduced judgment; may enhance a hypotensive response; inquire if patient has ingested alcohol or drugs prior to whirlpool.
Pregnancy	Maternal hyperthermia may harm the fetus; avoid full- or half-body immersion in very warm or hot whirlpools, especially during the first trimester.

Historically, chemicals have been added to whirlpool water to reduce infection and limit cross-contamination. The most common chemical additives are povidone-iodine (Betadine surgical scrub) diluted to 4 parts per million (ppm); sodium hypochlorite (bleach) diluted to 500 to 5,000 ppm; and chloramine-T (Chlorazene), which comes in prepackaged quantities based on the size of the whirlpool.[86] These additives have been shown to be cytotoxic to healthy tissue and their use is discouraged.

Clinical Controversy

Placing chemical additives in whirlpool water used to treat wounds is controversial, because in addition to beneficial antimicrobial effects, many additives are cytotoxic to human cells.

Health-care practitioners must carefully consider the advantages and disadvantages of chemical additives for their patients with open wounds when whirlpool treatment is indicated. Wounds contaminated with bacteria and foreign debris, such as animal bites, may benefit from short-term use of chemical additives in whirlpool water.[87] Chemical additives are contraindicated for patients with chemical wounds, very young patients, elderly patients, and anyone with hypersensitivity to these chemical additives.[86]

Nonimmersion Irrigation of Wounds

Pulsed lavage with suction (PLWS) is a hydrotherapy modality for the irrigation and debridement of open wounds. *Lavage* is the use of an electrically powered device that delivers wound irrigation under pressure.[86] The most common irrigants are saline and tap water. Moore and Cowman[88] performed a systematic review of the literature and found no difference in wound healing when using either saline or water. Pulsed lavage provides a controlled pressure of pulsations of irrigants to the wound. The pressure is maintained between 4 and 15 psi (pounds per square inch), depending on the amount of eschar and necrotic tissue in the wound and the patient's tolerance (Table 5-5). Concurrent suction applies a negative pressure to the wound bed during treatment to effectively remove the irrigants and facilitate removal of pathogens.[86]

PLWS is indicated for the treatment of wounds caused by arterial insufficiency, venous insufficiency, diabetes, pressure, small burns, surgery, and trauma.[89] Treatment with PLWS will help decrease bacteria and infection in the wound and promote granulation and epithelialization.[90] Precautions must be followed when treating bleeding wounds, facial tissues, and near sensitive tissues, such as major blood vessels and nerves. PLWS may be contraindicated on or near recent tissue grafts, flaps, or surgical procedures (check with the patient's surgeon). Use caution when using PLWS on patients taking anticoagulants because of the potential for hemorrhage and on insensate patients because of the danger of unperceived trauma to tissues.

Clinical Technique for PLWS

The use of PLWS for treating wounds begins with preparing the treatment area and the patient. PLWS is best performed in a private room with four walls and a door to limit cross-contamination. All supplies

Table 5•5	**PLWS: Frequency and Duration of Treatment**			
Frequency	**Daily**	**Twice Daily**	**3 Times Per Week**	**Discontinue**
Most wounds	X			
Greater than 50% Necrotic		X		
Purulent drainage		X		
Sepsis		X		
Full granulation base			X	
NPWT* being used			X	
No increased granulation for 1 week				X
No decreased necrotic tissue for 1 week				X
Wound closed				X

*Negative pressure wound therapy
Adapted with permission from Loehne, HB, PT. Management of Chronic Wounds, Wound Healing Treatment Interventions. Presented at American Physical Therapy Association Annual Conference in Baltimore, MD; June 13, 2009.

and the patient's personal items should be covered, as should any exposed tubes, ports, or other wounds not being treated. The patient should be positioned comfortably and all dressings removed from the wound. Towels or water-impermeable padding should be placed in the wound area to absorb any runoff of irrigants. Patients should wear a mask to limit inhalation of aerosolized irrigants and pathogens. Practitioners must wear protective devices, including gloves, shoe coverings, head coverings that include the ears, protective eyewear, gown, and mask.[86] The United States Department of Labor, Occupational Safety and Health Administration (OSHA) guidelines for infection control should be followed during PLWS treatments (available at http://www.osha.gov).

Consult the manufacturer's recommendations for proper operation of the pulsed lavage device (Fig. 5-16). Adjust the pressure between 4 and 15 psi based on the status of the wound being treated and patient comfort. Usually lower pressures are used initially to gauge patient's response and effectiveness of the chosen pressure. Increase pressure for wounds with tough eschar or excessive necrotic tissue. Decrease pressure if bleeding occurs or if directing the irrigants near a major or exposed vessel, nerve, tendon, bone, or lining of a cavity. Most treatments require 15 to 30 minutes. (See

Table 5-5 for recommended frequency and duration of treatments.) When the PLWS treatment is completed, the areas of intact skin should be dried with a towel and all single-use equipment properly disposed. The wound should be inspected and the effectiveness of the treatment documented.

PLWS has several advantages over whirlpool treatments for wound care. PLWS is portable and can be performed in the home. Morgan and Hoelscher[91] performed a retrospective cohort study that found treating wounds at home using pulsed lavage effectively removed necrotic tissue and promoted wound healing and was more cost-effective than in-hospital whirlpool treatments or surgical debridement. PLWS requires shorter treatment times and can be used to treat a small area rather than an entire extremity and may be less painful than whirlpool treatments. Disadvantages of PLWS include the cost associated with single-use attachments and the inability to treat large surface wounds such as extensive burns.

Assessment of Effectiveness and Expected Outcomes for Hydrotherapy

Clinical Decision-Making

The decision to include hydrotherapy in an intervention plan should be based upon the evidence for effectiveness. Practitioners must regularly consult the latest published literature to match their knowledge and expertise with the needs of the patient. Searches of databases for hydrotherapy enable the practitioner to base clinical decisions on available evidence of effectiveness. Key words or medical subject headings (MeSH) are helpful when searching databases for information on effectiveness of hydrotherapy.

Goals and Documentation

Goals of hydrotherapy should be clearly documented in the initial examination of the patient. The effectiveness of this therapy can be based on these goals and on response of the patient to each treatment. Outcomes can be determined by measuring the effect on impairments, which can include pain, joint ROM, strength, wound condition, edema, balance and coordination, and the assessment of function. Function may be a

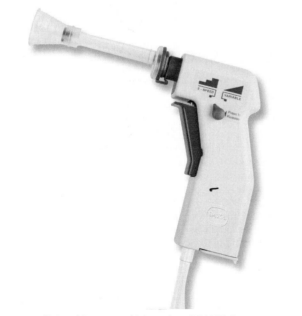

Fig 5•16 Pulsed lavage with suction (PLWS) for treatment of an open wound. *(Courtesy of DAVOL Company, Warwick, Rhode Island.)*

longer-term determination of the effectiveness of hydrotherapy interventions and an important concern for third-party payers. Functional inventories or questionnaires, such as the Functional Independence Measure (FIM), SF-36, and the Oswestry Low Back Pain Disability Questionnaire, may be helpful in assessing hydrotherapy effectiveness.

Documentation of hydrotherapy interventions should include the type of hydrotherapy performed, the parameters of the treatment, and the patient's response to the treatment.

Documentation Tips

Aquatic Therapy

- Water temperature
- Duration of the treatment
- Goals of pool therapy
- Movement or exercise techniques performed during therapy
- Assistive equipment used during therapy
- Means of entry and exit
- The patient's tolerance to the treatment, including vital signs
- Any adverse reactions
- Post-pool therapy changes in identified impairments or functional limitations

Whirlpool

- Type of whirlpool
- Body part immersed in water (partial or full immersion)
- Temperature of the water
- Agitation (mild, moderate, full) and whether directed at or away from body part
- Duration of treatment
- Passive (no movement during whirlpool) or active (movement or exercise during whirlpool)
- Patient response or tolerance for the treatment
- Post-whirlpool changes in identified impairments or functional limitations
- For wound care:
  - Additives placed in the water
  - Condition of wound pre- and post-whirlpool

Documentation of patient response to hydrotherapy should include any evidence of adverse reactions, including marked temperature changes of the patient's skin; changes in skin color such as erythema, blanching, or cyanosis; or changes in skin appearance such as excessive softening or wrinkling of skin. Open wounds should be closely inspected following whirlpool treatment, and documentation should be made of the wound's appearance and surrounding margins and of any changes in exudates and amount and type of necrotic tissue present in the wound. In addition, any change in the patient's pain, muscle spasm, ROM, strength, joint appearance, edema, coordination, orofacial control, endurance, functional level, and psychological state should be noted. Practitioners should be mindful that warm or hot water temperatures and full-body immersion have a tendency to cause transient weakness during or immediately following hydrotherapy interventions. Vital signs should be monitored and recorded during and immediately following hydrotherapy for any patient with a history of cardiac or pulmonary disease, to determine tolerance to the treatment.

Hydrotherapy in all its forms can be physically and psychologically therapeutic. However, practitioners must avoid indiscriminate use of this modality. Careful application of the principles of physics of water, knowledge of the physiological effects of water at various temperatures, and evidence of this modality's effectiveness for a given patient is essential for effective treatment. The advantages and disadvantages of hydrotherapy, including the cost of treatment, must be compared to other therapeutic interventions. Practitioners must be prepared to justify the choice of hydrotherapy as the best cost-effective intervention that is indicated for their patient.

☐ REFERENCES

1. Poyhonen T, Keskinen KL, Kyrolainen H, Hautala A, Savolainen J, Malkia E. Neuromuscular function during therapeutic exercise under water and or dry land. *Arch Phys Med Rehabil.* 2001;82:1446–1452.
2. Cole AJ, Eagleston RE, Moschetti M, Sinnett E. Aquatic rehabilitation of the spine. *Rehab Manag.* 1996;9:55–62.
3. Kurabayashi H, Machida I, Tamura K, Iwai F, Tamura J, Kubota K. Breathing out into water during subtotal immersion: a therapy for chronic pulmonary emphysema. *Am J Phys Med Rehabil.* 2000;79:150–153.
4. Martel GF, Harmer ML, Logan JM, Parker CB. Aquatic plyometric training increases vertical jump in female volleyball players. *Med Sci Sports Exerc.* 2005;37:1814–1819.
5. Takken T, van der Net J, Kuis W, Helders PJ. Aquatic fitness for children with juvenile idiopathic arthritis. *Rheumatology (Oxford).* 2003;42:1408–1414.
6. Volaklis KA, Spassis AT, Tokmakidis SP. Land versus water exercise in patients with coronary artery disease: effects on body composition, blood lipids, and physical fitness. *Am Heart J.* 2007;154:e1–e6.

7. Cider A, Schaufelberger M, Sunnerhagen KS, Andersson B. Hydrotherapy—a new approach to improve function in the older patient with chronic heart failure. *Eur J Heart Fail.* 2003;5:527–535.

8. Mannerkorpi K, Nyberg B, Ahlmen M, Ekdahl C. Pool exercise combined with an education program for patients with fibromyalgia syndrome. A prospective, randomized study. *J Rheumatol.* 2000;27:2473–2481.

9. Devereux K, Robertson D, Briffa NK. Effects of a water-based program on women 65 years and over: a randomised controlled trial. *Aust J Physiother.* 2005;51:102–108.

10. Silva LE, Valim V, Pessanha AP, et al. Hydrotherapy versus conventional land-based exercise for the management of patients with osteoarthritis of the knee: a randomized clinical trial. *Phys Ther.* 2008;88:12–21.

11. Belza B, Topolski T, Kinne S, Patrick DL, Ramsey SD. Does adherence make a difference? Results from a community-based aquatic exercise program. *Nurs Res.* 2002;51:285–291.

12. Eversden L, Maggs F, Nightingale P, Jobanputra P. A pragmatic randomised controlled trial of hydrotherapy and land exercises on overall well being and quality of life in rheumatoid arthritis. *BMC Musculoskelet Disord.* 2007;8:23.

13. Saggini R, Cancelli F, DiBonaventura V, Bellomo RG, Pezzatini A, Carniel R. Efficacy of two micro-gravitational protocols to treat chronic low back pain associated with discal lesions: a randomized controlled trial. *Eura Medicophys.* 2004;40:311–316.

14. Dale RB, Dale RB, MacDonald J, Messer L. Liquid assets: aquatic therapy offers benefits to a wide range of clinical populations. *Rehab Manag.* 2005;18:22–24.

15. Getz M, Hutzler Y, Vermeer A. Effects of aquatic interventions in children with neuromotor impairments: a systematic review of the literature. *Clin Rehabil.* 2006;20:927–936.

16. Brady B, Redfern J, MacDougal G, Williams G. The addition of aquatic therapy to rehabilitation following surgical rotator cuff repair: a feasibility study. *Physiother Res Int.* 2008;13:153–161.

17. Noh DK, Lim JY, Shin HI, Paik NJ. The effect of aquatic therapy on postural balance and muscle strength in stroke survivors—a randomized controlled pilot trial. *Clin Rehabil.* 2008;22:966–976.

18. Phillips VK, Legge M, Jones LM. Maximal physiological responses between aquatic and land exercise in overweight women. *Med Sci Sports Exerc.* 2008;40:959–964.

19. Waller B, Lambeck J, Daly D. Therapeutic aquatic exercise in the treatment of low back pain: a systematic review. *Clin Rehabil.* 2009;23:3–14.

20. Bartels EM, Lund H, Hagen KB, et al. Aquatic exercise for the treatment of knee and hip osteoarthritis. *Cochrane Database Syst Rev.* 2009;vol. 2.

21. Takeshima N, Rogers ME, Watanabe E, et al. Water-based exercise improved health-related aspects of fitness in older women. *Med Sci Sports Exerc.* 2002;34:544–551.

22. Gusi N, Tomas-Carus P, Hakkinen A, Hakkinen K, Ortega-Alonso A. Exercise in waist-high warm water decreases pain and improves health-related quality of life and strength in the lower extremities in women with fibromyalgia. *Arthritis Rheum.* 2006;55:66–73.

23. Jentoft ES, Kvalvik AG, Mendshoel AM. Effects of pool-based and land-based aerobic exercise on women with fibromyalgia/chronic widespread muscle pain. *Arthritis Rheum.* 2001;45:42–47.

24. Tomas-Carus P, Hakkinen A, Gusi N, et al. Aquatic training and detraining on fitness and quality of life in fibromyalgia. *Med Sci Sports Exerc.* 2007;39:1044–1050.

25. O'Neill DF. Return to function through aquatic therapy. *Athl Ther Today.* 2000; 5:14–16.

26. Colado JC, Tella V, Triplett NT, Gonzalez LM. Effects of a short-term aquatic resistance program on strength and body composition in fit young men. *J Strength Cond Res.* 2009; 23:549–559.

27. Hall J, Swinkels A, Briddon J, McCabe CS. Does aquatic exercise relieve pain in adults with neurologic or musculoskeletal disease? A systematic review and meta-analysis of randomized controlled trials. *Arch Phys Med Rehabil.* 2008; 89:873–883.

28. Thorpe DE, Reilly M. The effect of an aquatic resistive exercise program on lower extremity strength, energy expenditure, functional mobility, balance and self-perception in an adult with cerebral palsy: a retrospective case report. *J Aquatic Phys Ther.* 2000;8:18–24.

29. Edlich RF, Towler MA, Goitz RJ, et al. Bioengineering principles of hydrotherapy. *J Burn Care Rehabil.* 1987;8:580–584.

30. Kersey RD, West S, Kersey RD. Aquatic therapy. *Athl Ther Today.* 2005;10:48–49.

31. Hinman RS, Heywood SE, Day AR. Aquatic physical therapy for hip and knee osteoarthritis: results of a single-blind randomized controlled trial. *Phys Ther.* 2007;87:32–43.

32. Wang TJ, Belza B, Thompson FE, Whitney JD, Bennett K. Effects of aquatic exercise on flexibility, strength and aerobic fitness in adults with osteoarthritis of the hip or knee. *J Adv Nurs* 2007;57:141–152.

33. Keren O, Reznik J, Groswasser Z. Combined motor disturbances following severe traumatic brain injury: an integrative long-term treatment approach. *Brain Inj.* 2001;15:633–638.

34. Suomi R, Koceja DM. Postural sway characteristics in women with lower extremity arthritis before and after an aquatic exercise intervention. *Arch Phys Med Rehabil.* 2000;81:780–785.

35. McManus BM, Kotelchuck M. The effect of aquatic therapy on functional mobility of infants and toddlers in early intervention. *Pediatr Phys Ther.* 2007;19:275–282.

36. Yilmaz I, Yanarda M, Birkan B, Bumin G. Effects of swimming training on physical fitness and water orientation in autism. *Pediatr Int.* 2004;46:624–626.

37. Levine BA. Use of hydrotherapy in reduction of anxiety. *Psychol Rep.* 1984;55:526.

38. Robiner WN. Psychological and physical reactions to whirlpool baths. *J Behav Med.* 1990; 13:157–173.

39. Roehrs TG, Kartst GM. Effects of an aquatic exercise program on quality of life measures for individuals with progressive multiple sclerosis. *J Neurol Phys Ther.* 2004; 28:63–71.

40. Bovy P, Rodrique V. Rehabilitation after fracture of the femur in elderly patients. *Rev Med Liege.* 1997;52:577–581.

41. Templeton MS, Booth DL, O'Kelly WD. Effects of aquatic therapy on joint flexibility and functional ability in subjects with rheumatic disease. *J Orthop Sports Phys Ther.* 1996;23:376–381.

42. Takata S, Harada S, Mitsunobu F, et al. A patient with severe palindromic rheumatism and frequent episodes of pain. *Intern Med.* 2001;40:140–143.

43. Sukenik S, Flusser D, Abu-Shakra M. The role of spa therapy in various rheumatic diseases. *Rheum Dis Clin North Am.* 1999;25:883–897.

44. Balint G, Szebenyi B. Non-pharmacological therapies in osteoarthritis. *Ballieres Clin Rheumatol.* 1997;11:795–815.

45. Hall J, Skevington SM, Maddison PJ, Chapman K. A randomized and controlled trial of hydrotherapy in rheumatoid arthritis. *Arthritis Care Res.* 1996; 9:206–215.

46. Giancoli DC. *Physics.* 5th ed. Upper Saddle River, NJ: Prentice Hall; 1998.

47. Hecox B, Mehreteab TA, Weisberg J, Sanko J. *Physical Agents*. 2nd ed. Upper Saddle River, NJ: Pearson Prentice Hall; 2006.
48. Jamison LJ. The healing properties of water—how aquatic therapy can manage lymphedema. *Rehab Manage*. 2000; 13:58–62.
49. Jamison LJ. The therapeutic value of aquatic therapy in treating lymphedema comprehensive decongestive physiotherapy. *Rehab Manage*. 2000;13:58–60, 62.
50. McCulloch J, Boyd VB. The effects of whirlpool and the dependent position on lower extremity volume. *J Orthop Sports Phys Ther*. 1992;16:169–173.
51. Whitney SL. Physical agents: heat and cold modalities. In: Scully RM, Barnes MR, eds. *Physical Therapy*. Philadelphia: JB Lippincott; 1989.
52. Golland A. Basic hydrotherapy. *Physiotherapy*. 1981;67: 258–262.
53. Ruoti GR, Morris DM, Cole AJ. *Aquatic Rehabilitation*. Philadelphia: JB Lippincott; 1997.
54. Tuttle WW, Corleaux JF. The response of the heart to water of swimming pool temperature. *Res Q*. 1935;6:24–26.
55. Sussman C, Bates-Jensen BM. *Wound Care*. Gaithersburg, MD: Aspen; 1998.
56. Pariser G, Madras D, Weiss E. Outcomes of an aquatic exercise program including aerobic capacity, lactate threshold, and fatigue in two individuals with multiple sclerosis. *J Neurol Phys Ther*. 2006;30:82–90.
57. Peterson C. Exercise in 94 degrees F water for a patient with multiple sclerosis. *Phys Ther*. 2001;81:1049–1058.
58. Broach E, Dattilo J. The effect of aquatic therapy on strength of adults with multiple sclerosis. *Ther Recreation*. 2003;J 37: 224–239.
59. Wadell K, Sundelin G, Lundgren R, et al. Muscle performance in patients with chronic obstructive pulmonary disease—effects of a physical training programme. *Advances Physiother*. 2005;7:51–59.
60. Meyer K, Leblanc MC. Aquatic therapies patients with compromised left ventricular function and heart failure. *Clin Invest Med*. 2008;31:E90–E97.
61. Fallon RJ. Pseudomonas aeruginosa and whirlpool baths. *Lancet*. 1995;346:841.
62. Hollyoak VA, Freeman R. Pseudomonas aeruginosa and whirlpool baths. *Lancet*. 1995;346:644–645.
63. Hollyoak V, Boyd P, Freeman R. Whirlpool baths in nursing homes: use, maintenance, and contamination with *Pseudomonas aeruginosa*. *Commun Dis Rep CDR Rev*. 1995;5:R102–R104.
64. Resnick B. Encouraging exercise in older adults with congestive heart failure. *Geriat Nurs*. 2004;25:204–211.
65. Duffield MH, Skinner AT, Thompson AM. *Duffield's Exercise in Water*. Philadelphia: W.B. Saunders; 1983.
66. Campion MR. *Adult Hydrotherapy: A Practical Approach*. Oxford: Heinemann Medical; 1990.
67. Borrell PM, Parker R, Henley EJ, Masley D, Repinecz M. Comparison in vivo temperatures produced by hydrotherapy, paraffin wax treatment, and Fluidotherapy. *Phys Ther*. 1980;60:1273–1276.
68. Abramson DL, Tucks S, Zayak AM, Mitchel RE. The effects of altering limb position on blood flow, O_2 uptake and skin temperature. *J Appl Physiol*. 1962;17:191–194.
69. Niederhuber SS, Stribley RF, Koepke GH. Reduction of skin bacterial load with use of the therapeutic whirlpool. *Phys Ther*. 1975;55:482–486.
70. American Physical Therapy Association. Hydrotherapy/Therapeutic Pool Infection Control Guidelines. Alexandria, VA: American Physical Therapy Association Publication No. P-112; 1995.
71. Magness JL, Garrett TR, Erickson DJ. Swelling of the upper extremity during whirlpool baths. *Arch Phys Med Rehabil*. 1970;51:297–299.
72. Hoyrup G, Kjorvel L. Comparison of whirlpool and wax treatments for hand therapy. *Physiotherapy*. 1986;38:79–82.
73. Fiscus KA, Kaminski TW, Powers ME. Changes in lower leg blood flow during warm, cold and contrast water therapy. *Arch Phys Med Rehabil*. 2005;86:1404–1410.
74. Myrer JW, Drapre DO, Durrant E. Contrast therapy and intramuscular temperature in the human leg. *J Athl Train*. 1994; 29:318–322.
75. Higgins D, Kaminski TW. Contrast therapy does not cause fluctuations in human gastrocnemius intramuscular temperature. *J Athl Train*. 1998;33:336–340.
76. Smith K, Newton R. The immediate effect of contrast baths on edema, temperature, and pain in postsurgical hand injuries. *Phys Ther*. 1994;74(S):S157.
77. Cote DJ, Prentice WE, Hooker DN, Shields EW. Comparison of three treatment procedures for minimizing ankle sprain swelling. *Phys Ther*. 1988;68:1072–1076.
78. Kuligowski LA, Lephart SM, Giannantonio FP, Blanc RO. Effect of whirlpool therapy on the signs and symptoms of delayed-onset muscle soreness. *J Athl Train*. 1998;33:222–228.
79. Vaile J, Halson S, Gill N. Effect of hydrotherapy on the signs and symptoms of delayed onset muscle soreness. *Eur J Appl Physiol*. 2008;102:447–455.
80. Hamlin MJ. The effect of contrast temperature water therapy on repeated sprint performance. *J Sci Med Sport*. 2007;10: 398–402.
81. Epstein M. Cardiovascular and renal effects of head out water immersion in man. *Circ Res*. 1976;39:620–628.
82. Dolan MG, Thronton RM, Fish DR, Mendel FC. Effects of cold water immersion on edema formation after blunt injury to the hind limbs of rats. *J Athl Train*. 1997;32:233–237.
83. Basford JR. The physical agents. In: Grabois M, Garrison SJ, Hart KA, Lehmkuhl LD, eds. *Physical Medicine and Rehabilitation—The Complete Approach*. Malden, MA: Blackwell Science; 2000.
84. Toomey R, Grief-Schwartz R, Piper MC. Clinical evaluation of the effects of whirlpool and patients with Colles' fractures. *Physiother Can*. 1986;38:280–284.
85. Cohen A, Martin GM, Wakim KG. Effects of whirlpool bath with and without agitation on the circulation in normal and diseased extremities. *Arch Phys Med Rehabil*. 1949;30: 212–218.
86. Myers BA. *Wound Management Principles and Practice*. 2nd ed. Upper Saddle River, NJ: Pearson Prentice Hall; 2008.
87. Ogrin R. Current thoughts on the use of povidone-iodine (BETADINE) in wounds: Acute and chronic. *Australian J Podiatr Med*. 2002;36:13–19.
88. Moore Z, Cowman S. A systematic review of wound cleansing for pressure ulcers. *J Clin Nursing*. 2008;17:1963–1972.
89. Scott RG, Loehne HB. Treatment options: Five questions—and answers—about pulsed lavage. *Adv Wound Care*. 2000;13:133–134.
90. Haynes LJ, Brown MH, Handley BC, et al. PO-012-M: Comparison of Pulsavac and sterile whirlpool regarding the promotion of tissue granulation. *Phys Ther*. 1994;74:S4.
91. Morgan D, Hoelscher J. Pulsed lavage: promoting comfort and healing in home care. *Ostomy Wound Manage*. 2000;46:44–49.
92. Batavia M. *Contraindications in Physical Rehabilitation: Doing No Harm*. St. Louis, MO: Saunders Elsevier; 2006.

chapter 6

Electromagnetic Waves

Laser, Diathermy, and Pulsed Electromagnetic Fields

Enrico M. Dellagatta, PT, DPT, MEd | Thomas P. Nolan Jr., PT, DPT, OCS

The understanding of electromagnetic theory in the 19th century led to the development of the wireless telegraph and eventually to the development of radio, television, and cell phones. A whole new world of communication evolved that has profoundly changed the world we live in. The use of electromagnetic radiation, or waves, for therapeutic purposes began in the early 20th century when physicians began using high-frequency currents to heat muscles and joints.[1] The penetration of electromagnetic waves through body tissues enabled deeper heating than did applying superficial heating devices such as hot packs to the skin. Eventually, the development of devices that produce electromagnetic waves popularized what became known as *diathermy*. The use of electromagnetic waves (from the ultraviolet part of the electromagnetic spectrum) to treat skin problems also became popular during the 20th century. During the later part of the century, the development of lasers enabled the use of visible light (which is also an electromagnetic wave) for treatment purposes.

Lasers are a monochromatic beam of light from the visible part of the electromagnetic spectrum (Fig. 6-1). High-power lasers are used in surgery to cut and destroy tissue. Low-power lasers do not cut or destroy tissue and can be safely used for treating pain and inflammation and promoting soft tissue healing. Use of a low-power laser for patient interventions is known as *low-level laser therapy* (LLLT). The interest in low-power laser usage has increased dramatically since 2002, when the United States Food and Drug

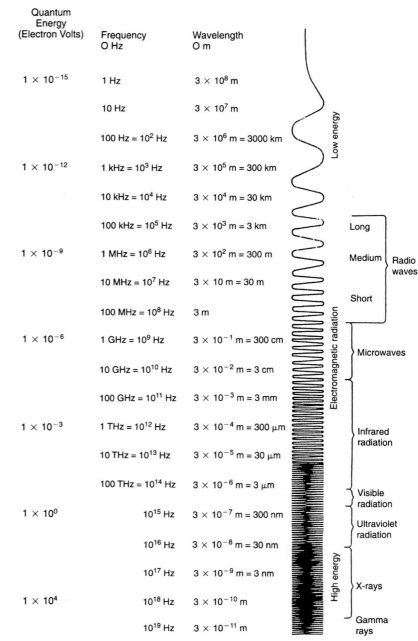

Fig 6•1 Electromagnetic spectrum of radiations organized by quantum energy, wavelength, and frequency. *(Adapted from Low, J., & Reed, A., eds. Electrotherapy Explained: Principles and Practice. Oxford: Butterworth-Heinemann, 1992:230.)*

Electric and magnetic fields—electromagnetic radiations

Administration approved its use for treating carpal tunnel syndrome.[2]

Diathermy is the application of electromagnetic waves to the body from the radio frequency (RF) part of the electromagnetic spectrum (see Fig. 6-1). It has been used primarily as a thermal modality, although pulsed diathermy or pulsed electromagnetic field (PEMF) devices produce little or no heating of tissues. The popularity of diathermy as a thermal modality decreased in the late 20th century. Health-care practitioners became concerned that diathermy's electromagnetic waves possibly posed a hazard for the patient and the practitioner. Diathermy devices were bulky and difficult to apply to patients, and there was a lack of evidence of effectiveness. The use of ultrasound to heat deep tissues gradually replaced the use of diathermy. Today, new diathermy devices are smaller and easier to apply, leakage of electromagnetic waves has been greatly reduced, and more studies are available addressing effectiveness of treatment. It is time for practitioners to take another look at diathermy as a possible effective clinical modality for their patients.

Ultraviolet (UV) light from the ultraviolet part of the electromagnetic spectrum has been shown to be an effective intervention for treating skin conditions and open wounds. Historically, practitioners have used portable ultraviolet lamps and booths equipped with ultraviolet lamps to provide treatments for skin conditions and wounds. The use of ultraviolet treatments by health-care practitioners has decreased because of advancements in the pharmacological treatment of skin disorders and the availability of ultraviolet lamps in nonmedical entities such as tanning salons. Ultraviolet will not be covered in this chapter; those interested are referred to Robertson et al.[3]

Electromagnetic Waves

Electromagnetic waves are waves of energy that are propagated through space. Accelerating electric charges produce electromagnetic waves of moving electric and magnetic fields. The electric and magnetic field strengths in an electromagnetic wave are illustrated in Figure 6-2. Notice that the electric and magnetic fields at any point of the electromagnetic wave are perpendicular to each other and to the direction of the wave's motion. These waves travel through space at the speed of light.[4]

Electromagnetic waves are grouped according to their quantum energy, frequency, and wavelength, known as the *electromagnetic spectrum* (see Fig. 6-1). Lower frequency waves are known as *radio waves*. These frequencies are used to transmit radio and television signals. Cellular phones, radar, and microwave ovens use higher frequencies in the "microwave" frequency range. Diathermy devices produce electromagnetic waves from either the shortwave or microwave frequency ranges. Lasers produce electromagnetic waves from the visible light frequency range. Much higher frequencies are used to produce ultraviolet light and x-rays for diagnostic purposes.

Electromagnetic waves of all wavelengths possess certain unique properties. They transport electrical and magnetic energy through space. Unlike sound waves, electromagnetic waves do not require a medium through which to travel and can travel through a vacuum unimpeded. Electromagnetic waves are composed of pure energy; therefore, they do not have mass. The electromagnetic waves themselves do not contain matter. However, they do have an effect on the matter through which they travel. This occurs because matter contains electric charges, which are interacted with, and influenced by, electromagnetic waves as they pass through the matter. The direction of propagation of radiant energy is normally a straight line. However, these waves of energy can be reflected, deflected, and absorbed by the media through which they travel.

KEY POINT! Regardless of the type of wave propagation, there is a fundamental relationship between frequency and wavelength, which is given by the equation $c = \lambda f$, where c is the speed of light, λ is the wavelength, and f is the frequency of an electromagnetic wave.[4]

All electromagnetic waves listed on the electromagnetic spectrum travel through space at the speed of light (3.0×10^8 m/s).[4]

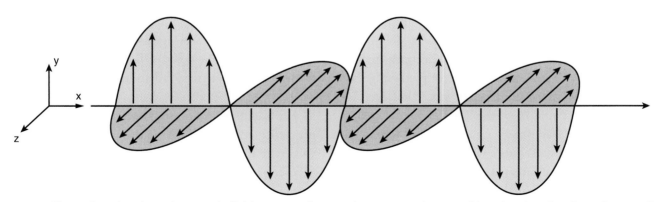

Fig 6•2 Alternating electric and magnetic fields surrounding an electromagnetic wave. Note that the electric and magnetic fields are perpendicular to each other and to the direction of the wave. *(Art concept by Sara Monath, PT student, Richard Stockton College of NJ.)*

The human body cannot detect most electromagnetic waves. Skin molecules can detect infrared waves because they resonate at infrared frequencies, resulting in absorption of energy and warming of the skin. The warming of the skin by the sun's rays is attributed to the infrared radiation produced by the sun. The eyes can detect wavelengths between 4 and 7×10^{-7} m, which is the visible light range of the electromagnetic spectrum.[4] Electromagnetic waves with frequencies higher than visible light, such as ultraviolet and x-rays, are not detected by the body and may be harmful to human tissues. A common example is sunburn, caused by damage to the skin from prolonged exposure to ultraviolet radiation from the sun.

Lasers

State of Events

Since 2002, when the FDA approved the medical use of low-level lasers, laser sales and clinical usage have increased geometrically. With this has come a gamut of professional opinion ranging from perfunctory acceptance to epistemological skepticism. Recent laboratory studies reaffirm the early physiological research that highlighted the ability of laser light to amplify cell metabolism. So the question is no longer whether therapeutic lasers have biological effects, but rather how they work and what conditions are they best suited to treat. Since it is now clear that therapeutic lasers have no undesirable effects in the hands of a qualified health-care practitioner, questions regarding the ability to manifest clinical changes linger.

History

The term *laser* is an acronym for "light amplification by stimulated emission of radiation." Lasers by definition generate a monochromatic beam of electromagnetic radiation.[4] Albert Einstein is credited for predicting the potential of stimulated emission in 1917; however, it was not until the middle of the 20th century that the first operational laser was created.[5,6] Bolstered by Schawlow and Townes's work with masers (microwave amplifiers by the stimulated emission of radiation), Theodore Maiman created a ruby laser in 1960 followed by the discovery of the helium-neon (HeNe) laser.[6–8] From 1960 to 1963, medical lasers continued to evolve with the development of the argon, carbon dioxide (CO_2), and neodymium: yttrium-aluminum-garnet (Nd: YAG) lasers.[9] In 1962, White and Rigden's discovery of visible red laser output at 623 nanometers (nm) spawned an ongoing interest in the photobiostimulation effect of low-intensity "cold" lasers.[10]

Since the inception of laser use, their utilization has depended on the operator's understanding of light-tissue interaction as well as the ability of the technology to deliver the light to the target tissue. Early use of lasers was limited by prohibitive cost, operational difficulties, and machine dependability. Cost, control, and precision of laser use dramatically improved in the mid-1980s with the development of semiconductor technology. Presently, lasers are a mainstay in ophthalmology, dermatology, otolaryngology, neurology, orthopedics, general surgery,[9] and most recently physical medicine and rehabilitation.[11]

While the evolution of lasers in physical medicine and rehabilitation has not paralleled that of the surgical lasers, the FDA's approval in 2002 of the 830 nm gallium aluminum arsenide (GaAlAs) laser for the treatment of carpal tunnel syndrome may prove to be a milestone for physical medicine practitioners.[11] Figure 6-3(A) illustrates the use of LLLT for treatment of carpal tunnel syndrome.

Physical Properties of Lasers

Laser light is created when photons stimulate the emission of other photons of equal wavelength and direction of travel. Light is electromagnetic energy that is transmitted through space either as a propagated wave or as small parcels of energy called *photons*. Light energy is quantified in two reciprocal forms of measurement: frequency (f) expressed in Hertz (Hz)—or cycles per second—and wavelength (λ), expressed in metric units of length. The color of light in the visible spectrum of electromagnetic radiation is determined by its wavelength.[4]

The addition of an energy source (thermal, electromagnetic, etc.) to an atom via the process of absorption will excite the particle from its ground state (E_1) to one of several tiers of higher energy (E_2). Spontaneous emission of light occurs when a quantum of energy representing the difference between the ground and excited state

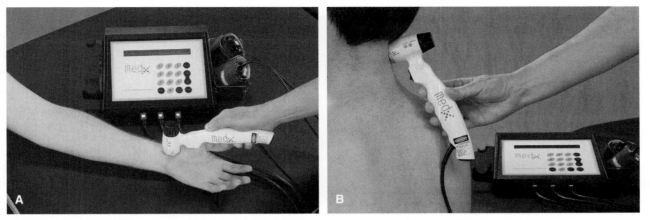

Fig 6•3 (A) Use of LLLT for treating carpal tunnel syndrome using a handheld wand. (B) Use of LLLT for treating cervical spine osteoarthritis using a handheld wand.

$(E_1 - E_2 + = E_\Delta)$ is released (Fig. 6-4). If the difference between E_1 and E_2 is the same for multiple particles, the output of esnergy and wavelength will be the same. Since the energy transition of most spontaneously emitted light is different, the output of the light is omnidirectional and of multiple wavelengths[4] (Fig. 6-5). A precondition for laser light known as *population inversion* is not achieved with spontaneous emission because the lifetime of the electrons in the excited state is insufficient to take them beyond the second energy tier.

Laser light is produced when a photon of E_Δ collides with an atom already in an elevated state E_2. This stimulated emission (Fig. 6-6) will produce a second photon whose wavelength and spatial and temporal orientation are the same. Repetitive collision of photons with atoms in the excited state E_2 and with the same spatial and temporal orientation produces light that is monochromatic, coherent, and collimated. Monochromatic light is of a singular wavelength and is one color (if within the viewable light spectrum). Because of its wavelength specificity, laser light is characteristically pure. Light purity is inverse to its wavelength, with the shorter wavelengths possessing greater purity.[4]

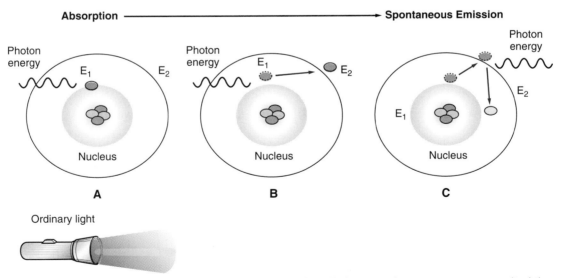

Fig 6•4 Spontaneous emission. (A) Atoms, ions, or molecules (E_1) while in ground energy state are excited through the process of absorption and elevated to a higher energy level (E_2). (B) The absorbed energy is released in the form of quantum energy as a function of the difference of (E_1) and (E_2). (C) Since ordinary light is composed of many wavelengths, the excited electrons randomly return to their respective ground state, causing a brief spontaneous emission of ordinary light.

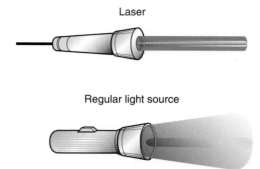

Laser

Regular light source

Fig 6•5 Schematic comparison of laser light to ordinary light.

Since laser light is wavelength and frequency specific, photons are temporally and directionally coherent. Spatial coherence allows the light to be directed through a focusing lens and directly propagated to a target tissue because of its directional stability. The high energy and coherency of laser light also pose potential hazards to the operator and recipient. When viewed directly, light beams from visible light lasers or near infrared lasers can cause retinal burns and scarring, leading to vision loss or even blindness.[12,13] When interfaced with tissue, laser may be absorbed, scattered, transmitted, or reflected (Fig. 6-7).

KEY POINT! The penetration depth of the laser in a given tissue is proportional to the inverse of the absorption coefficient (α).

A shallow layer of tissue with a high α results in high absorption of laser and ultimately intense heat at the tissue interface.[4,9,14]

Lasers consist of a few basic but integral components (Fig. 6-8). Laser light is created in a lasing cavity containing a medium such as CO_2 (high-powered laser) or helium-neon (HeNe; low-powered laser). A high-intensity flash lamp is used to raise the atoms, ions, or molecules of the medium to their upper energy state, creating a condition known as a *population inversion*. Light is repeatedly bounced between two parallel reflectors arranged at opposite ends of the lasing chamber, causing the excitation of more photons (amplification). Light traveling in other directions will escape the chamber and is lost as heat. One mirror is 100% reflective while the other is semipermeable and reflects a predetermined quantity of photons. A selected percentage of photons pass through the semipermeable reflector into a focusing lens where they become "usable output," or a laser beam. The atomic, ionic, or molecular structure of the lasing medium will determine the characteristic properties of its emitted light relevant to the electromagnetic spectrum (EMS).[4]

Diode lasers are a very efficient means of producing low-powered laser light. Semiconductors are formatted by a process called *doping*—adding a small amount of impurity as a silicon matrix. The valence of the diode is determined by the charge of the impurities added to the silicon to create the matrix. The charge can be either electropositive (p) or electronegative (n). As the electron crosses from the electronegative region to the electropositive region, a photon with energy proportionate to the n-p gap is emitted.[4] While diode lasers generally do not possess the linear power of a gas or solid-state laser, power necessary for surgical applications is generated from diodes that are arranged in linear or two-dimensional arrays.[14]

Power is the rate at which energy is being produced and is measured in watts (joules/sec) or as a smaller unit, such as the milliwatt (mW) or 10^{-3} watts (W).

Fig 6•6 Stimulated emission. If a photon strikes an electron in an upper quantum, a second photon of equal wavelength as well as temporal and spatial orientation is produced. Subsequent collisions of photons with excited electrons amplifies the photons yielding laser light.

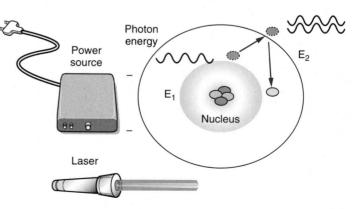

Absorption Stimulated Emission

Power source

Photon energy

E_1

E_2

Nucleus

Laser

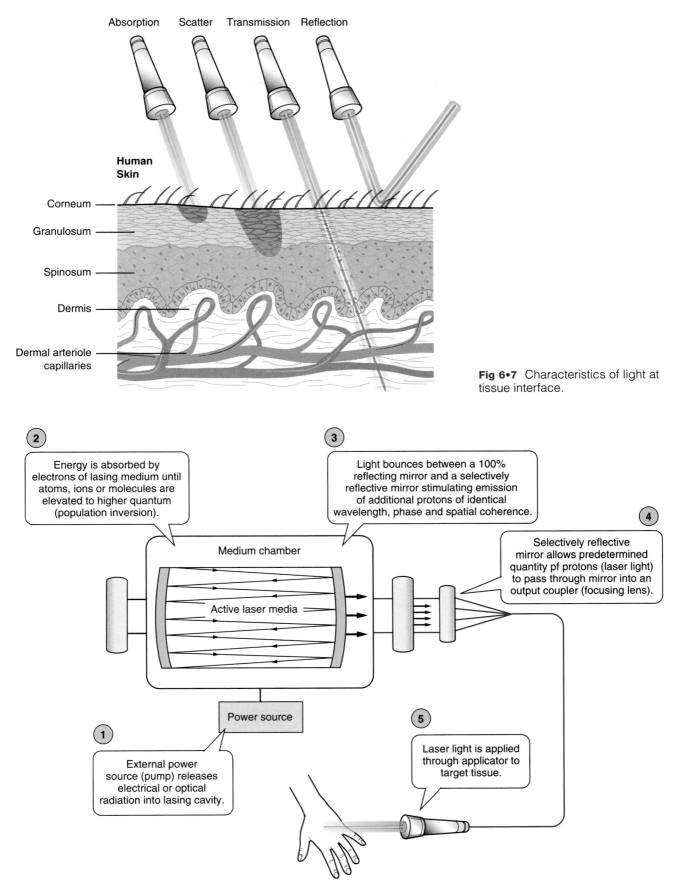

Absorption   Scatter   Transmission   Reflection

Human Skin

Corneum

Granulosum

Spinosum

Dermis

Dermal arteriole capillaries

Fig 6•7 Characteristics of light at tissue interface.

2 Energy is absorbed by electrons of lasing medium until atoms, ions or molecules are elevated to higher quantum (population inversion).

3 Light bounces between a 100% reflecting mirror and a selectively reflective mirror stimulating emission of additional protons of identical wavelength, phase and spatial coherence.

4 Selectively reflective mirror allows predetermined quantity pf protons (laser light) to pass through mirror into an output coupler (focusing lens).

Medium chamber

Active laser media

Power source

1 External power source (pump) releases electrical or optical radiation into lasing cavity.

5 Laser light is applied through applicator to target tissue.

Fig 6•8 Components of a gas/optical-powered laser delivery system.

Dosage is the average power multiplied by the time of the treatment. For instance, lasing continuously over a wound site for 15 seconds with a HeNe laser whose output is 1 mW per second would be 15 mW. Energy can also be expressed in terms of power density measured in W/cm² or in energy density measured in joules per centimeter squared (J/cm²). The same 1 mW HeNe laser lasing a wound with an area of 4 cm² has a power density of 0.25 mW/cm² or 1 mW/4 cm². Energy density, measured in J/cm² is *power* (W) multiplied by *time* (s) and divided by the area of irradiation (cm²). Lasing a 4 cm² wound at 1 mW for 4 seconds produces an energy density of 0.001 J/cm² or 1 mW/cm².[15,16]

Physiological Effects of Lasers

Unlike the thermal effect of surgical lasers, the effects of LLLT are more a function of photochemical activation of enzymes that catalyze the processing of molecular substrates. Early research describes ATP synthesis following 5 J/cm² of HeNe irradiation; this indicates a possible effect on the oxidative phosphorylative component of the mitochondrial membrane.[17] While generally accepted, this notion was refuted after HeNe irradiation of HeLa cells (a stable line of human malignant cells first cultured from patient Henrietta Lacks) demonstrated protein degradation.[18]

KEY POINT! Treatment outcomes for clinical applications of low-level lasers may vary, because the physiological effects depend upon wavelength differentiation, the timing of the application, and the particular type of cell irradiated.

It is generally accepted that the absorbing structures for the low-level laser wavelengths are hemoproteins. The identity of the photoreceptors responsible for the physiological conversion of laser light remains undetermined. Several studies have suggested that either elements in the mitochondrial cytochrome system or endogenous porphyrins (intermediate substance in the synthesis of hemoglobin) in the cell are the energy-absorbing chromophores in LLLT.[19,20] Since the tissue penetration of laser energy used in LLLT can be in the order of 5 to 10 mm, both superficial and deeper structures can be affected. However,

as the energy penetrates the tissues, there is a multiple scattering by both erythrocytes and microvessels; thus, both blood rheology and the distribution of the microvessels markedly influence final distribution of laser energy.[19]

A possible explanation for the conflicting outcomes may lie in the timing of the applications. In vitro studies using low-level radiation at 633 nm and 904 nm demonstrated increased cellular ATP synthesis and activation of calcium (Ca^{++}) at the cell membrane level.[21–23] The similarity of cellular outcome using both wavelengths of LLLT has led to the speculation that 633 nm photostimulation initiates early respiratory chain enzyme activity in the mitochondria, while 904 nm photostimulation of Ca^{++} activity at the membrane level occurs later in the respiratory chain.[21,23] Since both reactions are essential for the DNA and RNA synthesis leading to cell proliferation, it is thought that there is a latency period between excitation of receptor cells responsible for activating the oxidative enzymes throughout the electron transport system. During this period of "low" excitability, absorption of photons is ebbing. Since the excitation potential of cells may be longer or shorter than the pulse duration of the beam, optimal stimulation for some cells may be inefficient for others.

KEY POINT! The parameters of laser pulse rate, exposure timing, and simultaneous wavelengths are presently being researched to determine the most effective modes of stimulation for specific tissue types.

Early studies on multiple-wavelength, low-intensity laser radiation (MWLILR) demonstrated accelerated wound healing when compared to single wavelength stimulation.[24,25] Using HeLa cells irradiated with monochromatic light of 580 to 860 nm, Karu et al.[26] demonstrated active wavelength spectra for phototherapy. The authors concluded that there are four active regions of phototherapy but that the peak positions are not exact for all spectra.[26] Treatment with a combined wavelength (808 to 905 nm) low level laser for in vitro irradiation of two cell types (HeLa epithelial and TK6 lymphoblasts) demonstrated a greater proliferation of cells than did treatment with each wavelength individually.[27] Along with wavelength, cell type has been shown to be a determinant in cell growth. Laser-stimulated murine fibroblasts demonstrated greater proliferation than endothelial cells. Maximum cell proliferation was observed at 665 and 675 nm while fibroblastic growth was inhibited at 810 nm.[28]

Instrumentation and Clinical Application of Lasers

Laser is a special form of electromagnetic energy that is within the visible or infrared regions of the electromagnetic spectrum. Lasers are classified based on their beam wavelength and power and on their potential for causing fires, explosions, and bodily injury. Lasers fall in the range of optical radiation and are termed *mid-infrared, near infrared, visible light,* and *ultraviolet* (Fig. 6-9). Thermal or "hot" lasers, such as carbon dioxide (CO_2), holmium: yttrium-aluminum-garnet (holmium: YAG), and neodymium: yttrium-aluminum-garnet (Nd: YAG), range in wavelength from 10,600 nm (mid-infrared) to 1064 nm (near infrared). Since the power of the laser is wavelength dependent, a CO_2 continuous wave (CW) laser may produce 100 watts (W) while the superpulsed CO_2 laser may generate up to 10,000 W. Tissue responses to thermal lasers are elevation of temperature, dehydration of tissue, coagulation of protein, thermolysis, and evaporation.[9,14,29]

Lasers with power levels of 60 mW or less are termed *low power,* or *cold, lasers* and produce little to no thermal response. The effects of low-powered lasers (photobiostimulation) are a direct result of radiant energy imparted to the tissue rather than the small quantity of indirect thermal energy emitted.[14,16] Most contemporary low-powered lasers have multiple diodes and can be applied by stationary direct contact to singular or multiple points based on location, depth, and extent of the soft tissue lesion (Fig. 6-10).

The World Association of Laser Therapy (WALT) dosage recommendations for anti-inflammatory applications of GaAlAs and gallium arsenide (GaAs) lasers for tendinopathies and arthritis are shown in Table 6-1. WALT recommends beginning with the suggested dosages listed in the table followed by a 30% reduction when the inflammation subsides. These dosages were developed from ultrasonographic measurements of the depth and volume of the pathological tissue relative to the estimated penetration of the laser types. (It should be noted that these calculations were based on measurements of a Caucasian population. Skin color may affect laser penetration, and dosages may need to be increased for patients with darker skin.) WALT suggests a therapeutic window of +/- 50% of the suggested values.

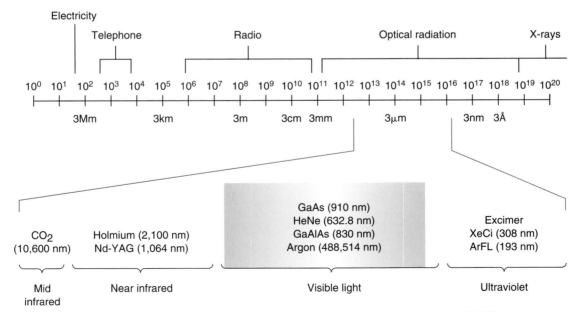

Fig 6•9 Visible light and infrared lasers positioned relevant to the electromagnetic spectrum (EMS).

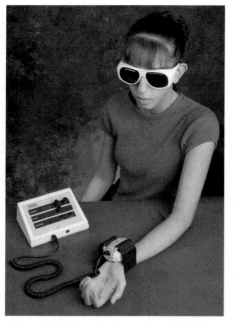

Fig 6•10 Treatment of carpal tunnel syndrome using LLLT with device strapped to patient's wrist. Note the protective goggles on the patient. *(NMA Duo Light 785 nm laser courtesy of National Medical Alliance/Current Therapeutics, 111 Canfield Avenue, Randolph, NJ 07869.)*

Clinical application of LLLT for open wounds often involves moving the laser over the injury. These techniques are generically similar with subtle variation. The "gridding" technique is a continuous series of vertical and horizontal strokes with the laser applicator over the length and width of a designated area. The aperture of the laser wand (the opening in the wand that emits the column of light) is held perpendicular to the wound's surface. The wound should be covered with a hydro-occlusive dressing that is free of convolutions and readily transparent. The wand's surface is held very close to or lightly touching the surface of the wound or wound covering. Each grid should have a surface area ranging between 1 to 1 1/2 cm². The suggested irradiation time for each grid is 20 seconds for HeNe and 10 seconds for GaAs or GaAlAs lasers.

The wound should be cleaned and debrided as needed, as eschar will reflect laser light and limit the absorption necessary for tissue photostimulation. If eschar is present, the operator may elect to apply the laser light to the tissues immediately surrounding the wound. Since wound tissue generally closes

Table 6•1 Recommended Anti-inflammatory Dosage for Low-Level Laser Therapy*

Points or cm²	Tendinopathies	Joules (780–820 nm)	Notes
2–3	Carpal tunnel	12	Minimum 6 joules per point
1–2	Lateral epicondylitis	4	Maximum 100 mW/cm²
1–2	Biceps tendon under coracohumeral ligament	8	
2–3	Supraspinatus	10	Minimum 5 joules per point
2–3	Infraspinatus	10	Minimum 5 joules per point
2–4	Trochanter major	10	
2–3	Patellar tendon	6	
2–3	Tract Iliotibialis	3	Maximum 100 mW/cm²
2–3	Achilles tendon	8	Maximum 100 mW/cm²
2–3	Plantar fasciitis	12	Minimum 6 joules per point
Points or cm²	**Arthritis**	**Joules**	
1–2	Finger PIP or MCP	6	
2–4	Wrist	10	
1–2	Humeroradial joint	4	
2–4	Elbow	10	
2–4	Glenohumeral joint	15	Minimum 6 joules per point
1–2	Acromioclavicular	4	
1–2	Temporomandibular	6	
2–4	Cervical spine	15	Minimum 6 joules per point
2–4	Lumbar spine	40	Minimum 8 joules per point
2–4	Hip	40	Minimum 8 joules per point
3–6	Knee medial	20	Minimum 5 joules per point
2–4	Ankle	15	

*Laser classes 3 or 3B, 780 to 860 nm GaAlAs; continuous or pulse output less than 0.5 W
Note: Daily treatment for 2 weeks or treatment every other day for 3 to 4 weeks is recommended.

circumference by granulating and differentiating from the outside in, the operator may stimulate the tissue at the periphery of the wound. Suggested application times for the "surround" technique is 30 seconds per 2 cm² of wound surface area with the HeNe laser and 20 seconds per 2 cm² wound surface area with a GaAs or GaAlAs laser.[9,14]

The "scanning" technique closely mimics gridding with the exception of the aperture being held less than 1 cm above the site. It should be noted that beam divergence will increase when the laser is not in full contact with the target surface. Movements are gridlike or analogous to the preferred motion for spray painting. Another clinical technique is "wanding," which is similar to scanning in that it does not contact the skin. However, the irradiating pattern is oscillatory rather than the spraylike pattern used when scanning.

Documentation Tips

The following should be documented in the patient's record when performing interventions with a laser:

- Location and surface area treated
- Dosage, expressed in joules/cm²
- Laser power (watts) multiplied by the treatment duration (seconds)
- Frequency and type of the laser (e.g., HeNe 633 nm)
- Use mode (continuous or pulsed)
- Patient's response to the intervention

Indications for the Use of Lasers

Wound Healing

Although there has been much research regarding the use of LLLT to treat chronic and surgical wounds, the body of evidence has been inconclusive because of variability in methodologies, reporting, equipment calibration, and design controls. Despite the dearth of systematic research protocol, increased wound closure, tensile strength, and collagen content has been noted with the use of LLLT for soft tissue wound healing. Animals with loose areolar skin, such as rabbits, rats, and mice, appeared more responsive to LLLT than studies using pigs, whose skin more closely resembles that of humans.[30–32] LLLT at 670 nm produced an accelerated inflammatory, proliferative, and maturation phase of Sprague-Dawley rats with controlled full-thickness skin

wounds.[33] HeNe (633 nm) irradiation of both diabetic and nondiabetic rats produced less intense inflammatory markers (inflammatory cells, vessels, and fibroblasts) than a control group.[34]

In a comparison of animal and human clinical studies, wound healing was accelerated in the group treated with LLLT. Other outcomes included decreased dependency on drugs, accelerated functional recovery, and earlier return to work.[35] Two separate meta-analyses indicated positive response to augmentation of collagen synthesis and increases in wound tensile strength along with reduced healing time.[36,37]

Clinical Controversy

Evidentiary affirmation of effectiveness of LLLT remains limited due in part to small study size, short follow-up time periods, heterogeneity of dosage, and issues of frequency and duration of treatment. Confounding clinical issues such as these may in fact originate in the laboratory or with in vitro studies, which indicate that the physiological effects of LLLT vary with wavelength differentiation, timing of the application relevant to respiratory chain activity, and the particular type of cell irradiated.

Bone Regeneration and Fracture Healing

Studies on the effect of LLLT on fracture healing continue to be equivocal.[38–41] A preponderance of research involving bone healing has come from the field of dentistry. Pinhiero et al.[42] studied the effect of an 830 nm laser on the repair of standardized femoral bone defects of three groups of Wistar albino rats that were grafted with inorganic bovine bone (Genox). The laser irradiated, Genox group demonstrated superior bone formation and collagen fibers around the graft site at 15 days postgraft.[42,43] Using Wister albino rats, Genox, and an 830 nm laser, Gerbi and colleagues[44] noted improved collagen formation in the early stages of bone healing (15 days) along with an increase of well-organized bone trabeculae at 30 days postonset.

When compared to the conventionally used ultrasonic therapy, laser irradiation at 780 nm (GaAlAs) increased bony formation by proliferation of osteoblast quantity, surface area, and volume, whereas ultrasound enhanced bone repair by promoting bony resorption. When the bone was stressed, the laser-assisted bone formation load failure was higher in the laser group than in the ultrasound group.[45] In a study by Kazem-Shakouri and colleagues,[46] findings were consistent for early stage bone healing but were not consistent for load-bearing capability. Despite the promise of these and other studies, there remains equivocation regarding the quality of research.[47,48]

Herpes Simplex Wounds

Patients with recurring herpes simplex virus (HSV) receiving HeNe (633 nm) and Acyclovir demonstrated reduced frequency and decreased duration of relapse as compared to patients treated with HeNe LLLT or Acyclovir alone. The authors concluded that HeNe and Acyclovir produced a therapeutic synergism.[49] In a randomized, double-blind, placebo-controlled study, patients with perioral herpes simplex irradiated with laser at 690 nm experienced a significantly lower recurrence of herpes simplex outbreak.[50] Subsequent research confirms the positive effects of LLLT in the treatment of HSV 1 or 2.[51–55]

Epicondylitis

Several studies evaluated the effectiveness of 904 nm low-level laser therapy in the management of epicondylitis. Lam and Cheing[56] noted greater improvement of mechanical pain threshold, maximum grip strength, and pain at maximum grip strength subjectively in all but two subsections of the Disabilities of the Arm, Shoulder, and Hand (DASH) questionnaire.

The use of LLLT for epicondylitis has been compared to adjunctive procedures, such as counterpressure bracing or plyometric exercises. In a randomized, controlled, single-blind trial, Oken and colleagues[57] found that LLLT produced longer lasting relief than bracing alone. Additionally, laser was more effective than the combination of bracing and ultrasound at improving grip strength. When LLLT and exercise was compared to polychromatic noncoherent light and exercises, both were found to relieve pain and improve function immediately following treatment.[58]

An early meta-analysis[59] "lightly" cited the consideration of LLLT in treating epicondylitis. Bjordal et al.[60] reviewed 18 randomized, placebo-controlled trials of which 12 of the RCTs satisfied 50% or more of the methodological criteria. Using Egger's graphical analysis to filter publication bias, they determined that LLLT

at doses of 904 nm (and possibly 632.9 nm) applied directly to the lateral elbow tendon insertions offered short-term pain relief and less disability. These findings were consistent for LLLT alone or in concert with an exercise regimen.

Tendinopathies

Bjordal et al.[61] examined the anti-inflammatory effect of 904 nm laser on Achilles tendonitis. Patients with bilateral Achilles tendonitis had both Achilles tendons irradiated at 5.4 joules per point (power density of 20 mw/cm²) in random, blinded order. The test group demonstrated reduced prostaglandin E_2 levels along with increased pressure pain threshold. Recreational athletes with Achilles tendinopathy treated with 820 nm LLLT and eccentric exercises demonstrated decreased pain on the 100 mm visual analog scale at 4 weeks, 8 weeks, and 12 weeks postintervention as compared to the eccentric exercises/placebo group. A similar pattern was noted for morning stiffness, active dorsiflexion, palpable tenderness, and crepitation.[62] A systematic review meta-analysis of 25 controlled clinical trials showed positive effects for an effective window of dosage consistent with recommended guidelines. Subjects with lateral epicondylitis, treated with LLLT, showed higher grip strength than those in control groups. Subjects with Achilles tendinopathy receiving LLLT exhibited 13.6 mm less pain (100 mm VAS) than the control group.[63]

Studies have investigated the effects of LLLT for subacromial impingement syndrome (SAIS). Evidence regarding the effectiveness of LLLT for SAIS remains convoluted because of variability in the designs of the studies and characteristics of the subjects, such as age and activity levels. Michener and colleagues[64] reported the benefits of laser when utilized in isolation rather than in combination with therapeutic exercise. Andres and Murrell[65] noted inconsistent results with LLLT in combination with ultrasound and iontophoresis in the treatment of tendinopathy.

In a randomized study, Stergioulas[66] examined the efficacy of LLLT in patients with frozen shoulder using 810 nm laser. When compared to a placebo group, the laser group demonstrated a decrease of overall night pain, decreased shoulder pain index, and Croft Shoulder Disability Questionnaire scores. Post-treatment follow-up at 8 and 16 weeks using the DASH questionnaire

CASE STUDY 6•1   SELECTING LOW-LEVEL LASER THERAPY (LLLT) FOR LATERAL EPICONDYLITIS

A 34-year-old female is a cashier at a local supermarket. After working a double shift, she noted extreme soreness (pain rating 77 mm/100 mm VAS) at the lateral epicondyle of her right elbow. Upon testing dynamometry, the patient presented with a 50% disparity in grip strength and 35% disparity of composite (sum of flexion + extension + supination + pronation) elbow strength.

CLINICAL DECISION-MAKING

1. Does the patient have a dysfunction, limitation, or problem that can be improved with the use of low-level laser therapy?
   Answer: Yes, symptoms indicate a recently acquired acute inflammation of the lateral elbow tendon insertions.

2. Is the patient appropriate for LLLT (i.e., do any of the general precautions or contraindications to LLLT apply to the patient, or are there any specific considerations regarding applying LLLT to this patient)?
   Answer: The patient is not pregnant, epileptic, or febrile. She is devoid of hemorrhaging/infectious lesions or cancers. Her elbow has mature epiphyseal plates. Laser stimulation will not be in proximity to genitalia, the vagus nerve, or the mediastinum.

3. What are the specific goals to be achieved with the use of LLLT?
   Answer: Initially, pain relief sufficient enough to initiate eccentric exercises with elastic band. Once exercise has been initiated, LLLT will be utilized to prevent further bouts of acute inflammation.

4. What specific type of LLLT would be appropriate for the patient?
   Answer: Gallium aluminum arsenide laser (GaAlAs) at 780 to 820 nm.

5. Can you select the specific parameters of LLLT that are appropriate for the patient?

Answer: Delivery to two points at the lateral epicondyle at a maximum of 100 mW/cm^2 (0.1 J/cm^2).

6. What are the proper application procedures for LLLT?
   Answer: Inform the patient of the purpose of the procedure. Be sure to explain the difference between LLLT and surgical lasers. A brief demonstration may serve to reinforce the benign nature of the procedure. Set the laser to the appropriate dosage. This may be preset on the device or determined by setting the device timer for the dosage according to the number and power of the diodes (e.g., 1 diode delivering 100 mW/sec = 100 millijoules/sec or 0.1 J/sec). Using this diode, it would take 1 second to deliver 1 joule. Since most dosages are calculated in J/cm^2, lasing 10 seconds over a 1 cm^2 area would amount to a 1 J/cm^2 dosage.
   Pretreatment: Ask the patient to point to the painful location and rate the level of discomfort. Next, confirm the location of pain by palpation. If necessary, retest with Cozen, Mills, and "handshake" tests. The patient is requested to wear protective eye glasses during the treatment.
   During Treatment: Position the patient in a manner that affords greatest access to the affected area as well as comfort. Depending on the level of resting pain, the position may be with the upper extremity supported with a cushion or pillow in either a supine or sitting position. Depending on the nature of the equipment, the laser diode(s) is handheld or attached to the application site(s).
   Post-Treatment: Remove the diode(s) and inspect the application site(s). Ask the patient to once again rate their pain.

were also lower than the control group. Two other studies found LLLT did not augment a comprehensive home exercise program or supervised progressive resistance program for subjects with frozen shoulder.[67,68]

Carpal Tunnel Syndrome

The 830 nm GaA1As laser was initially approved by the FDA for treating only carpal tunnel syndrome (CTS). Effects of LLLT on CTS were believed to be relief of pain, increased active ROM, increased strength, and improved tolerance of functional activities. Weintraub[69] treated 30 hands with CTS using the GaAlAs laser. Five points along the median nerve were treated with 8 J/point at 33-second intervals. Subjects felt no discomfort or heat sensation. Complete resolution of pretreatment symptoms and abnormal physical findings was achieved in 77% of the hands.[69] Figure 6-3A demonstrates clinical application of LLLT to the carpal tunnel. The usual dosage is 6 joules per point delivered at 2 or 3 points overlying the median nerve in the carpal tunnel (see Table 6-1).

Pulsed (25% duty cycle) ultrasound delivered at 1 MHz, 1.0 W/cm² for 15 minutes was more effective than 830 nm laser delivered at 9 J/point over 15 visits.[70] In a double-blind, randomized, controlled study by Irvine and colleagues,[71] 15 patients with CTS were irradiated with 6 J/point using a 860 nm GaAlAs laser. They found no significant difference in functional outcomes between the test and sham groups. GaAlAs laser and placebo therapy both improved pain and functional hand scores in patients with rheumatoid arthritis and CTS.[72] In other studies, patients with CTS treated with LLLT demonstrated significant improvement of sensory and motor nerve latencies, pain assessment, and grip strength.[73–75]

Arthritis

Some studies indicate that there may be beneficial effects of low-level laser treatments for arthritis. Basirnia and colleagues[156] used an 810 nm pulsed infrared diode laser on five periarticular tender points in 29 patients with knee osteoarthritis once per day for a total of 12 sessions. The authors reported significant improvement in pain relief and quality of life in 70% of patients following the 12 LLLT treatments. Trelles and colleagues[157] used an 830 nm infrared continuous-wave gallium aluminum arsenide diode laser with an output power of 60 mW to treat 40 patients with knee osteoarthritis. They used a power density of 18 J/cm² per session, for two sessions per week for 8 weeks. A significant reduction in pain level and increased knee joint mobility occurred in 33 of the patients (82%). LLLT may also be beneficial in patients who have neck or back pain caused by osteoarthritis. Oezdemir and colleagues[158] applied LLLT to the cervical spine in 60 patients with radiologically diagnosed osteoarthritis. Pain, paravertebral muscle spasm, lordosis angle, and cervical spine ROM improved significantly compared to a placebo group. Figure 6-3B demonstrates the use of a handheld wand to deliver LLLT to the cervical spine.

Contraindications and Precautions for Lasers

The classification of lasers is based on their potential for causing immediate damage to the eye or skin and for causing fires. Class I lasers are typically enclosed and pose no danger to users. CD players and laser printers are examples of class I lasers. Class II lasers emit radiation in the visible portion of the EMS. The blink reflex (0.25 seconds when exposed to laser light) is sufficient to protect the eye against deleterious effects. It should be noted that chronic exposure to light from class II lasers, such as a laser pointer, may cause damage to the eyes.[13] Class IIIa lasers such as the HeNe laser (not exceeding 5 mW) will not produce injury with momentary viewing. Class IIIb lasers (HeNe lasers above 5 mW but not exceeding 500 mW) may cause injury with direct viewing of the beam or specular reflections. Class IV lasers, which include all lasers with power levels greater than 500 mW, pose eye, skin, and fire hazards. Operators of lasers should consult the American National Standards Institute (ANSI) guidelines.[76]

Lasers, unlike ordinary light, emit a beam that is completely focused on the fovea of the eye. Absorption of the energy can produce a burn that causes partial or complete loss of vision.

KEY POINT! As a precautionary measure, goggles with an appropriate optical density (OD) rating should be worn by practitioners and patients during laser therapy.

The goggles should have an obvious imprint of the optical density and the wavelength (or laser type) for which they are to be used. It should not be assumed that a single pair of goggles is appropriate for all wavelengths.[13]

LLLT is not recommended for patients with epilepsy, fever, malignancy, areas of decreased sensation, or infected tissue. Anatomically, the gonads, epiphyseal plates of children, sympathetic ganglia, vagus nerve, and mediastinum should be avoided.

Contraindications to LLLT are irradiation during pregnancy, over the open fontanelles of children, over cancerous lesions, over the cornea, over endocrine glands, and over hemorrhaging lesions.

Assessment of Effectiveness of Lasers

The benchmark analytical tool for clinical decision-making for using LLLT is a systematic review or meta-analyses of the literature. In 2002, when the FDA approved laser treatment for carpal tunnel syndrome, only in vitro laboratory studies were available; blinded, random, controlled clinical studies were not available. The rationale for clinical usage of lasers was often predicated on the abundance of in vitro studies validating the physiological effects of laser-irradiated tissue. Due to its novelty, the same could not be said of clinical outcomes due to issues of machine quality, study design, and user competence. The advent of the semiconductor diode laser, improved study design, and increased user contact time has significantly advanced the volume and quality of randomized controlled trials during the past decade.

A systematic review with meta-analysis of the use of LLLT for lateral elbow tendinopathy that included 13 randomized controlled trials (730 patients) found that pain relief as measured on a 100 mm visual analog scale showed a weighted mean difference of 10.2 mm (95% CI: 3 to 17.5). Negative results were noted for trials treating acupuncture points as well as laser irradiation using wavelengths of 820, 830, and 1,064 nm. Significant pain relief was noted with irradiation of lateral elbow tendon with 904 nm lasers (four trials) and with 632 nm wavelength (one trial). The LLLT doses in this subgroup ranged between 0.5 and 7.2 joules. Follow-up data from this subgroup 3 to 8 weeks after the end of treatment found pain free grip strength, pain pressure threshold, and sick leave were significantly improved (p less than 0.02).[60]

A Cochrane Review of nonspecific low back pain was deemed to have insufficient data to determine the clinical effect of LLLT for treating low back pain. The authors cited the need for "rigorous randomized, controlled trials to establish parameters such as lengths of treatment, wavelengths, and dosage."[77] Mixed results were noted in a systematic review of nonpharmacological therapies. Four trials indicated a positive effect of LLLT (compared to sham treatment) in the treatment of low back pain. Other trials within the review showed no effect or an effect similar to exercise or combined LLLT and exercise.[78]

A Cochrane systematic review of LLLT treatment of rheumatoid arthritis noted a positive effect for short-term relief of pain and morning stiffness. However, the meta-analysis was unable to discern data regarding the effects of wavelength, treatment duration, dosage, and application site over nerves versus joints.[79] LLLT was no better than a placebo in reducing pain or morning stiffness or improving the functional status of patients with osteoarthritis of the hands.[80] The use of LLLT was not substantiated in several reviews of wound healing.[81]

The clinical use of LLLT has become more prominent as a physical agent in the treatment of musculoskeletal conditions. Laboratory studies continue to substantiate the positive effect of low-level laser stimulation on the inflammatory process. More randomized, controlled clinical studies are needed to identify the conditions that respond best to LLLT treatment, those that do not respond, and the optimal dosage and treatment frequency for each condition. More information on laser therapy can be found at websites listed in Box 6-1.

Clinical Controversy (LLLT)

As with many new therapies in the formative phase, evidence-based information may be as much a source of consternation as confirmation. Reviews of clinical studies often cite a lack of valid or robust conclusions supporting the use of LLLT. Recently, these evidentiary reviews have come under reverse scrutiny by laser researchers for a publication bias.[82,83] While this process is necessary and will ultimately improve the body of evidence, health-care professionals must evaluate current information and decide, beyond the "do no harm" level of engagement, how effective this physical agent can be as an adjunct therapy or primary intervention. The 5th Congress of the World Association of Laser Therapy has authored study designs for both random, controlled trials and systematic reviews of laser research literature.[84,85]

Box 6•1 Recommended Websites for Laser Therapy

http://www.laser.nu	Laser World-Swedish Medical Laser Society
http://walt.nu	World Association of Laser Therapy
http://www.naalt.org	North American Association for Laser Therapy

Diathermy

The term *diathermy* literally means to "heat through."[1] Historically, the term has been applied to modalities that cause heating of deeper tissues such as muscles and joints. This chapter will limit the term to the use of electromagnetic waves from the radio frequency or microwave frequency ranges of the electromagnetic spectrum.

Physical Principles of Diathermy

Diathermy is the application of electromagnetic waves in the radio frequency range of the electromagnetic spectrum to the tissues of the body. The most common form of diathermy in use today uses 27.12 MHz frequency waves from the short wavelength range of radio frequency waves and is commonly referred to as *shortwave diathermy* (SWD). A less common type of diathermy is microwave diathermy (MWD), which uses electromagnetic waves from the microwave range of the electromagnetic spectrum. The frequency most commonly used for microwave diathermy is 2,450 MHz.

In response to great demands for the use of various frequencies for communication purposes in the United States, the Federal Communications Commission (FCC) has carefully regulated frequencies that can be utilized for television and radio transmission, radar, and medical applications. Approved frequencies for diathermy are listed in Table 6-2.

Diathermy can be delivered continuously or through regular pulses or bursts of radio frequency energy. Pulsed shortwave diathermy (PSWD) uses a timing circuit to electronically interrupt the 27.12 MHz waves, resulting in bursts of pulse trains containing a series of high-frequency sine wave oscillations emitted from the PSWD treatment applicator. Each pulse train has a preset duration, or "on time," and is separated from successive pulse trains by an "off time" that is determined by the pulse repetition rate or frequency (Fig. 6-11). Depending on the device, the pulse frequency can be varied from 1 to 7,000 pulses per second and is selected with a pulse-frequency control on the equipment-operation panel. Pulsed radio frequency waves, delivered to the patient at a very low intensity, that do not create heat in the tissues is often referred to as *pulsed electromagnetic fields* (PEMF) or *pulsed radio frequency energy* (PRFE).

The radio frequency waves produced by diathermy devices will pass through the tissues of the body and initially are not detected. Gradually, absorption of energy by the tissues may cause an increase in tissue temperature, depending on the intensity of the waves and whether the waves are continuous or pulsed. Patients may perceive a feeling of warmth as the tissue temperature rises. Generally the closer the diathermy applicator is to the patient's skin, the greater the effect on the tissues.

Diathermy can affect deeper tissues of the body than superficial modalities such as hot packs, because radio frequency waves can travel through superficial tissues. There is minimal reflection of waves at tissue interfaces and on bone, so there is no accumulation of energy at these interfaces, such as occurs with ultrasound.

Therapeutic Diathermy Devices: Delivery of Radio Frequency Waves to the Patient

Shortwave and microwave diathermy generators require an electrical source that provides an alternating current (available from an electrical outlet). There are two types of shortwave diathermy: the electric field or capacitive method and the magnetic field or inductive method.

Capacitive Method

The capacitive method involves using an applicator system that requires making the patient's tissues part of the dielectric of a capacitor (Fig. 6-12). This technique, also called the *electric field method,* affects tissues primarily by applying an oscillating electric field. When performing the capacitive method of SWD to heat tissues that are beneath a thick layer of subcutaneous fat, care must

Table 6•2	Radio Frequencies Approved by the FCC for SWD/MWD and PEMF	
Frequency (MHz)	**Wavelength**	**Type of EM RADIATION**
13.56	22 m	SWD/PEMF
27.12*	11 m	SWD/PEMF
40.68	7.5 m	SWD/PEMF
915.00	33 cm	MWD
2450.00	12 cm	MWD

*Most widely used frequency for SWD and PEMF

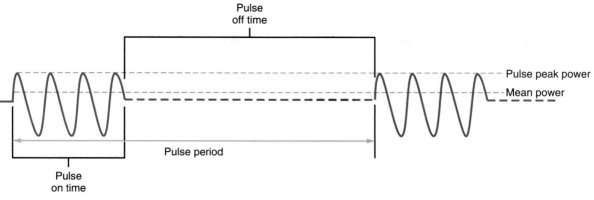

Pulse off time

Pulse peak power

Mean power

Pulse period

Pulse on time

Fig 6•11 Pulsed shortwave diathermy (PSWD). The 27.12 MHz frequency wave is interrupted to create bursts (pulses) of waves, separated by a period of no bursts ("off-time"). The amount of energy delivered to the tissues depends on the *mean power*, which is determined by the pulse peak power, pulse frequency, and pulse duration. *(Art concept by Sara Monath, PT student, Richard Stockton College of NJ.)*

be taken when positioning the treatment applicators. Subcutaneous fatty tissue may be heated considerably more than muscle when both tissues are exposed to the SWD electric field. One explanation for this is the presence of numerous blood vessels that pervade the thick layer of fat tissue. These blood vessels contain blood, which has a high conductivity and is therefore preferentially heated.

Another factor that must be considered is the superficial location of subcutaneous fat in relation to deeper muscle tissue. Air-spaced plates have a glass or plastic guard surrounding each metal plate (electrode) to prevent contact between the electrode and the patient's skin. A severe electrical burn may occur if either the

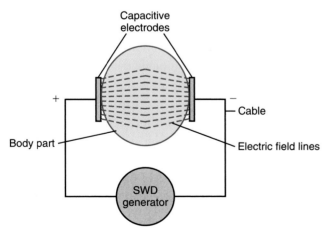

Fig 6•12 Capacitive method of diathermy. The body part is placed between two electrodes and becomes part of the electric field. The relative field density is greater closer to the electrodes. *(Illustration by Sara Monath, PT student, Richard Stockton College of NJ.)*

therapist's or the patient's skin contacts the bare metal plate of the diathermy device. A single layer of terry-cloth toweling should be placed between the plate guards and the patient's skin to prevent concentration of the electric field on perspiration that may accumulate on the skin.

Most plates are manually movable through a distance of about 3 cm within the guard. In some older models, the plate is not movable, but the plate guard can be manually adjusted so the plate-to-skin distance is 1 to 2.5 cm. The guard should be about 1 to 3 inches (2 to 10 cm) from the skin for optimal heating, and the metal plate should be as far away from the skin as the guard allows (2.5 cm). Proper positioning of the plate and guard in relation to the skin provides for an increased relative heating depth of the tissues and effective absorption of thermal energy. When applied correctly to patients whose subcutaneous fat layer is less than 1 cm thick, the capacitive-field technique may be capable of delivering energy into tissue depths that correspond to the depths heated with inductive applicators. Most SWD devices maintain constant power output with changes in plate-skin distance. Power or dosage is determined by the patient's subjective perception of heat. The closer the plates are to the skin, the greater the heat sensation. Air-spaced plates should always be positioned so the distance between any part of the two plates is at least as great as the plate's diameter. As the plate-to-skin distance increases, heat perception decreases, allowing for the power output to be increased so more heating can reach deeper tissues.

Air-spaced plates may be positioned in two different arrangements that produce different tissue heating patterns: contraplanar or coplanar. In the contraplanar arrangement, the plates are placed on each side of the body part so that the body part is between the plates. In this arrangement, tissue heating will be proportional to the impedance that each type of tissue offers to the oscillating molecules. Fat will be heated more than muscle or bone because it has a higher impedance. A coplanar arrangement requires that the plates be positioned parallel on the same body surface, rather than placing the body part between the plates (Fig. 6-13). In this arrangement, both superficial and deep tissues are parallel to the two applicator plates. Tissues that receive more heating in a parallel plate arrangement are those with low impedance (higher conductivity). Thus, muscle tissue will be selectively heated because the current takes the path of least resistance in more highly conductive tissue. The coplanar method may be more beneficial when treating problems of the lumbar or thoracic paravertebral musculature.

Inductive Method

The inductive method involves using an inductive applicator in which an oscillating magnetic field induces oscillating "eddy" currents in the tissues (Fig. 6-14). This approach is also called the *magnetic field method*. Because of the high-frequency radio waves used with diathermy, the electromagnetic energy can be transmitted through "wireless airwaves" to the patient with an airspace or insulating material placed between the applicator and the skin surface.

Once the magnetic field enters the body part, an electrical current is induced within the tissues having the lowest impedance. The induced electrical eddy

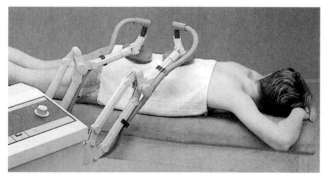

Fig 6•13 Coplanar arrangement of capacitive diathermy electrodes.

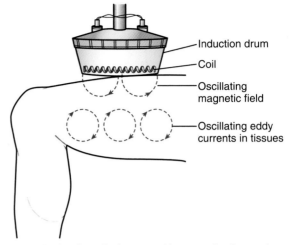

Fig 6•14 Inductive diathermy with monode drum placement over tissues creates a magnetic field that induces oscillating eddy currents in the tissues. *(Art concept by Sara Monath, PT student, Richard Stockton College of NJ.)*

currents alternate in direction with changes of the magnetic field. Thus, the greatest density of eddy current activity, and therefore the greatest amount of heating, occurs in low-impedance tissues containing the highest electrolyte content, such as skeletal muscle and blood.

Two types of coil applicators can be used to deliver the magnetic field energy to the patient: drums or sleeves. Drum applicators consist of a coil-shaped cable that is contained within two types of rigid plastic insulator housings. The treatment surface of the plastic applicator serves the same function as the plate guard of the air-spaced plate applicator—to space the inductive coil away from the skin.

A monode is a drum used to treat a single body surface and requires a single layer of terry-cloth toweling to create additional spacing and moisture absorption from the skin (Fig. 6-15). The diplode is a hinged drum that allows one or more body part surfaces to be treated simultaneously. The diplode consists of a rectangular induction coil contained within an insulator housing that also serves to space the coil away from the patient's skin. Because of the coil's closer proximity to the treatment surface within the diplode, approximately 1 cm of terry-cloth toweling is recommended to separate the applicator from the patient's skin; this will prevent excessive surface heating and will absorb perspiration.

The induction sleeve is shaped to fit around a body part such as the elbow and forearm, providing a circumferential treatment effect (Fig. 6-16).

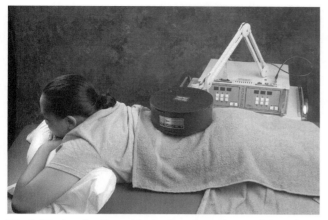

Fig 6-15 Application of induction drum (monode) to the low back. A single layer of towel is placed between the skin and the surface of the drum.

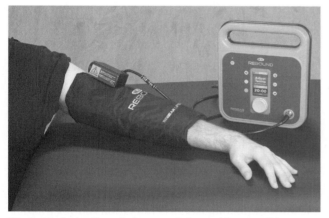

Fig 6•16 Induction diathermy delivered by a coil in a sleeve shaped to fit the body part. *(Rebound System courtesy of GameReady, 1201 Marina Village Parkway, Suite 200, Alameda, CA 94501.)*

Some diathermy devices have external cables that connect the applicator to the console and deliver the electromagnetic (EM) energy from the high-frequency oscillating circuit to the applicator. Cables on older devices may not be adequately shielded and may emit radiation in all directions when the applicators are energized. In this case, care must be taken to prevent the cables from directly contacting the patient or any metal or synthetic materials.

Microwave Diathermy

The generation of electromagnetic waves in the microwave frequency range requires a device called a *magnetron*. A magnetron generates alternating current at a high power level that is transmitted to an antenna housed inside an emitter (drum or applicator) that directs the electromagnetic field to the body part to be treated. Microwave ovens used for heating and cooking food use a magnetron similar to those used for diathermy. Frequencies allotted for microwave diathermy (MWD) in the United States are listed in Table 6-2. In Europe, Australia, and New Zealand, 434 MHz is also approved for medical use.[3]

Application of MWD to the patient requires proper alignment of the emitter in relationship to the body part to be treated. Placing the emitter at a right angle to the body part ensures microwaves will be applied perpendicular to the skin's surface and will limit reflection of waves. Some emitters are placed at a small distance from the skin's surface with an air gap between the emitter and the skin. Other emitters are designed to be placed in contact with the skin.

MWD can be used to treat a more focused area of the body than SWD can provide. However, the thermal effects are usually not as deep as SWD. This is because microwaves are partially reflected from tissue layers, resulting in standing waves that concentrate the energy absorption in superficial tissues.[3] There is an increased risk of damage to superficial tissues because of this greater absorption of energy. Microwaves have a greater frequency than shortwaves; therefore, a higher intensity of energy is delivered to the tissues. MWD is used in medicine for hyperthermia of malignant tumors. However, it is currently not commonly used for therapeutic rehabilitation purposes.

Pulsed Shortwave Diathermy (PSWD)

Today, most modern diathermy devices are either pulsed shortwave diathermy or have both continuous and pulsed modes. Most PSWD devices use the inductive method with a drum electrode. Bursts of electromagnetic waves are created by interrupting the flow of continuous waves generated by the device. The burst (also known as *pulse*) duration is preset by the device's manufacturers in a range from 40 to 400 microseconds (μsec). The practitioner can adjust the burst or pulse frequency, which usually ranges from 1 to 1,000 bursts per second (also called *pulses per second,* or pps). The peak pulse power (the power in watts delivered during a pulse) ranges between 100 and 1,000 W in most devices that provide PSWD. If the pulse duration is 400 μs (0.4 ms) and the peak power and pulse frequency are known, the mean power is easily calculated. For example, at a peak pulse power of 800 W, if the pulse frequency is 200 pps, then the pulse period (the pulse on-time plus the pulse off-time) may be calculated as the pulse period (ms) ÷ pulse frequency, or in this case 1,000 ÷ 200 = 5 ms (see Fig. 6-11). In this example, the percentage of time during which the pulsed short-wave output is delivered is 0.4 ÷ 5 = 8%. This is some-times called the *duty cycle.* Consequently, the mean power is 8% of 800 W, or 64 W. Generally, with most PSWD devices, the highest mean power output that can be delivered is lower than the power delivered (80 to 120 W) during most continuous SWD treatments.

Pulsed Electromagnetic Fields (PEMF)

There is some confusion in the literature about the use of the term *pulsed electromagnetic fields,* or PEMF. Some publications use this term to indicate application of pulsed shortwave diathermy at an intensity that may cause heating of tissues. Other publications use PEMF to describe electromagnetic waves delivered at a very low intensity and that do not cause heating of tissues. Bassett[112] limited PEMFs to devices that deliver low-energy *magnetic* fields that cause nonthermal effects on tissues, such as promotion of bone healing. In this chapter, PEMF will be limited to those devices that deliver very low-intensity electromagnetic waves that do not heat tissues. The use of magnetic fields for ther-apeutic purposes is discussed in Chapter 15.

PEMF devices have been in use since the 1950s, when the FCC approved the Diapulse device for thera-peutic purposes.[111] These devices generate PEMFs by an induction coil aerial that is placed on the skin's sur-face. Average power is typically limited to 1 W or less. There are portable devices available that are battery powered and can be worn by the patient (Fig. 6-17). These devices are primarily used to promote tissue heal-ing, presumably by nonthermal facilitation of cellular metabolism and ionic fluctuation.

Physiological Effects of Diathermy

The frequencies of electromagnetic waves used for diathermy applications are *not* capable of depolarizing motor nerves or eliciting a contractile response from innervated or denervated skeletal muscle. Excitation of a nerve or muscle using currents with minimal amplitude requires pulses of about 0.1 ms (millisecond) duration

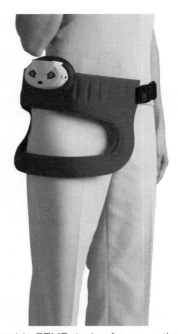

Fig 6•17 Portable PEMF device for promotion of bone healing. *(Courtesy of Orthofix Orthopedics North America, 1720 Bray Central Drive, McKinney, Texas.)*

or longer. The pulse duration at 27.12 MHz would only be 36 nanoseconds (36,310[29] seconds); therefore, exci-tation of these tissues, resulting in depolarization, does not occur because the wavelength (duration) of each cycle of the high-frequency alternating current does not last sufficiently long to cause migration of ions through cellular membranes of nerve or muscle.

KEY POINT! Electromagnetic waves in the radio fre-quency range are nonionizing radiation, which means that there is insufficient energy concentration to dis-lodge orbiting electrons from atoms. Therefore, these waves will not induce mutations.

Electromagnetic energy from the radio frequency part of the spectrum provides energy that may or may not be perceived by the skin. Regardless of whether it is perceived by the body, radio frequency energy delivers only a fraction of the energy level required to produce ionization in tissue. For example, the energy at a frequency of 100 MHz (in the FM radio frequency band) is approximately 300 million times too weak to produce ionization.[86] Therefore, radio frequency electromagnetic waves will not induce mutations or the uncoupling of DNA single strands that result from ionizing x-ray radiation therapy used in cancer treatment.

Thermal Effects

The goal of most diathermy treatments is to increase the temperature of body tissues. The amount of energy delivered to the patient will depend on the type of diathermy (continuous or pulsed); the proximity of the electrode, drum, or emitter to the patient's skin; and the duration of the treatment. The ability of a diathermy device to raise tissue temperature depends on the device's power output, measured in watts (W). The power output range for most SWD devices is 55 to 500 W, which is sufficient to raise the temperature of most tissues to a range of 37.5°C to 44°C (99.5°F to 111.2°F). The range of peak (instantaneous) pulse power for most pulsed shortwave devices is 100 to 1,000 W. However, the potential for producing a heating effect with these devices depends on the mean power delivered to the tissues with successive bursts of pulse trains. The highest mean power that can be delivered with PSWD devices is lower than the usual power output delivered during continuous SWD treatments.

The thermal effects of diathermy on tissues will result in similar physiological responses discussed in Chapter 3. One key difference is the greater depth of heating that occurs with diathermy compared to superficial thermal modalities. How is heat produced in body tissues when radio frequency waves from a diathermy device are directed at a body part? Tissues contain large numbers of ions, and when these charge carriers are exposed to an oscillating electromagnetic field, the ions are accelerated first in one direction and then in the other. As a result of the increased ionic motion, ions collide with nearby molecules, increasing their random motion, which in turn leads to increased internal kinetic energy and heat generation in the tissues (Fig. 6-18A).[3] Additional significant heating occurs because many tissues, especially muscle and blood, are primarily composed of water. Although water molecules are electrically neutral, they are also polar or have polarity because one end of the molecule is positively charged while the other end is negatively charged. Because it has ends of opposite charge, the water molecule is called a *dipole*. When exposed to the high-frequency oscillating electric field, the polar water molecules undergo dipole rotation, and in the process of spinning, they collide with other molecules, increasing

random motion and heat generation (Fig. 6-18B). Other atoms and molecules that are not electrically charged (nonpolar) may have the paths of their orbiting electrons shifted by the oscillating electric field, which results in a back-and-forth oscillation of their electron cloud. This distortion of the electron cloud allows for only minimal friction and movement between adjacent molecules, which in turn results in minor heating (Fig. 6-18C). Ward[87] believed increased ionic motion is the most efficient mechanism for converting high-frequency current into heat.

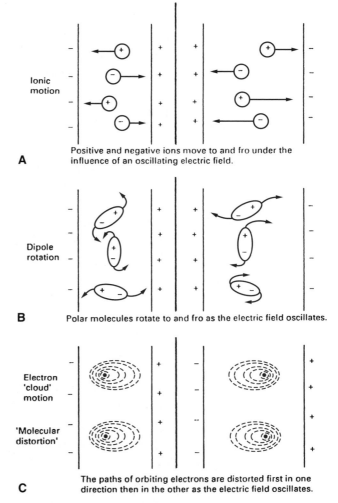

A Positive and negative ions move to and fro under the influence of an oscillating electric field.

B Polar molecules rotate to and fro as the electric field oscillates.

C The paths of orbiting electrons are distorted first in one direction then in the other as the electric field oscillates.

Fig 6•18 Effects of electromagnetic waves on ions and molecules in tissues of the body. (A) Back-and-forth motion (oscillations) of ions results in collisions that produce heat. (B) Rotation of dipoles (water molecules) results in increased random motion of adjacent molecules and produces heat. (C) Distortion of atoms and molecules that are not charged results in increased random motion of adjacent molecules, which may cause some heat. *(Modified from Robertson, Ward, Low, and Reed. Electrotherapy Explained, Principles and Practice. 4th ed. Oxford, UK: Butterworth Heinemann Elsevier; 2006)*

The patterns of heating of capacitive and inductive SWD are different because they introduce electromagnetic energy into tissues differently. Inductive SWD heating is produced mainly by inducing currents in the tissues (see Fig. 6-14). A strong magnetic field enters the body and generates small, circular electrical (eddy) currents in the target tissue that alternately change direction with fluctuations of the magnetic field. The magnetic field passes easily through the tissues and tends to be more intense close to the treatment applicator and less intense as the field spreads into deeper tissues.

Inductive SWD will effectively elevate the temperature of deep tissues (such as muscle) without causing an unsafe rise in skin or fat tissue temperature.[1] There is less heating of subcutaneous fat and more heating of superficial muscle.[88] The amount of heating will occur in tissues having the lowest impedance and the greatest eddy current density or activity. Inductive SWD is particularly effective for heating tissues with high conductivities and high electrolyte content, particularly those well perfused with blood, such as muscle. High temperatures are also produced in areas surrounding joints. This method of application causes less heating in fat, bone, or collagen tissues than the capacitive technique because these tissues have lower conductivity than muscle. The amount of heating occurring in a specific tissue is based on Joule's law and can be calculated using the following equation:

$$H = I^2 Rt$$

where H is the amount of heating, I^2 is the current squared, R is the resistance, and t is time.

Capacitive SWD requires placing the patient's tissues between the electrodes (plates) of the device. The plates, intervening air, and body part form a capacitor that can store an electrical charge (see Fig. 6-12). The charge of the high-frequency electric field oscillates from one plate to the other, resulting in tissue heating. There are factors other than ion oscillation, dipole rotation, and electron-cloud distortion that explain how capacitive diathermy heats tissues. Tissue heating by ionic oscillation depends on tissue conductivity; however, heating by dipole rotation and electron-cloud distortion depends on ease of depolarization of polarizable molecules. The amount of depolarization is characterized by a property of insulators known as the *dielectric*

constant, which is the ratio of the capacity of a material (tissue) to that of free space. Generally, tissues that have high dielectric constants, such as skin and muscle, are good conductors, while tissues with low dielectric constants, such as fat and bone, have low conductivity (Table 6-3). Electrical conductivity is inversely related to resistance. Fat tissue has low electrical conductivity and has high electrical, or ohmic, resistance. Muscle has a higher dielectric constant than fat; therefore, muscle has greater conductivity than fat tissue. The variance in conductivities of the tissues in a given body part tends to cause an electromagnetic field to refract when passing through various tissue interfaces near the body surface and between deeper tissue layers. This spreads the field and the area of heating within the tissues.

Tissues with higher dielectric constants, such as skin and skeletal muscle, have a greater percentage of water, which is a polarizable dipole. Tissues with a greater number of dipoles will hold more charge for a given voltage across the treatment applicator plates. Therefore, one would expect capacitive SWD to have a greater heating effect on muscle, since it has a greater amount of water dipoles. However, the rate of fatty tissue heating is greater than muscle with capacitive SWD, because the field intensity is highest close to the electrodes, and fatty tissue is closer to the electrodes than muscle. Other reasons that the capacitive method does not heat muscle as well as the inductive method is the vascular system cools muscle by heat transfer more efficiently than it cools fat tissue, and the heat capacity of muscle is much higher than fat tissue.[3] Figure 6-19 shows a comparison of the heating effects of capacitive and inductive diathermy.

Table 6·3	**Dielectric Constants and Conductivities of Select Tissues and Materials***	
Tissues/Materials	**Dielectric Constants (e)**	**Conductivity (s)**
0.9% saline/blood	80	11.7
Muscle/skin	85–100	0.7–0.9
Bone marrow	7–8	0.02–0.04
Fat tissue	11–13	0.04–0.06
Distilled water	80	2×10^4
Oil	2	10^{11}
Metals	—	10^4–10^7

*Values are given for tissues and materials at 37°C and 50 MHz. The values are temperature and frequency dependent. The unit for conductivity is siemens per meter (S/m).

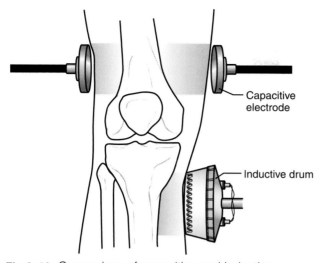

Fig 6•19 Comparison of capacitive and induction diathermy on heating of tissues. Note that capacitive tends to heat superficial fat tissue greater than inductive, and inductive heats deeper muscle tissue greater than capacitive. *(Art concept by Sara Monath, student PT at Richard Stockton College of NJ.)*

The effectiveness of SWD to heat muscle tissue has been demonstrated by published research studies. Draper as well as other researchers[89–92] used induction PSWD (800 bursts per second [bps], 400 μsec burst duration, 48 W average RMS power) for 20 minutes and successfully increased muscle temperature as much as 4°C (39.2°F) after 15 minutes of treatment. Mitchell[93] used the same parameters for PSWD and demonstrated an increase in muscle temperature up to 2°C (35.6°F) at a depth of 2.5 cm.

Heating of tissues can be demonstrated by monitoring changes in circulation. Millard[94] studied the effects of SWD heating on skin blood flow and showed that clearance of radioactive sodium increased nearly 150% after exposure, resulting in an average temperature rise of 5.3°C (41.5°F). Muscle clearance rates increased by 36%, with a muscle temperature rise of 5.2°C (41.3°F). Mayrovitz and Larsen[95] demonstrated increased microvascular blood perfusion in a group of subjects who received 40 minutes of PSWD (600 pps, 65 μsec pulse duration, 35 W average power) to their forearms. Harris[96] demonstrated a 100% increase in circulation in knee joints following SWD application, based upon radio-sodium clearance from the joints. Increased muscle blood flow following 10 minutes of condenser field SWD (80 W) was demonstrated by Karasuno and colleagues.[97] They found blood flow increased greater with SWD than another group that received electric hot packs.

Effects on Tissue Flexibility

The combination of heat and prolonged low-load stretch (PLLS) has been shown to effectively increase tissue elasticity and facilitate connective tissue flexibility and joint ROM. Peres and colleagues[98] applied PSWD (800 pps, 400 μsec pulse duration, 48 W average RMS power) to the musculotendinous junction of the triceps surae for 20 minutes, with PLLS added for the last 5 minutes of the treatment. An ice bag was applied to the musculotendinous junction for 5 minutes following the 20-minute diathermy treatment. Subjects who received PSWD, PLLS, and ice had greater immediate and net ROM increases than subjects who received PLLS alone.

Draper and colleagues[99] found that subjects with tight hamstrings who received PSWD (800 pps, 400 μsec pulse duration, 48 W average RMS power) to their hamstrings for 10 minutes prior to and 5 minutes during stretching of the hamstrings had greater flexibility (increased knee extension) than subjects who received sham diathermy and stretching. Diathermy may help increase tissue flexibility without stretching. Robertson and colleagues[100] applied SWD for 15 minutes to the lower leg by placing two capacitive pads parallel to the leg and close to the skin and perpendicular to the top of a plinth. Subjects did not perform stretching during or after the treatment. Ankle dorsiflexion ROM increased 5.2% after SWD compared to 2% for subjects who received hot packs and −0.4% for the control group.

Muscle Strength

Applying diathermy to muscle tissue may affect muscle contraction. Currier and Nelson[101] compared the effects of exercise (riding an ergometer for 5 minutes) and shortwave diathermy (applied to the low back for 20 minutes) on motor nerve conduction velocity of the peroneal nerve. Motor nerve conduction velocities increased for both conditions; however, exercise caused a greater increase in conduction rate than diathermy. Chastain[102] used an isokinetic dynamometer to measure the isometric strength of the quadriceps in subjects who received inductive SWD for 20 minutes. Initially, isometric strength decreased an average of 2.15 newton meters (Nm). After 30 minutes, strength increased an average of 14.1 Nm, and after 90 minutes the strength levels for each subject fluctuated. Practitioners need to consider possible changes in muscle strength following diathermy treatments and adjust the timing of exercise programs and quantification of muscle strength. The application of diathermy immediately preceding exercise may augment exercise performance. Cetin and colleagues[103] found that applying physical modalities, including capacitive SWD, before isokinetic exercise in patients with symptomatic osteoarthritis of the knees led to improved exercise performance and function.

Pain

Reduction of pain by diathermy can most likely be explained by the well-known analgesic effects of heat (see Chapter 3). McCray and Patton[104] compared the effects of inductive SWD to moist hot packs on the sensitivity of trigger points in the neck, shoulders, and back. SWD was more effective at relieving pain at trigger points than moist heat. In a study by Cetin and colleagues,[103] women with pain caused by osteoarthritis of the knees were relieved by a combination of capacitive SWD, hot packs, and isokinetic exercise. Laufer and colleagues[105] were unable to demonstrate any effect on pain in patients with osteoarthritis in the knees who received either PSWD at 300 pulses per second (300 μsec pulse duration, mean power 18 W), PSWD at 110 pulses per second (82 μsec pulse duration, mean power 1.8 W), or sham diathermy. Pain was assessed by the WOMAC arthritis index questionnaire. Interestingly, the group who received PSWD at 300 pps reported a "comfortable feeling of warmth" despite the low mean power (18 W).

In another study, Santiesteban and Grant[106] applied PSWD (700 pulses per second, 95 μsec pulse duration, pulse peak power of 120 W) to patients following foot surgery. Individuals receiving PSWD had significantly shorter hospitalization and fewer analgesic medications compared to a control group that did not receive PSWD. In addition, Balogun and Okonofua[107] reported a case study of a woman with an 8-year history of pelvic inflammatory disease; nine treatment sessions of SWD delivered by electrodes placed on the abdomen and lumbar region was effective in relieving abdominal pain.

Some pain relief may be secondary to nonthermal mechanisms. Wagstaff and colleagues[108] compared the effects of inductive SWD, PSWD at 82 pulses per second (mean power 23.2 W), and PSWD at 200 pulses per second (mean power 23.4 W) applied to subjects with low back pain. All three groups had a significant relief of pain, with both PSWD groups achieving more significant pain relief than the SWD group. The groups that received PSWD had either no heating or very low (barely perceptible) heating of tissues, because the mean power levels were lower than the usual mean power needed to cause perceptible heating (believed to be around 38 W). PEMF, which does not heat tissues, has been shown to help control pain in patients with idiopathic trigeminal neuralgia[109] and to decrease pain and increase mobility of the temporomandibular joint in patients with temporomandibular joint arthralgia.[110]

Tissue Healing

Diathermy has been shown to promote healing of soft tissues and bone.[111–116] Increases in tissue temperature that occur with thermal-level SWD and MWD can increase circulation, which explains improved tissue healing rates. Effects on tissue regeneration were demonstrated by Hill and colleagues[117] using PSWD at a mean power of 48 W for 10 minutes. This resulted in increased fibroblast proliferation, and PSWD at a mean power of 6 W for 10 minutes increased chondrocyte proliferation. In a study by Mayrovitz and Larsen,[118] evidence for nonthermal effects on healing was demonstrated using PSWD that increased local microvascular perfusion around the perimeter of ulcers in patients with diabetes. PEMFs using a Diapulse device have been shown to accelerate healing of pressure ulcers.[119,120] Studies by Bassett[121] and Sharrad[113] demonstrated effective promotion of fracture healing by PEMFs. Portable battery-operated "bone stimulators" are in common use today for promoting healing of nonunion or delayed-union fractures and arthrodeses.

Clinical Application of Diathermy

Preparation of Patient and Device

The decision to use diathermy requires knowing the physiological effects of this modality (discussed earlier in this chapter), indications and contraindications based on published evidence (to be discussed later in this chapter), and the advantages and disadvantages of this modality compared to other devices with similar effects (such as ultrasound). The practitioner should thoroughly explain the effects of diathermy to the patient, including any possible negative effects, and allow the patient to choose whether to receive the treatment. Steps to follow for preparing the patient and the device for treatment are listed in Box 6-2.

Dosage

Dosage is a measure of the amount of energy delivered to the body that is absorbed and converted into heat. Dosimetry is the measurement of this energy transfer in calories per unit time. An average value of the energy absorbed by the body is called the *specific absorption rate* (SAR), which is expressed in watts per kilogram (W/kg). Dosimetry measurements require small temperature probes to be inserted into or through the skin to measure the heat produced by the energy transfer that takes place during a diathermy treatment.

Box 6•2 | Preparation of Patient and Device for Diathermy

Treatment

1. Choose appropriate device depending on goals of treatment (CSW, PSWD, PEMF)
2. Describe expected effects, including any possible negative effects, to patient
3. Position patient comfortably on a nonmetal table or chair
4. Remove all metal from area to be treated (including jewelry and body piercings)
5. Remove clothes from area to be treated
6. Inspect skin for color, perspiration, irritation, growths, and vascularity
7. Place a cotton or terry-cloth towel on skin to absorb perspiration during treatment (not needed for PEMF)
8. Position applicator appropriately in relation to patient's skin:
   - Capacitive plates: both must be placed an equal distance from the skin surface, about 1 to 3 inches (2 to 10 cm) from the skin, parallel to skin surface
   - Inductive drum: directly over tissues to be treated, almost touching towel on skin
   - Microwave drum: parallel to patient's skin, about 1 to 3 inches (2 to 10 cm) away
9. Choose appropriate parameters for treatment (see text)
10. Tell patient not to move body part during treatment (moving body part will affect distance of skin to plate or drum and may alter delivery of energy to patient)
11. Activate device and adjust intensity based on patient's response
12. Instruct patient to inform practitioner immediately if he or she cannot tolerate treatment

---

Temperature probes cannot be inserted into patient's tissues in clinical practice; therefore, it is not possible to measure the amount of electromagnetic energy transferred from a diathermy device to the patient's tissues.

KEY POINT! ▶ Practitioners must use the patient's subjective heat-sensation response as a guide for dosage during diathermy treatments.

Individuals with a documented or a potential sensory deficit must be tested for pain and temperature sensation before beginning treatment to determine if they are capable of reporting changes in cutaneous heat sensation. Based on Joule's law, the maximum tissue temperature reached regardless of the heat modality depends on the square of the intensity, the tissue impedance, and the duration of the heat treatment. The amount of tissue temperature elevation depends on several factors, including the adequacy of blood perfusion through the tissues. Poor blood perfusion, such as arterial insufficiency of the lower extremities, may not allow for adequate heat dissipation when heat from any source is applied directly to the poorly perfused tissues. When tissues are adequately perfused, the body's thermoregulatory mechanism increases heat removal from the local tissue until a new higher-temperature steady state is reached, thus avoiding tissue damage from excessive heat. It is essential to frequently monitor the patient during the first 10 minutes of tissue heating with diathermy to determine the amount of heating that is occurring in the tissues and the patient's tolerance of it.

The extent of biological reactions elicited during diathermy interventions depends on the tissue temperature reached during and at the end of a treatment. The practitioner needs to estimate the intensity and duration (dosage) required to increase tissue temperature to the therapeutic range (between 37.5°C and 44°C [99.5°F and 111.2°F]). This requires knowing which stage of healing (acute, subacute, or chronic) the patient is in, the location of the target tissues, the approximate thickness of overlying tissues, and the patient's tolerance. The practitioner then chooses the intensity that will most likely achieve effective tissue heating, which may be no heating at all if the choice is nonthermal PSWD or PEMF. Some diathermy devices display intensity on a linear scale of arbitrary units, such as

0 to 10. The correlation of this scale with power (watts) may be described in the device manual. The amount of power delivered to the patient will be an estimate based on the value displayed by the device and the patient's response. See Table 6-4 for a suggested dosage scheme based on the patient's response to diathermy.

Continuous diathermy power output is labeled as *peak power,* and pulsed diathermy power output is labeled as *mean power.* Mean power values that are greater than 38 W may produce a tissue heating effect that elicits physiological responses from absorbed thermal energy. PSWD devices produce heat in tissues the same way heat is produced in tissues by continuous SWD—that is, by increasing random motion and kinetic energy between atoms, ions, and molecules. Whether PSWD induces heat in tissues depends on three parameters: (1) peak pulse/burst power, (2) pulse/burst frequency, and (3) pulse/burst duration. These parameters are used to calculate the mean power output. The heating effect of a PSWD device is related to the magnitude of the mean power output. Adjusting the pulse/burst frequency will affect the mean power output and the thermal sensation experienced by the patient. Murray and Kitchen[122] found a significant correlation between pulse/burst frequency and the ability to feel a thermal sensation during PSWD application to the thigh. Low mean power values less than 38 W will cause minimal heating of tissues that may or may not be perceptible. Mean power values between 38 and 80 W are appropriate for subacute inflammatory conditions and correspond to dose II causing a mild heat sensation (see Table 6-4). Mean power values between 80 and 300 W may be used in late subacute conditions in which the signs and symptoms of inflammation are

almost resolved (dose III, a moderate heat sensation). Dose IV (vigorous heating) requires higher mean wattages above 300 W, which may not be possible for PSWD devices and may require continuous SWD. Practitioners should check the patient's response to treatment about every 5 minutes to adjust the dosage level (if needed) to maintain a comfortable, well-tolerated heat sensation.

Duration and Frequency of Treatments

There is general agreement in the literature that the treatment duration of a SWD application should be about 20 minutes to achieve effective heating of tissues. Starkey[123] recommends 20 to 30 minutes of SWD for moderate intensities and about 15 minutes for vigorous heating. The treatment duration for PSWD depends on the mean power output determined by the parameters selected for the treatment and whether the goal is a thermal or nonthermal treatment. Draper and colleagues[89,91] applied PSWD at 800 Hz and a mean power output of 48 W for 20 minutes to the triceps surae. Peak muscle temperature increases at 3 cm below the skin occurred at 15 minutes and slightly declined at 20 minutes of treatment. Duration for treatments with either nonthermal PSWD or PEMF vary widely in the literature, from 30 minutes[124,125] to 3 hours,[126] although many of these treatments were described as "magnetotherapy" with intensity measured in gauss or micro-teslas (see Chapter 15).

The frequency of diathermy treatments and the number of treatments needed to achieve a positive outcome are based on the injury's stage of healing, the urgency of the need for treatment, the patient's availability for treatment sessions, and the availability of the equipment and a practitioner to provide the treatment. Acute conditions such as soft tissue trauma can be treated two or three times daily with either dose I or II for 15 minutes each. This may be possible in some clinic settings, such as in-patient care settings or sports team treatment rooms, where the patient, practitioner, and the equipment may be readily available. Subacute and chronic conditions are typically treated with once-per-day or every-other-day diathermy. Discontinuation of diathermy treatments is based on the treatment's goals. Diathermy should be discontinued if the treatment goal is met, if no response is

Table 6•4	**Dosages for Diathermy Treatments**	
Dose	**Response***	**Suggested Clinical Use**
Dose I	Nonthermal	Acute injuries (sprains, strains, etc.)
Dose II	Mild heat sensation	Subacute injuries and inflammation
Dose III	Moderate heat sensation	Pain, muscle spasm, chronic inflammation
Dose IV	Vigorous heating	Increase blood flow, heating of collagen fibers for stretching of soft tissues

*Based upon patient's report of perception of tissue heating

achieved after one to five treatments, or if adverse effects or patient intolerance occurs. It is difficult to judge the number of treatments needed to achieve treatment goals; more research is needed to establish these guidelines.

Documentation

Consistent and accurate documentation of the treatment parameters and the patient's response to treatment is important for justification of continued diathermy treatments, insurance reimbursement, and outcomes assessment. Practitioners are encouraged to collect and analyze outcomes data and publicize effective and ineffective responses to diathermy interventions.

Documentation Tips

- Type of diathermy: SWD, MWD, PSWD, or PEMF
- Method: capacitive, induction drum or sleeve, flexible pads or cables
- Body part exposed to the electromagnetic waves
- Patient's position during treatment
- Duration of treatment
- Peak power in watts (W) for SWD and MWD
- Pulse/burst frequency and duration and mean power for PSWD and PEMF
- Dosage (I through IV) or type (nonthermal, mild, moderate, or vigorous heating)
- Other modalities or procedures performed
- Patient response (positive or negative comments, affect on pain, skin color changes, sweating, or other responses to treatment)
- Goals of treatment and outcomes

Indications for Diathermy

SWD, MWD, and PSWD

Most of the indications for thermotherapy described in Chapter 3 also apply to SWD, MWD, and thermal-level PSWD. There are two primary advantages of using diathermy for thermotherapy: Diathermy provides a greater depth of heating than superficial thermal modalities, and it can heat a larger area (greater amount of tissue) than ultrasound. These advantages make diathermy the best choice for heating large joints such as the knee or shoulder or large areas of muscle such as the hamstrings.

The research literature includes many studies that support the use of diathermy for therapeutic interventions, but some studies found that diathermy was ineffective (Tables 6-5 and 6-6). Literature reviews published since 1995 are listed in Table 6-7.

Heating of shortened tissues may enhance collagen extensibility in fibrous muscle or joint capsule contractures[127] when followed by stretching. Muscle guarding and pain, which occur as a result of injury to tendons and joint structures; degenerative joint disease; bursitis; sacroiliac strains; and ankylosing spondylitis may be relieved by SWD applications to the muscles in spasm.[128]

Joint structures may be selectively heated by SWD when the joint is covered by a thin layer of soft tissue (such as the elbow). Vigorous heating of a synovial joint should be done only for chronic conditions, such as a joint contracture or an advanced degenerative (quiescent) stage of rheumatoid arthritis. The goal of treatment is to improve joint ROM by decreasing stiffness and improving resilience of contracted soft tissues. In the subacute stage of traumatic arthritis, SWD at dose level II may be beneficial in joints that have a thin soft tissue cover to improve blood circulation, thereby aiding in the resolution of edema and hemorrhage.

Very mild heating at dose I using SWD or PSWD may be effective for recurring inflammatory conditions to improve blood flow and facilitate diffusion of oxygen and metabolite clearance.[127] Lehmann and Lehmann and colleagues[127,128] advocated the use of SWD to induce low heating to produce a mild physiological response for late-stage traumatic arthritis, chronic pelvic inflammatory disease, epicondylitis, degenerative joint disease, ankylosing spondylitis, and other chronic arthritic conditions.

Clinical Controversy

Practitioners often have a range of thermal modalities to choose for their patients. Superficial thermal modalities are usually readily available and generally easy to apply; however, their depth of heating is limited to superficial tissues except in areas of the body that have thin soft tissue covering such as fingers, hands, toes, and feet. Effective heating of deeper tissues such as muscles and joints in most areas of the body requires either ultrasound or diathermy. Ultrasound is available to most practitioners, but it may not be the best choice for heating large muscles and joints. Diathermy may be

Table 6•5 **Effective Applications of Diathermy**[98–100, 103, 104, 107, 108, 111, 116, 134, 159–161]

Condition	Variables	Type of Diathermy	Reference/Type of Study
OA (knees)	Pain disability index scores	SWD	Cetin et al. 2008 (RCT)
OA (knees)	Synovial sac thickness	SWD	Jan et al. 2006 (RCT)
Calcific tendinopathy	Pain, ROM, disability index scores, presence of calcium deposits on x-ray	MWD	DiCesare et al. 2008 (CS)
Joint ROM	Ankle dorsiflexion	PSWD	Seiger & Draper 2006 (CSR)
Joint ROM	Ankle dorsiflexion	SWD	Robertson et al. 2005 (RCT)
Joint ROM	Ankle dorsiflexion	PSWD	Peres et al. 2002 (RCT)
Hamstring flexibility	ROM of knee with hip at 90°	PSWD and long-duration stretching	Draper et al. 2004 (RCT)
RA	Pain scale joint stiffness	MWD	Usichenko 2003 (RCT)
Acute muscle injury	Pain (VAS) ultrasonography	MWD	Giombini et al. 2001 (RANC)
Acute ankle sprain	Swelling subjective improvement	PSWD	Pennington 1993 (RCT)
Chronic pelvic inflammatory disease	Pain	SWD	Balogun & Okonofuna 1988 (CS)
Low back pain	Pain (VAS)	SWD and PSWD	Wagstaff et al. 1986 (RANC)
Painful trigger points	Pain and sensitivity	SWD	McCray et al. 1984 (RANC)

Key: *RCT*, randomized controlled trial; *CS*, case study; *CSR*, case series; *RANC*, randomized allocation of subjects, no control.

Table 6•6 **Ineffective Applications of Diathermy**[162–167]

Condition	Variables	Type of Diathermy	Reference/Type of Study
Neck disorders	Pain questionnaire	PSWD	Dziedzic et al. 2005 (RCT)
Joint ROM	Ankle dorsiflexion (retention of gains in ROM following stretching)	PSWD	Brucker et al. 2005 (FRM)
OA (knees)	WOMAC Index	PSWD	Laufer et al. 2005 (RCT)
OA (knees)	Joint inflammation knee ROM	PSWD	Callaghan et al. 2005 (RCT)
Hamstring flexibility	Sit and reach ROM	PSWD and short-duration stretching	Draper et al. 2002 (RCT)
Ankle sprain	Pain, swelling, time to full weight-bearing	PSWD	McGill 1988 (RCT)
Ankle sprain	Ankle ROM, swelling, gait	PSWD	Barker et al. 1985 (RCT)

Key: *RCT*, randomized controlled trial; *FRM*, 2x4 factorial design with repeated measures.

Table 6•7 **Published Literature Reviews: Diathermy Applications**[115, 168, 169, 170]

Type of Diathermy	# of Studies Reviewed	Conclusions	Reference
SWD	3	Less effective than spinal manipulation for LBP; no difference: SWD vs. sham SWD	Chou and Huffman 2007
MWD	NS	Effective for short-term care of musculoskeletal injuries	Giombini et al. 2007
PEMF	2*	No clinically important benefit for OA of the knee or cervical spine	Hulme et al. 2002
SWD and PSWD	11	Equivocal findings; studies had poor methodological quality	Marks et al. 1999
PSWD	9	Effective for ankle sprains only at higher peak and mean powers and longer treatment durations	Low 1995

*A third study included in this review used pulsed electric stimulation, not PEMF.
Key: *NS*, not specified

the more effective modality for heating deep, large areas of tissue; however, the cost of diathermy devices and practitioner bias or lack of knowledge of the literature may preclude its clinical usage.

Continuous shortwave techniques may be used for selective heating of pelvic organs in chronic inflammatory pelvic diseases.[107,127] This treatment produces a significant increase in vascularity and blood flow, which causes increased cardiac output in women. As a result of the improved vascularity, antibiotic levels to inflamed tissues may be enhanced.

Allberry[129] and Barnett[130] reported positive results with SWD in enhancing the drying of blisters from herpes zoster and in alleviating the associated pain. Both

CASE STUDY 6•2   SELECTING PULSED SHORTWAVE DIATHERMY (PSWD) FOR AN ATHLETE WITH TIGHT HAMSTRINGS

A 21-year-old female field hockey player has a history of several right leg hamstring strains. Measurement of right knee extension ROM with the right hip flexed at 90° finds 30° limitation from full extension, compared to left knee, where extension ROM with the hip flexed at 90° is 15° from full extension. She has been performing frequent stretching exercises for the right hamstrings with minimal change in ROM.

CLINICAL DECISION-MAKING

1. Does the patient have a dysfunction, limitation, or problem that can be improved with the use of PSWD?
   Answer: Yes, the thermal effects of PSWD can help relax the hamstrings and soften tropocollagen bonds to facilitate stretching of the musculotendon complex.

2. Is the patient appropriate for PSWD? Do any of the general precautions or contraindications to PSWD apply to the patient, or are there any specific considerations regarding the application of PSWD to this patient?
   Answer: She had one contraindication: metal jewelry piercing of the umbilicus, which she was able to remove prior to the treatment. She also had one precaution: menstruation. She was informed that there was a slight chance that PSWD could increase menstrual flow because of the proximity of the pelvic cavity to the treatment area.

3. What are the specific goals to be achieved with the use of PSWD?
   Answer: Decrease tightness of hamstrings to facilitate stretching.

4. Do you have the specific type of diathermy that would be appropriate for this patient?
   Answer: Yes, a diathermy device with an induction drum (monode or diplode) and pulsed selection is available.

5. What specific parameters of PSWD would be appropriate for this patient?
   Answer: Appropriate parameters for PSWD for this patient are frequency of 800 bursts (pulses) per second, burst (pulse) duration of 400 µsec, peak pulse power of 150 W, and mean power of 48 W, for at least 15 minutes.

6. What are the proper application procedures for PSWD for this patient?
   Answer: A single layer of terry-cloth towel should be placed over the posterior thigh and the induction drum placed over the proximal or distal hamstrings. Ideally, stretching of hamstrings should occur during PSWD, for at least the last 5 minutes of the treatment, and immediately after the treatment. Prolonged stretching has been shown to be more effective than short-term stretching.
   Pretreatment: Determine the type of diathermy application technique to be used for this athlete and any precautions or contraindications. Inspect skin of posterior thigh for any irritation, infection, or broken skin. Explain the treatment to the patient, including goals of treatment. Instruct her in proper positioning during the treatment and to monitor heating effects and report any discomfort immediately.
   During treatment: Monitor the amount of tissue heating by asking her to report amount of thermal sensation and any discomfort. Remind her not to move her leg during the treatment.
   Post-treatment: Inspect skin of posterior thigh (mild to moderate reddening of skin is normal). Continue stretching of hamstrings and measure any change in knee extension with the hip at 90°.

---

reports emphasized the importance of applying mild heating within a few days of the rash's onset, preferably on the first day if possible. Daily 20-minute applications at the level of the involved dorsal root ganglia are recommended until pain is decreased or the scabs fall off.

PEMF

The literature supports the use of nonthermal pulsed electromagnetic fields for promoting superficial wound and bone healing (see Chapter 14). A systematic review published by McCarthy and colleagues[131] analyzed five randomized, controlled trials of PEMF (defined as "electromagnetic fields with on and off effect of pulsing to produce athermal effects") and reported that PEMF does not significantly decrease pain of knee osteoarthritis. More studies are needed to determine if the nonthermal effects of PEMF are effective for other clinical problems.

Precautions and Contraindications for Diathermy

Practitioners who choose diathermy (including PEMF) for their patients must be aware of precautions and contraindications for using this modality. (See Table 6-8 for a list of these precautions and contraindications). The thermal effects of diathermy are contraindicated whenever heating of tissues may cause harm (see Chapter 3 for precautions and contraindications for heating of tissues). Any significant tissue heating should be avoided if acute inflammation is present, if there is a tendency for hemorrhage, if perfusion is restricted by vascular compromise, or if the patient is febrile or has insensate skin that prevents accurate reporting of heat sensation.

Metals

A unique concern for diathermy is the presence of metal on or in the patient or in the area of the treatment field. Metals are highly conductive, and electromagnetic waves will take the path of least resistance and pass through metal more readily than body tissues.

Table 6•8 Precautions and Contraindications for Diathermy

Precaution/Contraindication	Explanation
Any metallic object on the patient or within the electromagnetic field	Contraindicated because metals can overheat and burn tissue
Metals in the tissues of the body	Precaution for PSWD over small metals, such as screws or metal fragments; contraindication for SWD and MWD
Intrauterine contraceptive devices with copper	Diathermy may cause slight heating of device but not a contraindication
Cancerous tissues	Contraindication because heating of tissues may promote growth and spread of cancer (malignancy)
Impaired sensation	Precaution because patient may not be able to recognize overheating of tissues (contraindication for patients with total loss of sensation)
Impaired circulation	Precaution because tissues may not be able to respond to increased metabolic demands caused by heating of tissues (contraindication for patients with severe circulatory impairment)
Hemorrhage or increased tendency of hemorrhage	Contraindication because heating of tissues may exacerbate or cause hemorrhage
Cardiac pacemakers, implanted stimulators, including any device with lead wires attached or unattached	Electromagnetic waves from diathermy can interfere with the function of these devices and cause malfunction and damage to tissues
Acute injury or inflammation	Contraindicated for thermal diathermy because heating of tissues may exacerbate swelling and inflammation and damage tissue
Pregnancy	Contraindicated because the effects on the fetus are unknown and may be harmful
Joints or organs containing high levels of fluid, including the eyes or testes	Contraindicated because thermal diathermy can rapidly heat fluids in these structures, possibly causing injury
Synthetic materials such as clothing, pillows, and bed coverings	Contraindicated because thermal diathermy may overheat these materials, which can burn tissues
Head, face, or TMJ for patients wearing contact lenses	Contraindicated because thermal diathermy may cause overheating of perforations in lens, which may damage the eye
Unconscious patients or patients who are mentally confused	Contraindicated because patient is unable to determine amount of heating occurring in tissues; confused patients may not be able to maintain position during treatment.
Over growing epiphyses in children	Some authors are concerned about the effect of electromagnetic waves on cell growth of epiphysis; consider it a precaution.
Obese patients	Precaution or contraindication, depending on amount of subcutaneous adipose tissue that may overheat during diathermy, particularly capacitive diathermy
Over moist clothes, dressings, or accumulations of perspiration on the skin	Thermal diathermy will heat fluids faster, which may cause burns.
Use of diathermy near other medical electrical devices, especially near patients who have electrodes attached to their skin	Electromagnetic waves from diathermy devices may interfere with the function of these devices and may exacerbate the intensity of stimulation under electrodes.
Over the low back or pelvis in women who are menstruating	A precaution because diathermy may increase menstrual flow.
Atrophic, infected, or damaged skin	Use caution when applying thermal diathermy because of possible sensation and circulatory impairments of skin, intolerance to heat, or spread of infection. Severe conditions are a contraindication.

Patients receiving diathermy should lie on nonmetallic tables or sit on nonmetallic chairs. Metal objects within the immediate treatment area should be removed, including metal jewelry or piercings on the patient; clothing that contains metal zippers, hooks, buttons, or fasteners; or braces or devices that contain metal. The presence of imbedded metal in a patient receiving diathermy is a precaution but may not be a contraindication, depending on the size and shape of the object. Scott[132] explained how metal acts as a "shunt" of the electric field and produces little or no heating in the metal but causes great dissipation of the heat in the tissues at the ends of the shunt. Therefore, the metal itself is unlikely to cause burning of tissues; however, the tissues at the end of the shunt may be burned. The longer the metal, the greater the shunting effect and the greater the chance of tissue damage. Small pieces of metal imbedded in body tissues are unlikely to cause tissue burning. The presence of larger metal objects imbedded in tissues, such as screws and plates for internal fixation of fractures and prostheses with metallic components, is common in patients who may benefit from the deep heating effects of diathermy.

Draper and colleagues[133] performed PSWD (27.12 MHz, 400 μsec, 800 pps, 48 W for 20 minutes) using a monode induction coil applicator over the elbow of a 39-year-old woman who had an internal fixation with metal screws and a titanium plate in the joint. The patient reported a gentle, warm feeling and no discomfort, and the physician who later removed the hardware reported no evidence that the metal implants had overheated.

Seiger and Draper[134] reported on a case series of patients with surgical metal implants in ankles that received PSWD (27.12 MHz, 400 μsec, 800 pps, 48 W for 20 minutes). All the patients reported a mild vibration and no pain or burning, and all had improvement in ankle ROM without any evidence of harmful effects attributable to PSWD. The authors advise caution when applying PSWD over metal implants in peripheral joints. No studies have shown whether continuous SWD and MWD are safe over metal implants, so using these forms of diathermy should still be considered a contraindication. Copper-bearing intrauterine contraceptive devices contain a small amount of metal that does not overheat when exposed to diathermy.[135-137] Applying diathermy to the pelvis or low back of patients who have these devices is not contraindicated.

Implanted Electronic Devices

No form of diathermy should be used on patients who have implanted electronic devices, such as pacemakers, defibrillators, or neurostimulators. Wires attached to these devices can act as antennas and cause significant tissue damage. Wires are sometimes left in the body after these devices are removed, so practitioners must be certain that no wires remain before using diathermy on these patients.[138]

Practitioner Exposure to Electromagnetic Fields

There is concern about the electromagnetic fields created by diathermy devices and their effect on practitioners and others who may be in proximity of the device during treatment. There are many factors that determine the amount of electromagnetic field exposure to practitioners during diathermy treatments, including type of diathermy, size and placement of electrodes on the patient, output intensity, and the practitioner's location in relationship to the active diathermy device.[139,140] The use of diathermy is not believed to be harmful to practitioners if they follow the safety guidelines for limiting exposure to electromagnetic fields.[141-144] The guidelines include maintaining a distance of 1 to 2 m (3.28 to 6.56 ft) from active SWD devices and .5 to 1 m (1.64 to 3.28 ft) from active PSWD devices.[140,145,146]

Pregnancy

Diathermy should not be performed on pregnant patients because the effects of maternal hyperthermia and electromagnetic fields on fetal development are not known and may be harmful.[138] Female practitioners who are pregnant must consider the effects of exposure to electromagnetic fields on their fetus. Some studies have found weak correlations between practitioner exposure to electromagnetic fields from diathermy treatments and spontaneous abortions and congenital malformations.[147-150] Ouellet-Hellstrom and Stewart[151] found a correlation between MWD and miscarriages but no correlation between SWD and miscarriages. At this time, because of the uncertainty of the research, female health-care practitioners of child-bearing age who are or may be pregnant can set up diathermy devices for patient treatments but should not remain in the treatment area when the diathermy device is on.

Specific Organs and Tissues

Organs and tissues with high fluid volume have a higher conductivity and will heat greater than surrounding tissues when exposed to electromagnetic fields from diathermy devices. This may result in overheating and tissue damage, so it is best to avoid exposing the eyes, testes or ovaries, fluid-filled joints, and internal organs to diathermy.[138] Some references recommend not applying diathermy over epiphyseal tissues because of the possibility of adversely affecting the growth plate; however, this has not been confirmed by research using human subjects. Diathermy over cancerous tissues is contraindicated because of the danger of increasing blood flow to the cancer cells and promoting malignancy.[138,152]

Synthetic Materials

Practitioners must use caution when exposing any synthetic materials (such as nylon, foam rubber, or plastics) on or in the patient to electromagnetic fields from diathermy devices. Synthetic clothing should be removed from the treatment area, and pillows and table coverings made from these materials should be removed. Internal synthetic devices may overheat and cause tissue damage. Scott[153] warned that electromagnetic fields can overheat contact lenses in the eyes. Riambau and colleagues[154] reported a case in which a patient who had a Vanguard endograft repair of an abdominal aortic aneurysm had a thrombosis of the left limb of the endograft following a MWD treatment for lumbar pain.

Other Concerns

Application of capacitive diathermy to obese patients must be performed cautiously or not at all because of excessive heating of fat tissue that may lead to burns. Inductive diathermy is a better choice for obese patients because of less heating of fat tissue. Patients who are mentally impaired (dementia, effects of medications) or who have sensory deficits may be unable to communicate to the practitioner any discomfort caused by the diathermy. These patients must be monitored carefully during the treatment, or it may be best to avoid diathermy if communication or sensation is significantly impaired.

Diathermy treatments to the low back or pelvis of a female patient during menstruation may temporarily increase menstrual flow. This is not a contraindication to diathermy; however, patients should be informed that this may occur. If increased menstrual flow is a concern, then low-intensity diathermy, such as PSWD or PEMF, can be used. Employing diathermy devices in the vicinity of other electronic medical devices (such as EKG, EEG, TENS, and computer-controlled devices) may interfere with these devices' function and should be avoided.[138] This type of equipment should be at least 3 to 5 meters (about 10 to 16 feet) away from any active diathermy devices.[152]

Clinical Decision-Making: When Is Diathermy the Treatment of Choice?

A patient presents with a condition that is an indication for diathermy. How does a practitioner determine which type of diathermy is best? Or would ultrasound be a better choice? Is diathermy a cost-effective alternative to other interventions for this condition?

Conditions that may benefit from deep heating of tissues will require either ultrasound or diathermy, since superficial thermal modalities will not significantly heat tissues that are more than 1 to 3 cm below the skin's surface. (See Table 6-9 for a comparison of ultrasound and diathermy.) Ultrasound primarily heats dense collagen tissue such as tendons, ligaments, and joint capsules, and the area of tissue heating is limited to a small area about twice the size of the sound head. Diathermy heats tissues with high fluid content such as muscle and will heat a much larger area than ultrasound. The type of diathermy will depend on the treatment's goal. Vigorous heating of tissues will require SWD (or MWD if available). Inductive diathermy is more effective in heating muscle and will heat fat tissue less than capacitive diathermy. If mild or moderate heating is desired, then PSWD is a good choice. Acute conditions require PSWD with a mean power intensity less than thermal range, or they may require PEMF, which will not heat tissues.

Table 6•9 Comparison: Diathermy and Ultrasound

Clinical Aspects	SWD/PSWD	Ultrasound
Type of energy	Electromagnetic	Mechanical
Depth of tissue heating	3–5 cm	2–3 cm
Type of tissue heated	Muscle, fat, skin	Mostly dense, high-collagen tissues (tendons, tissue interfaces)
Rate of tissue heating	Constant	Fluctuates with movement of sound head
Area affected	About 200 cm² (using induction drum)	About 2 to 15 cm (depending on size of sound head)
Heat retention	Moderate	Minimal
Treatment time	15–30 minutes	5–15 minutes
Practitioner attendance during treatment	Unattended	Attended
Average cost of device*	$6,000–8,000	$1,500–3,000

*Based on quotes from three biomedical companies, in U.S. dollars

Today's diathermy devices are safer, technologically superior, and easier to use than devices used during the 20th century. Now diathermy can be delivered using a portable device that uses a sleeve containing an inductive cable. The patient places the wrist, ankle, or knee inside the sleeve (see Fig. 6-16). Other portable devices provide both SWD and PSWD using large rubber pad electrodes or a monode drum.

Unfortunately, this author has found a continued bias against the use of diathermy in the United States despite new technologically advanced devices available from biomedical companies. The use of diathermy is more common in other countries, such as Ireland, the UK, Australia, and Canada.[144] A survey of 46 physiotherapy departments in National Health Service hospitals in England published by Shah and Farrow in 2007[155] found that 93.5% had PSWD devices, 30.4% had SWD devices, and none had MWD devices. PSWD was used more frequently than SWD, with 32.6% of the departments using PSWD 4 to 5 days per week.

The higher cost of diathermy devices (compared to ultrasound devices and most superficial thermal modalities) may affect the clinical decision to use this modality for patient treatment. Practitioners need to consider the advantages of diathermy compared to other modalities, such as greater depth of heating, larger area treated, and longer duration of thermal effect, and diathermy does not require constant practitioner presence during the treatment. Multiple patients can receive diathermy treatment while the practitioner is attending to other patients. Consideration of these advantages, weighed against the disadvantages of diathermy discussed previously, will enable the practitioner to make a wise decision regarding the use of this modality for patient treatment.

▢ REFERENCES

1. Guy AW, Lehman JF, Stonebridge JB. Therapeutic Applications of Electromagnetic Power. *Proc IEEE.* 1974; 62:55–75.
2. Department of Health and Human Services, Food and Drug Administration, Section 510k # k010175 Notification of Premarket Approval. February 6, 2002.
3. Robertson V, Ward A, Low J, Reed A. *Electrotherapy Explained: Principles and Practice.* 4th ed. Oxford, UK: Butterworth Heinemann Elsevier; 2006.
4. Giancoli DC. *Physics.* 6th ed. Upple Saddle River, NJ: Prentice Hall; 2005.
5. Calder N. *Einstein's Universe.* New York: Greenwich House; 1982.
6. Goldman L. *Biomedical Aspects of Laser.* New York: Springer-Verlag; 1967.
7. Kroetlinger M. On the use of laser in acupuncture. *Internat J of Acupunct and Electrother Res.* 1980;5:297.
8. Lengyell B. *Laser Generation of Lightly Stimulated Emission.* New York: John Wiley & Son; 1962.
9. Fuller TA. Physical considerations of surgical lasers. *Obstet Gynecol Clin North Am.* 1991;18:391–405.
10. Caspers K. Laser stimulation in therapy. *Int Z Phys Med Rehabil.* 1997;18:426.
11. U.S. Department of Health and Human Services, Food and Drug Administration. http://www.fda.gov/medicaldevices/productsandmedicalprocedures/deviceapporvalsandclearances'inmedicaldevices. Accessed November 2, 2009.
12. AORN. Recommended practices for laser safety in practice setting. *AORN J.* 1989;155–158.
13. Elson L, ed. *Practical Laser Safety in Oral and Maxillofacial Surgery.* New York: Thieme Medical Publishers; 1997.
14. Snyder-Mackler L, Seitz L, eds. *Therapeutic Uses of Light in Rehabilitation.* Philadelphia: FA Davis; 1990.
15. Basford JR. Low-energy laser therapy: controversies and new research findings. *Lasers Surg Med.* 1989;9:1–5.
16. Cameron M. *Physical Agents in Rehabilitation.* Philadelphia: WB Saunders; 1999.
17. Passerella S CE, Molinari S. Increase of proton electrochemical potential and ATP synthesis in rat liver mitochondria irradiated in vitro by Helium-Neon laser. *FEBS Lett.* 1984; 175: 95–99.

18. Loevschall H, Arenholt-Bindslev D. Effect of low level diode laser irradiation of human oral mucosa fibroblasts in vitro. *Lasers Surg Med.* 1994;14:347–354.

19. Abergel RP, Meeker CA, Lam TS, Dwyer RM, Lesavoy MA, Uitto J. Control of connective tissue metabolism by lasers: recent developments and future prospects. *J Am Acad Dermatol.* 1984;11:1142–1150.

20. Karu T. Molecular mechanisms of the therapeutic effects of low intensity laser radiation. *Lasers Life Sci.* 1989;2:53–74.

21. Findl E, ed. *Membrane Transduction of Low Energy Level Fields and Ca++ Hypothesis.* New York: Plenum Press; 1987.

22. Lam T. Laser stimulation of collagen in human skin fibroblast cultures. *Laser Life Sci.* 1986;11:1142–1150.

23. Smith K. The photobiological basis of low level laser radiation. *Laser Ther.* 1991;3:19–24.

24. Becker J. [Biostimulation of wound healing in rats by combined soft and middle power lasers]. *Biomed Tech (Berl).* 1990;35:98–101.

25. Rezvan M. Prevention of x-ray induced dermal necrosis by treatment with multi-wavelength light. *Lasers Surg Med.* 1992;12:288–293.

26. Karu TI, Kolyakov SF. Exact action spectra for cellular responses relevant to phototherapy. *Photomed Laser Surg.* 2005;23:355–361.

27. Mognato M, Squizzato F, Facchin F, Zaghetto L, Corti L. Cell growth modulation of human cells irradiated in vitro with low-level laser therapy. *Photomed Laser Surg.* 2004;22:523–526.

28. Moore P, Ridgway TD, Higbee RG, Howard EW, Lucroy MD. Effect of wavelength on low-intensity laser irradiation-stimulated cell proliferation in vitro. *Lasers Surg Med.* 2005;36:8–12.

29. Alster TS, Kauvar AN, Geronemus RG. Histology of high-energy pulsed CO_2 laser resurfacing. *Semin Cutan Med Surg.* 1996;15:189–193.

30. Abergel R, Castel JC, Dwyer RM, Uitto J. Biostimulation of wound healing by lasers: experimental approaches in animal models and in fibroblast cultures. *J Dermatol Surg Oncol.* 1987;13:127–133.

31. Hunter J, Leonard L, Wilson R, Snider G, Dixon J. Effects of low energy laser on wound healing in a porcine model. *Lasers Surg Med.* 1984;3:285–290.

32. Posten W, Wrone DA, Dover JS, Arndt KA, Silapunt S, Alam M. Low-level laser therapy for wound healing: mechanism and efficacy. *Dermatol Surg.* 2005;31:334–340.

33. Gal P, Vidinsky B, Toporcer T, et al. Histological assessment of the effect of laser irradiation on skin wound healing in rats. *Photomed Laser Surg.* 2006;24:480–488.

34. Rabelo SB, Villaverde AB, Nicolau R, Salgado MC, Melo Mda S, Pacheco MT. Comparison between wound healing in induced diabetic and nondiabetic rats after low-level laser therapy. *Photomed Laser Surg.* 2006;24:474–479.

35. Simunovic Z, Ivankovich AD, Depolo A. Wound healing of animal and human body sport and traffic accident injuries using low-level laser therapy treatment: a randomized clinical study of seventy-four patients with control group. *J Clin Laser Med Surg.* 2000;18:67–73.

36. Woodruff LD, Bounkeo JM, Brannon WM, et al. The efficacy of laser therapy in wound repair: a meta-analysis of the literature. *Photomed Laser Surg.* 2004;22:241–247.

37. Enwemeka CS, Parker JC, Dowdy DS, Harkness EE, Sanford LE, Woodruff LD. The efficacy of low-power lasers in tissue repair and pain control: a meta-analysis study. *Photomed Laser Surg.* 2004;22:323–329.

38. Chen J, Zhou Y. Effect of low level carbon dioxide laser irradiation on biochemical metabolism of rabbit mandibular bone. *Laser Ther.* 1989;1:83–87.

39. Niccoli-Filho W, Okamoto T. The effect of exposure to continuous Nd:YAG laser radiation on the wound healing process after removal of the teeth (a histological study on rats). *Stomatologiia (Mosk).* 1995;74:26–29.

40. Tang XCB. Effect of CO_2 laser irradiation on experimental fracture healing: a transmission electron microscopy study. *Lasers Surg Med.* 1987;7:36–45.

41. Trelles MA, Mayayo E. Bone fracture consolidates faster with low-power laser. *Lasers Surg Med.* 1987;7:36–45.

42. Pinheiro AL, Limeira Junior Fde A, Gerbi ME, Ramalho LM, Marzola C, Ponzi EA. Effect of low level laser therapy on the repair of bone defects grafted with inorganic bovine bone. *Braz Dent J.* 2003;14:177–181.

43. Pinheiro AL, Limeira Junior Fde A, Gerbi ME, et al. Effect of 830-nm laser light on the repair of bone defects grafted with inorganic bovine bone and decalcified cortical osseous membrane. *J Clin Laser Med Surg.* 2003;21:301–306.

44. Gerbi ME, Pinheiro AL, Marzola C, et al. Assessment of bone repair associated with the use of organic bovine bone and membrane irradiated at 830 nm. *Photomed Laser Surg.* 2005;23:382–388.

45. Lirani-Galvao AP, Jorgetti V, da Silva OL. Comparative study of how low-level laser therapy and low-intensity pulsed ultrasound affect bone repair in rats. *Photomed Laser Surg.* 2006;24:735–740.

46. Kazem-Shakouri S, Soleimanpour J, Salekzamani Y, Oskuie MR. Effect of low-level laser therapy on the fracture healing process. *Lasers Med Sci.* 2009;28.

47. Salmos J, Gerbi ME, Braz R, Andrade ES, Vasconcelos BC, Bessa-Nogueira RV. Methodological quality of systematic reviews analyzing the use of laser therapy in restorative dentistry. *Lasers Med Sci.* 2009;8.

48. Pinheiro AL, Gerbi ME. Photoengineering of bone repair processes. *Photomed Laser Surg.* 2006;24:169–178.

49. Velez-Gonzalez M, Urrea-Arbelaez A, Nicholas M, et al. Treatment of relapse in herpes simplex on labial and facial areas and of primary herpes simplex on genital areas and "area pudenda" with low-power He-Ne laser or Acyclovir administered orally. In: Karu TI, Young AR, eds. Effects of Low-Power Light on Biologic Systems. *Proc, SPIE.* 1996; 2630:43–50.

50. Schindl A, Neumann R. Low-intensity laser therapy is an effective treatment for recurrent herpes simplex infection. Results from a randomized double-blind placebo-controlled study. *J Invest Dermatol.* 1999;113:221–223.

51. Marotti J, Aranha AC, Eduardo Cde P, Ribeiro MS. Photodynamic therapy can be effective as a treatment for herpes simplex labialis. *Photomed Laser Surg.* 2009;27:357–363.

52. Ferreira Dde C, Martins FO, Romanos MT. [Impact of low-intensity laser on the suppression of infections caused by Herpes simplex viruses 1 and 2: in vitro study]. *Rev Soc Bras Med Trop.* 2009;42:82–85.

53. Navarro R, Marquezan M, Cerqueira DF, Silveira BL, Correa MS. Low-level-laser therapy as an alternative treatment for primary herpes simplex infection: a case report. *J Clin Pediatr Dent.* 2007;31:225–228.

54. Rallis TR. Low-intensity laser therapy for recurrent herpes labialis. *J Invest Dermatol.* 2000;115:131–132.

55. Lacour J. [Low-power laser and recurrent labial herpes]. *Ann Dermatol Venereol.* 2000;127:652–656.

56. Lam LK, Cheing GL. Effects of 904-nm low-level laser therapy in the management of lateral epicondylitis: a randomized controlled trial. *Photomed Laser Surg.* 2007;25:65–71.

57. Oken O, Kahraman Y, Ayhan F, Canpolat S, Yorgancioglu ZR, Oken OF. The short-term efficacy of laser, brace, and

ultrasound treatment in lateral epicondylitis: a prospective, randomized, controlled trial. *J Hand Ther.* 2008;21:63–67.

58. Stasinopoulos D, Stasinopoulos I, Pantelis M, Stasinopoulou K. Comparing the effects of exercise program and low-level laser therapy with exercise program and polarized polychromatic non-coherent light (bioptron light) on the treatment of lateral elbow tendinopathy. *Photomed Laser Surg.* 2009; 27: 513–520.

59. Stasinopoulos DI, Johnson MI. Effectiveness of low-level laser therapy for lateral elbow tendinopathy. *Photomed Laser Surg.* 2005;23:425–430.

60. Bjordal JM, Lopes-Martins RA, Joensen J, et al. A systematic review with procedural assessments and meta-analysis of low level laser therapy in lateral elbow tendinopathy (tennis elbow). *BMC Musculoskelet Disord.* 2008;9:75.

61. Bjordal JM, Lopes-Martins RA, Iversen VV. A randomised, placebo controlled trial of low level laser therapy for activated Achilles tendinitis with microdialysis measurement of peritendinous prostaglandin E2 concentrations. *Br J Sports Med.* 2006;40:76–80.

62. Stergioulas A, Stergioula M, Aarskog R, Lopes-Martins RA, Bjordal JM. Effects of low-level laser therapy and eccentric exercises in the treatment of recreational athletes with chronic Achilles tendinopathy. *Am J Sports Med.* 2008;36:881–887.

63. Tumilty S, Munn J, McDonough S, Hurley DA, Basford JR, Baxter GD. Low level laser treatment of tendinopathy: a systematic review with meta-analysis. *Photomed Laser Surg.* 2010;28:2–16.

64. Michener LA, Walsworth MK, Burnet EN. Effectiveness of rehabilitation for patients with subacromial impingement syndrome: a systematic review. *J Hand Ther.* 2004;17:152–164.

65. Andres BM, Murrell GA. Treatment of tendinopathy: what works, what does not, and what is on the horizon. *Clin Orthop Relat Res.* 2008;466:1539–1554.

66. Stergioulas A. Low-power laser treatment in patients with frozen shoulder: preliminary results. *Photomed Laser Surg.* 2008;26:99–105.

67. Yeldan I, Cetin E, Ozdincler AR. The effectiveness of low-level laser therapy on shoulder function in subacromial impingement syndrome. *Disabil Rehabil.* 2009;31:935–940.

68. Bal A, Eksioglu E, Gurcay E, Gulec B, Karaahmet O, Cakci A. Low-level laser therapy in subacromial impingement syndrome. *Photomed Laser Surg.* 2009;27:31–36.

69. Weintraub MI. Noninvasive laser neurolysis in carpal tunnel syndrome. *Muscle Nerve.* 1997;20:1029–1031.

70. Bakhtiary AH, Rashidy-Pour A. Ultrasound and laser therapy in the treatment of carpal tunnel syndrome. *Aust J Physiother.* 2004;50:147–151.

71. Irvine J, Chong SL, Amirjani N, Chan KM. Double-blind randomized controlled trial of low-level laser therapy in carpal tunnel syndrome. *Muscle Nerve.* 2004;30:182–187.

72. Ekim A, Armagan O, Tascioglu F, Oner C, Colak M. Effect of low level laser therapy in rheumatoid arthritis patients with carpal tunnel syndrome. *Swiss Med Wkly.* 2007;137:347–352.

73. Evcik D, Kavuncu V, Cakir T, Subasi V, Yaman M. Laser therapy in the treatment of carpal tunnel syndrome: a randomized controlled trial. *Photomed Laser Surg.* 2007;25:34–39.

74. Shooshtari SM, Badiee V, Taghizadeh SH, Nematollahi AH, Amanollahi AH, Grami MT. The effects of low level laser in clinical outcome and neurophysiological results of carpal tunnel syndrome. *Electromyogr Clin Neurophysiol.* 2008;48:229–231.

75. Yagci I, Elmas O, Akcan E, Ustun I, Gunduz OH, Guven Z. Comparison of splinting and splinting plus low-level laser therapy in idiopathic carpal tunnel syndrome. *Clin Rheumatol.* 2009;28:1059–1065.

76. Institute ANS. American National Standard for the Safe Use of Lasers. Z136.1. ANSI: Laser Institute of America; 1996.

77. Yousefi-Nooraie R, Schonstein E, Heidari K, et al. Low level laser therapy for nonspecific low-back pain. *Cochrane Database Syst Rev.* 2008(2):CD005107.

78. Chou R, Huffman LH. Nonpharmacologic therapies for acute and chronic low back pain: a review of the evidence for an American Pain Society/American College of Physicians clinical practice guideline. *Ann Intern Med.* 2007;147:492–504.

79. Brosseau L, Robinson V, Wells G, et al. Low level laser therapy (classes I, II and III) for treating rheumatoid arthritis. *Cochrane Database Syst Rev.* 2005(4):CD002049.

80. Brosseau L, Wells G, Marchand S, et al. Randomized controlled trial on low level laser therapy (LLLT) in the treatment of osteoarthritis (OA) of the hand. *Lasers Surg Med.* 2005; 36:210–219.

81. Samson D, Lefevre F, Aronson N. Wound-healing technologies: low-level laser and vacuum-assisted closure. *Evid Rep Technol Assess (Summ).* 2004;111:1–6.

82. Bjordal J. Letter to the editor: inadequate statistical analysis hides significant effect of low level laser therapy in carpel tunnel syndrome. *Photomed Laser Surg.* 2007;25:530–531.

83. Bjordal JM, Lopes-Martins RA, Klovning A. Is quality control of Cochrane reviews in controversial areas sufficient? *J Altern Complement Med.* 2006;12:181–183.

84. Consensus agreement on the design and conduct of clinical studies with low level laser therapy and light therapy for musculoskeletal pain and disorders. Guaruja, Brazil: World Association of Laser Therapy; 2004.

85. Standard for the design and conduct of systematic reviews with low level laser therapy for musculoskeletal pain and disorders. Guaruja, Brazil: World Association of Laser Therapy at the 5th World Congress; 2004.

86. Wilkening GM, Sutton CH. Health effects of nonionizing radiation. *Environ Med.* 1990;74:489–507.

87. Ward AR. *Electricity Fields and Waves in Therapy.* Marrickville, NSW, Australia: Science Press; 1986.

88. Guy AW. Biophysics of high frequency currents and electromagnetic radiation. In: Lehman JF, ed. *Therapeutic Heat and Cold.* 3rd ed. Baltimore: Williams & Wilkins; 1982:199–277.

89. Draper DO, Knight K, Fujiwara T, Castel JC. Temperature change in human muscle during and after pulsed short-wave diathermy. *J Orthop Sports Phys Ther.* 1999;29:13–22.

90. Garrett CL, Draper DO, Knight KL. Heat distribution in the lower leg from pulsed short-wave diathermy and ultrasound treatments. *J Athl Train.* 2000;35:50–55.

91. Draper DO, Castel CJ, Knight K, Fujiwara T, Darrow H. Temperature rise in human muscle during pulsed short wave diathermy: Does the modality parallel ultrasound? (abstract). *J Athl Train.* 1997;32:S36.

92. Castel JC, Draper DO, Knight K, Fujiwara T, Garrett C. Rate of temperature decay in human muscle after treatments of pulsed short wave diathermy. *J Athl Train.* 1997;32:S34.

93. Mitchell SM, Trowbridge SM, Fincher AL, Cramer JT. Effect of diathermy on muscle temperature, electromyography, and mechanomyography. *Muscle Nerve.* 2008;38:992–1004.

94. Millard JB. Effect of high frequency currents and infra-red rays on the circulation of the lower limb in man. *Ann Phys Med.* 1961;6:45.

95. Mayrovitz HN, Larsen PB. Effects of pulsed electromagnetic fields on skin microvascular blood perfusion. *Wounds.* 1992;4:197–202.

96. Harris R. Effect of shortwave diathermy on radio-sodium clearance from the knee joint in the normal and in rheumatoid arthritis. *Phys Med Rehabil.* 1961;42:241.

97. Karasuno H, Morozumi K, Fujiwara T, Goh AC, Yamamoto I, Senga F. Changes in intramuscular blood volume induced by continuous short wave diathermy. *J Phys Ther Sci.* 2005;17:71–79.

98. Peres SE, Draper DO, Knight KL, Ricard MD. Pulsed short-wave diathermy and prolonged long-duration stretching increase dorsiflexion range of motion more than identical stretching without diathermy. *J Athl Train.* 2002;37:43–50.

99. Draper DO, Castro JL, Feland B, Schulthies S, Eggett D. Shortwave diathermy and prolonged stretching increase hamstring flexibility more than prolonged stretching alone. *J Orthop Sports Phys Ther.* 2004;34:13–20.

100. Robertson VJ, Ward AR, Jung P. The effect of heat on tissue extensibility: a comparison of deep and superficial heating. *Arch Phys Med Rehabil.* 2005;86:819–825.

101. Currier DP, Nelson RM. Changes in motor conduction velocity induced by exercise and diathermy. *Phys Ther.* 1969; 146–152.

102. Chastain PB. The effect of deep heat on isometric strength. *Phys Ther.* 1978;58:543–546.

103. Cetin N, Aytar A, Atalay A, Akman MN. Comparing hot pack, short-wave diathermy, ultrasound, and TENS on isokinetic strength, pain, and functional status of women with osteoarthritic knees: a single-blind, randomized, controlled trial. *Am J Phys Med Rehabil.* 2008;86:443–451.

104. McCray RE, Patton NJ. Pain relief at trigger points: a comparison of moist heat and shortwave diathermy. *J Orthop Sports Phys Ther.* 1984;5:175–178.

105. Laufer Y, Zilberman R, Porat R, Nahir AM. Effect of pulsed short-wave diathermy on pain and function of subjects with osteoarthritis of the knee: a placebo-controlled double-blind clinical trial. *Clin Rehabil.* 2005;19:255–263.

106. Santiesteban AJ, Grant C. Post-surgical effect of pulsed shortwave therapy. *J Am Podiatr Assoc.* 1985;75:306–309.

107. Balogun JA, Okonofua FE. Management of chronic pelvic inflammatory disease with shortwave diathermy. *Phys Ther.* 1988;68:1541–1545.

108. Wagstaff P, Wagstaff S, Downey M. A pilot study to compare the efficacy of continuous and pulsed magnetic energy [short-wave diathermy] on the relief of low back pain. *Physiotherapy.* 1986;72:563–566.

109. Van Zundert J, Brabant S, Van de Kelft E, Vercruyssen A, Van Buyten JP. Pulsed radiofrequency treatment of the gasserian ganglion in patients with idiopathic trigeminal neuralgia. *Pain.* 2003;104:449–452.

110. Al-Badawi EA, Mehta N, Forgione AG, Lobo SL, Zawawi KH. Efficacy of pulsed radio frequency energy therapy in temporomandibular joint pain and dysfunction. *Cranio.* 2004; 22:10–20.

111. Pennington GM, Danley DL, Sumko MH. Pulsed, non-thermal, high frequency electromagnetic energy (DIAPULSE) in the treatment of grade I and grade II ankle sprains. *Military Med.* 1993;158:101–104.

112. Bassett CA. Fundamental and practical aspects of therapeutic uses of pulsed electromagnetic fields (PEMFs). *Crit Rev Biomed Eng.* 1989;17:451–529.

113. Sharrad WJW. A double blind trial of pulsed electromagnetic fields for delayed healing of tibial fractures. *J Bone Joint Surg.* 1990;72B:347–355.

114. DiCesare A, Giombini A, Dragoni S, et al. Calcific tendinopathy of the rotator cuff. Conservative management with 434 MHz local microwave diathermy (hyperthermia): a case study. *Disabil Rehabil.* 2008;30:1578–1583.

115. Giombini A, Giovannini V, Di Cesare A, et al. Hyperthermia induced by microwave diathermy in the management of muscle and tendon injuries. *Brit Med Bull.* 2007;83:379–396.

116. Walker NA, Denegar CR, Preische J. Low intensity pulsed ultrasound and pulsed electromagnetic field in the treatment of tibial fractures: a systematic review. *J Athl Train.* 2007; 42:530–535.

117. Hill J, Lewis M, Mills P, Kielty C. Pulsed short-wave diathermy effects on human fibroblast proliferation. *Arch Phys Med Rehabil.* 2002;83:832–836.

118. Mayrovitz HN, Larsen PB. A preliminary study to evaluate the effect of pulsed radio frequency field treatment on lower extremity peri-ulcer skin microcirculation of diabetic patients. *Wounds.* 1995;7:90–93.

119. Itoh M, Montemayor JS, Matsumoto E, et al. Accelerated wound healing of pressure ulcers by pulsed high peak power electromagnetic energy (Diapulse). *Decubitus.* 1991; 2:24–28.

120. Salzberg CA, Cooper-Vastola SA, Perez FJ, et al. The effect of non-thermal pulsed electromagnetic energy (Diapulse) on wound healing of pressure ulcers in spinal cord injured patients: a randomized, double-blind study. *Wounds.* 1995;7:11–16.

121. Bassett CA. The development and application of pulsed electromagnetic fields (PEMFs) for ununited fractures and arthrodeses. *Orthop Clin North Am.* 1984;15:61–87.

122. Murray CC, Kitchen S. Effect of pulse repetition rate on the perception of thermal sensation with pulsed shortwave diathermy. *Physiother Res Int.* 2000;5:73–85.

123. Starkey C. *Therapeutic Modalities.* 3rd ed. Philadelphia: FA Davis; 2004.

124. Cheing GLY, Wan JWH, Lo SK. Ice and pulsed electromagnetic field to reduce pain and swelling after distal radius fractures. *J Rehabil Med.* 2005;37:372–377.

125. Sutbeyaz ST, Sezer N, Koseoglu BF. The effect of pulsed electromagnetic fields in the treatment of cervical osteoarthritis: a randomized, double blind, sham-controlled trial. *Rheumatol Int.* 2006;26:320–324.

126. Mackenzie D, Veninga FD. Reversal of delayed union of anterior cervical fusion treated with pulsed electromagnetic field stimulation: a case report. *South Med J.* 2004;97: 519–524.

127. Lehmann JF. *Therapeutic Heat and Cold.* 4th ed. Baltimore: Williams & Wilkins; 1990.

128. Lehmann JF, Warren CG, Scham SM. Therapeutic heat and cold. *Clin Orthop.* 1974;99:207.

129. Allberry J. Shortwave diathermy for herpes zoster. *Physiotherapy.* 1974;60:386.

130. Barnett M. SWD for herpes zoster. *Physiotherapy.* 1975; 61:217.

131. McCarthy CJ, Callaghan MJ, Oldham JA. Pulsed electromagnetic energy treatment offers no clinical benefit in reducing the pain of knee osteoarthritis: a systematic review. *BMC Musculoskelet Disord.* 2006;7:51.

132. Scott BO. Shortwave diathermy. In: Licht S, ed. *Therapeutic Heat and Cold.* 2nd ed. Baltimore, MD: Waverly Press; 1965: 279–309.

133. Draper DO, Castel CJ, Castel D. Low-watt pulsed shortwave diathermy and metal-plate fixation of the elbow. *Athl Ther Today.* 2004;9:28–32.

134. Seiger C, Draper DO. Use of pulsed shortwave diathermy and joint mobilization to increase ankle range of motion in the presence of surgical implanted metal: a case series. *J Orthop Sports Phys Ther.* 2006;36:669–677.

135. Sandler B. Heat and the U.U.C.D. *Br Med J.* 1973;25:458.

136. Nielsen NC, Hansen R, Larsen T. Heat induction in copper-bearing IUDs during shortwave diathermy. *Acta Obstet Gynecol Scand.* 1979;58:495.

137. Heick A, Espesen T, Pederson HL, Raahauge J. Is diathermy safe in women with copper-bearing IUDs? *Acta Obstet Gynecol Scand*. 1991;70:153–155.

138. Batavia M. *Contraindications in Physical Rehabilitation: Doing No Harm*. St. Louis, MO: Saunders Elsevier; 2006.

139. Al-Mandeel MA, Watson T. Pulsed and continuous shortwave therapy. In: Watson T, ed. *Electrotherapy Evidence-Based Practice*. 12th ed. Philadelphia: Churchill Livingstone Elsevier; 2008:137–160.

140. Shields N, O'Hare N, Gormley J. An evaluation of safety guidelines to restrict exposure to stray radiofrequency radiations from short-wave diathermy units. *Phys Med Biol*. 2004;49:2999–3015.

141. Martin JC, McCallum HM, Strelley S, Heaton B. Electromagnetic fields from therapeutic diathermy equipment: a review of hazards and precautions. *Physiotherapy*. 1991;77:3–7.

142. McDowell AD, Lunt MJ. Electromagnetic field strength measurements on megapulse units. *Physiotherapy*. 1991;77:805–809.

143. Lerman Y, Jacubovich R, Caner A, Ribak J. Electromagnetic fields from shortwave diathermy equipment in physiotherapy departments. *Physiotherapy*. 1996;82:456–458.

144. Shields N, Gormley J, O'Hare N. Short-wave diathermy: current clinical and safety practices. *Physiother Res Int*. 2002;7:191–202.

145. Martin CJ, McCallum H, Heaton B. An evaluation of radiofrequency exposure from therapeutic diathermy equipment in the light of current recommendations. *Clin Phys Physiol Meas*. 1990;11:53–63.

146. Belanger AY. *Evidence-Based Guide to Therapeutic Physical Agents*. Baltimore, MD: Lippincott Williams & Wilkins; 2003.

147. Taskinen H, Kyyrönen P, Hemminki K. Effects of ultrasound, shortwaves, and physical exertion on pregnancy outcome in physiotherapists. *J Epidem Comm Health*. 1990;44:196–201.

148. Larsen A. Congenital malformations and exposure to high-frequency electromagnetic radiation among Danish physiotherapists. *Scand J Work Environ Health*. 1991;17:318–323.

149. Larsen A, Olsen J, Svane O. Gender specific reproductive outcome and exposure to high frequency electromagnetic radiation among physiotherapists. *Scan J Work Environ Health*. 1991;17:324–329.

150. Lerman Y, Jacubovich R, Green MS. Pregnancy outcome following exposure to shortwaves among female physiotherapists in Israel. *Am J Ind Med*. 2001;39:499–504.

151. Ouellet-Hellstrom R, Stewart WF. Miscarriages among female physical therapists who report using radio-and microwave-frequency electromagnetic radiation. *Am J Epidemiology*. 1993;138:775–786.

152. Docker M, Bazin S, Dyson M, et al. Guidelines for the use of continuous shortwave therapy equipment. *Physiotherapy*. 1992;78:755–757.

153. Scott B. Effect of contact lenses on shortwave field distribution. *Br J Opthalmol*. 1956;40:696.

154. Riambau V, Caserta G, Garcia-Madrid C. Thrombosis of a bifurcated endograft following lower-back microwave therapy. *J Endovasc Ther*. 2004;11:334–338.

155. Shah SGS, Farrow A. Investigation of practices and procedures in the use of therapeutic diathermy: a study from the physiotherapists' health and safety perspective. *Physiother Res Int*. 2007;12:228–241.

156. Basirnia A, Sadeghipoor G, Esmaeeli DG. The effect of low power laser therapy on osteoarthritis of the knee. *Radiol Med (Torino)*. 1998;95:303–309.

157. Trelles MA, Rigau J, Sala P, Calderhead G, Ohshiro T. Infrared diode laser in low reactive-level laser therapy (LLLT) for knee osteoarthritis. *Laser Ther*. 1991;3:149–153.

158. Oezdemir F, Birtane M, Kokino S. The clinical efficacy of low-power laser therapy on pain and function in cervical osteoarthritis. *Clin Rheum*. 2001;20:181–184.

159. Jan MH, Chai HM, Wang CL, Lin YF, Tsai LY. Effects of repetitive shortwave diathermy for reducing synovitis in patients with knee osteoarthritis: an ultrasonographic study. *Phys Ther*. 2006;86:236–244.

160. Usichenko TI, Ivashkivsky OI, Gizhko VV. Treatment of rheumatoid arthritis with electromagnetic millimeter waves applied to acupuncture points—a randomized double blind clinical study. *Acupunct Electro Res*. 2003;28(1–2):11–18.

161. Giombini A, Casciello G, Di Cesare MC, Di Cesare A, Dragoni S, Sorrenti D. A controlled study on the effects of hyperthermia at 434 MHz and conventional ultrasound upon muscle injuries in sport. *J Sports Med Phys Fitness*. 2001;41:521–527.

162. Dziedzic K, Hill J, Lewis M, Sim J, Daniels J, Hay EM. Effectiveness of manual therapy or pulsed shortwave diathermy in addition to advice and exercise for neck disorders: A pragmatic randomized controlled trial in physical therapy clinics. *Arth & Rheum*. 2005;53:214–222.

163. Brucker JB, Knight KL, Ribley MD, Draper DO. An 18-day stretching regimen, with or without pulsed shortwave diathermy, and ankle dorsiflexion after 3 weeks. *J Athl Train*. 2005;40:276–280.

164. Callaghan MJ, Whittaker PE, Grimes S, Smith L. An evaluation of pulsed shortwave on knee osteoarthritis using radioleucoscintigraphy: a randomized, double blind, controlled trial. *Joint Bone Spine*. 2005;72:150–155.

165. Draper DO, Miner L, Knight KL, Ricard MD. The carry-over effects of diathermy and stretching in developing hamstring flexibility. *J Athl Train*. 2002;37:37-42.

166. McGill S. The effects of pulsed shortwave therapy on lateral ligament sprain of the ankle. *New Zealand J Physiother*. 1988;16:21–24.

167. Barker AT, Barlow PS, Porter J, et al. A double-blind clinical trial of low power pulsed shortwave therapy in the treatment of a soft tissue injury. *Physiotherapy*. 1985;7:500–504.

168. Hulme J, Welch V, deBie R, Judd M, Tugwell P. Electromagnetic fields for the treatment of osteoarthritis. *Cochrane Database Syst Rev*. 2002;Issue 1 (Art. No.: CD003523).

169. Marks R, Ghassemi M, Duarte R, Van Nguyen JP. A review of the literature on shortwave diathermy as applied to osteoarthritis of the knee. *Physiotherapy*. 1999;85:304–316.

170. Low J. Dosage of some pulsed shortwave clinical trials. *Physiotherapy*. 1995;81:611–616.

chapter 7

Spinal Traction

Charles Hazle, PT, MS, PhD

Foundations of Traction

The practice of using traction—applying tensile forces to the long axis of the spine—to treat patients with spinal pain has been advocated for centuries. Modern support for traction stemmed largely from the British physician James Cyriax, who in the 1940s recommended using traction to treat patients with disc lesions.[1] Practitioners from Cyriax's time and spanning to the present day, including Australian physiotherapist Geoffrey Maitland, also proposed traction to be of value in treating patients with spinal disorders.[2,3] The rationale for this intervention may have evolved, but the fundamental concept has remained remarkably consistent over the years.

However, in the current evidence-guided era, traction has been closely examined for efficacy in patient care. Many practitioners continue to cite traction as an essential clinical modality, often based on anecdotal patient care experiences, even though objective evidence of its value remains in question. In this chapter, traction will be described in terms of possible physiological and biomechanical effects. We will also discuss clinical trials, variations on traditional uses, and the conventions often used by practitioners.

Biomechanical and Physiological Effects of Traction

Cervical Spine

One of the purported effects of traction is increasing the space between vertebrae. The theorized value of intervertebral separation is for normalizing morphology and the disc's position and increasing the dimensions of the intervertebral foramen containing the spinal nerve root.

Imaging studies in vivo and with cadaveric specimens have investigated the effect of traction on the spaces between vertebrae and the intervertebral foramen. One study using fresh cadaveric human specimens[4] and one using live humans[5] yielded near identical results. The dimensions of the intervertebral foramina were measured with computed tomography (CT) and radiography, respectively. In both studies, traction with the cervical spine in a neutral position significantly increased foraminal size. Combined cervical flexion and traction did not increase foraminal size greater than either flexion or traction alone. Other studies have documented a decrease in pressure[6] and an increase in volume[7] of the intervertebral foramen with flexion of the cervical spine; this is often the basis for including flexion when applying cervical traction.

In live humans, cervical intervertebral disc spaces were observed to increase with traction of almost 30 pounds when the cervical spine was positioned in neutral and flexion. Similar changes in the intervertebral disc spaces were not observed while traction was administered in extension. Separation of the zygapophyseal joints was achieved only with traction in extension. In this study, the investigators reported traction in a position of cervical extension was, however, intolerable for many subjects.[7]

The effect of traction on the disc has been of primary interest in other investigations. CT was used to assess cervical disc herniations in 13 subjects before and immediately following 20 minutes of traction.[8] Following traction, the mean area of the disc herniation was reduced and disc space was increased. Further, the spinal canal area was increased, and the longitudinal dimension of the cervical spinal column was greater. The duration of these effects was not measured.

Multiple studies have examined the effect of traction on the musculature surrounding the cervical spine. Results of these investigations have been varied; elevated[9,10] and diminished[11,12] levels of muscle activity have been observed, and in some cases the traction had no effect.[13] One study observed an increase in blood flow in the musculature commensurate with lessening pain associated with the use of traction.[14]

Lumbar Spine

The effects of traction on lumbar spine vertebral alignment and the level of trunk muscle activity have been evaluated by several investigators. In one study,[15] trunk muscle activity in 29 asymptomatic subjects was found to increase initially with the application of traction but quickly subside to prior levels. Whether traction was continuous or intermittent yielded no difference in the observations of muscle activity.

More than 60 years ago, Cyriax proposed that negative pressure created by traction in effect draws in a protruding disc, reducing the extension of disc tissue beyond the vertebral body margin.[1] Intradiscal pressures have been observed to increase during active lumbar traction (distractive force by the subject's effort).[16] This is consistent with observations that intradiscal pressure increases with trunk muscle activation even with concurrent distractive force applied to the lumbar spine.[17]

Of relevance to possibly decreasing nerve root compression in radicular disorders arising from disc herniations, a reduction of disc material beyond the borders of the vertebral bodies was noted in 21 of 30 subjects as measured by CT. The reduction effect was greatest in patients with median herniations and lowest among those with lateral herniations.[18] These measurements were completed before and during the application of lumbar traction. The investigators did not attempt to measure the persistence of these changes after traction.

Box 7•1 | **Biomechanical and Physiological Effects of Traction: Synopsis of Literature**

Cervical Spine

- There is evidence that intervertebral foramina dimensions increase during traction application. Whether this can be further influenced by positioning in flexion or lateral flexion is not established.
- Limited evidence suggests that disc herniation extension tends to be reduced when measured immediately after traction.
- Evidence is conflicting as to the effects of traction on the activity of cervical spine musculature.
- The duration of any observed biomechanical or physiological effect is not known.

Lumbar Spine

- During passive traction, intradiscal pressures can reduce or become negative. Traction from patient-generated forces may increase intradiscal pressures. These pressures are thought to rapidly return to their prior state when traction ends.
- The expanse of herniated disc material is suggested to reduce in some subjects during traction. Most single-observation studies suggest the effect is temporary. A cumulative effect with repeated traction sessions may occur.

The disc dimensions of a group of 24 subjects with confirmed lumbar disc herniations who received traction for treatment were compared by CT with a control group of 22 subjects who had disc herniations but did not receive traction. Otherwise, both groups received the same treatment with physical therapy modalities and medications over a course of 15 sessions. Those subjects receiving traction demonstrated a substantially greater reduction of the total area of herniated disc material as measured by CT.[19]

KEY POINT! The lasting effect of the change in anatomical relationships caused by traction remains in question.

Prior to use of sophisticated imaging analyses, a cadaveric study of traction[20] determined the elongation induced during traction did not continue beyond 30 minutes after treatment. Similarly, another study[21] demonstrated that a return to pretraction relationships occurred after only 10 minutes after traction.

Pain occurring distal to the knee with straight leg raising (SLR) was measured before and after traction in a group of subjects with positive SLR below 45° of hip flexion.[22] An increase in SLR was observed immediately following lumbar traction at magnitudes of 30% and 60% of body weight, compared to no increase in SLR in subjects who received no traction and traction at 10% of body weight. Duration of the effect was not measured (Box 7-1).

Basic Applications of Clinical Traction

The application of traction for mechanical neck and back pain syndromes has many approaches. Individual practitioner and patient care experiences often serve as the stimulus for the development of clinical traction techniques, which are subsequently propagated by convention. The lack of substantial data to support particular utilization guidelines has allowed for numerous permutations in the elemental practice of applying tension to the spine for symptom relief. To adequately understand traction and its uses, this chapter provides details on the basic features more commonly available on modern traction devices.

Components of the Traction Table

Traction tables allow patients to receive treatment of the cervical and lumbar spine in relative comfort (Fig. 7-1). The table is adjustable in height by a hand or foot control switch. At one end of the table is the traction unit, consisting of an electric motor and a control panel. The traction unit usually produces the tensile force via a cable that extends from the electric motor. The cable is attachable to the traction harnesses, which directly contact the patient. With the evolution of computer technology, the control panels of traction units have become increasingly sophisticated. Many modern models have touch-screen features and the capacity to adjust numerous variables in the delivery of traction (Fig. 7-2). Treatment duration, cycle times, tension levels, and progressive or regressive steps in tension can be programmed into the session with these controls.

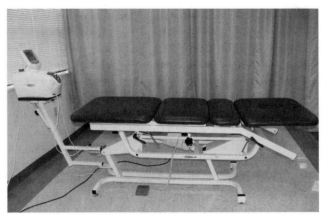

Fig 7•1 Traction table.

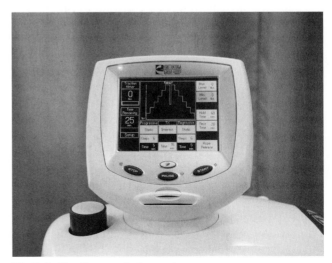

Fig 7•2 Traction control panel.

Most traction tables also have a split top. The table surface, having multiple segments, can be separated to minimize friction when applying traction to the lumbar spine. The section of the table nearest the motor can be unlocked so it glides within tracks that are set on rollers on the table's frame (Fig. 7-3). This allows the patient's pelvis and lower extremities to be moved while the trunk is stabilized on the nongliding sections of the table. Thus, traction can be more accurately administered to the lumbar spine by significantly reducing the friction provided by the patient's superincumbent body weight. The nongliding segments of the table sometimes have adjustable tilting features to create more options for traction or to facilitate patient comfort with positioning.

Manufactured traction tables now routinely have a removable harness unit that allows traction to be applied to the cervical spine (Fig. 7-4). These harnesses usually snap-fit or pressure-fit into a latch mechanism on the motorized portion of the traction table. The occipital harnesses have mobile and stationary portions. Adjustable padded wedges on the harness directly contact the patient's head and neck along with a flat padded area for the occiput. The wedges fit snugly against the posterolateral aspects of the patient's cranium and are often capable of being approximated toward the patient's midline with a screw knob adjustment to prevent slipping during traction. The padded wedges are affixed to the movable segment of the harness, which slides along the stationary portion via the tension produced by the traction motor. Occipital harnesses usually have a strap that can be tightened over the patient's forehead to secure the head in the harness (Fig. 7-5). The need to secure the patient's head firmly

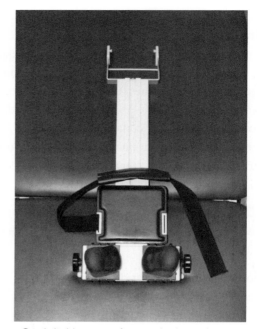

Fig 7•4 Occipital harness for cervical traction.

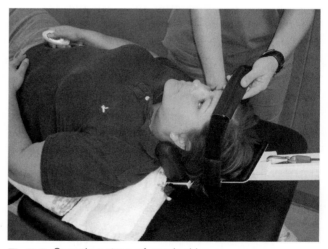

Fig 7•5 Securing strap of cervical harness.

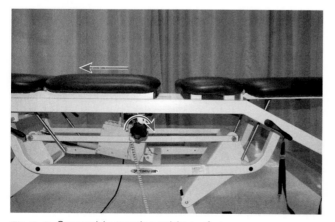

Fig 7•3 Separable traction table surface.

is greater with higher amounts of tension, as the potential for the harness to slip increases. At lower levels of tension, practitioners often avoid using the strap so the patient can be more comfortable.

Another feature of traction tables is a patient-controlled safety switch (Fig. 7-6). Patients receiving traction usually have intervals of indirect supervision, so their safety is enhanced with a manually activated switch that allows them to immediately release the traction while sounding an alarm for assistance. Patients who occasionally experience anxiety with an unfamiliar intervention are often comforted by knowing they are ultimately in control of

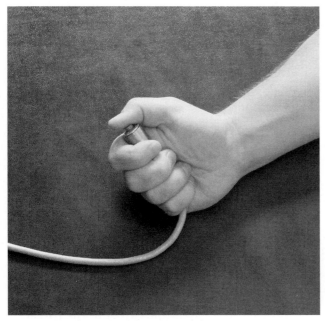

Fig 7•6 Patient-controlled safety switch.

the traction unit. Similarly, if patients experience discomfort while receiving traction, response time by the practitioner to render assistance can be reduced or effectively eliminated by activation of the switch.

Traction tables represent significant capital equipment investments for most clinical settings and are often used for many years. At the time of this publication, the price range for traction tables was approximately $4,000 to $19,000, depending on the features and options included.

Cervical Spine Traction: Procedures and Practice

Essential Elements

When describing the setup of cervical traction, the term *harness* may not be an ideal descriptor as current clinical apparatuses are considerably different from older devices. In the 1980s, the portion of the equipment directly contacting the patient usually consisted of straps that encircled the patient's occiput and chin in order to gain purchase on the head for a superiorly oriented force. However, practitioners grew concerned about the force being applied to the mandible and through the temporomandibular joints, so occipital-contact-only harnesses became more popular and are now universally used. These devices are generally accepted as being more comfortable for all patients in

addition to avoiding compressive force through the temporomandibular joints.

The typical preparatory steps for a cervical traction treatment session include the following:

- The cervical harness is first attached to the motorized unit (Fig. 7-7).
- The cable is slackened from the motor and then linked to the mobile portion of the harness (Fig. 7-8). Any slack in the cable is then removed without changing the position of the mobile portion of the harness (Fig. 7-9).

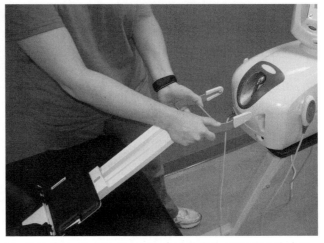

Fig 7•7 Step 1: Attachment of occipital-contact-only harness to motor.

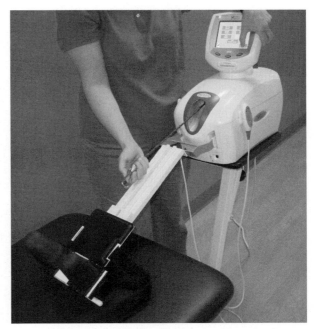

Fig 7•8 Step 2: Slackening of cable to allow attachment of mobile portion of harness.

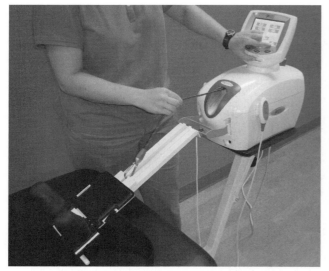

Fig 7•9 Step 3: Removal of cable slack.

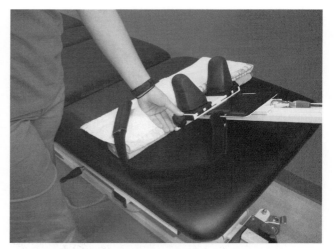

Fig 7•11 Step 4: Opening of the harness to accommodate the patient.

- Patient comfort and relaxation during cervical traction are promoted as much as possible. For this reason, practitioners will often place small, well-insulated hydrocollator packs against the inferior edge of the harness upon which the patient will lie (Fig. 7-10). Most patients find the warming sensation from the hydrocollator packs across the upper thoracic and scapular regions relaxing, although the packs probably have negligible therapeutic value. Caution must be taken to prevent the hydrocollator packs from overheating the patient's upper back. This is particularly a concern in older patients who perhaps have less ability to dissipate heat.
- The harness is opened, and the patient is asked to lie supine on the table with the head placed on the flat padded area of the harness (Fig. 7-11).

Proper positioning of the patient in the harness is important for comfort (Fig. 7-12). If the padded wedges are positioned too high relative to the patient's mastoid processes, slippage may occur during the traction session. In addition, patients become uncomfortable if the wedges compress on the posterior cranium from being positioned too high. Careful positioning of the harness and padded wedges usually allows the wedges to contact more along the inferior aspect of the cranium.

- The padded wedges are then approximated toward the midline to securely fit the harness to the patient's occiput (Fig. 7-13). Caution must be used to not overtighten this adjustment,

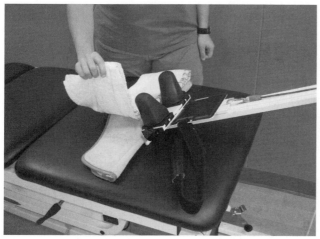

Fig 7•10 Placement of small hydrocollator pack (optional).

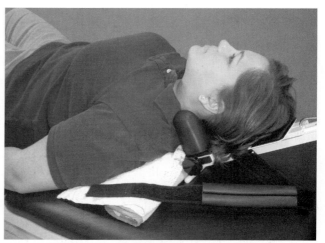

Fig 7•12 Step 5: Positioning of the patient in the cervical harness.

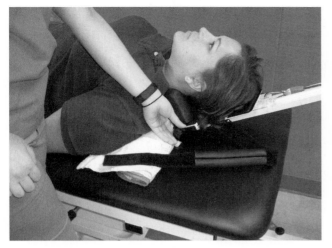

Fig 7•13 Step 6: Adjustment of padded harness wedges to patient.

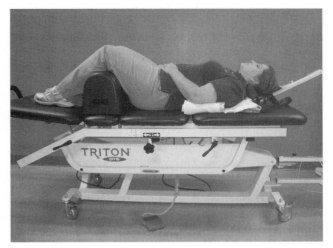

Fig 7•15 Step 7: Positioning the patient's upper and lower extremities for comfort in cervical traction.

which would cause an uncomfortable compressive sensation on the patient's neck.

- The angle of the traction harness is adjusted, if necessary, for the relative amount of cervical flexion and any desired lateral flexion. This is usually accomplished by adjusting the table height relative to the fixed height motor and control unit (Fig. 7-14).

- Support from one or two pillows or sometimes a bolster is placed under the patient's knees to promote comfort. Some practitioners support under the arms proximally with small rolled towels. This enhances patient comfort, particularly in those with excessive thoracic kyphoses or remarkably protracted scapulae (Fig. 7-15).

- Practitioners will discuss with the patient the sensations and responses they should expect while receiving traction. The patient should be instructed to notify the clinician immediately if pain increases or if the patient becomes uncomfortable in any way during the session. It is recommended to have the patient verbalize his or her understanding of these instructions.

- The patient is provided with an aid to call for assistance or is shown the safety switch (Fig. 7-16).

- The settings of the traction unit are programmed into the control panel and traction is initiated.

- The prudent clinician will directly observe the traction unit mechanics and the patient response

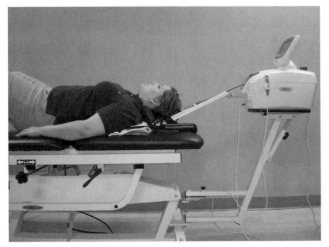

Fig 7•14 Step 8: Angle of cervical traction.

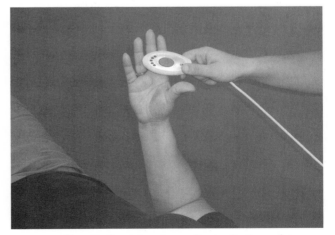

Fig 7•16 Step 9: Providing the patient with the safety switch or another aid to call for assistance.

when the session begins. A minimum of 2 to 3 minutes of observation is recommended. This is further opportunity to ensure the patient's comfort, assess an immediate response, and reinforce with the patient expected and unintended responses during the treatment session.

Mechanical Preparation

In addition to patient comfort, the arrangement of the table and harness angle is also a variable in the effects of cervical traction. This is particularly in reference to the angle of cervical spine flexion as measured by the harness relative to the horizontal table surface (see Fig. 7-14). Many practitioners, however, have methods of choosing the angle of application or the line of pull for the cervical traction harness, such as selecting the angle depending on the level of the cervical spine that is most symptomatic. For example, the lower cervical spine levels are often treated with greater amounts of flexion while the middle and upper levels may be treated with considerably less flexion.

Other practitioners choose a more simplistic approach of asking the patient to report the angle of greatest comfort and adjust the table height accordingly. In addition to the sagittal plane angle, some practitioners will elect to use a lateral flexion angle, presumably to have greater distractive effect on the side of the cervical spine with greater involvement, in the presence of asymmetrical or unilateral symptoms (Fig. 7-17). Most traction tables now have the option of setting the motor and control unit at angles in the patient's coronal plane to achieve traction in lateral cervical flexion. Whether a particular arrangement of the cervical harness results in better patient outcomes has not been validated but remains a convention. The angle of traction should be based on each patient's condition and comfort.

Traction Dosage and Decision-Making

In addition to the angle of traction, several other variables are at the discretion of the practitioner. The amount of tension, the duration of the treatment, and the timing of the cycle with intermittent traction may all be manipulated by the practitioner. These variables may collectively be considered traction dosage (Box 7-2). Again, the use of accepted, if not substantiated, practices

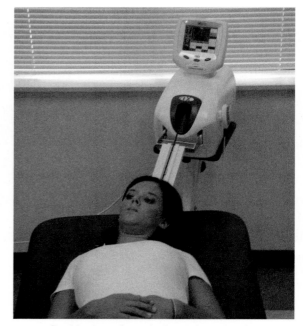

Fig 7•17 Positioning of cervical traction with right-side bias induced by lateral flexion to left.

are generally seen in reference to these parameters. Practitioners often view traction dosage as analogous to the grading of manually applied mobilizations to the spine.

As previously described, comfort is a foremost consideration with patients receiving traction. As a rule, the amount of tension applied to the cervical spine should not cause or increase symptoms. In the presence of peripheral symptoms, possibly of nerve-root origin, practitioners generally agree that distal symptoms warrant particular observation for changes during and immediately following traction. If the patient reports any increase of upper extremity symptoms during a

---

Box 7•2	**Variables at Practitioner's Discretion in Delivery of Cervical Traction**

- Static or intermittent
- Angle of application
- Dosage
  - Amount of tension
  - Duration of traction
  - Cycle
    - Total cycle duration
  - Proportion of time of maximum vs. minimum tension
  - Inclusion of ascending or descending steps at initiation or conclusion

treatment session, whether pain or paresthesia, traction should immediately cease. Similarly, if there is an increase of symptoms after traction, the practitioner should reconsider the traction dosage or determine if traction is an appropriate treatment option at that time. The practitioner's assessment of the acuity and irritability of the patient's condition is part of this reasoning process. Mechanical pain syndromes characterized by pain that is quickly and easily increased with minimal movement or provocation generally suggest very conservative traction dosages initially. Symptoms not highly irritable or acute may tolerate greater dosages. Thus, the practitioner is challenged to find a threshold that has a beneficial effect without applying excessive force or provoking symptoms.

KEY POINT! When the decision is made to use traction, most practitioners will choose a conservative traction dosage for the first application; this will establish a favorable, or at least neutral, patient response to the initial treatment.

Within the context of the patient having been recently evaluated, perhaps with provocative maneuvers, assessing the patient's response during and subsequent to the first traction session requires caution. It is common for the patient to report a modest pulling or stretching sensation within or immediately adjacent to the spine during treatment. This is not an indication to stop or alter treatment. Indeed, frequently patients will describe this stretching or pulling sensation favorably, with the feeling often diminishing over the course of the traction session. Practitioners often hypothesize that the reduction of this stretching or pulling sensation may indicate an improvement of soft tissue extensibility. Thus, such a response is generally viewed as favorable.

Tension amounts will range between 10 and 25 pounds for the upper limit of intermittent cervical traction.[23–26] Although continuous and intermittent traction are possible on most tables, the majority of practitioners will use intermittent traction, cycling between two levels of tension for the duration of the session. Practitioners often use a lower level of tension that is approximately one-half that of the upper level. If continuous traction is chosen, less tension and total duration than the upper level of intermittent traction are typically chosen.

With cervical traction applied in the supine position, as opposed to the older practice of seated traction with a vertical pull, the weight of the head is less of a factor in the net amount of tension applied to the cervical spine. However, the angle of the traction harness may be a factor in the tension applied. A greater angle of cervical flexion will increase the vertical force component of the head's weight, whereas the vertical component will be negligible with a low flexion angle. Thus, to achieve a comparable net traction on the cervical spine, the amount of tension programmed into the traction unit may need to be relatively larger to compensate for a greater flexion angle. The practitioner may elect to increase the tension setting by an increment of 2 or 3 pounds at the greater flexion angle and then reassess the patient's response for comfort and symptom reduction.

The duration of the treatment session is usually 10 to 20 minutes as determined by the overall dosage and the acuity and irritability of the patient's condition. In the absence of well-established criteria, this is arbitrary, as is the timing of the cycles with intermittent traction. A cycle proportion of 30 seconds at the greater tension to 10 seconds at the lower tension of intermittent traction is common, but wide variation of this occurs due to therapist preference. With this proportion along with total time being substantial variables at the practitioner's discretion, caution is to be used when selecting these amounts based on the individual patient characteristics.

Patients receiving traction will also occasionally experience a rebound effect, with them feeling better during traction but then having a symptom increase that remains for minutes or hours afterward. When a rebound effect occurs, detailed communication between the practitioner and patient is required for accurate interpretation. A brief, transient increase of centrally located symptoms after traction may be a one-time localized tissue response or may be an indication for less traction dosage while continuing with the original plan of care. Conversely, an increase of symptoms lasting several hours, particularly including distal symptoms, demands the practitioner reconsider the decision to use traction. However, when interpreting this feedback from the patient, the practitioner must also consider concurrent interventions being administered, along with the patient's activities and behaviors following the first traction session. Thus, practitioner-patient communication is paramount in appropriate decision-making with traction.

After a traction session ends, it is common practice to release the tension from the harness, loosen the harness from its closure on the neck, and allow the patient to rest for approximately 5 minutes before rising. The patient should also be allowed to rest briefly in sitting after returning from supine to minimize the effect of any positional hypotension. A patient reporting dizziness or feeling faint during or immediately after traction or upon returning to sitting demands close observation and a check of vital signs. Such a response requires the symptoms to subside before the patient rises from the table. A prolonged response may warrant a medical consultation for underlying conditions, and the practitioner should reconsider using traction as an intervention in this particular patient.

KEY POINT! Among those practitioners who use cervical traction, there is consensus that it cannot be a sole intervention for patients with cervical spine mechanical pain syndromes. Use of therapeutic exercise and manual therapy techniques are clearly supported by evidence[27] for patients with cervical spine dysfunction and are often used in concert with cervical traction.

Before deciding to use traction in subsequent sessions, the practitioner should carefully interpret the patient's response to the prior session. If the patient reports temporary or lasting symptom relief, particularly with peripheral pain or paresthesia, and greater function, this suggests a possible benefit. Other objective evidence indicating favorable responses to cervical traction can include an increase in cervical range of motion (ROM), increased ability to complete specific daily activities (especially involving the upper extremities), improved upper extremity reflexes, increased upper extremity strength (i.e., grip), or normalization of previously observed sensory losses.

Lumbar Spine Traction: Procedures and Practice

Essential Elements

Traction for the lumbar spine of patients with mechanical dysfunction has a longer history of usage than does traction for patients with cervical spine syndromes. Lumbar traction is commonly used in some facilities; however, there is limited evidence for effectiveness and lack of agreement on treatment parameters.

After choosing to use traction, the first thing the practitioner must decide is whether to apply traction while the patient is prone or supine. No well-developed criteria exist to guide this decision. Some practitioners have a preference for using one position exclusively, unless patient comfort or poor response suggests the alternative. Other practitioners will place patients in their most comfortable position. If the patient's symptoms are less severe when lying prone, then the practitioner may use the prone position for traction. Alternately, supine traction may be chosen if the patient gets the most relief from lying supine with hips and knees flexed. Another factor may be age. For example, older patients, perhaps more likely to have mechanical pain associated with degenerative changes of the posterior elements of the lumbar spine, are thought to typically respond favorably to a flexed, supine position.

Mechanical Preparation

Once the patient's position is determined, the traction table and harnesses can be set with the following considerations:

- During supine positioning, well-insulated hydrocollator packs are often used under the patient's back (Fig. 7-18). There is no known direct clinical benefit from the heat application. Because of the superincumbent body weight and little

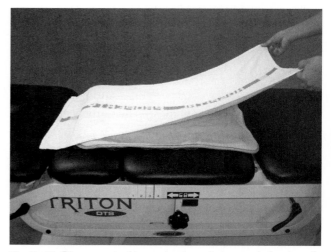

Fig 7•18 Placement of large hydrocollator pack (optional).

flexibility for adjustment once traction has begun, particular caution must be employed to avoid burning or overheating the patient. Older individuals with less ability to dissipate heat may require additional layers of insulation and more frequent monitoring during treatment. If used, the hydrocollator packs are placed on the table surface, and the pelvic and thoracic harnesses are set (Fig. 7-19). Given the lack of clinical benefit and increased risk of thermal injury, this use of hydrocollator packs is generally discouraged.

- The patient's lumbar spine is positioned over the separation between mobile and stationary segments of the table (Fig. 7-20). This allows the distraction to be more localized to the lumbar spine when the gliding portion of the table is released.

- The patient is asked to lie supine on the harnesses, and the lower extremities are positioned for comfort with the hips and knees partially flexed; support is placed under the knees. Many practitioners prefer a "90-90 position" in which a stool is placed under the calves of the supine patient, resulting in the hips and knees each being positioned at approximately 90 degrees of flexion (Fig. 7-21). Other options include use of a bolster under the flexed knees to achieve a comfortable position for the patient (Fig. 7-22).

- Precise placement of the harnesses is important for patient comfort. The traditional pelvic

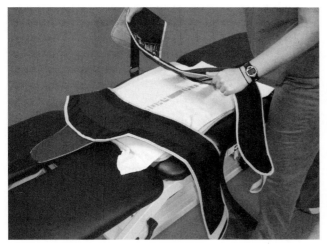

Fig 7•19 Step 1: Placement of the pelvic and thoracic harnesses for lumbar traction.

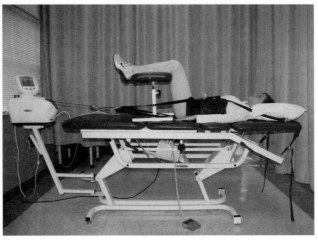

Fig 7•21 Step 3: Positioning for "90-90" lumbar traction.

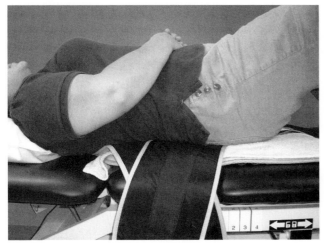

Fig 7•20 Step 2: Positioning of the target area of traction over the table separation.

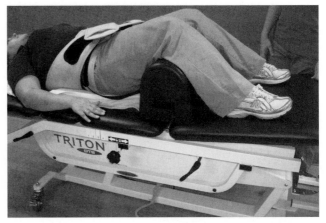

Fig 7•22 Step 3, alternative: Positioning for traction in supine with a bolster under the knees.

harness with two securing straps requires that the upper of the two straps securing the harness be placed above the patient's iliac crests. The lower strap will ideally be below the iliac crests but above the greater trochanters. Thus, each strap on the pelvic harness will be seated against a bony prominence when traction is applied, minimizing the likelihood of slipping (Fig. 7-23). The thoracic harness is best placed below the widest lateral dimension of the rib cage. Thus, when traction is applied, the thoracic harness will also seat against the bony prominences at the flare of the rib cage. Some newer lumbar traction harnesses have only one securing strap (Fig. 7-24).

Clothing can sometimes interfere with the function of the thoracic harness. Multiple layers of clothing, synthetic materials offering minimal friction, or bulky garments can all compromise the thoracic harness's position. The straps on both harnesses are clasped and tightened (Fig. 7-25). The extent of tightening is dependent on the amount of traction tension to be used. Larger amounts of tension require the straps to be firmly secured, whereas more modest traction tension does not require the straps to be as tight. The goal is patient comfort while also preventing the harnesses from slipping from their optimal placements on the patient's body. For female patients, a rolled towel placed vertically between the breasts before closing the thoracic harness may help prevent discomfort from the harness.

- Once the harnesses are secured, slack in the anchoring straps of the thoracic harness is removed to minimize any upper body movement. The cable is drawn from the motorized unit (Fig. 7-26) and attached to the pelvic harness (Fig. 7-27). The sequence of some steps may vary, depending on the particular traction unit and harnesses being used. In all cases, the harnesses are secured first around the patient before slack is removed from the other harness attachments.

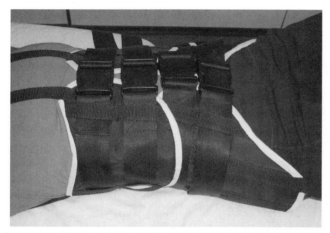

Fig 7•23 Step 4: Overlap of thoracic and pelvic harnesses with both seating against bony prominences.

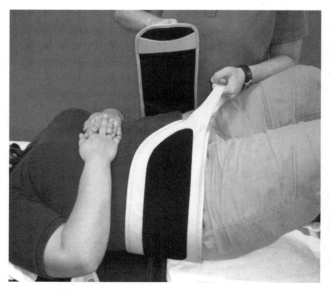

Fig 7•24 Traction harness with a single strap.

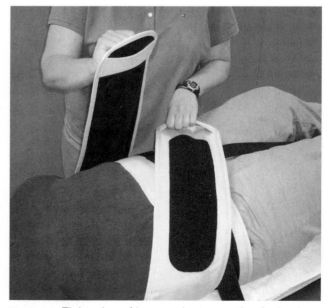

Fig 7•25 Tightening of harness in preparation for lumbar traction.

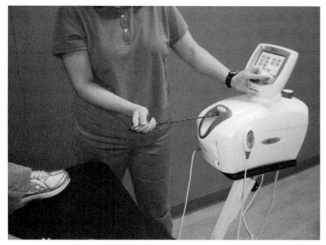

Fig 7•26 Step 5: Slackening of cable to allow attachment to the harness.

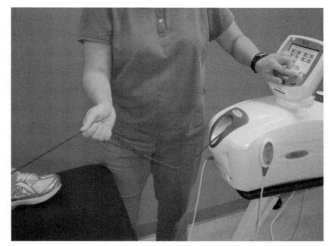

Fig 7•28 Step 7: Removal of cable slack.

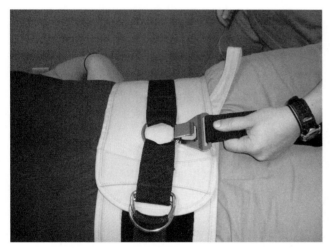

Fig 7•27 Step 6: Attachment of cable to pelvic harness.

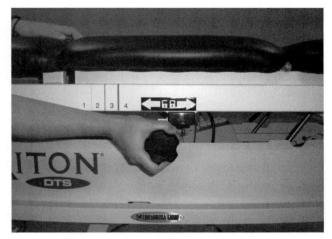

Fig 7•29 Step 8: Release of table lock.

- Once the patient is positioned and the harnesses are secured, the slack in the cable between the harness and motor is removed (Fig. 7-28).
- Next, the table surface lock is released, allowing the segments underlying the lumbar spine and pelvis to separate once the traction tension increases (Fig. 7-29).
- The traction parameters are programmed into the control panel and traction is initiated.
- The prudent practitioner will closely observe the patient and apparatus over two to three cycles of intermittent traction, assuring the harnesses are secured and do not slip. Avoid allowing the thoracic harness to slip up and sit against the axillae. Some patients may have body shapes that make

it challenging to secure harnesses enough to avoid slippage during traction.

With prone positioning, the harnesses are similarly placed on the table such that the lower lumbar segments or the lumbosacral junction align with the splits of the tabletop's segments (Fig. 7-30). Usually, this allows the patient's face to fit comfortably in the opening of the table's head segment. The tilt of this segment is often adjusted for greater patient comfort. The inability to communicate face-to-face with the patient during prone traction requires diligence on the practitioner's part to ensure the patient is not having an unfavorable response.

Some practitioners prefer to immediately apply manual mobilizations to the lumbar spine or encourage

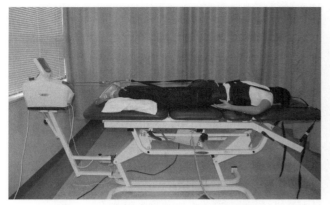

Fig 7•30 Positioning for prone lumbar traction.

the patient to complete extension exercises immediately after traction and before weight-bearing through the spine. This may be accomplished more easily with prone traction, as only the belts being loosened and the table surfaces being secured are necessary to proceed. If these interventions are chosen to follow supine traction, a nearby table can be brought next to the traction table, allowing the patient to roll prone onto the second table. As described in the section on cervical traction, a rest period following the release of traction is usually warranted before proceeding with another procedure.

With prone or supine positioning, the table height and the angle of the traction unit relative to the table can be adjusted, but these do not appear to exert the same effect as in the cervical spine. Without the stationary arm of the cervical traction harness providing for greater angulation of the tension, only minor variation of the traction tension is possible with lumbar traction arrangements.

Traction Dosage and Decision-Making

The variables in lumbar traction tension are similar to those described previously for the cervical spine. Additionally, the practitioner must determine whether supine or prone positioning is preferable. Positioning of the lower extremities may also be a consideration because this influences the alignment of the lumbar spine during traction. Collectively, total duration, cycle time, and amount of tension can be considered the traction dosage. Values are usually set conservatively to establish patient tolerance, particularly with conditions judged to be highly irritable or acute. Use of tension up to approximately one-half of the patient's body weight

is common practice, although this may not occur at the time of the initial treatment session. Similar to cervical traction, a cycle proportion of approximately 30 seconds at the maximum tension to 10 seconds at the lower tension is typical, although this is subject to practitioner preference. Manipulation of these variables can significantly increase or decrease total traction dosage (Box 7-3).

Communication between the practitioner and patient at the time of the traction session about expectations and responses is a necessity. Further communication at the time of the next visit is essential to assess the patient's response before beginning treatment again. A reduction in pain, particularly with lower extremity symptoms, along with increased ambulatory or sitting tolerances are indications of a positive response to lumbar traction. Additional evidence of a positive response is increased SLR, along with improvement in deficits in reflexes or sensation. Assessment of the patient's response to traction must always be made within the context of concurrent interventions and the patient's activities or behaviors.

Patient Safety

Generally, patients will not be directly supervised during the entire treatment period. Therefore, it is essential patients have a call system they can use if they need assistance during the traction session. Even though the patient safety switch is available, some practitioners prefer a bell or similar audible call method patients can use if they merely need to make minor adjustments or

---

Box 7•3	**Variables at Practitioner's Discretion in Delivery of Lumbar Traction**

- Supine or prone position
- Positioning of lower extremities that influences lumbar spine alignment
- Static or intermittent
- Angle of application
- Dosage
  - Amount of tension
  - Duration of traction
  - Cycle
    - Total cycle duration
    - Proportion of time of maximum vs. minimum tension
    - Inclusion of ascending or descending steps at initiation or conclusion

if they have a question and do not need to immediately terminate the traction treatment.

KEY POINT! The patient and practitioner must communicate about expectations and anticipated responses from traction to ensure no harm is done and the experience for the patient is favorable.

Patients must understand that they should alert the practitioner if there are any undesirable responses during treatment. Questions should be asked and answered before a patient's first traction experience. The practitioner must ensure the patient understands that traction should be a comfortable experience, rather than one to be endured for later benefit. If the patient's symptoms worsen, particularly if they are referred or radicular in nature, the patient should contact the practitioner or other clinical staff immediately. Similarly, the practitioner or other clinical staff must frequently assess the patient's comfort and response during the traction session. Patients with highly acute or irritable conditions require meticulous observation to ensure they are not having an adverse response to the traction.

When a lumbar traction session has ended, it is mandatory to secure the lock for the traction table segments immediately after releasing the tension. A sudden shift of the mobile portion of the table while the patient is on it or when rising from it can cause injury or negate the benefit of the traction.

Indications for Traction

There are no clearly established indications for using traction to treat the cervical or lumbar spine for mechanical pain syndromes. Historically, the trend has been to use traction more prominently in the overall treatment plan when patients present with signs and symptoms consistent with radiculopathies. As classification schemes for patients with cervical or lumbar spine syndromes have evolved, some have included a subgroup of patients for whom traction is a preferred or optional intervention.

The initial proposal of a treatment-based classification for low back pain contained a subgroup of patients for whom traction was suggested as the preferred intervention.[28] This categorization was largely based on patients experiencing distal symptoms when they performed movement in any direction. However, more recent descriptions of the treatment-based classification system[29,30] have not as clearly identified a traction

subgroup designation. The presence of symptoms distal to the knee, particularly when worsened with extension movements, along with a crossed straight-leg raise and neurological deficits, were cited in one study as possible indicators for traction.[31] Many clinicians will consider traction for patients with lumbar spine syndromes when peripheral symptoms, including radicular signs, are not reduced by movement or position testing in a manner similar to that initially proposed by Delitto et al.[28] Additionally, the reduction of symptoms with manually applied traction may be another criterion used in decision-making, although this has yet to be validated (Fig. 7-31).

Similarly, a recently published impairment-based classification system for neck pain[27] cites traction as a preferred intervention for those patients presenting with radiating upper extremity symptoms. Evidence for this designation includes provocation of upper extremity symptoms with foraminal compression, such as Spurling's maneuver (Fig. 7-32); reduction of those symptoms with manual traction (Fig. 7-33); and possible accompaniment of neurological involvement with upper extremity sensory, motor, and reflex deficits. Most recently, a clinical prediction rule for identifying patients most likely to benefit from cervical traction has been proposed.[32] The identifying characteristics included peripheralization of pain with lower cervical mobility testing, a positive shoulder abduction test, age of 55 or older, reduction of symptoms with manual distraction, and a positive upper limb tension test. The reported statistical support for this clinical prediction rule was very robust; however, validation of this clinical prediction rule remains to be completed.

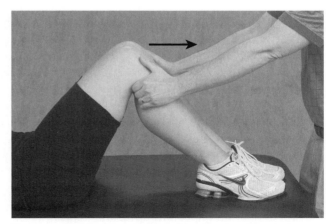

Fig 7•31 Application of manual lumbar traction during examination.

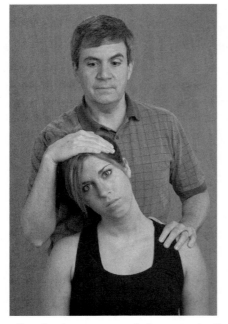

Fig 7•32 Spurling's maneuver during examination.

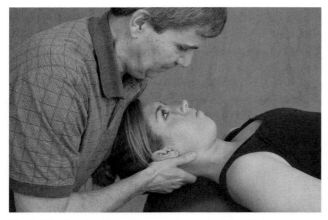

Fig 7•33 Application of manual cervical traction during examination.

KEY POINT! Clearly and definitively delineating the criteria for who might respond most favorably to traction has yet to occur. In the absence of clear practice guidelines, practitioner discretion is the largest variable in traction usage. The evolution of evidence supporting manual therapy and exercise suggests those interventions be considered as a concurrent first option, rather than traction for many patients with cervical and lumbar spine clinical syndromes.[27,33,34] For patients who have success with those interventions, traction should be considered a second-line or complementary intervention.

Contraindications for Traction

Before using traction on the spine, practitioners must screen patients for conditions that may cause poor responses or for which definitive contraindications exist. Cervical traction is contraindicated in patients with acute cervical spine trauma, particularly recent whiplash-associated disorders. Connective tissue diseases or rheumatologic disorders that can result in tissue laxity or joint hypermobility/instability are specific contraindications for the cervical spine. Foremost among these is rheumatoid arthritis, which is often characterized by asymptomatic subluxations of the upper cervical spine.[35–39] Ankylosing spondylitis, although characterized by rigidity and ossification in the lumbar and thoracic spine regions, may lead to upper cervical instability and is also a specific contraindication.[35,36,40–42]

Other diseases and disorders known to affect bone integrity, such as osteoporosis and osteopenia, are also contraindications for traction. Similarly, traction is contraindicated in patients with histories of steroid use or consumption of other medications that tend to weaken or demineralize bone. Localized hypermobility or instability in the region of interest is also a contraindication.

Traction is also contraindicated in patients having received surgical stabilization or decompression of the spine or in patients having received spine implants or prosthetic discs. The structural integrity of those devices or the bone-implant material interface may be threatened with the traction force.

Patients having undergone cervical spine discectomy often will have also received interbody fusions at the involved segment and thus would be inappropriate to receive traction. Traction may not be strictly contraindicated in a patient with a remote history of a simple lumbar discectomy on a single level, but the practitioner should be careful when deciding which treatment option is appropriate. Given the altered anatomy following discectomy, the practitioner must contemplate the proposed benefit from traction as opposed to other therapeutic options.

Because of multiple unknowns and the potential risks, lumbar traction during pregnancy is to be avoided. Use of cervical traction during pregnancy may not be absolutely contraindicated, but consideration

CASE STUDY 7•1   CERVICAL TRACTION

A 38-year-old male arrives at physical therapy with primary complaints of left neck, periscapular, and arm pain. He also describes paresthesia distal to the left elbow, extending into the first and second digits. He is unable to identify a specific event precipitating these symptoms but noted them gradually increasing the day after moving a household appliance 1 week ago. Upon questioning, he specifically denies any trauma to his cervical spine. His occupation is manager of several multiunit apartment buildings. He reports an inability to complete both the more physically demanding aspects of his job as well as the desk and computer-based responsibilities.

Upon clinical examination, cervical active ROM is observed to be severely pain-limited in all planes, particularly with extension, left rotation, and left lateral flexion. His upper extremity reflexes are 2+, except for the left biceps, which are at 1+. Muscle testing across the upper extremities yields grades of 5/5 on the right. Left upper extremity muscle tests are all pain-limited to 4+/5, except for the left biceps 4/5. Grip strength on his dominant right side is 105 pounds and the left is 27 pounds. Light touch sensory ability is diminished at the pad of the left second digit. Spurling's maneuver on the right is negative but on the left elicits an increase of distal paresthesia. Manually applied traction reduces the left periscapular and proximal arm pain. Left upper limb tension testing is highly provocative of symptoms in the arm and forearm with full positioning limited to 30° of full extension during the test.

CLINICAL DECISION-MAKING

1. Does the patient have a problem that can be improved with the use of traction?
   Answer: Although specific indications for traction remain unclear, the examination findings are noteworthy. Given that manual traction reduced his symptoms, adding it to his treatment regimen may be warranted, particularly since no other position or measure has offered pain relief over the past week.

2. Is the patient appropriate for application of traction? Do any of the general precautions or contraindications to traction apply, or are there any specific considerations regarding application of traction to this patient?
   Answer: The patient denies any medical history that would contraindicate the use of traction. The examination findings and his history since the onset suggest his condition to be highly acute and irritable. The presence of multiple indications of peripheral neurological deficit requires close observation and careful decision-making.

3. What are the specific goals to be achieved with the use of traction?
   Answer: The immediate goal for this patient would be to reduce the pain, which is theorized to be of nerve root origin. Pain relief would allow the patient to resume restorative sleep and perhaps return to a portion of his job duties. A reduction of pain will also enhance his ability to complete the therapeutic exercise and other active interventions planned for home and in subsequent clinical visits.

4. What specific type of traction is appropriate for the patient?
   Answer: The evidence is limited, but intermittent traction at the angle of cervical flexion offering the lowest level of peripheral symptoms is a reasonable starting point from which to begin a trial of traction. This may be adjusted during the course of traction and after the first treatment, based on his response.

5. What specific parameters of traction would be appropriate for the patient?
   Answer: The apparent level of acuity and irritability of his condition demands caution with the initial trial of mechanical traction. Traction dosage on the first day should be modest. As such, a reasonable trial with intermittent traction may be cycling between 12 and 6 pounds for 30 and 10 seconds, respectively. The initial total treatment time may be as little as 10 minutes. These variables, however, are subject to adjustment during the course of the traction session. Given his level of pain and inability to participate in daily demands, a follow-up visit the next day may be warranted.

6. What are the effective and safe application procedures for traction related to this patient?
   Answer: A dramatic improvement with one session of traction is unrealistic. Perhaps the first objective is to establish his tolerance to the chosen intervention. It is imperative to assess the patient's status during and immediately following the first session of traction. An increase of symptoms peripherally is to be specifically avoided. If this occurs during the traction, the treatment should stop immediately. His response for the next several hours following traction will be, in part, basis for determining the direction of his care at his next visit. A cumulative effect of pain reduction with subsequent applications is expected. Failure for this to occur indicates the need for medical consultation and diagnostic imaging, particularly if the neurological deficits persist.

CASE STUDY 7•2 LUMBAR TRACTION

A 46-year-old male arrives at physical therapy with primary complaints of right low back, buttock, thigh, and calf pain of 2 weeks' duration. He describes the onset of these symptoms subsequent to lifting a spool of wire into a truck at his construction job. He reports difficulty with maintaining any position for greater than 30 minutes duration, particularly sitting. He specifically denies any change in bowel or bladder function since the onset of these symptoms.

Upon examination, pain grossly limits his lumbar ranges of motion in all planes with provocation of distal symptoms at the end of the available range in each direction. Side-gliding of his lumbar spine is severely limited with distal symptoms in the left and a firm barrier to the right. He is intolerant of testing the S1 motor distribution in standing on the right because of pain. In supine, muscle testing across the lower extremities is particularly remarkable for ankle eversion on the right at 4/5 with no other deficits observed. Muscle stretch reflexes are 2+, except the right ankle 1+. Straight leg raising on the right causes distal symptoms at 30° and is negative on the left. Decreased light touch sensation is noted for the great toe of his right foot. Attempts at repeated movement testing of the lumbar spine and eliminating the block to right side-gliding result only in an increase of the lower extremity symptoms. Upon the application of manual lumbar traction, he reports a modest reduction of his back and lower extremity symptoms.

CLINICAL DECISION-MAKING

1. Does the patient have a problem that can be improved with the use of traction?

   Answer: At the time of this examination, manually applied traction is the only procedure that reduces the patient's symptoms, particularly those in his lower extremity. All of the other attempts to centralize or reduce his pain worsen his symptoms. His outcome is difficult to project given the acuity and apparent irritability of his condition accompanying neurological deficits that suggest radiculopathy. Based on the examination findings, however, a trial of traction to assess his response is the best option to start his process of recovery.

2. Is the patient appropriate for traction? Do any of the general precautions or contraindications to traction apply, or are there any specific considerations regarding application of traction to this patient?

   Answer: Upon review of his history and overall health status, there are no indications that traction is inappropriate to use in his treatment. Given the severity of his condition and apparent nerve root involvement,

caution will be required. The specific traction dosage on the first attempt will be modest to assess his tolerance, and he will require close supervision during traction. Additionally, he will require close observation in the period immediately following traction and before he leaves the clinic to assess his response for future treatments.

3. What are the specific goals to be achieved with the use of traction?

   Answer: With conditions suggesting radicular pain, a reduction of peripheral symptoms is usually an early objective. If these symptoms can be decreased, he will become a candidate for other interventions not currently tolerated, which may accelerate his progress. These would include manual therapy, self-mobilization exercise, and higher demand exercise consistent with his functional demands at work.

4. What specific type of traction is appropriate for the patient?

   Answer: With his most comfortable position being supine with his hips and knees flexed, the initial trial would logically incorporate that positioning. He gained relief with the manually applied traction as his hips were flexed approximately 45° and his knees flexed approximately 90°. Thus, replicating that position for the first attempt would be logical and could be accomplished with a bolster under his knees. There is no evidence to support either static or intermittent traction being superior overall or with subgroups of particular clinical presentations. With any sustained mechanical stresses apparently being poorly tolerated, the preferred initial arrangement is intermittent traction.

5. What specific parameters of traction would be appropriate for the patient?

   Answer: Given the acuity and apparent irritability of his condition, the initial trial of traction will require caution. The initial treatment, to assess his response and attempt to establish a tolerance level, will be at 25% of his body weight and for a shorter than usual period of 10 minutes. With his body weight at 200 pounds, the traction unit will be set at 50 pounds at the maximum tension and 25 pounds for the minimum tension. The time settings will be programmed for 10 total minutes with 30 seconds at maximum tension and 10 seconds at the minimum tension. Because of his condition's acuity and apparent irritability, two progressive and two regressive steps are also being programmed into the traction control unit.

CASE STUDY 7-2 cont. from p. 190

6. What are the effective and safe application procedures for traction related to this case example?

Answer: Using traction with this patient is only the first step into what will evolve into a multimodal treatment approach. Provided he responds favorably to the traction on the first visit, the traction parameters will be progressed at the time of his second visit and perhaps subsequent visits to greater amounts of tension and longer duration. If symptoms are reduced, his response to repeated movements will be reassessed with the objective of advancing his self-treatment regimen to include self-mobilization procedures, most likely in a lumbar extension orientation. Exercises to activate the musculature supporting the lumbopelvic complex will also be incorporated early in his rehabilitation and progressed according to his tolerance and the quality of his recruitment patterns. He may also become a candidate to receive manual therapy at some point in his treatment. As his distal symptoms diminish, traction would likely be discontinued. The overarching concept is that traction in this patient's care is an early treatment to reduce pain and facilitate an increased tolerance to other interventions.

must be given to hormonal influences potentially affecting tissue laxity.

If the patient reports pain in the spine that cannot be determined in the initial examination to be of mechanical origin, the practitioner should suspect potentially serious pathology. The inability to find movements or positions that relieve pain may be indicative of a serious health condition beyond the scope of physical therapy. As such, further medical consultation or additional diagnostic testing may be warranted rather that using traction as a treatment. Similarly, patients who report histories of cancer should have a thorough diagnostic evaluation, including imaging, before receiving traction (Box 7-4).

Precautions

Individuals with claustrophobia may not be well suited to receive mechanical traction, particularly for the lumbar spine. The sensation of being enclosed in the harnesses and confined on the table may precipitate anxiety that will not allow the patient to participate in traction. Similarly, if the traction table is located in a small room in the clinic, the effect may be magnified. For this reason, many practitioners prefer to place their traction tables in a curtained area within an open part of the clinic. With some patients, the curtain partition, perhaps even partly opened, allows enough relaxation for the treatment to be well tolerated.

Patients with chronic obstructive pulmonary disease (COPD) or other respiratory disorders may also find the harnesses uncomfortable and may be compromised by the supine position. Being able to secure the harnesses adequately while permitting the patient to relax and breathe comfortably may be difficult. In some patients, traction may not be appropriate due to their distress.

Home Traction

An outgrowth of the benefit and sometimes transient symptom relief of clinical traction is the availability of a variety of home traction units. These units are often available over the counter or from some retail outlets. Other more sophisticated traction devices are available only through health-care providers or upon prescription from a physician.

Cervical Spine

Recently, portable equipment closely replicating clinical models have become available (Fig. 7-34). These

---

Box 7•4	**Contraindications for Mechanical Traction**

- Acute cervical trauma, including whiplash-associated disorders
- Osteoporosis or osteopenia
- Use of steroids or other medications that tend to weaken bone
- Rheumatologic disorders affecting connective tissue, including rheumatoid arthritis and ankylosing spondylitis
- Joint hypermobility/instability
- Pregnancy (lumbar traction)
- Prior surgical stabilization or decompression
- Spinal implants/prosthetic discs
- Nonmechanical pain

devices usually have an occipital harness capable of gliding on a small, stable frame. The traction is provided by a manually operated pneumatic pump that includes a gauge for quantifying tension. The patient lies supine and is positioned in the harness similar to the larger clinical models. Some home models have adjustable harnesses, where the patient can turn a knob to adjust the pads. Other models have self-adjusting pads that seat against the occiput once traction is initiated. The patient achieves the traction effect by activating the manual pump, causing the harness to glide along the frame away from the base. An intermittent mechanical traction effect can be achieved by cycling the pressure up to a designated amount (usually replicating the amount found beneficial during clinical treatment), sustaining that pressure for a time interval (e.g., 1 minute), then releasing the pressure by a valve on the pump. Multiple cycles of this sequence can be completed. Manipulating the variables for home traction on one of these models can closely simulate that achieved on clinical traction tables.

Perhaps the simplest and least expensive apparatus, improvised many decades ago, is still available for cervical spine traction. A water-weighted bag attached to a cord that courses over a pulley that provides tension to a harness worn on the head can provide a modest traction effect for the cervical spine. These devices, used while sitting, must first overcome the weight of the head to apply traction to the neck. Additionally, there is the risk that pressure through the mandible can cause or exacerbate temporomandibular joint dysfunction. Use of one of these models to achieve intermittent traction is not easily accomplished, and static traction may be more practically completed, particularly if the patient is unassisted during the home traction session.

Lumbar Spine

Home lumbar traction units were largely impractical and of questionable effectiveness until recently, when the design features successful in home cervical spine traction units were incorporated into lumbar spine units. A similar pneumatic pumping device is used to separate two surfaces on which the patient can lie, secured by harnesses (Fig. 7-35). The traction tension is often considerably less than that produced by clinical models, but it may be sufficient to have a modest effect or complement clinical traction. These units are usually compact and are self-contained in a carrying case. Patients with high levels of pain may have difficulty administering home lumbar traction without assistance. Positioning on the floor is required; thus, the associated mobility demands and the need to self-tighten the harnesses may prove difficult for someone with significant pain-limiting impairments. Lifting and carrying the home lumbar traction unit may offer a similar challenge.

Most of the pneumatic traction units, whether for the cervical or lumbar spine, have safety valves to prevent potentially injurious tension levels.

The usual intent of providing patients with home traction units is to enhance the effect achieved clinically and empower the patient toward recovery. Once a beneficial dosage is identified in the clinical setting, tension amounts and durations for home treatment usually approximate those used on the automated equipment. Alternately, individuals may attempt self-treatment at their own discretion or possibly by their physician's choice without clinical supervision.

The practitioner should guide the patient carefully through the process of home traction, completing the

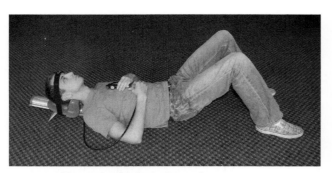

Fig 7•34 Home cervical traction unit.

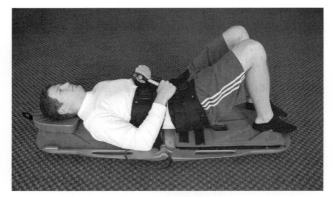

Fig 7•35 Home lumbar traction unit.

steps with the home unit while still under clinical supervision. Patient education to avoid causing injury with a home unit is important. Instructions detailing traction dosage and frequency should be provided to the patient. In addition, instruct patients to take particular safety measures, such as using a timer with an alarm to avoid falling asleep in the traction unit. Prolonged single-session use from patients falling asleep during home traction has been known to significantly exacerbate pain. To minimize the risk of pain worsening from home traction unit use, practitioners must require patients to verbalize their understanding and demonstrate appropriate use of home traction before they initiate self-treatment. Similarly, specific questioning of the response to home traction and any necessary problem-solving are essential in subsequent visits.

Home units are usually purchased, although some medical equipment providers will allow rental. The simple water bag home cervical traction units are available for as little as $20. Currently, the more sophisticated pneumatic versions emulating clinical models are approximately $400 to $500. The pneumatic lumbar home traction models are approximately $450 to $600. Because of this, home traction should not be recommended for patients unless clear benefit is demonstrated from clinical use and several sessions are anticipated for maximum benefit.

Patient Outcome Evidence

Despite traction having been a widely used intervention for neck and back pain for decades, strong evidentiary support for its use is lacking. The many studies evaluating traction are methodologically deficient and may not offer meaningful results. Additionally, many of the studies possessing the best research design do not correlate well to routine clinical practice. Thus, the ability to generalize the results in patient care scenarios may be limited.

Multiple studies have used simulated traction or traction at presumably ineffective levels of tension for comparisons against traction at greater and potentially therapeutic levels of tension.[24,43–47] While such methods allow allocation concealment to a greater degree, the actual differences in interventions between the groups may be minimized.

Other studies use traction as the sole intervention,[25,43] which does not replicate the generally accepted standard of care. In routine clinical practice, patients receiving traction will frequently have complementary interventions, such as manual therapy, exercises for key muscle recruitment and strengthening, and neural mobilization.[23,27,48–50] However, using multiple interventions makes it different to separate the effects of each intervention, including traction. To get strong evidence in a study, the preferred study design is to isolate the independent variable of interest. The interaction between interventions or synergistic effects of various treatments, however, may not be appreciated in the results of such study designs.

Perhaps the most frequent methodological issue is the heterogeneity of groups receiving traction. Practitioners have long sought to delineate particular patient characteristics that would predict those responding best to traction. Despite robust design, many studies have combined patients with various clinical presentations in the groups being compared.[24,43–46,51–53] Thus, potential benefit in subsets of patients with neck or back pain syndromes receiving traction may not be recognized. The effort to identify patients most likely to benefit from traction has been a clear direction in recent research.

Auto-traction is a form of patient-powered traction similar to passive traction that has been used as the variable of interest in several studies.[44,53] Given the well-documented activation of spinal-supporting musculature with simple limb movements and more complex motor patterns,[54–62] self-traction may be completely ineffective in achieving distraction of spinal structures. In a previously mentioned study,[16] activation of the patient's musculature when performing self-traction easily precluded any distractive effects on the spine. Further, intradiscal pressures have been observed to increase during self-traction attempts.[16,17] Thus, considering auto-traction to be equivalent to passive traction within this review of evidence is probably inappropriate.

A small number of clinical trials, representative of clinical practice, yield conflicting results.[46,63] Case series have been published suggesting value in traction, particularly in patients presenting with signs and symptoms consistent with radiculopathies.[23,48,49] However, the absence of control, or comparison, groups limits the ability to assess the effect of traction as the key variable. The outcomes of patients receiving traction cannot be easily differentiated from those patients receiving alternative interventions or from the natural history of the disorders.

Recently published systematic reviews and suggested practice guidelines[64–66] have concluded there is minimal evidence for the use of traction in the treatment of neck and back pain. These conclusions, however, must be considered within the context of the inadequacy of the research and are generalized for populations, not particular individuals who may respond favorably to the use of traction.

KEY POINT! Sound clinical reasoning and problem-solving, based on individual patient factors, remain incumbent on the practitioner in the application and assessment of mechanical traction in a multimodal approach for the treatment of spinal pain syndromes.

The cumulative evidence for benefit from cervical spine traction in mechanical neck pain syndromes is moderately greater than that for the lumbar spine. While evidence-based practice and clinical guidelines can guide practitioners in the clinical reasoning process of patient care, this does not minimize the importance of personal experience and clinical judgment.

Documentation Tips

For documentation of traction treatment, describing the variables as listed in Box 7-2 and Box 7-3 is appropriate. Additionally, describing the patient's responses to traction during the treatment session and immediately afterward while still under observation is recommended.

Clinical Controversies

Spinal Decompression

Spinal decompression has been marketed intensely in recent years as a new method of addressing back and neck pain while yielding remarkable results. Popular media advertising through radio, newspaper, and Internet sites have often been used to promote decompression as a "novel approach" in the treatment of spinal disorders. Spinal decompression is performed on equipment that imparts cyclical longitudinal force on the spine, while the patient lies supine on a tablelike device with a motorized unit (Fig. 7-36). According to the U.S. Food and Drug Administration (FDA), spinal decompression is described differently than traction largely because of a technicality. In the application process for equipment approval, manufacturers must label the equipment according to its presumed effects. Spinal decompression is labeled separately from traction on 510(k) applications to the FDA for marketing medical devices. Also, decompression has been granted a Current Procedural Terminology (CPT) code apart from traction. These technical differences allow marketers to distinguish decompression from traction in media campaigns.

Advocates of decompression claim physiological and biomechanical effects greater than traction, particularly on the intervertebral disc. Decreased or negative levels of intradiscal pressure have been measured in vivo during decompression.[67] Three case series suggested noteworthy improvement levels in patients receiving decompression and are frequently the sources of statistics used in marketing campaigns.[68–70] A systematic review of the clinical trials using decompression reveals that six of the seven studies report no difference in outcomes with spinal decompression; one investigation reported less pain but no change in disability of the subjects.[71] Additionally, a preponderance of the studies

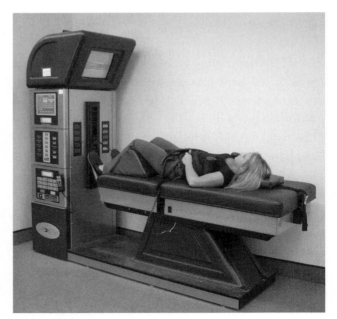

Fig 7•36 Lumbar spinal decompression unit.

evaluating spinal decompression has been of relatively poor quality.

Manufacturers and some professional groups openly promote decompression services as a means of increasing practice revenue. Assistant staff members, typically without substantive training in treating spinal disorders, are often used to administer the decompression to patients over a course of approximately 20 visits without requiring the time and effort of the supervising practitioner. As discussed among some practitioners, decompression's primary benefit to the practitioner is the increase in cash-paying patients. Strategies emphasizing the aesthetic qualities of decompression devices are often used in marketing to the public without regard to evidence of efficacy.[72] The lack of evidence in the current literature has led to the conclusion that spinal decompression has not been validated to be a superior intervention to traction.[66,73]

Inversion

One method of providing a distractive effect on the low back that does not require a clinical setting is the use of inversion devices, which allow gravity-facilitated traction. Home inversion equipment is available without prescription or assignment by practitioners. With many of these devices, the individual sits in a frame and then secures the lower extremities and pelvis with straps. The device can be unlocked and the person can invert body position such that the upper trunk weight is distracted from the secured pelvis and lower extremities. Inversion is remarkably simple and documented to increase lumbar intervertebral space immediately following the procedure.[74]

However, the inverted position can have other unintended effects. Major increases in intraocular pressure leading to optic nerve dysfunction have been observed.[75,76] In addition, significant alterations in blood pressure of the individual in the device has been observed.[77–79] Anxiety while inverted has also been reported to be common.[80] Inversion would not be an ideal choice for persons with histories of dizziness or vertigo. The physical demands to safely invert one's own body and then carefully return to an upright position are also a necessity for this process and may not be easily accomplished by some persons, particularly those in significant pain. Thus, safety and adverse effects are an issue, particularly when these devices are used without assistance.

■ REFERENCES

1. Cyriax J. The treatment of lumbar disk lesions. *Br Med J.* 1950;2:1438–1438.
2. Maitland G, Hengeveld E, Banks K, English K. *Maitland's Vertebral Manipulation.* 7th ed. Oxford, England: Butterworth-Heinemann; 2005.
3. Maitland G. *Vertebral Manipulation.* London: Butterworth & Company; 1964.
4. Humphreys SC, Chase J, Patwardhan A, Shuster J, Lomasney L, Hodges SD. Flexion and traction effect on C5-C6 foraminal space. *Arch Phys Med Rehabil.* 1998;79(9):1105–1109.
5. Vaughn HT, Having KM, Rogers JL. Radiographic analysis of intervertebral separation with a 0 degree and 30 degree rope angle using the Saunders cervical traction device. *Spine.* 2006;31(2):E39–E43.
6. Farmer JC, Wisneski RJ. Cervical spine nerve root compression. An analysis of neuroforaminal pressures with varying head and arm positions. *Spine.* 1994;19(16):1850–1855.
7. Yoo J, Zou D, Edwards T, Bayley J, Yuan H. Effect of cervical spine motion on the neuroforaminal dimensions of human cervical spine. *Spine.* 1992;17(10):1131–1136.
8. Sari H, Akarirmak Ā, Karacan I, Akman H. Evaluation of effects of cervical traction on spinal structures by computerized tomography. *Adv Physiother.* 2003;5(3):114–121.
9. Delacerda FG. Effect of angle of traction pull on upper trapezius muscle activity. *J Orthop Sports Phys Ther.* 1980;1(4):205–209.
10. Murphy MJ. Effects of cervical traction on muscle activity. *J Orthop Sports Phys Ther.* 1991;13(5):220–225.
11. Lee MY, Wong MK, Tang FT, Chang WH, Chiou WK. Design and assessment of an adaptive intermittent cervical traction modality with EMG biofeedback. *J Biomech Eng.* 1996;118(4):597–600.
12. Nanno M. [Effects of intermittent cervical traction on muscle pain. Flowmetric and electromyographic studies of the cervical paraspinal muscles]. *Nippon Ika Daigaku Zasshi.* 1994;61(2):137–147.
13. Jette DU, Falkel JE, Trombly C. Effect of intermittent, supine cervical traction on the myoelectric activity of the upper trapezius muscle in subjects with neck pain. *Phys Ther.* 1985;65(8):1173–1176.
14. Tesio L, Franchignoni FP. Autotraction treatment for low-back pain syndromes. *Crit Rev Phys Rehabil Med.* 1995;7(1):1–9.
15. Hood CJ, Hart DL, Smith HG, Davis HC. Comparison of electromyographic activity in normal lumbar sacrospinalis musculature during continuous and intermittent pelvic traction. *J Orthop Sports Phys Ther.* 1981;2(3):137–141.
16. Andersson GB, Schultz AB, Nachemson AL. Intervertebral disc pressures during traction. *Scand J Rehabil Med Suppl.* 1983;9:88–91.
17. Schultz A, Andersson G, Ortengren R, Haderspeck K, Nachemson A. Loads on the lumbar spine. Validation of a biomechanical analysis by measurements of intradiscal pressures and myoelectric signals. *J Bone Joint Surg Am.* 1982;64(5):713–720.
18. Onel D, Tuzlaci M, Sari H, Demir K. Computed tomographic investigation of the effect of traction on lumbar disc herniations. *Spine.* 1989;14(1):82–90.

19. Ozturk B, Gunduz OH, Ozoran K, Bostanoglu S. Effect of continuous lumbar traction on the size of herniated disc material in lumbar disc herniation. *Rheumatol Int.* 2006;26(7):622–626.

20. Twomey LT. Sustained lumbar traction. An experimental study of long spine segments. *Spine.* 1985;10(2):146–149.

21. Colachis SC, Jr., Strohm BR. Effects of intermittent traction on separation of lumbar vertebrae. *Arch Phys Med Rehabil.* 1969;50(5):251–258.

22. Meszaros TF, Olson R, Kulig K, Creighton D, Czarnecki E. Effect of 10%, 30%, and 60% body weight traction on the straight leg raise test of symptomatic patients with low back pain. *J Orthop Sports Phys Ther.* 2000;30(10):595–601.

23. Cleland JA, Whitman JM, Fritz JM, Palmer JA. Manual physical therapy, cervical traction, and strengthening exercises in patients with cervical radiculopathy: a case series. *J Orthop Sports Phys Ther.* 2005;35(12):802–811.

24. Klaber-Moffett J, Hughes G, Griffiths P. An investigation of the effects of cervical traction. part 1: clinical effectiveness. *Clin Rehabil.* 1991;4:205–211.

25. Zylbergold RS, Piper MC. Cervical spine disorders. A comparison of three types of traction. *Spine.* 1985;10(10):867–871.

26. Caldwell JW, Krusen EM. Effectiveness of cervical traction in treatment of neck problems: evaluation of various methods. *Arch Phys Med Rehabil.* 1962;43:214–221.

27. Childs JD, Cleland JA, Elliott JM, et al. Neck pain: Clinical practice guidelines linked to the International Classification of Functioning, Disability, and Health from the Orthopedic Section of the American Physical Therapy Association. *J Orthop Sports Phys Ther.* 2008;38(9):A1–A34.

28. Delitto A, Erhard RE, Bowling RW. A treatment-based classification approach to low back syndrome: identifying and staging patients for conservative treatment. *Phys Ther.* 1995;75(6):470–485; discussion 85–89.

29. Fritz JM, Brennan GP, Clifford SN, Hunter SJ, Thackeray A. An examination of the reliability of a classification algorithm for subgrouping patients with low back pain. *Spine.* 2006;31(1):77–82.

30. Pinto D, Cleland J, Palmer J, Eberhart SL. Management of low back pain: a case series illustrating the pragmatic combination of treatment- and mechanism-based classification systems. *J Man Manip Ther.* 2007;15(2):111–122.

31. Fritz JM, Lindsay W, Matheson JW, et al. Is there a subgroup of patients with low back pain likely to benefit from mechanical traction? Results of a randomized clinical trial and subgrouping analysis. *Spine.* 2007;32(26):E793–E800.

32. Raney NH, Petersen EJ, Smith TA, et al. Development of a clinical prediction rule to identify patients with neck pain likely to benefit from cervical traction and exercise. *Eur Spine J.* 2009;18(3):382–391.

33. Gross AR, Goldsmith C, Hoving JL, et al. Conservative management of mechanical neck disorders: a systematic review. *J Rheumatol.* 2007;34(5):1083–1102.

34. Gross AR, Hoving JL, Haines TA, et al. A Cochrane review of manipulation and mobilization for mechanical neck disorders. *Spine.* 2004;29(14):1541–1548.

35. Martel W, Page JW. Cervical vertebral erosions and subluxations in rheumatoid arthritis and ankylosing spondylitis. *Arthritis Rheum.* 1960;3:546–556.

36. Sharp J, Purser DW. Spontaneous atlanto-axial dislocation in ankylosing spondylitis and rheumatoid arthritis. *Ann Rheum Dis.* 1961;20(1):47–77.

37. Zikou AK, Alamanos Y, Argyropoulou MI, et al. Radiological cervical spine involvement in patients with rheumatoid arthritis: a cross sectional study. *J Rheumatol.* 2005;32(5):801–806.

38. Roche CJ, Eyes BE, Whitehouse GH. The rheumatoid cervical spine: signs of instability on plain cervical radiographs. *Clin Radiol.* 2002;57(4):241–249.

39. Neva MH, Hakkinen A, Makinen H, Hannonen P, Kauppi M, Sokka T. High prevalence of asymptomatic cervical spine subluxation in patients with rheumatoid arthritis waiting for orthopaedic surgery. *Ann Rheum Dis.* 2006;65(7):884–888.

40. Lee JY, Kim JI, Park JY, et al. Cervical spine involvement in longstanding ankylosing spondylitis. *Clin Exp Rheumatol.* 2005;23(3):331–338.

41. Lee HS, Kim TH, Yun HR, et al. Radiologic changes of cervical spine in ankylosing spondylitis. *Clin Rheumatol.* 2001;20(4):262–266.

42. Ramos-Remus C, Gomez-Vargas A, Guzman-Guzman JL, et al. Frequency of atlantoaxial subluxation and neurologic involvement in patients with ankylosing spondylitis. *J Rheumatol.* 1995;22(11):2120–2125.

43. Beurskens AJ, de Vet HC, Koke AJ, et al. Efficacy of traction for nonspecific low back pain: 12-week and 6-month results of a randomized clinical trial. *Spine.* 1997;22(23):2756–2762.

44. Walker L, Svenkerud T, Weber H. Traksjonbehandling ved lumbago–ischias: en kontrollsert undersolske med Spina–trac. *Fysioterapeuten.* 1982;49:161–163, 177.

45. van der Heijden GJ, Beurskens AJ, Koes BW, Assendelft WJ, de Vet HC, Bouter LM. The efficacy of traction for back and neck pain: a systematic, blinded review of randomized clinical trial methods. *Phys Ther.* 1995;75(2):93–104.

46. Shakoor MA, Ahmed MS, Kibria G, et al. Effects of cervical traction and exercise therapy in cervical spondylosis. *Bangladesh Med Res Counc Bull.* 2002;28(2):61–69.

47. Brewerton D, Nichols P, Logue V, et al. Pain in the neck and arm: a multi-centre trial of the effects of physiotherapy. *Br Med J.* 1966;1(5482):253–258.

48. Browder DA, Erhard RE, Piva SR. Intermittent cervical traction and thoracic manipulation for management of mild cervical compressive myelopathy attributed to cervical herniated disc: a case series. *J Orthop Sports Phys Ther.* 2004;34(11):701–712.

49. Waldrop MA. Diagnosis and treatment of cervical radiculopathy using a clinical prediction rule and a multimodal intervention approach: a case series. *J Orthop Sports Phys Ther.* 2006;36(3):152–159.

50. Cleland JA, Fritz JM, Whitman JM, Heath R. Predictors of short-term outcome in people with a clinical diagnosis of cervical radiculopathy. *Phys Ther.* 2007;87(12):1619–1632.

51. Kogstad OA, Karterud S, Gudmundsen J. Cervicobrachialgia. A controlled trial with conventional therapy and manipulation. *Tidsskr Nor Laegeforen.* 1978;98(16):845–848.

52. Werners R, Pynsent PB, Bulstrode CJK. Randomized trial comparing interferential therapy with motorized lumbar traction and massage in the management of low back pain in a primary care setting. *Spine.* 1999;24(15):1579.

53. Bihaug O. Autotraksjon for ischialgpasienter: en kontollert sammenlikning mellom effekten av Auto–traksjon–B og isometriske ovelser ad modum Hume endall og enkins. *Fysioterapeuten.* 1978;45:377–379.

54. Hodges PW, Richardson CA. Relationship between limb movement speed and associated contraction of the trunk muscles. *Ergonomics.* 1997;40(11):1220–1230.

55. Hodges PW, Richardson CA. Feedforward contraction of transversus abdominis is not influenced by the direction of arm movement. *Exp Brain Res.* 1997;114(2):362–370.

56. Hodges PW, Gandevia SC. Changes in intra-abdominal pressure during postural and respiratory activation of the human diaphragm. *J Appl Physiol.* 2000;89(3):967–976.

57. Falla D, O'Leary S, Fagan A, Jull G. Recruitment of the deep cervical flexor muscles during a postural-correction exercise performed in sitting. *Man Ther.* 2007;12(2):139–143.

58. Hides JA, Stanton WR, McMahon S, Sims K, Richardson CA. Effect of stabilization training on multifidus muscle cross-sectional area among young elite cricketers with low back pain. *J Orthop Sports Phys Ther.* 2008;38(3):101–108.

59. Hides JA, Richardson CA, Jull GA. Multifidus muscle recovery is not automatic after resolution of acute, first-episode low back pain. *Spine.* 1996;21(23):2763–2769.

60. Van K, Hides JA, Richardson CA. The use of real-time ultrasound imaging for biofeedback of lumbar multifidus muscle contraction in healthy subjects. *J Orthop Sports Phys Ther.* 2006;36(12):920–925.

61. Dankaerts W, O'Sullivan P, Burnett A, Straker L. Altered patterns of superficial trunk muscle activation during sitting in nonspecific chronic low back pain patients: importance of subclassification. *Spine.* 2006;31(17):2017–2023.

62. Richardson CA, Snijders CJ, Hides JA, Damen L, Pas MS, Storm J. The relation between the transversus abdominis muscles, sacroiliac joint mechanics, and low back pain. *Spine.* 2002;27(4):399–405.

63. Young IA, Michener LA, Cleland JA, Aguilera AJ, Snyder AR. Manual therapy, exercise, and traction for patients with cervical radiculopathy: a randomized clinical trial. *Phys Ther.* 2009;89(7):632–642.

64. Graham N, Gross A, Goldsmith CH, et al. Mechanical traction for neck pain with or without radiculopathy. *Cochrane Database Syst Rev.* 2008;(3).

65. Chou R, Qaseem A, Snow V, et al. Diagnosis and treatment of low back pain: a joint clinical practice guideline from the American College of Physicians and the American Pain Society. *Ann Intern Med.* 2007;147(7):478–491.

66. Gay RE, Brault JS. Evidence-informed management of chronic low back pain with traction therapy. *Spine J.* 2008;8(1):234–242.

67. Ramos G, Marin W. Effects of vertebral axial decompression (VAX-D) on intradiscal pressure. *J Neurosurg.* 1994;81:350–353.

68. Gionis T, Groteke E. Spinal decompression. *Orthopedic Technol Rev.* 2005;5:36–39.

69. Gose E, Naguszewski W, Naguszewski R. Vertebral axial decompression therapy for pain associated with herniated or degenerated discs or facet syndrome: an outcome study. *Neurol Res.* 1998;20:186–190.

70. Naguszewski W, Naguszewski R, Gose E. Dermatomal somatosensory evoked potential demonstration of nerve root decompression after VAX-D therapy. *Neurol Res.* 2001;23:706–714.

71. Macario A, Pergolizzi JV. Systematic literature review of spinal decompression via motorized traction for chronic discogenic low back pain. *Pain Pract.* 2006;6(3):171–178.

72. Kaplan E. Decompression is more than traction. *The American Chiropractor.* 2008;March:24–28.

73. Tyburski M, Akuthota V. Motorized lumbar traction devices: what's the evidence? *Spine Line.* 2006;November/December:36–39.

74. Kane MD, Karl RD, Swain JH. Effects of gravity-facilitated traction on intervertebral dimensions of the lumbar spine. *J Orthop Sports Phys Ther.* 1985;6(5):281–288.

75. Sanborn GE, Friberg TR, Allen R. Optic nerve dysfunction during gravity inversion: visual field abnormalities. *Arch Ophthalmol.* 1987;105(6):774–776.

76. Friberg TR, Sanborn G. Optic nerve dysfunction during gravity inversion pattern reversal visual evoked potentials. *Arch Ophthalmol.* 1985;103(11):1687–1689.

77. Ballantyne BT, Reser MD, Lorenz GW, Smidt GL. The effects of inversion traction on spinal column configuration, heart rate, blood pressure, and perceived discomfort. *J Orthop Sports Phys Ther.* 1986;7(5):254–260.

78. Haskvitz EM, Hanten WP. Blood pressure response to inversion traction. *Phys Ther.* 1986;66(9):1361–1364.

79. Souza SA. Cardioperipheral vascular effects of inversion on humans. *Phys Ther.* 1987;67(5):680–687.

80. Guvenol K, Tuzun C, Peker O, Goktay Y. A comparison of inverted spinal traction and conventional traction in the treatment of lumbar disc herniations. *Physiother Theory Pract.* 2000;16(3):151–160.

chapter 8

Intermittent Pneumatic Compression

Ellen Lowe, PT, MHS | James W. Bellew, PT, EdD

Physical Principles

Compression is the application of external mechanical pressure to the body for therapeutic purpose. It has been used in rehabilitation for years and for a variety of reasons. The *Guide to Physical Therapist Practice*[1] cites intermittent pneumatic compression (IPC) as an appropriate intervention for a variety of practice patterns.

Intermittent pneumatic compression is most commonly used to control or minimize edema, but it also has a variety of other applications. These include reducing lymphedema, improving venous circulation, healing stasis ulcers, reducing orthostatic hypotension, healing wounds, and preventing thrombophlebitis. It can also help reduce contractures and control hypertrophic scarring. Studies have shown that intermittent pneumatic compression can produce hemodynamic alterations in venous flow and systemic circulation.[2-15] Changes in central venous pressure, pulmonary pressure, and pulse pressure have been noted as a result of the application of intermittent pneumatic compression. Tissue compression can increase the pressure of the fluid in the interstitial spaces to a higher pressure than that in the blood or lymph vessels. This change in pressure gradient allows the fluid to flow out of the interstitial tissues and back into the venous and lymphatic vessels for drainage.

Indications for Intermittent Pneumatic Compression

Edema

Edema is a local or generalized condition in which the body tissues contain an excessive amount of fluid. It may result from increased permeability of the capillary walls, increased capillary pressure due to venous obstruction or heart failure, lymphatic obstruction, disturbances in renal functioning, reduction of plasma proteins, inflammatory conditions, fluid and electrolyte disturbances, or any condition that causes increased pressure in the blood or lymph vessels or decreased pressure in the interstitial tissues.

Edema occurs when the venous or lymphatic vessels are impaired. Patients undergoing rehabilitation frequently experience this complication. It can produce a variety of problematic effects on patient recovery, such as occupying joint space and decreasing range of motion (ROM). Edema located near a nerve can produce pain. Edema also decreases the effectiveness of the lymphatic drainage system, making a patient more prone to infection. If edema cuts off the blood flow to tissues, as in the case of compartment syndrome, it can lead to necrosis. Therefore, it is important to treat edema as aggressively as possible to minimize its deleterious effects. Intermittent pneumatic compression is one modality frequently employed to do this.[14–16]

KEY POINT! *Inflammation* is the body's initial response to injury or harmful stimuli. It is mediated by histamine release with an increase in capillary permeability and movement of plasma and leukocytes from the blood volume into the interstitial space. Increased inflammatory fluid in the interstitial space causes *swelling*, which when accumulated is termed *edema*. Edema is clinically apparent when there is approximately a 30% increase above the normal fluid volume in the interstitial space. Thus, edema is an abnormal accumulation of fluid in the interstitial spaces. Edema is termed subacute when it persists beyond 2 weeks and chronic when it persists beyond 3 months after an injury.

Traumatic Edema

Trauma is a common cause of edema. When IPC is used to reduce traumatic edema,[17] it should be done only when the patient has passed the acute stage and is in the subacute or chronic stage of healing. Premature application of IPC can result in increased bleeding.

KEY POINT! IPC for edema secondary to trauma should not be applied during the acute stage of healing. IPC is indicated for the post-acute and chronic stages of healing.

Venous Stasis Ulcers

Venous stasis ulcers are areas of tissue breakdown and necrosis that can occur when venous circulation is impaired. Roughly 1% of the people in industrialized countries will suffer from a venous stasis ulcer at some time. Studies have shown that IPC can be beneficial in healing this condition.[18–21] IPC devices mechanically increase venous return and are shown to stimulate fibrinolysis and increase skin perfusion pressure, which may assist tissue oxygenation and promote healing.

Stump Reduction in Amputated Limbs

The distal portion of the stump of amputated limbs tends to swell following surgery, especially when in a gravity-dependent position. This edema can inhibit stump healing and delay fitting for a prosthesis. IPC helps to decrease edema and healing time.

Prevention of Deep Vein Thrombosis

Deep vein thrombosis (DVT) can be a serious complication of immobilization following surgery or prolonged illness. If circulation is poor, the blood may move slowly enough to allow coagulation and the formation of a thrombus. The use of IPC has been shown to reduce the incidence of DVT formation in postoperative and immobilized patients.[5,22–27] IPC assists blood flow into deeper vessels and the femoral veins. Venous distension decreases, and the chance of DVT formation is lowered. It should be noted that the use of IPC is a preventive measure. After the presence of DVT is suspected or confirmed, IPC is contraindicated.

Wound Healing

IPC may lead to a more favorable environment for wound healing by promoting small vessel circulation, reducing edema, and oxygenating ischemic tissue.[2,4,6–8,28–31]

Arterial Insufficiency

IPC can augment arterial flow and microcirculation by contributing to an arteriovenous (A-V) pressure gradient.[11]

Lymphedema

Lymphedema can occur when lymph flow is impeded or when lymphatic vessels are impaired. If lymphatic fluid exceeds transport capacity of the lymphatic system, lymph fluid accumulates in the interstitial tissues. This fluid causes tissue channels to increase in size and number, reduces oxygen to tissues, interferes with wound healing, and promotes infection. IPC has been shown to be effective in decreasing lymphedema and increasing fluid movement through the lymph system; however, protein absorption is not facilitated.[15,22,24,32,34-43]

The use of IPC for lymphedema, especially in patients who have undergone a mastectomy, does have its opponents.[4,33,44] Some feel that scar tissue and blockage present from surgery or radiation impede the flow of lymphatic fluid, and the increased volume of fluid driven back into the lymph system can encourage swelling at the site of the injured nodes and cause trauma to the already damaged tissues.

Contraindications

Acute Pulmonary Edema

Pulmonary edema refers to the buildup of fluid in the lungs caused by back pressure in the lung veins. It is a complication of several disorders of the heart, including heart attack and heart valve disease. It can also occur as a result of exposure to high altitude. As pressure in the pulmonary veins increases, fluid is forced out of the veins and into the air spaces of the lungs (called the *alveoli*). This affects the lungs' ability to exchange oxygen and carbon dioxide in the alveoli. Application of IPC can return interstitial edema back to the venous circulation—increasing the stress on the heart and lungs, which are already compromised.

Congestive Heart Failure

Congestive heart failure, or *heart failure,* refers to any condition in which the heart is unable to adequately pump blood throughout the body or to prevent blood from backing up into the lungs. These conditions cause shortness of breath (dyspnea), fatigue, weakness, and swelling (edema) of the legs and sometimes the abdomen. As with acute pulmonary edema, application of IPC can increase stress on the heart and lungs.

Recent or Acute Deep Vein Thrombosis

Deep vein thrombosis refers to the formation of a thrombus (blood clot) within a deep vein, commonly in the thigh or calf. The blood clot can either partially or completely block the flow of blood in the vein. Due to the increased venous flow and the intermittent forces applied by IPC, applying IPC to an area with DVT can cause the thrombus to dislodge from a vein wall, travel to the heart or lung, and block an artery.

Uncontrolled Hypertension

Compression may elevate blood pressure and increase vascular load to the heart.

KEY POINT! Pharmacologically controlled hypertension should be considered a precaution to IPC therapy. Monitoring blood pressure during and after compression therapy is recommended to observe the hemodynamic response to compression.

Acute Fracture

In the cases of acute and unstable bone fracture, changes in pressure could cause movement and delay healing.

Acute Local Dermatological Infections

Contact with the stockinette or the IPC sleeve as well as perspiration can cause spread of infection.

General Description and Operation of the Unit

Equipment

Intermittent pneumatic compression is applied using a device that includes the control box and pump, the hose(s), and the compression sleeve (Figs. 8-1 and 8-2). The control box varies in equipment. In some models, the operator can control the parameters of on:off time as well as pressure; in other models, the on:off time is preset. The hoses attach from the control/pump to the limb compression sleeve. In single-chamber pumps, there is usually only one hose. The multichamber pumps have multiple hoses, usually three. They are frequently color-coded with the controls and the sleeve to ensure proper sequencing of the inflation. A variety of sizes of compression sleeves are available. Selection is made by choosing the sleeve whose size most closely corresponds to the size of the area being treated.

Intermittent pneumatic compression can be applied using equipment with either a single chamber or multiple chambers. Multichamber pumps inflate chambers sequentially, beginning in the distal portion of the sleeve and then moving proximally. It is believed that this sequencing serves to move the fluid proximally and out of the affected limb. It is frequently reported

that the multichamber device using a sequential pattern is more effective than the single-chamber device.[20,45]

KEY POINT! Wraps, such as short or long stretch wraps; gradient compressive stockings, such as JOBST stockings; and certain taping techniques represent additional forms of compression (Fig. 8-3).

Clinical Parameters

One of the most difficult aspects of applying IPC is the lack of established parameters for treatment.[46] This lack of protocol has contributed to a disparity in outcomes in research literature.

The clinical parameters of IPC that can be adjusted include inflation pressure, on:off time, and total treatment time. As stated earlier, there is little agreement in the literature as to optimal settings for application. Most IPC devices are supplied with manufacturer's guidelines that usually contain a wide range of options for safe application. Additionally, many facilities have policies and procedures that address guidelines for applying IPC.

Inflation pressure is the maximum pressure reached during the period of inflation. It is generally accepted that inflation pressure should not exceed diastolic blood pressure minus 10 mm Hg. Pressures above this limit are believed to have the potential to collapse blood vessels. It should be noted that 10 mm Hg below diastolic blood pressure is a maximum, not necessarily the recommended pressure. In patients with hypertension, the "10 mm Hg below diastolic pressure" number might well exceed recommended pressures.

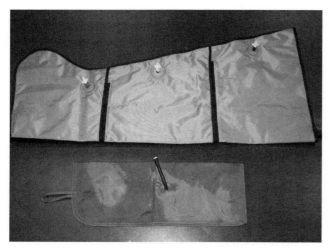

Fig 8•1 Multi- and single-chamber sleeves for application of IPC.

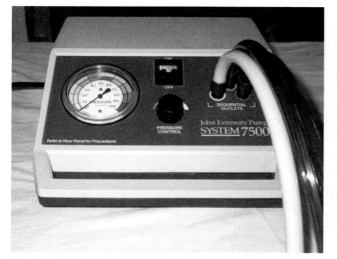

Fig 8•2 IPC pump.

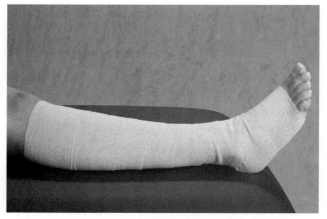

Fig 8•3 Low stretch and elastic bandages are common clinical forms of compression.

A recent study by Segers et al.[47] found significant discrepancies between the target pressure indicated by the controller on the ICP device and the pressure measured inside the cuff chambers. Actual pressure in the most distal chamber was up to 80% higher than that indicated by the controller. These authors recommend that IPC devices be used at much lower target pressures (less than 30 mm Hg) than those applied in clinical practice.

Arterial capillary pressure is generally about 30 mm Hg, so any pressure above that amount should be useful in assisting an arteriovenous (AV) pressure gradient and encouraging the absorption of edema. Nicolaides et al.[20] found that pressure higher than 35 mm Hg did not increase venous peak flow of the limbs.

On:off time sequence refers to the ratio of time that the machine is inflated and the time the machine is deflated. In some machines, this parameter is preset. Recommendations in the literature for on:off times vary significantly; however, patient comfort is the most important determining factor.

Total treatment time is the length of time (duration) the treatment device is applied. In clinical practice, this is frequently a convenience-based time determined by availability of equipment and space. Total treatment time is usually between 45 minutes and 1 hour. Recommendations in the literature vary from 45 minutes

up to 4 hours. (See Tables 8-1 and 8-2 for treatment guidelines provided by two of the major manufacturers of IPC units for clinical application of IPC.)

KEY POINT! Exercise and the repetitive activation of skeletal muscle act as a pump mechanism for the venous system. The deep veins of the legs, which are contained within the calf muscle fascia, are dependent upon this mechanism. Low stretch bandages assist the musculoskeletal pump by causing an increased pressure against the veins because the bandages do not yield to the muscle movement.

Preparation for IPC Treatments

Patients will need to remain in one position for the duration of the treatment, so they must be positioned comfortably with maximum access to their environment. Positioning to allow reading, viewing television, or even computer access will occupy patients during treatment and help alleviate boredom. Patients should empty their bladder prior to initiating treatment. Fluid returning to the circulation is filtered through the kidneys, and urinary urgency is not uncommon. Trips to the restroom can result in delay or interruption of the treatment.

A treatment table with appropriate height and size to accommodate the area being treated is essential. The

Table 8•1 Treatment Guidelines for IPC Recommended by the Jobst Institute

Indications	Pressure (mm Hg)	Recommended Treatment Periods	Inflation Time (On)	Deflation Time (Off)
Postmastectomy lymphedema	30–50	Two treatments per day for 3 hours	80–100 seconds	25–30 seconds
Edema of lower extremities	30–60	Two treatments per day for 3 hours	80–100 seconds	25–30 seconds
Peripheral edema and venous stasis ulceration	85	One treatment period of 2½ hours, three times per week	80–100 seconds	30 seconds
Stump reduction	30–60	Three treatment periods per day for 4 hours	40–60 seconds	10–15 seconds
Hand edema	30–50	Two treatment periods a day of 30 minutes to 1 hour each	Flexed position: 5–10 minutes	Extended position: 5–10 minutes

Table 8•2 Treatment Guidelines for IPC Recommended by Huntleigh Technology

Indications	Pressure (mm Hg)	Minimum/Day	Total
Venous ulcers	50	Two 2-hour periods	As necessary (not less than 6 weeks)
Edema (venous)	40–80	Two 2-hour periods	4–8 weeks
Lymphatic edema	70–90	2 hours	As necessary (not less than 6–8 weeks)
Traumatic edema	50	2 hours	As necessary
Stump forming	20–50	1 hour	4–6 weeks

patient should feel that all body parts are supported and will not slide off the edge of the table with minimal movement or position shifting. Pillows, wedges, or other supports should be used to keep the area being treated in a comfortable position and elevated above the level of the heart. An elevated position is an important adjunct to the compression and can encourage venous return (Fig. 8-4).

Treatment cuffs or sleeves come in a variety of sizes and shapes. When selecting a cuff for a patient, use the smallest one that will provide adequate coverage to the treatment area. Apply a stockinette or a similar product to the limb to cover the area under the treatment cuff to absorb perspiration.

Treatment Application Guidelines

First, review the patient's history and check for any condition that would contraindicate compression therapy. All jewelry and clothing in the treatment area should be removed. The entire limb should be exposed to allow for a complete examination of the limb prior to applying the compression sleeve. Measure and record the patient's blood pressure to create a baseline for comparison during treatment and to establish a maximum pressure guideline. Circumferential measurements of the limb must be determined and recorded prior to and after each treatment session. These are most easily documented and compared if recorded in a chart or table format. Select landmarks that can be easily located and will not change as edema decreases. References to bony landmarks are generally most easily reproducible. Measurements are most accurate if performed by the

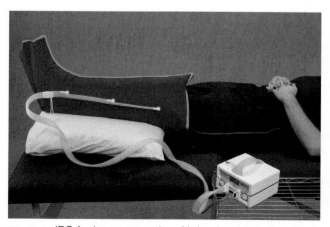

Fig 8•4 IPC for lower extremity with leg in elevated position.

same examiner using the same measurement technique for each treatment session. Measurements are generally taken every 10 cm from the landmark. The same landmarks should be used before and after treatment and in subsequent treatments to allow for accurate assessment of changes. Volumetric measurements may also be used.

If there is an open wound in the treatment area, it should be covered with a dressing, such as a sterile gauze pad or Telfa pad, and secured in place. The limb to be treated should be clean and dry. The limb's skin sensation and the patient's mentation must also be assessed, because patients with impaired sensation or decreased awareness may not realize when there is too much pressure over a nerve or bony area or be able to notify staff if there is a problem.

Before applying the sleeve to the limb, a stockinette should be placed over the limb. Wrinkles in the stockinette should be smoothed out because these can cause restriction and discomfort. After the sleeve is applied over the stockinette, the hose to the pump and the sleeve should be connected. In units with multiple hoses, be sure that the hose is inserted into the proper location to ensure proper inflation sequence in units with sequential chamber inflation. The hoses and receptacles are frequently color-coded to avoid confusion. After the hoses are attached, set the appropriate parameters on the dials on the pump. The patient must be given a bell or call button to alert the practitioner during treatment if any discomfort or unusual sensations occur. Monitor the patient's blood pressure during treatment, and modify or end treatment if there is a significant change in pressure.

The treatment should be terminated while the limb is still in an elevated position. To terminate treatment, turn the pressure dial to the off or "0" position and turn the power off. Disconnect the tubing from the machine and treatment sleeve, and remove the treatment sleeve from the patient. Remove the stockinette and assess the skin for any pressure or reddened areas. Repeat the circumferential measurements and record. If indicated, ROM or other exercises may be performed with the extremity elevated, if possible. Following appropriate exercise, application of a compression garment or elastic compression wrap will help maintain the effects of the treatment. The intervention session should be clearly documented.

Following treatment, provide assistance as needed to help the patient to a standing position. Slight dizziness or unsteadiness is not uncommon because of the circulatory changes that may occur with prolonged immobilization. If these symptoms are prolonged or severe, another form of treatment may need to be considered. Also instruct the patient in an appropriate home treatment program (see list of instructions in Box 8-1).

Possible Complications of Treatment

- Swelling in other areas may occur as a result of fluid returning to the circulation. This is often controlled with elevation and gentle active exercise.
- Stiffness of joints within the treatment area sometimes occurs as a result of prolonged immobilization in one position. This generally resolves quickly and is not a cause for concern unless it lasts longer than about 15 to 30 minutes. If stiffness persists, try an alternative, better-supported position.
- Shortness of breath may indicate fluid overload in the lungs or pulmonary embolism. Monitor shortness of breath closely and contact the physician if this persists.
- Numbness or tingling in the distal extremity may indicate DVT or nerve irritation or nerve damage. Stop treatment and assess immediately if your patient complains of numbness or tingling.[48]

Intermittent Pneumatic Compression: Evidence of Effectiveness

Considerable evidence to support the effectiveness of IPC is found in the literature. IPC has been shown to improve lymph return and reduce edema.[20,49] Studies demonstrate that it can decrease venous stasis and treat venous ulcers—even longstanding, chronic ones—that had not healed with other treatment methods.[18–21,50,51] It has also been shown to increase mobility and decrease pain following injury.[17,49] The use of IPC has been shown to reduce the incidence of DVT formation in postoperative and immobilized patients.[5,22–27] Furthermore, patients generally expressed satisfaction with pneumatic compression devices, and some studies reported higher compliance than with other compression methods.[52]

Although the effectiveness of intermittent pneumatic compression has been demonstrated, there is a lack of research to document ideal treatment protocols. Parameters vary widely among studies. Questions persist regarding the required treatment time, frequency, pressure, and on:off ratio. Time and frequency range from treatment five times per week for 45 minutes[51] to daily treatment for 4 hours.[53] Protocols regarding pressure and on:off times are also lacking. Although manufacturers provide recommendations, they vary widely and fail to provide reliable data to support their recommendations. A prospective, randomized study to evaluate these parameters has not been reported. Until these studies are available, clinicians will need to use an empirical approach to determine the protocols they will use.

Documentation Tips

The following should be documented with application of IPC, preferably in a table format for ease of comparison of response to each treatment session:

- Blood pressure taken before, during, and after each treatment session
- Circumferential measurements before and after treatment
- Limb sensation and mobility
- Area treated
- Size and description of wound (if present)
- Position of patient during treatment
- Inflation pressure
- On:off ratio
- Total treatment time
- Response to treatment

Box 8•1 | **Post-IPC Treatment Instructions**

After treatment, instruct your patient to do the following:
- Note return of edema (time, location, amount)
- Elevate the extremity as much as possible
- Apply compression (compressive wrap or garment)
- Engage in active movement as possible

CASE STUDY 8•1 INTERMITTENT PNEUMATIC COMPRESSION

Harold is a 61-year-old male with chronic venous insufficiency. He presents to the clinic with swelling of both lower extremities and complaints of pain with the swelling. He has a history of hypertension that is controlled by medication and painful osteoarthritis in both hands. The patient's blood pressure as recorded today is 140/75. Patient has been referred for reduction of edema.

CLINICAL DECISION-MAKING

1. Does the patient have a problem that can be improved with the use of intermittent pneumatic compression?
   Answer: Yes, the patient has venous insufficiency with bilateral swelling in the legs.

2. Is the patient appropriate for application of IPC (i.e., do any of the general precautions or contraindications to IPC apply, or are there any specific considerations regarding application of IPC to this patient)?
   Answer: The patient has hypertension that is controlled by medication. Nevertheless, as a precaution, it is prudent that the maximal pressure not exceed 10 mm Hg less than the diastolic pressure (i.e., not to exceed 65 mm Hg in this case). However, this is a maximal pressure and not necessarily the optimal pressure to be used. A lesser maximal pressure is recommended for the initial applications.

3. What are the specific goals to be achieved with the use of IPC?
   Answer: Sequential intermittent compression reduces edema by increasing circulation. It moves excessive fluid from the tissues into the normal drainage pattern.

4. Do you have the specific type of intermittent pneumatic compression that is appropriate for the patient?
   Answer: A mechanical intermittent pneumatic compression pump will be used.

5. What specific parameters of intermittent pneumatic compression would be appropriate for the patient?
   Answer: For venous insufficiency of the lower extremities:
   Pressure: 30 to 65 mm Hg (not to exceed diastolic BP minus 10 mm Hg). The distal pressure will be the greatest and set around 30 mm Hg, decreasing in the chambers moving proximally.
   On:off times: A 3:1 ratio. In this case, a 90-second on time and a 30-second off time will be used.
   Duration: 45 to 60 minutes per session
   Frequency: Two sessions per day

6. What are the proper (i.e., effective and safe) application procedures for intermittent pneumatic compression related to this case example?
   Answer: Harold should be positioned supine with his legs elevated approximately 30°. Stockinette or an IPC sleeve should be placed on the patient's leg prior to applying the compressive sleeves. Attach the hoses, select the appropriate compression for each chamber, and observe at least one cycle. Monitor the patient's blood pressure during and after the application.

☐ REFERENCES

1. American Physical Therapy Association: *Guide to Physical Therapist Practice.* 2nd ed. Alexandria, VA: American Physical Therapy Association; 2001.
2. Abu-Own A, Cheatle T, Scurr JH, Coleridge Smith PD. Effects of intermittent pneumatic compression of the foot on the microcirculatory function in arterial disease. Eur J Vasc Surg. 1993;7:488–492.
3. Eze AR, Comerata AAJ, Cisek PL, et al. Intermittent calf and foot compression increases lower extremity blood flow. *Am J Surg.* 1996;172:130–135.
4. Janssen H, Trevino C, Williams D. Hemodynamic alterations in venous blood flow produced by external pneumatic compression. *J Cardiovasc Surg.* 1993;34:441–447.
5. Knight MT, Dawson R. Effect of intermittent pneumatic compression of the arms on deep venous thrombosis in the legs. *Lancet.* 1976;2:1265–1268.
6. Lawrence D, Kakkar W. Graduated external compression of the lower limb: a physiological assessment. *Br J Surg.* 1980;67:119–121.
7. Liu K, Chen L, Seaber AV, et al. Influences of inflation rate and duration on vasodilatory effect by intermittent pneumatic compression on distant skeletal muscle. *J Orthop Res.* 1999;17:415–430.
8. Liu K, Chen L, Seaber A, et al. Intermittent pneumatic compression of legs increases microcirculation in distant skeletal muscle. *J Orthop Res.* 1999;17:17–23.
9. Lurie F, Awaya DJ, Kistner RL, Eklof B. Hemodynamic effect of pneumatic compression and the position of the body. *J Vasc Surg.* 2003;37:137–142.
10. Miranda F, Perez MC, Castiglioni ML, et al. Effect of sequential intermittent pneumatic compression on both leg lymphedema volume and on lymph transport as semi-quantitatively evaluated by lymphoscintigraphy. *Lymphology.* 2001;34:135–141.
11. Morris RJ, Woodcock JP. Effects of supine intermittent compression on arterial inflow to the lower limb. *Arch Surg.* 2002;137:1269–1274.
12. Ricci MA, Fisk P, Knight S, Case T. Hemodynamic evaluation of foot venous compression devices. *J Vasc Surg.* 1997;6:803–808.

13. Thordarson DB, Greene N, Shepherd L, Perlman M. Facilitating edema resolution with a foot pump after calcaneus fracture. *J Orthoped Trauma.* 1999;13:43–46.

14. Allenby F, Calnan JS, Flug JJ. The use of pneumatic compression in the swollen leg. *J Physiol.* 1973;231:65P–66P.

15. Leduc O, Leduc A, Burgeois P, Belgrado J. The physical treatment of upper limb oedema. *Cancer.* 1988;83:2835–2839.

16. Roper TA, Redford S, Tallis RC. Intermittent compression for the treatment of the oedematous hand in hemiplegic stroke: a randomized control trial. *Age Ageing.* 1999;28:9–13.

17. Airaksinen O, Kolari PJ, Herve R, Holopainen R. Treatment of posttraumatic oedema in lower legs using intermittent pneumatic compression. *Scand J Rehabil Med.* 1988;20:25–28.

18. Allsup, DJ. Use of intermittent pneumatic compression device in venous ulcer disease. *J Vasc Nurs.* 1994;12:106–111.

19. McCulloch JM, Marler KC, Neal MB, Phifer TJ. Intermittent pneumatic compression improves venous ulcer healing. *Adv Wound Care.* 1994;7:22–25.

20. Nicolaides AN, Fernandes E, Fernandes J, Pollock AV. Intermittent sequential pneumatic compression of the legs in the prevention of venous stasis and postoperative deep venous thrombosis. *Surgery.* 1980;87:69–76.

21. Vowden K. The use of intermittent pneumatic compression in venous ulceration. *Br J Nurs.* 2001;10:491–509.

22. Fort CW. Get pumped to prevent DVT. *Nursing.* 2002;32:50–52.

23. Hooker JA, Lachiewicz PF, Kelley SS. Efficacy of prophylaxis against thromboembolism with intermittent pneumatic compression after primary and revision of total hip arthroplasty. *J Bone Joint Surg.* 1999;81:690–696.

24. Hull RD, Faskob GE, Gent M. Effectiveness of intermittent pneumatic leg compression for preventing deep vein thrombosis after total hip replacement. *JAMA.* 1990;263:2313–2317.

25. King CA. Thromboembolitic prophylaxis with use of aspirin, exercise and graded elastic stockings or intermittent compression devices in patients managed with total hip arthroplasty. *AORN J.* 2000;72:1077–1079.

26. Soderhal DW, Henderson SR, Hansberry KL. A comparison of intermittent pneumatic compression of the calf and whole leg in preventing deep venous thrombosis in urological surgery. *J Urol.* 1997;157:1774–1776.

27. Woolston ST. Intermittent pneumatic compression prophylaxis for proximal deep vein thrombosis after total hip replacement. *J Bone Joint Surg.* 1996;78:1735–1740.

28. Fermor B, Weinberg JB, Pisetsky DS, Misukonis MA. The effects of static and intermittent compression on nitric oxide production in articular cartilage explants. *J Orthop Res.* 2001;19:729–732.

29. Montori VM, Kavros SJ, Walsh EE, Rooke TW. Intermittent compression pump for nonhealing wounds in patients with limb ischemia: the Mayo Clinic experience (1998–2000). *Intl Angiol.* 2002;21:360–366.

30. Wanderlinch RP, Armstrong DG, Harkless LB. Is intermittent pulsatile pressure a valuable adjunct in healing the complicated diabetic wound? *Ostomy Wound Manage.* 1998;44:70–77.

31. Armstrong DG, Nguyen HC. Intermittent pneumatic compression promoted healing in foot infections. *Arch Surg.* 2000;1405–1409.

32. Brennan M, Miller L. Overview of treatment options and review of the current role and use of compression garments, intermittent pumps and exercise in the management of lymphedema. *Cancer.* 1998;83:2821–2827.

33. Dini D, Del Mastro L, Gozza A, et al. The role of pneumatic compression in the treatment of post mastectomy lymphedema: a randomized phase III study. *Ann Oncol.* 1998;9:187–190.

34. Franzeck UK, Spiegel I, Fischer M, et al. Combined physical therapy for lymphedema evaluated by fluorescence microlymphography and lymph capillary pressure measurements. *J Vasc Res.* 1997;34:306–311.

35. Harris SR, Hugi MR, Olivotto IA, Levine M. Clinical practice guidelines for the care and treatment of breast cancer. *Can Med Assoc J.* 2001;164:191–200.

36. Kim-Sing C, Basco VE. Postmastectomy lymphedema treated with the Wright linear pump. *Can J Surg.* 1987;30:368–370.

37. Lachmann EA, Rook JL, Tunkel R, Nagler W. Complications associated with intermittent pneumatic compression. *Arch Phys Med Rehabil.* 1992;73:482–485.

38. Megans A, Harris SR. Physical therapist management of lymphedema following treatment for breast cancer: a critical review of its effectiveness. *Phys Ther.* 1998;78:1302–1311.

39. Newman AV, Ciccone CD. Can a comprehensive lymphedema management program decrease limb size and reduce the incidence of infection in a woman with postmastectomy lymphedema? *Phys Ther.* 2002;82:133–135.

40. Newman, G. Which patients with oedema are helped by intermittent external pneumatic compression therapy? *J R Soc Med.* 1988;81:377–379.

41. Pappas CH, O'Donnell TF Jr. Long-term results of compression treatment for lymphedema. *J Vasc Surg.* 1992;16:555–564.

42. Richmand DM, O'Donnell TF Jr, Zelikovski A. Sequential pneumatic compression for lymphedema: a controlled trial. *Arch Surg.* 1985;129:1116–1119.

43. Pohjola RT, Kolari PJ, Pekanmaki K. Intermittent pneumatic compression for lymphoedema: a comparison of two treatment modes. *Prog Lymphol.* 1988;11:583–586.

44. Foldi, E. Massage and damage to lymphatics. *Lymphology.* 1995;28:1–3.

45. Kamm R, Butcher R, Froelich J, et al. Optimization of indices of external pneumatic compression for prophylaxis against deep vein thrombosis: radionuclide gated imaging studies. *Cardiovasc Res.* 1986;20:588–596.

46. Whitelaw GP, Oladipo OJ, Shah BP, et al. Evaluation of intermittent pneumatic compression devices. *Orthopedics.* 2001;24:257–261.

47. Segers P, Blegrado J, Leduc A, et al. Excessive pressure in multichambered cuffs used for sequential compression therapy. *Phys Ther.* 2002;82:1000–1008.

48. McGrory BJ, Burke DW. Peroneal nerve palsy following intermittent sequential pneumatic compression. *Orthopedics.* 2000;23:1103–1105.

49. Valtonen EJ. Syncardial massage for treating extremities swollen by traumata, vein diseases, or idiopathic lymphoedema. *Acta Chir Scand.* 1967;133:363–367.

50. Morey KR, Watson AH. Team approach to treatment of post-traumatic stiff hand: case report. *Phys Ther.* 1986;66:225–228.

51. Pekanmaki K, Kolari PJ, Kiistala U. Intermittent pneumatic compression treatment for post-thrombotic leg ulcers. *Clin Exp Dermatol.* 1987;12:350–353.

52. Berliner E, Ozbilgin B, Zarin DA. A systematic review of pneumatic compression for treatment of chronic venous insufficiency and venous ulcers. *J Vasc Surg.* 2003;37(3):539–544.

53. Coleridge-Smith PD, Sarin S, Hasty J, Scurr JH. Sequential gradient pneumatic compression enhances venous ulcer healing: a randomized trial. *Surgery.* 1990;108:871–875.

chapter 9

Foundations of Electrotherapy

James W. Bellew, PT, EdD

Overview of Electrotherapy

Electrotherapy may seem challenging and difficult to comprehend. This chapter will set the foundations to make electrotherapy understandable and, more importantly, clinically useful. Although there are many uses of electrotherapeutics across the many areas of rehabilitation, there is but one shared purpose: stimulation to elicit or facilitate some desired therapeutic response. Whether electrical stimulation (ES) is used to activate skeletal muscle for strengthening or improving volitional movement, relaxing skeletal muscle to facilitate functional activity, decreasing pain, improving circulation, or facilitating tissue healing, all are based on the stimulation of tissues via electric current.

This chapter will delineate the steps to learning ES in a way that will be user-friendly, trying to minimize confusion as you develop new terminology. This can be likened to learning to drive a car; if you are taught to drive in one brand of car, you are likely to be successful if you use those same skills when driving a comparable vehicle; therefore, effectiveness is based on a competent knowledge and application of basics.

The overall purpose of this chapter is to address the fundamental principles of electricity and electrical charge that underlie the therapeutic effects for which electricity is used. This chapter and the following will present not only the "how," but the "when," "why," and "what" of electrotherapy. Chapters 11 and 12 present more specific applications of clinical electrotherapy.

Principles of Electricity: Making The Physics Make Sense

To discuss clinical applications of electrotherapy without first addressing the fundamentals of electricity is like asking someone to play a game without telling them how. Without some prior knowledge and understanding of the basic rules and strategy of the game, it may look like someone is playing the game, but the outcome will eventually reveal the lack of knowledge. So it is with clinical electrotherapy—without an understanding of the fundamentals, clinical effectiveness is less likely. A functional and useful understanding of electrotherapy must include and begin with the basics.

Charge

Charge is the fundamental property of electromagnetic force and serves as the underlying mechanism by which living cells communicate with one another. Charge is obtained by the addition or removal of electrons and is measured in coulombs (C) or microcoulombs (μC). A net gain of electrons results in a negative charge, whereas a net loss of electrons results in a positive charge.[1] Although atoms are composed of positive protons and negative electrons, the concept of charge is specific to the net gain or loss of electrons (Fig. 9-1). An atom that becomes positively charged does so by the loss of electrons, not by the addition of protons. A positively charged body has lost electrons, whereas a negatively charged body has gained electrons. An atom that has gained or lost an electron is termed an *ion,* and the process of changing the electrical state of an atom or object is termed *ionization.*[2]

Four fundamental properties of electrical charge explain how charge is used for therapeutic purposes:

1. There are two types of charge—positive and negative.
2. Like charges repel while opposite attract.
3. Charge is neither created nor destroyed.
4. Charge can be transferred from one object to another.[2]

Polarity and the Electric Field

Charge is either negative or positive and is described by polarity, with *polarity* referring to the net charge of the

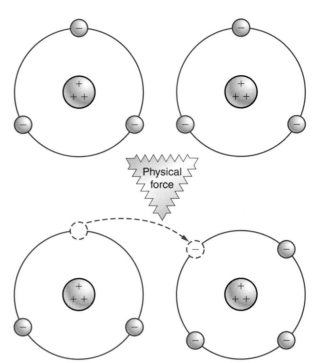

Fig 9•1 "Charge" is conferred by transfer of electrons. Addition of electrons results in net negative charge, whereas loss or removal results in net positive charge.

Clinical Principles in Practice: Principles of Charge in the Clinic

Clinical application of the fundamental properties of electrical charge is seen during iontophoresis. A clinician chooses to treat a patient with dexamethasone sodium phosphate, a negatively charged anti-inflammatory drug that is delivered transcutaneously via electrical current (e.g., iontophoresis). Knowing that like charges repel, the practitioner attaches the negative end of a circuit to the electrode containing the drug. The force of electrical charge will "push" or repel the negatively charged medicine away from the negative electrode and into the tissue requiring treatment.

object. In a simple circuit, one electrode is the positive pole and one is the negative pole. The pole with net negativity is termed the *cathode,* and the pole with net positivity is the *anode.*[1] A common household battery serves as a simple example of charge and polarity (Fig. 9-2). One pole has a concentration of electrons and the other has a deficiency.

Keeping in mind the second fundamental concept of electricity—that like charges repel and opposite charges attract—the force created by the separation of charge may be one of attraction, or repulsion and represents the *electrical field.* Magnets offer a good example of a

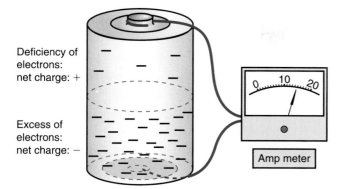

Fig 9•2 A common household battery. The separation of charge creates a concentration gradient. When connected, current flows between the poles.

force field. If the north pole of one magnet and the north pole of another are slowly brought near each other, the magnets begin to repel each other (Fig. 9-3). If you attempt to join the magnets, the resisting force is an example of a force field. The larger the magnets, the larger and stronger the force field is. For the clinician in the "Clinical Principles in Practice" example earlier, too little charge may limit the amount of dexamethasone delivered to the patient. And too much charge could result in adverse effects.

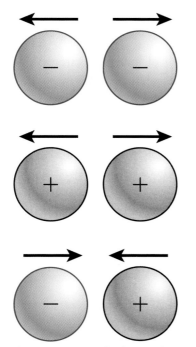

Fig 9•3 Like charges are repelled away from each other. Opposite charges are attracted to move closer to each other.

Voltage

The force of attraction or repulsion created by an electric field represents potential energy. The greater the force, the greater the potential energy. This force is termed *voltage* and represents the driving force that moves electrons.[1] The unit of electrical force is the *volt* (or millivolt).

A voltage force is best explained when considering the interaction of two magnets or two charged bodies as one approaches the other. When a larger magnet or charged body with a greater polarity or charge approaches another stationary magnet or charged body with the same but smaller polarity or charge, the force field exerted by the larger body on the smaller body increases as the distance between the two decreases. At some point, the repulsive force overcomes the inertia acting on the smaller body, and the smaller body is repelled away from the larger. The force of the electrical field that caused the smaller body to move is the voltage force. Voltage may also be referred to as the *electromotive force* or *electrical potential energy*.[1]

KEY POINT! Electricity produced by a power plant is delivered to homes miles away. This requires a considerable amount of work. To deliver electricity over this distance, a large amount of voltage is required. This is why you often see warning signs reading "High Voltage."

The change in electrical potential energy and the distance charges are moved represents the effects of a voltage force. Voltage can be thought of as the force that pushes charge. Keeping with the fundamental principle of electrical charge, voltages are created whenever oppositely charged particles are separated or when like charges are brought closer together. In terms of conventional electricity for purposes of power, these charged particles are the electrons that are moved within a powered machine and wires. In our biological system, however, voltage forces are created by the uneven distribution of charged particles, resulting in regions that are more or less negative or positive to adjacent regions. In tissues, these charged particles are ions, such as sodium (Na^+), potassium (K^+), and chloride (Cl^-).[3] In conventional circuits and electrical generators used to deliver power to our homes and electrotherapeutic devices, the charged, flowing particles are electrons. This text focuses on the electrophysiological and therapeutic effects of electrical stimulation on the human body, thus the terms *ions* and *electrons* will be used in place of *charged particles* (Box 9-1).

In our bodies, voltage forces are created when a separation of ions creates a concentration gradient.[3] The separation of charges across the phospholipid cell membrane is an ideal example of a voltage force. The greater concentration of sodium (Na^+) outside the cell versus inside the cell reflects a separation of charge *and* a concentration gradient. Because this concentration gradient separates charged ions (i.e., Na^+), the gradient is also referred to as an electrochemical gradient. It is this separation of charge across the cell membrane, and thus electrical potential, that sets up the ability for the cell to depolarize and initiate or transmit electrical signals.

Conductors and Insulators

For ions or electrons to move freely, they require materials that permit such movement. Materials in which ions or electrons move freely are termed *conductors*. Metals and water are examples of conductors. In the human body, tissues such as muscle, nerve, and bodily fluid serve as conductors (Fig. 9-4). In part, this reflects the high water content and presence of ions in these tissues.

Materials in which charged particles are not free to move or do not move easily are termed *insulators*. Rubber and plastic are typical materials considered to be insulators. Often conductors and insulators exist

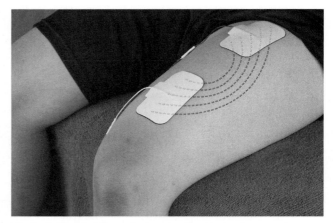

Fig 9•4 Current flows between electrodes by passing through biological tissues, which serve as conductors. This allows current to reach the peripheral nerves and muscles.

together both in everyday life and in biological examples. Take, for instance, an extension cord used in our homes: The metal wire inside conducts current to our appliances while the plastic coating insulates the current, preventing it from entering our body and shocking us. In the human body, fat is an insulator and does not allow ions or electrons to move freely.

Current

The movement of ions or electrons in a conductor in response to a voltage force is termed *current*. The flow of current is directly proportional to the magnitude of the driving force (i.e., the voltage). Current is the quantity or amount of ions or electrons flowing at a given time and is designated by the universal symbol I.[1] The international unit for current is the ampere (amp or A), but most therapeutic applications of current use milliamperes (10^{-3}; mA, thousandths of an ampere) or microamperes (10^{-6}; uA, millionths of an ampere). See Box 9-2.

Box 9•1 | **Hands-On Learning**

To better understand the role ions have in the creation of electrical current, place the lead wires of an electrotherapy device into a small bowl, making sure the leads are separated and do not touch. (Do not submerse the device in the water!) A device with a visible amp meter or output for monitoring current flow is preferred. (Note: A volt meter is not the same as an amp meter and may not work in this example.) First, pour distilled water into the bowl. After turning on the device, increase the amplitude. What happens? Nothing! Note that the meter does not move, indicating that no current is flowing. If your device lacks a meter, you may hear a warning beep indicating the lack of a complete circuit and no current flow. Why is this? The answer: Distilled water has had all ions removed, so there are no charged particles to move in the bowl. Now add salt to the water and watch the amp meter register flow of current. This occurred because the salt (NaCl) dissociated into sodium (Na^+) and chloride (Cl^-), allowing charged particles to move. The movement of ions represents flow of current.

Clinical Principles in Practice: Human Tissue as Conductors and Insulators

While treating a patient with low back pain, a clinician chooses electrical stimulation to help activate the lumbar muscles in order to lessen the pain. The patient is obese with a large amount of lumbosacral adipose tissue that does not conduct current well. For current to penetrate deep enough to stimulate the nerves of the lumbar muscles, the clinician increases the intensity of the current. Because adipose tissue is a better insulator than a conductor, it resists the current and results in an uncomfortable stinging sensation at the electrodes as the high current activates nociceptors.

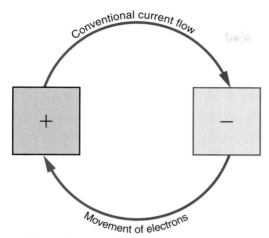

Fig 9•5 Flow of current versus flow of electrons.

Ohm's Law: Resistance, Capacitance, and Impedance

So far, we have described current as the free or unresisted flow of ions or electrons in a conductor in response to a voltage. The magnitude of current flow is directly proportional to the voltage force and quantity of charge moving. Rarely, if ever, does current flow in biological tissues without some kind of resistance. *Resistance* is opposition to the flow of current and comes in many forms in the body (Box 9-3).[1]

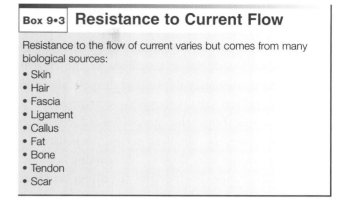

Box 9•3 **Resistance to Current Flow**

Resistance to the flow of current varies but comes from many biological sources:

- Skin
- Hair
- Fascia
- Ligament
- Callus
- Fat
- Bone
- Tendon
- Scar

The relationship between resistance and the flow of current is given in Ohm's law: $I = V/R$, where current (I in amperes) is directly proportional to the voltage force (V) pushing the current and inversely proportional to resistance (R) to the voltage force.[2] The standard international unit of resistance is the *ohm*. From a more clinical view, Ohm's law tells us that the more resistance there is to the flow of current, the less current there will be. Being aware of factors that affect biological resistance is important when applying ES for therapeutic use. Calloused skin, for example, presents high resistance, so the flow of current through an area such as the heel may be greatly reduced. This knowledge can impact applications, such as iontophoresis, when trying to move ions across the skin into the plantar fascia.

Capacitance and *impedance* are properties of current flow and are related to resistance. Capacitance is the degree to which electrical charge is stored in a system containing conductors and insulators, such as the human body.[1] Capacitance arises from the storage of charge in an insulator that is within a field of current. Because current does not pass freely across an insulator, the electrical potential across the insulator increases the electrical potential energy of the molecules of the insulator. This storage of electrical energy in the insulator reflects capacitance. When current flow ceases, the energy stored in the insulator flows back through the conductors (Box 9-4). The clinical significance of capacitance is seen in some devices that have a capacitor. Most modern stimulating devices linearly decrease the flow of current once the application has ended. This gradual decrease in current allows the capacitor to discharge stored charge. If the clinician abruptly terminates the application by unplugging or turning off the device before the current has decreased, the current

Box 9•2 **What Direction Does Current Flow?**

By convention, flow of current is designated as flowing from positive to negative. However, the astute student may notice that this is inconsistent with the laws of mass action and concentration gradients. If current is the movement of electrical charge and electrical charge is defined by gain or loss of electrons, the law of mass action tells us that movement should occur from high concentration (areas of more electrons or negativity) to low concentration (areas of less electrons or more positivity; see Fig. 9-5). Then the flow from a greater concentration of electrons to one of lesser electrons must be from negative to positive. But this is opposite. Indeed, this is how electrons move, but it remains that current is designated as flowing from positive to negative despite being contrary to scientific law. The details underlying this inconsistency are varied, but scientific lore has it that scientists studying electrical charge noted movement of "electric fluid" but were uncertain as to what exactly was moving, how, and in what direction. Out of attempts to describe their observations, they were forced to designate a direction of the movement and to arbitrarily designate the place from which flow seemed to originate as "positive" and the place to which flow appeared to go as "negative." This designation of the direction of current flow remains despite counterexplanation.

stored in the capacitor can freely flow through the electrodes. This is often perceived as a very brief and often uncomfortable surge in the stimulation's intensity.

Impedance is a form of resistance to the flow of current but is frequency-dependent. Impedance more accurately reflects the voltage-to-current ratio, as it incorporates both the properties of resistance and capacitance. In simplest terms, impedance is the resistance to the flow of alternating current, whereas resistance is specific to direct current. Clinically, gels and adhesive conductive agents on electrodes serve to decrease impedance between the electrode and skin.

Currents and Waveforms

Terminology used to describe electrotherapy can seem confusing; however, most of this is due to inconsistency in the terms and language used to describe electrotherapy and procedures. Greater understanding and increased comfort with the language of electrotherapy is readily achieved if some basic fundamental terms are used. In addition, a clinically competent understanding of the terminology of currents and waveforms is easily obtained if you keep in mind that these currents and waveforms are merely modifications of the two most fundamental electrical currents: direct current (DC) and alternating current (AC).

From the standpoint of electrophysics (a branch of physics from which electrotherapy comes), there are only two types of electrical current: direct current and alternating current. While these currents can be used for therapeutic purposes, the most common form of current used in electrotherapeutics is pulsed current,

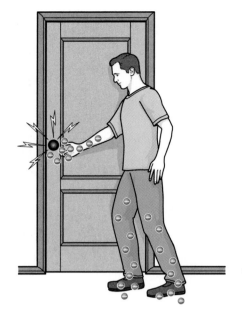

Fig 9•6 Electrons are transferred, resulting in accumulation of charge and flow when a circuit is completed.

or pulsatile current, and this is the terminology we will use in this text. In regards to applied science, pulsed current is the third major class of electrical current. (Terminology and descriptions used in this text are consistent with the American Physical Therapy Association, or APTA, and section on Electrophysiology and Wound Care.[1])

The Basic Currents

Understanding electrical currents is easy when visualizing their specific parameters. Consider a graphical depiction of each current and the specific ways in which each would be described or drawn. When you begin to use terms to explain the shape, magnitude, and duration of currents, you are describing the current *waveform*. The waveform is simply a depiction of the characteristics that represent a given current. A good example of a waveform can be shown on the Etch A Sketch (Fig. 9-7).

All currents have parameters in the vertical (*y* coordinate) and horizontal (*x* coordinate) directions (Fig. 9-8). Parameters in the horizontal axis are used to describe and quantify time or duration characteristics of current (in milli- or microseconds), whereas parameters in the vertical axis are used to describe or quantify magnitude or intensity (in milli- or microamps or milli- or microvolts).

Box 9•4	**Static Shock: Why Does It Happen?**

When acted upon by external forces, such as heat, friction, chemical, electrical, or other physical forces, the number of electrons may be altered. Rubbing your feet on the carpet results in a transfer of electrons from the floor to your body via friction. These electrons are temporarily stored in your body, which acts as a capacitor. When you touch a metal object, it acts as a conductor, creating a circuit, and the stored electrons flow freely from you into a metal object (see Fig. 9-6). The physical effect is a surprising shock!

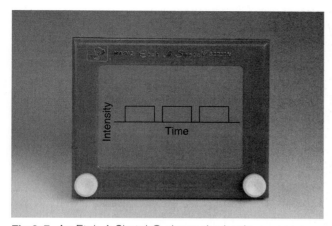

Fig 9•7 An Etch A Sketch® shows the basic *x-y* components of waveforms representing time and amplitude of current.

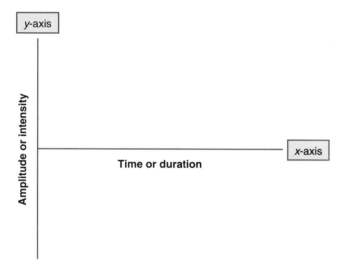

Fig 9•8 Basic *x-y* axes for time and amplitude. Time may be in seconds (sec), milliseconds (msec, 10⁻³), or microseconds (μsec, 10⁻⁶). Intensity may be in volts (V), millivolts (10⁻³, mV), microvolts (10⁻⁶, μV), amperes (amp), milliamps (10⁻³, mA), or microamps (10⁻⁶, μA)

Direct Current

Direct current is the continuous unidirectional flow of ions or electrons for at least 1 second[1] (Fig. 9-9). Here, the term *direction* implies flow from positive to negative or negative to positive. The most common or familiar source of DC is the household battery. When the poles are connected in a circuit, such as when putting batteries in a device, current will flow. Variations of DC exist, but to accurately be called DC, they must remain unidirectional and uninterrupted for a period of time.[1] Other forms of DC include *interrupted DC,* where the

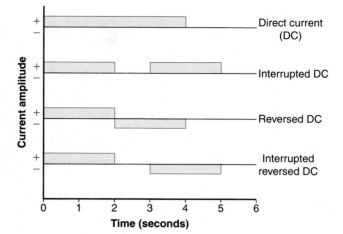

Fig 9•9 Direct current (DC) comes in many forms with conventional DC most commonly used.

direction of flow ceases after 1 second before resuming in the same direction for at least 1 second; *reversed DC,* where the flow ceases after 1 second before resuming in the opposite direction for at least 1 second; and *interrupted reversed DC,* which is a combination of both.

When using DC, one of the electrodes will be the anode (positive) and one will be the cathode (negative). This will remain so unless the direction of current reverses, as in reversed DC. The most common clinical uses of DC are for iontophoresis (Fig. 9-10) and wound care, both of which are covered in Chapter 10.

Alternating Current

In contrast to DC, *alternating current* (AC) is the uninterrupted bidirectional flow of ions or electrons and

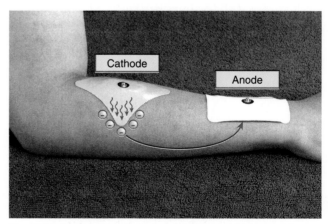

Fig 9•10 Iontophoresis uses direct current to move ions. Negatively charged ions placed under the cathode will be "pushed" or repelled into the tissue.

must change direction at least one time per second[1,4] (Fig. 9-11). The rate at which AC switches direction is termed *frequency* and is described with the international unit *hertz* (Hz) or in the unit *cycles per second* (cps). The most common or familiar source of AC is the electricity coming from the wall outlets in our homes, supplying electricity to most appliances (e.g., your cell phone charger uses an AC source). Clinical use of pure sinusoidal AC is not common; however, modulated forms of AC, such as burst modulated AC (i.e., Russian current) and amplitude modulated AC (i.e., interferential current), are commonly used and will be discussed later this chapter.

KEY POINT! ▸ Think about it: AC must change direction at least one time per second. If it does not, then what type of current would it be? DC.

Pulsed Current

Because the electrophysiological effects of DC or AC are not well suited for most electrotherapeutic applications, a third category of current has been designated: *pulsed current* (PC). Pulsed current, sometimes termed *pulsatile* or *interrupted current*, is the uni- or bidirectional flow of ions or electrons that periodically ceases for a small period of time before the next electrical event.[1] Some sources use the terms *pulsed DC* or *pulsed AC*. However, these terms are not preferred.

The definition of *PC* reflects flow of current that ceases before the next "event." This event is a *pulse*—an isolated electrical event separated from the next by a period of time termed the *interpulse interval*. Referring back to the *x-y* coordinate system, the duration (*x* coordinate) and amplitude (*y* coordinate) of the pulse give the time and magnitude of the voltage or current of the

pulse, respectively. Descriptions of PC refer to the shape or configuration of the pulses (Box 9-5). Common forms of pulsed current include square, rectangular, and triangular pulses (Fig. 9-12).

The generation of two or more consecutive pulses separated from the next series of consecutive pulses is termed a *burst*, and the time between bursts is the *interburst interval*[1] (Fig. 9-13). The frequency at which bursts are generated is the *burst frequency*, while the frequency of the underlying AC waveform in the burst is termed the *carrier frequency*.[1,5,6] In some cases, the uninterrupted generation of pulses at a fixed frequency is used. This is termed a *train* of pulses and is different from bursts in that there is no interruption of the pulses at a set frequency (i.e., bursts). The practical use of burst and carrier frequency is presented later in this chapter.

KEY POINT! ▸ Think about it: What is the longest duration a pulse can have and still be termed a pulse? Less than 1 second.

Pulsed current may be monophasic or biphasic, with a *phase* being the flow of current in one direction for a

---

Box 9•5 **Pulsed Current vs. DC: Effects on Muscle Stimulation**

PC is used for stimulating skeletal muscle for strengthening and activity. Because PC is a series of pulses, muscle fibers can be stimulated frequently, resulting in tetanic contraction. But what will happen if using DC? Won't this result in a tetanic contraction because DC flows continuously? No! DC will depolarize the muscle and cause a single twitch, but only one. To get a tetanic contraction, the muscle must depolarize and repolarize before depolarizing again. The time between successive pulses of pulsed current allows the muscle fibers to repolarize so they can be depolarized again. DC results in a sustained state of depolarization. The muscle cannot repolarize until the DC temporarily ceases.

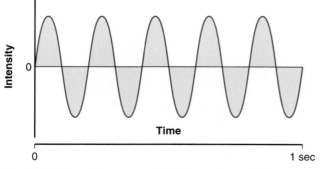

Fig 9•11 Alternating current (AC) as a sinusoidal waveform.

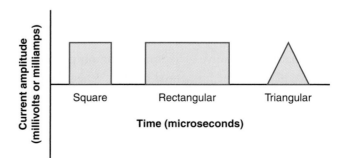

Fig 9•12 Pulsed current comes in many shapes, including square, rectangular, and triangular waveforms.

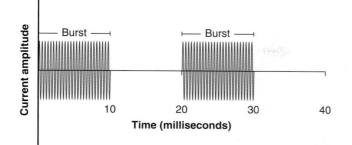

25 cycles in 10 msec = 2500 Hz carrier frequency

2 bursts in 40 msec = 50 bursts per second

Fig 9•13 Burst and carrier frequency: In this figure, a 2,500 Hz AC carrier frequency is delivered in bursts. The figure shows 10 msec bursts with 25 cycles per burst and 10 msec between bursts. Twenty-five cycles in 10 msec equates to 2,500 Hz. Two bursts in 40 msec equate to a burst frequency of 50 bursts per second (bps).

short period of time[1] (Fig. 9-14). A *monophasic* pulse deviates from the isoelectric line in only one direction, depending on what direction the current initially flows before ceasing (i.e., returning to the isoelectric line). With monophasic pulses, ions or electrons move briefly in only one direction before stopping. *Monophasic pulsed current* (MPC) is the delivery of repeated monophasic pulses separated from each other by an *interpulse interval*; it is produced by intermittently interrupting a DC current source. In contrast, a *biphasic* pulse is one that deviates from the isoelectric line first in one direction, then in the other direction from the isoelectric line. *Biphasic pulsed current* (BPC), therefore, is the delivery of repeated biphasic pulses separated from the next pulse by an interpulse interval and is produced by intermittently interrupting an AC current source. By definition, with monophasic pulsed current, a *pulse* and a *phase* are synonymous.

Accordingly, the term *monophasic* cannot be used to describe AC.

When further describing and differentiating pulsed waveforms, similarity in amplitude and duration of each phase must be considered. *Amplitude,* often referred to as *intensity,* is the magnitude of current or voltage with respect to the isoelectric or baseline on the *x-y* current-time plot (Fig. 9-15). Amplitude is reported in units of current (amps, milliamps, or microamps) or voltage (in volts, millivolts, or microvolts) and can be described in terms of a single phase or both phases. Most uses of ES use milliampere amplitude. The highest current or voltage reached in a phase of a monophasic pulse or in any one phase of a biphasic waveform is termed the *peak amplitude.* The highest value measured from the peak of the first phase to the peak of the second phase of a biphasic waveform is termed the *peak-to-peak amplitude.* For monophasic waves, there is no peak-to-peak value.

KEY POINT! Pulse duration is the total time elapsed from the beginning to the end of a single pulse, including the interphase (intrapulse) interval. If the phase durations of the biphasic pulse are 150 µsec each and the interphase interval is 50 µsec, the total pulse duration is 350 µsec.

The time-dependent characteristics used to describe waveforms reflect the *x* coordinate when plotting waveforms (see Fig. 9-15). *Phase duration* is the time from the beginning of one phase to its end. *Pulse duration* is the time from the beginning to end of all phases plus the interphase interval within one pulse. The *interphase interval* (or intrapulse interval) is the time between phases of a single pulse, whereas the *interpulse interval* is the time between successive pulses.[1] Phase and pulse duration are most commonly reported in milliseconds (msec) or microseconds (µsec).

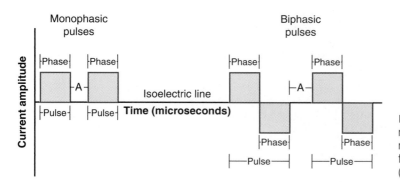

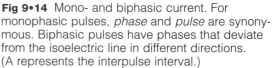

Fig 9•14 Mono- and biphasic current. For monophasic pulses, *phase* and *pulse* are synonymous. Biphasic pulses have phases that deviate from the isoelectric line in different directions. (A represents the interpulse interval.)

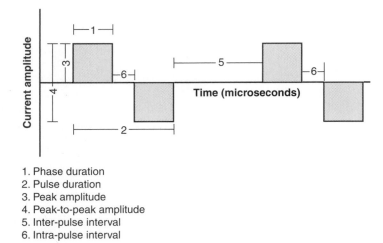

1. Phase duration
2. Pulse duration
3. Peak amplitude
4. Peak-to-peak amplitude
5. Inter-pulse interval
6. Intra-pulse interval

Fig 9•15 Amplitude and time (duration) characteristics of pulsed current.

KEY POINT! Pulse duration is often labeled *pulse width* on many devices. This terminology is not preferred, as pulse duration is a unit of time, whereas *width* implies a unit of linear measure.

Modulation of Pulsed Current

Modulation of pulsed current is widely used in electrotherapeutics to impart a variety of different effects. The duration that a series of pulses or bursts is delivered is termed the *on-time,* and the duration or time between a series of pulses or bursts is the *off-time*. The percentage of the on-time to the total time (on-time plus off-time) multiplied by 100% is termed the *duty cycle*.[1] Duty cycle is a commonly reported parameter of pulsed currents, but some confusion can arise from the use of this term. Because duty cycle is a relative measure of the "on" to "total" time, a variety of combinations can result in the same duty cycle. For example, a clinical application for muscle strengthening may use an on-time of 10 seconds with an off-time of 40 seconds. The duty cycle of this application would be 10 seconds (on-time) divided by 50 seconds (total-time) multiplied by 100%, or 20%. However, the same duty cycle also accurately describes any on-time and off-time ratio of 1 on to 4 off. Thus, applications of 1 second on and 4 seconds off, 15 seconds on and 60 seconds off yield the same duty cycle of 20%. The significance here is that the use of duty cycle does not always accurately reflect the specific on- and off-times. This can lead to errors when using ES in follow-up visits. This can be avoided if actual on- and off-times are individually documented in absolute seconds instead of expressed as duty cycle.

Amplitude Modulation

Modulation of the amplitude characteristics of pulsed current is used for differing effects. Often it is necessary to slowly increase the amplitude of a current to the desired intensity. Take, for example, stimulating muscle after an injury. A gradual increase in current amplitude and muscle activation may be more tolerable and ultimately beneficial than a rapid increase and abrupt muscle contraction. In contrast, a rapid rise in amplitude, and thus muscle stimulation, may be used to quickly stimulate the tibialis anterior when assistance with ankle dorsiflexion is desired for toe clearance during the swing phase of gait.

Ramp refers to the progressive increase or decrease in amplitude (Fig. 9-16). When the amplitude is progressively increased, it is called *ramp-up*, and when amplitude is decreased, it is called *ramp-down*. The terms *rise time* and *fall time* are used to describe the time required

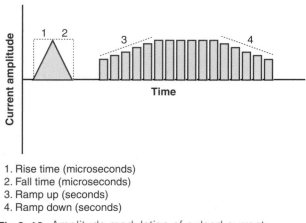

1. Rise time (microseconds)
2. Fall time (microseconds)
3. Ramp up (seconds)
4. Ramp down (seconds)

Fig 9•16 Amplitude modulation of pulsed current: Ramps, rise time, and fall time.

for the leading edge of a single phase to reach peak amplitude and the time required for the trailing edge of a single phase to return to the isoelectric line, respectively. Ramps are specific to the increase or decrease in the amplitude of a series of pulses.

It is important to understand how the use of ramp times affects the total current delivered to the patient. Because current is still being delivered to the patient during both the ramp up and down times, they should be considered part of the on-time. Long ramp times can greatly reduce the total amount of current delivered to the patient and thus greatly impact the overall therapeutic effect. For example, Figure 9-17 shows two series of pulses, each with an on-time of 10 milliseconds. Series A has a ramp-up time of 1 second and no ramp-down. Series A reaches peak amplitude in 1 second and maintains that amplitude for the duration of the on-time—9 seconds in this example. In contrast, series B has a ramp-up of 4 seconds and a ramp-down of 2 seconds. Thus, series B is at peak amplitude for only 4 of the 10 seconds as opposed to 9 seconds in series A. Since series A is at peak amplitude longer than B, the total amount of current delivered to the patient is greater in series A.

It is important to read the user's manual for electrotherapeutic devices so the clinician understands how ramps are incorporated into the total on- and off-times. For example, some manufacturers include ramp-down time in the off-time. However, this is problematic, because current is still being delivered during the ramp-down and should be considered on-time (Fig. 9-18). In this case, the off-time may not accurately reflect a period when there is no current. Still other manufacturers extend the total on-time to include the ramp-up. Thus, as an example, a 3-second ramp-up may be

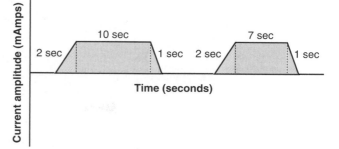

Fig 9•18 How ramp times are incorporated with the total on-time varies by devices. For example, suppose a 10-second on-time is desired with a 2-second ramp-up and a 1-second ramp-down. The image on the left indicates that the ramps are separate from the 10-second on-time. This equates to 13 total seconds of on-time, 30% longer than initially selected. In contrast, the image on the right shows that the ramps are included as part of the total on-time. This then means the current is at peak amplitude for only 70% of the total on-time.

added to a selected on-time of 10 seconds, resulting in a total on-time of 13 seconds. If the clinician is not aware of these variations and nuances in the manufacturer specifications, clinical outcomes following treatment may vary greatly.

Phase and Pulse Charge

When the amplitude and time-dependent characteristics are considered together, waveforms can then be viewed in terms of the "area under the curve," or the integrated sum of current amplitude and duration. This represents the total charge delivered in each phase or pulse (Fig. 9-19). *Phase charge* is the charge within one phase of a pulse, and *pulse charge* is the cumulative charge of all phases within a single pulse.[1] For monophasic pulses, phase charge and pulse charge are synonymous. For biphasic waveforms, determining average current delivered is not as easy and requires

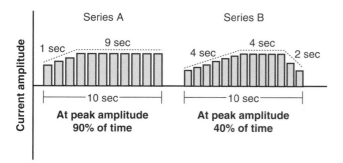

Fig 9•17 Effect of ramps on total current delivered.

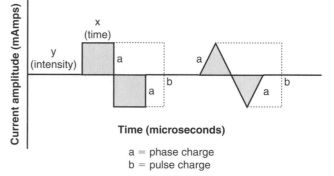

a = phase charge
b = pulse charge

Fig 9•19 Phase and pulse charge.

further consideration. Note that the area under the curve can be increased by increasing either the pulse amplitude or duration, or both.

Clinical Principles in Practice: Pulse Charge

Using a handheld TENS unit with controls for pulse duration and amplitude, set the pulse duration and frequency as low as possible. Apply the electrodes to the extensor muscles of your forearm. Then begin by increasing the intensity of the device until you notice small but easily observed muscle twitches. Now leave the intensity alone. Slowly increase the pulse duration. What effect is observed? The increase in the stimulus intensity is the result of increasing the total pulse charge (area under the curve) by increasing pulse duration, not amplitude.

For biphasic waveforms, if the sum of current amplitude and duration of the first phase (i.e., phase charge) are identical to the second, the phases are termed *symmetrical*. If the amplitude and duration characteristics between the two phases of the biphasic waveform differ in any manner, the phases are termed *asymmetrical*.[1] If the phases of a biphasic waveform are not symmetrical, then it is necessary to determine if the integrated sums of the phases are equal (i.e., have equal phase charges). Despite not being symmetrical in shape, the area under the curve (i.e., phase charge) can be equal or unequal. If the area under the curve of the first phase is equal to that of the second phase, the phases are termed *balanced*. In this case, the average charge is zero because equal amounts of current flow in both directions of the biphasic wave. If the phases are not of equal area, they are termed *unbalanced*. In this case, the average charge is not zero and the total pulse charge will have the polarity of the phase with greater charge. Thus, one electrode will maintain a net negative charge and the other a net positive charge.

The significance of symmetry, asymmetry, and balance lies in the potential for delivering a current with a net charge or polarity. This can be thought of again as using area under the curve. If the phases of a biphasic waveform are symmetrical or asymmetrical but balanced, the net charge of the current is zero.[1] This means there is no sustained polarity, or no sustained positive or negative pole, since equal amounts of current flow in each direction and the direction is constantly changing. If, however, the phase charges of a biphasic waveform

are asymmetrical and unbalanced, more current is generated in one direction than the other. This results in a net charge. The pole with the greater area under the curve determines the current's net charge. In this case, there will not be an average of zero charge but rather a net accumulation of charge with a polarity of the phase with greater quantity. In Figure 9-20, three biphasic currents are shown: one with phase charges of $+15$ μC and -15 μC, one with phase charges of $+15$ μC and -6 μC, and a third with phase charges of $+6$ μC and -15 μC. The first results in a current with zero net charge, as the $+15$ and -15 balance each other out. However, the asymmetrical phases of the middle example will result in a pulse with a net charge of $+9$ μC while the third example will result in a net charge of -9 μC. In this case, one electrode will remain more negative than the other while one remains more positive as long as the current flows. When the current has zero net charge, there is no sustained polarity and each electrode alternates equally from being the anode or cathode according to the frequency. With unbalanced waveforms, one electrode will maintain a great negativity and the other positivity; in this case, there is a true anode and cathode, depending on the net charge under each.

There are only three commonly used currents that do not result in zero net charge and thus can result in

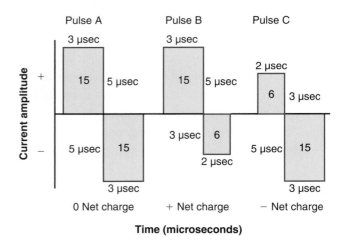

Total charge in each phase is in microcoulombs (μC)

Fig 9•20 The combination of amplitude and duration creates an "area under the curve" that represents the total charge delivered. Pulse A is symmetrical and balanced with equal amounts of charge in each phase, resulting in zero net charge. Pulses B and C are asymmetrical and unbalanced, resulting in net charge.

the accumulation of charge with a specific polarity: DC, monophasic pulsed current, and asymmetrical unbalanced biphasic current. The significance of not having zero net charge is that biological tissues respond differently when anodal and cathodal stimulation are sustained at an electrode. These reactions are presented in the "Electrochemical Effects" section of this chapter.

Most therapeutic uses of monophasic pulsed current and asymmetrical unbalanced waveforms incorporate interphase and interpulse intervals long enough to minimize any polar effects while still allowing for therapeutic benefit. Monophasic pulsed current is commonly used in wound care specifically for the effects seen at each pole (see Chapter 14 for treatment details). In contrast, DC does not have such intervals. Thus, charge continues to accumulate at each electrode. Without attention to amplitude, the polar effect of DC can be quite dramatic and potentially harmful. In fact, reactions ranging from itching to skin burns can occur. However, electrotherapeutic devices that use these three currents typically have lower peak amplitudes, lower frequencies, and long interphase and interpulse intervals, essentially allowing the charge to dissipate without damaging tissue.

KEY POINT! Many clinical electrical devices offering symmetrical biphasic or asymmetrical balanced waveforms have lead wires with a black and red or white lead. To those unfamiliar with principles of electrical waveforms, this would seem to indicate a cathode and anode, respectively. However, neither of these waveforms result in a net charge or polarity, so the designation of a cathode and anode is meaningless.

Besides the amplitude and time characteristics used to describe pulsed current, other descriptors aid in describing and differentiating waveforms and, thus, therapeutic effects (Box 9-6 and Fig. 9-21). *Frequency* is the term used to describe the number of pulses occurring in 1 second and is reported as pulses per second (pps). Earlier it was stated that frequency, in hertz (Hz), is used to describe the number of times AC switches direction in 1 second. However, hertz and pulses per second are both used to describe the frequency of pulsed current. A lesser used derivative of frequency (but still relevant to the discussion of electrotherapy) is *period*.

Box 9•6	**Describing Pulsed Current: The Bottom Line**

When describing pulsed current, three *basic* characteristics need to be specified:
- The waveform type and shape (e.g., symmetrical biphasic square)
- The pulse frequency (e.g., 50 hertz)
- The pulse duration (e.g., 400 microseconds)

Figure 9-21 shows a flow diagram of the various waveforms and the key parameters to be considered with each.

Period is the inverse of frequency and is calculated as $1/f$. In other words, the period is the time from one point on a waveform to the identical part on the next pulse. For example, a pulsed current occurring one thousand times per second (1,000 Hz) has a period of 1/1,000, or 0.001. Thus a new pulse occurs every 1 msec.

KEY POINT! Oftentimes, an electrotherapeutic device or current used for pain control, edema control, or muscle performance enhancement will be described by its frequency as high, medium, or low. There remains no universally accepted definition of these terms; therefore, their use is not recommended.

Clinical Principles in Practice: Frequency

Delivering pulses more or less frequently can have a dramatic effect. Using a TENS unit and the electrodes over the wrist extensor muscles, set the pulse duration and frequency as low as possible. Increase the intensity until a small but visible muscle twitch occurs. Now slowly increase the frequency. What happens? Delivery of more frequent pulses increases the total amount of charge delivered per unit time, and the response of the muscle is greater. The increased muscle response is directly related to the increased frequency of pulses delivered.

Physiological Response to Electrical Current

The effects of ES are variable and are based on the specific type of current applied, the parameters of those currents, and the dosage. There are three general electrophysiological effects that occur with the delivery of electrical current: chemical, thermal, and physical.

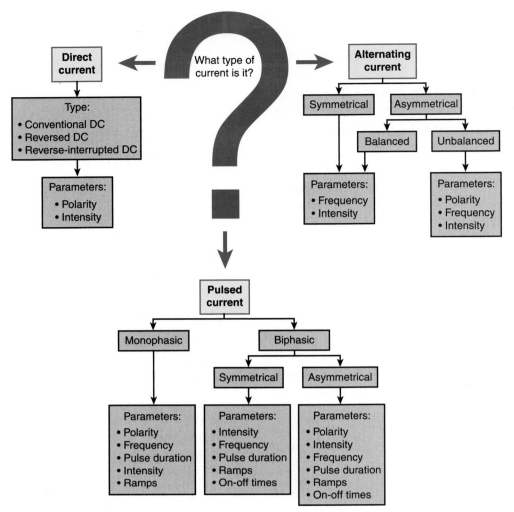

Fig 9•21 Classification of waveforms and key parameters.

Electrochemical Effects

The flow or movement of electrical current through the body is due to the movement of ions in the fluid component of bodily tissues. Excluding blood, our body's extracellular fluid environment is largely salt water due to the concentrations of sodium and chloride (sodium chloride; $NaCl$). In response to electrical stimulation, $NaCl$ is split into Na^+ and Cl^- ions. Like magnets do when they come close to other magnets, the Na^+ and Cl^- ions move according to the principles of charge or electricity. Thus, the positively charged Na^+ will migrate toward the cathode and the negatively charged Cl^- will move toward the anode (Box 9-7).

At the cathode, Na^+ joins with water to form sodium hydroxide, an alkaline reaction. This results in a localized area of pH greater than the pH of 7.4 of extracellular fluid. At the anode, Cl^- joins with water in an acidic reaction to form hydrochloric acid (HCl), thereby creating a localized acidic environment with pH less than 7.4. The localized accumulation of Na^+ at the cathode secondary to an applied electrical field causes water to move with Na^+ via ionohydrokinesis.[7] The local increase in water at the cathode results in a

Box 9•7	Localized Effects of Sustained Charge[7]	
	Anode (+)	Cathode (−)
Attracts	Cl^-	Na^+
Forms	HCl	$NaOH$
Process	Sclerotic	Sclerolytic
Effect	Skin hardens	Skin softens*

* Increases risk of electrical burn and tissue damage to DC.

decrease in the protein density of the local tissue, thereby softening the tissues and imparting a sclerolytic effect. In contrast, the localized accumulation of Cl⁻ at the anode results in an acidic effect, a decrease in local water content with subsequent increase in protein density, and a hardening, or sclerotic, effect.[7]

KEY POINT! To remember the local effects of charge, it may be helpful to remember the following: If your car breaks down and you don't have AAA, you might have to take a CAB (anode attracts acid and cathode attracts base).

If the current is DC or monophasic pulsed current, the Na^+ and Cl^- ions will continue to accumulate at the cathode and anode, respectively, as long as the current continues to flow. If the current is alternating or biphasic and changing directions at a specific frequency, then Na^+ and Cl^- moves back and forth between the electrodes. Recall that with AC and biphasic currents, each electrode alternates being the cathode or anode as the direction of current flow changes. Adverse effects of ES resulting from acidic or alkaline reactions at the electrode-skin interface are more common with DC current and, to a lesser extent, monophasic pulsed currents.

KEY POINT! Most monophasic pulsed currents (e.g., high-volt pulsed current [HVPC]) have such short pulse durations and long interpulse intervals that any charge accumulated at the electrode-skin interface dissipates before causing lasting adverse polar effects.

Electrothermal Effects

The laws of thermodynamics tell us that energy is neither created nor destroyed but rather exchanged, and during this exchange, some energy will be lost in the form of heat. As charged particles move through a conductor, the friction encountered by the particles results in microvibration of the conductor's elements.[2] This friction and vibration reflect kinetic energy created by moving parts, and heat is a product of this energy. The amount of heat produced in biological tissues depends on the amount of current flowing, the resistance to the current, and the duration the current flows.

Because the skin resists the transcutaneous delivery of current, accumulation of heat at the skin is a concern. Superficial hair, calloused skin, dried skin caused by alcohol cleansers, and lotions and oils increase skin resistance; shaving hair and removing lotions and oils reduces skin resistance. The redness noted under electrodes following stimulation is the most common result of the thermal or electrochemical effects of current.

Electrothermal heating is of greater concern when using DC current than with AC or pulsatile current. This is due to the nature of the currents. Because DC is a continuous flow of current in one direction, it is necessary to keep the current amplitude low so as to avoid overheating the tissue. Most clinical applications using DC current will be less than 5 mA, permitting applications of several minutes. AC currents pose less risk of burn, because current does not flow in one direction for very long. Pulsatile current poses significantly less risk of heating because the interpulse intervals result in a lower average current. The most common clinical sign of adverse electrothermal effects is redness of the skin lasting longer than a few hours.

Electrophysical Effects

The ability to depolarize and propagate electrical signals is what allows nerve and muscle cells to be excitable and to communicate with each other. An understanding of the electrophysical effects of current must begin at the cell. The electrophysical responses underlying the therapeutic effects of electrical stimulation are based on activation, or depolarization, of cells. The specific types of cells stimulated will differ based on several factors, including electrode location, current type and amplitude, and the integrity of the patient's neuromuscular system.

At rest, living cells maintain a separation of charge across the cell membrane such that a net negativity exists in the intracellular environment. This separation of charge represents an electrical potential, or, in other words, a voltage difference. The separation of charge is maintained by the selective permeability of the cell membrane to specific ions within the intra- and extracellular environments—chiefly sodium (Na^+) and potassium (K^+).[3] The resting membrane is relatively, but not completely, impermeable to Na^+, which is held in greater concentration outside the cell. In contrast, the resting membrane is significantly more permeable to K^+, which is held in greater concentration inside the cell. However, driven by concentration gradients, small amounts of Na^+ leak into the cell and K^+ leaks out of the cell. Adenosine triphosphate (ATP)–driven Na-K^+ pumps help to maintain the separation of ions by transporting 3 Na^+ out of the cell to every 2 K^+ back into the cell. The resultant effect of 3 Na^+ out to 2 K^+ in is a net negativity on the inside of the cell and the creation of an electrical potential. This potential across the cell membrane is termed the *resting membrane potential* (RMP) and varies for different types of cells based on the relative permeability to Na^+ and K^+. For neuronal cells, the RMP of the membrane (the neurolemma) is roughly –70 mV, whereas the RMP of the membrane of skeletal muscle (the sarcolemma) is closer to –90 mV and that of cardiac myocytes is –85 mV.[3]

The separation of charge across the cell membrane by the Na-K^+ pump results in the cell's polarization. So what is the significance of being polarized? In order to be depolarized, the cell membrane must have been polarized. In the presence of a chemical, thermal, physical, or electrical stimulus, the permeability of the cell membrane to Na^+ is increased, resulting in a reduction in the RMP. The process of depolarization reflects a reduction of the RMP and movement of ions across the cell membrane; the fundamental physiological effect of electrical stimulation is depolarization of the cell membrane.[3]

When applying this information to the clinical use of ES, it should be noted that electrodes are used to deliver therapeutic currents. As current flows from positive to negative between electrodes, the concentration of negatively charged ions or electrons at the cathode induces the depolarization of the cell membrane that, when a critical threshold of depolarization is reached, will depolarize the cell; this precipitates the process of depolarization along the cell membrane. Because the RMP of the neurolemma has a threshold for activation at –70 mV, the application of electrical stimulation elicits its electrophysical effects by first depolarizing the nerve. This is a key point when discussing the differences between using ES to activate innervated muscle versus using ES to activate denervated muscle. More details of using ES to stimulate innervated and denervated muscle are presented in Chapter 11.

Clinical Controversy

It is a common misconception that electrical stimulation to contract muscle works by directly stimulating the muscle fibers. This is not accurate, assuming the muscle maintains normal innervations. The nerve, with an RMP of –70 mV, will depolarize before the muscle cell with an RMP of –90 mV. Activation of innervated skeletal muscle occurs by first depolarizing the nerve and then propagating the stimulus along the motor axon, across the neuromuscular junction, and the across the sarcolemma.

Response of Excitable Tissues to Stimulation

For an electrical stimulus to depolarize the cell and elicit an action potential, it must be of sufficient strength and duration. If strength (e.g., current amplitude) and duration (e.g., pulse duration) are insufficient, the cell is not depolarized and the generation and propagation of action potentials is not initiated. The "stimulus" is an electrical pulse or, more commonly, a series of pulses. The relationship between stimuli of sufficient amplitude and duration to successfully depolarize the cell is such that stimuli of increasingly shorter duration require a nonlinearly increasing amplitude. For nerve and muscle cells, there is not a single strength and duration but rather a range of stimulus combinations with varying strength and duration capable of depolarizing the cell and thus generating action potentials. If these combinations were determined and plotted for a given nerve, the graphic depiction would yield a strength-duration curve (S-D curve) (Fig. 9-22). The line of the

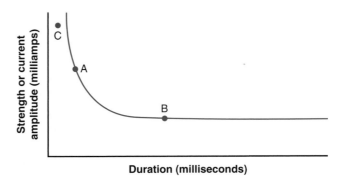

Fig 9•22 Strength-duration curve. Points A and B represent two combinations of stimulus amplitude and duration capable of eliciting a motor response. The stimulus point C is incapable of eliciting a response, as the pulse duration is too short despite the greater intensity.

curve reflects stimuli of minimally sufficient strength or amplitude and duration to stimulate the tissue.

The various combinations of strength and duration in Figure 9-22 reflect the assortment of parameter options that can be used to stimulate the given nerve or muscle. Both stimulus A and B are capable of exciting the cell, but stimulus B, with a much lower amplitude, may be more comfortable to the patient. Furthermore, as can be seen from the S-D curve, stimuli of very short duration cannot bring the cell to depolarization despite the amplitude (see stimulus C). Stimuli exceeding the minimal strength and duration capable of depolarizing the cell are termed *suprathreshold stimuli*. In contrast, stimuli with amplitude and duration not capable of depolarizing the cell are termed *subthreshold stimuli*.

Earlier in this chapter, the amplitude and duration of a pulse were used to draw a visual representation of the waveform. The area under the curve, termed the *phase charge*, was shown to increase by increasing the amplitude or the duration of the stimulus. The S-D curve is the physical manifestation of this principle, as each point on the S-D curve represents a different combination of stimulus (pulse) strength and duration that can stimulate tissue. Consider Figure 9-22 again: Moving from left to right on the curve, as the intensity of the stimulus is decreased, the tissue may still be excited by increasing the duration. In contrast, as the duration of a pulse is decreased, the amplitude must increase to excite the tissue.

Testing of all the possible combinations of strength and duration capable of exciting a tissue is not feasible, as most clinical devices have a limited pulse duration. The S-D curve reflects the graphical plot of each nerve or muscle tested during strength duration testing. From the S-D curve, two objective pieces of information are derived. *Rheobase* is the minimum strength (mA) of a stimulus of very long duration that is capable of eliciting a minimally detectable motor response (Fig. 9-23). Once rheobase is determined, it is possible to determine chronaxie—the duration (μsec or msec) of a stimulus two times the rheobase strength capable of eliciting a minimally detectable motor response. Chronaxie can be used to assess the integrity of the tissue, as healthy innervated tissue should have a chronaxie less than 1 msec. Prolonged chronaxie, often 10- to 20-fold longer, is indicative of denervation or other

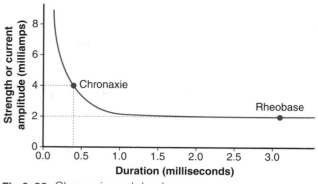

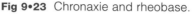

Fig 9·23 Chronaxie and rheobase.

pathology involving the excitability of the tissue.[4] Technological advances in neurodiagnostics have rendered S-D testing obsolete, but nevertheless, observing a tissue's response to stimuli of varying strength and duration is valuable in understanding tissue responses to electrical stimulation (Box 9-8).

Using a stimulus with an amplitude or duration greater than that minimally capable of eliciting an action potential will not alter or change the action potential. Action potentials are generated in an "all-or-nothing" manner, so a stimulus with an amplitude or duration greater than minimally required will not generate a larger or bigger action potential, and no action potential will be generated if the minimally required amplitude and duration are not reached.

Box 9·8	Using a TENS Unit for a Modified Strength-Duration Curve

If you have a TENS unit with manual controls for pulse duration and intensity, you can perform a modified strength-duration curve. (Most clinical stimulators do not have a pulse duration long enough to complete a full S-D curve.) Place two small electrodes of one channel of the TENS unit on your wrist extensors or arm. Set the pulse duration as high as possible and set the frequency at 3 to 5 Hz. Then slowly increase the intensity, looking for a small but visible motor response (i.e., twitches). Note the intensity required to elicit this response. Now slowly decrease the pulse duration approximately 20% and note what happens. The motor response will diminish. To return the motor response to the prior level, you must increase the intensity. Repeat this process of decreasing the pulse duration by 20% and noting the increase in intensity required to maintain the motor response as a small but visible motor twitch. If you plot these combinations of pulse duration and intensity, you will have performed a modified S-D test and experienced firsthand the relationship between stimulus strength and duration.

KEY POINT! When failing to elicit a motor response, a common misconception is that the patient is denervated when in fact the device used probably does not offer a combination of strength and duration capable of eliciting a motor response. Further neurodiagnostic testing may be needed for patients who show abnormal or absent responses to stimulation.

The S-D curve is based on the stimulus parameters capable of eliciting a minimally detectable motor response, but different nerve types have their own combinations of strength and duration needed for excitation. When a nerve is excited, the excitatory response is dependent on the stimulus parameters but also on two other key factors: nerve size and location of the electrodes. Most applications of clinical electrical stimulation involve stimulation of a peripheral nerve. Peripheral nerves are commonly termed *mixed peripheral nerves* to reflect the various nerve subtypes contained within a peripheral nerve. Nerve fibers within a peripheral nerve differ in diameter and in their resistance to excitation.[8] In the presence of a stimulus of sufficient strength and duration, nerve fibers with the greatest diameter and lowest resistance will depolarize first. The largest of the nerve fibers within a mixed peripheral nerve are the A-alpha (A-α) carrying motor and proprioceptive signals; thus, these are first to be depolarized (Table 9-1). To excite the smaller diameter A-β fibers (touch and pressure sensation) and even smaller diameter A-δ (pain and temperature) and C fibers (pain), stimuli of progressively greater amplitude and duration are required. In comparison, to directly depolarize the muscle membrane of a denervated muscle, stimuli of significantly greater amplitude and duration are required.

Although larger diameter nerve fibers are more easily excited, the location of the fibers to the electrodes will affect the order of recruitment. The fibers closest to the electrode will be excited before those fibers farther away (Fig. 9-24). But among those fibers that are stimulated, the largest will still be excited before the smaller. Fibers deeper or farther from the stimulating current can be stimulated by increasing the amplitude of the stimulus. Thus, A-β sensory nerves of the superficial dermis are activated before the larger diameter A-α, which lie deeper. This largely explains why you feel the stimulus before a motor response is noted.

The strength-duration relationship describes the amplitude and duration characteristics of a single stimulus (i.e., pulse) capable of depolarizing the cell and eliciting a single action potential. However, single action potentials do not lead to purposeful muscle activity. The tension created in a muscle fiber twitch from a single action potential will completely decrease unless followed by a subsequent action potential. If the frequency of action potentials is increased, the

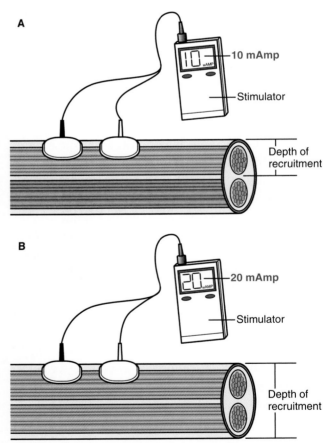

Fig 9•24 (A) With stimulation to a mixed peripheral nerve, large-diameter fibers will be recruited before smaller-diameter fibers. (B) Increasing the stimulus amplitude will recruit more fibers, as the electrical stimulus is able to reach and depolarize a greater number of nerve fibers.

Table 9•1	**Differentiation of Mixed Peripheral Nerve**	
	Function	**Diameter**
Type A		
Alpha (α)	Proprioception, motor	12–20 *um*
Beta (β)	Touch, pressure	5–12 *um*
Delta (δ)	Pain, temperature	2–5 *um*
Type C		
Dorsal root	Pain	0.4–1.2 *um*

subsequent muscle fiber twitches will occur before the previous one has decreased, resulting in increased tension. *Twitch summation* refers to the addition, or summation, of tension in individual muscle fibers, thereby resulting in greater whole muscle tension. This occurs because the duration of a fiber twitch may be less than 100 to a few 100 milliseconds, whereas an action potential can be generated every 1 to 5 milliseconds, allowing action potentials to come before the muscle fibers have completely relaxed. Longer duration and greater muscle tension occurs with increasing frequency of stimulation, so even though a single action potential in a muscle fiber generates twitch tension, greater tension can be realized by increasing the frequency of stimulation.[3] The relationship between stimulation frequency and muscle force is called the *force-frequency relationship*. When the muscle fibers are stimulated so frequently that the tension generated in the fibers does not have time to decrease between action potentials, the tension is sustained; this is termed *tetany*.

Levels of Response to Electrical Stimulation

There are three levels of response to therapeutic electrical stimulation: sensory, motor, and noxious (although, most of the time, we are not trying to produce noxious stimulation). With stimuli of relatively low amplitudes that can still excite the nerve, the first perception of an electrical stimulus is often described as pins and needles or tapping secondary to excitation of A-β fibers in the superficial dermis. If the amplitude and duration of the stimulus is increased, excitation of the A-α fibers (alpha motor neurons) will occur and a motor response will be elicited. The magnitude of the motor response is proportional to the intensity of the stimulus (up to a point); thus, the initial motor response may appear as fasciculations or small twitches in the muscle. With increasing amplitude, the motor response will increase to a more full and robust contraction. Further description of the effect of muscle fiber recruitment and therapeutic effects of ES appears in Chapter 11.

With further increases in amplitude or duration beyond that capable of eliciting sensory and motor responses, the A-δ and C fibers are excited, eliciting the perception of pain. This is the third level of response to electrical stimulation. Eliciting a noxious-level response

Clinical Principles in Practice: Electrode Placement

When you attempt to elicit a muscle contraction, your patient reports the onset of strong tingling and then pain, but you do not see a motor response. What could be the cause of this? If the electrodes are not placed over areas of A-α nerves (i.e., motor tissue), the stimulus is incapable of eliciting a motor response because there is little to no motor tissue in the area stimulated. Relocation of the electrodes to regions where the alpha motor neurons exist or to areas of more depolarizable muscle tissue will yield the desired motor response.

is sometimes used for therapeutic purposes, as will be described in Chapter 10.

The first time most students and patients use therapeutic electrical stimulation, it is common to see a low tolerance level to stimulation. Upon subsequent applications, tolerance usually improves, allowing use of stimulus parameters suitable for the clinical goals to be achieved. If a patient is unable to tolerate the stimulus parameters required to elicit the necessary therapeutic effect, the efficacy of this treatment is greatly compromised. For example, when using stimulation to improve the strength of skeletal muscle, the patient must be able to tolerate an intensity that is sufficient to activate the muscle at a level consistent with eliciting adaptation. If the patient is unable to tolerate the stimulus needed to elicit an appropriate motor response, an alternative approach to facilitate muscle activation should be selected. The first attempt at using ES can be considered a familiarization session, allowing the patient an opportunity to experience the stimulus while you fully explain the anticipated sensations and effects. In addition, to completely educate your patient regarding their experience, you must undergo therapeutic ES yourself.

Therapeutic Currents by Name: Variations of the Basic Currents

Once you choose to include ES in the intervention plan, you must then determine the stimulus characteristics, including the type of waveform, to elicit the desired response, whether that is motor activation (e.g., muscle contraction), sensory stimulation (e.g., a "buzzing sensation" with no muscle contraction), or something else. Most units in clinical settings today are multiwaveform devices offering more than one type of current waveform and thus more than one type of potential response or effect. Even though all waveforms are derived from DC, AC, or pulsed current, variations in the specific parameters of these three currents are what differentiates the many therapeutic currents used today. By modulating previously described basic parameters of current, a myriad of waveforms and subsequent electrobiophysical effects are possible. Therefore, it is critical to understand currents and waveforms in order to maximize the potential of electrotherapeutics.

Much confusion is created by the various and inconsistent use of waveform names, in part due to the industry's enthusiasm in marketing equipment and trying to claim the "leading edge" with a new current or feature. When discussing electrotherapeutics, inconsistency in terminology leads to confusion and, more often, miscommunication and misunderstanding. Therefore, it is recommended that waveforms be described by the specific parameters that constitute the waveform rather than terms or names perpetuated by clinical lingo. Often times, these clinical names are fleeting, coming and going like fashion trends. To help the clinician decide which waveform to use and how to differentiate them, the more popular or common

waveforms will be described here using their popularized names with some description as to their clinical use. Greater explanation of their clinical use and evidence for use will be presented in later chapters addressing specific therapeutic applications.

Russian Current

Perhaps the most widely recognized waveform in clinical use today is Russian current, named after Dr. Yakov Kots, a Russian exercise physiologist credited for popularizing this waveform in the 1970s. Touting strength gains up to 40% in elite Russian Olympic athletes, Kots's claims were significant because they represented gains in healthy individuals, something previously unrealized. Significant gains in muscular strength and power beyond that accompanying training were attributed to use of the Russian current, thus increasing its popularity.[9] Russian current is simply a variation of alternating current. Conventional Russian current as described by Kots is a 2,500 Hz alternating sinusoidal current that is interrupted and delivered in short bursts. This is termed *burst modulation* and is a defining characteristic of Russian current. The bursts are delivered at 50 bursts per second with a burst duration of 10 msec and an interburst interval of 10 msec (Fig. 9-25). The

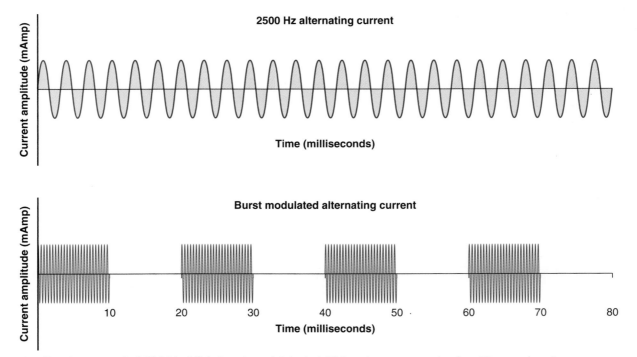

Fig 9•25 Russian current: 2,500 Hz AC is burst modulated at 50 bursts per second using 10-msec bursts.

frequency of the sine wave that is interrupted into bursts is called the *carrier frequency* (most commonly 2,500 Hz). Within each 10-msec burst, there are 25 complete cycles of AC. This results in a waveform with a therapeutic, or treatment, frequency of 50 Hz and 400 μsec cycle duration (i.e., 1/2,500 cycles per second), which is well suited for activating skeletal muscle.

The original Russian 10/50/10 protocol calls for 10-second contraction time and 50-second off-time for 10 repetitions.[9] Because the burst duration is equal to the interburst interval, Russian current is often described as having a 50% duty cycle. This duty cycle is different than defined earlier, which was on-time divided by total-time × 100%. The 50% duty cycle of Russian current is a "relative" duty cycle, sometimes referred to as *Russian duty cycle,* while the actual duty cycle of a 10-second on/50-second off protocol would be 16.7% (10/60 × 100%). The 50% relative duty cycle and 400-μsec pulse duration are two of the proposed benefits of burst modulated AC for muscle strengthening. Simply stated, when Russian current is "on," it is on for a long time. However, the evidence for burst modulated AC (i.e., Russian current) versus other waveforms for muscle strengthening remains inconclusive.[9–12] In 2009, Ward[13] reported that the evidence for Russian current ranges from a single case study reporting increased strength[14] to evidence of no increase in strength.[15] Only two studies have examined whether Russian current is the best form of AC current for increasing strength, and both studies found a 1,000 Hz carrier frequency elicited greater torque than 2,500 Hz. Data also indicated that burst durations of 2 to 5 msec may be better suited for muscle stimulation in comparison to the 10-msec burst duration of conventional Russian current.[16,17]

> **KEY POINT!** A variation on Russian current is "Aussie" current—a 1,000 Hz burst modulated AC current delivered in 4-msec bursts. Greater torque production and decreased rate of muscle fatigue have been reported with the Aussie current compared to conventional 2,500 Hz, 10-msec burst waveform of Russian current.[6,18]

Clinical Principles in Practice: Using Russian Current in the Clinic

A patient is referred for strengthening of the quadriceps following right total knee arthroplasty. Assessment reveals 4– strength of the right quadriceps. The clinician chooses to use Russian current waveform to stimulate the quadriceps to facilitate strengthening. A device offering Russian current is selected, and the quadriceps are stimulated for 10-second contractions with 50-second rest periods between the 10 maximal contractions used in this session.

High-Volt Pulsed Current

High-voltage currents gained popularity in the 1970s with interest in using currents of high amplitude. High-volt pulsed current (HVPC), also known as *high volt* or *high volt pulsed galvanic,* is a twin-peaked monophasic pulsed current waveform with peak voltage typically reaching 150 to 500 V, a short pulse duration typically lasting 50 to 100 μsec, and a frequency of 1 to 120 Hz[20] (Fig. 9-26). However, the term *galvanic,* traditionally given to interrupted DC, is no longer preferred, as it does not accurately reflect the waveform characteristics of HVPC.

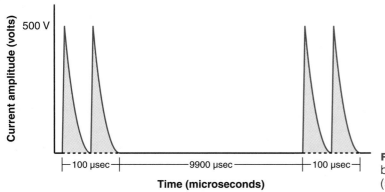

Fig 9•26 High-volt pulsed current is characterized by a high peak intensity and short pulse duration (shown at a frequency of 100 Hz).

Because use of high-voltage pulses necessitates very short pulse durations in order to avoid tissue damage, HVPC uses a twin peak pulse with an almost instantaneous rise time and immediate exponential fall-time—thus the name "twin-peak" monophasic.[19] The short pulse duration, typically up to 100 microseconds, and long interpulse interval result in a low relative duty cycle, often 1% or less.[21,22] This long interpulse interval permits use of high-peak voltages yet results in a much lower average current over the entire duty cycle.[20] The product is a high-peak voltage but overall low average treatment voltage.

KEY POINT! To understand the high-intensity voltage and short pulse duration of HVPC, think about touching a very hot stove. The high heat of the stove can be very dangerous, but if you touch it very quickly and infrequently, there is little to no risk of burn. However, if you touch the stove for longer time and more frequently, you may burn yourself.

HVPC is a monophasic waveform, which means one electrode will accumulate negative charge (cathode) and the other will accumulate positive charge (anode). One electrode is placed over the treatment area; this is the active, or treatment, electrode. The other electrode is placed at some site away from the treatment site; this is the reference, or dispersive, electrode. Most devices on the market offering HVPC will allow you to select the polarity of the active, or treatment, electrode as either positive or negative. The dispersive, or reference, electrode consequently becomes the other polarity. Some modern and many older versions of HVPC devices use a dispersive electrode that is much larger in relation to the active electrodes (Fig. 9-27). This and the ability to choose a polarity of the current are classic telltale signs that the device generates a monophasic pulsed current and is likely a HVPC unit, but the best way to tell is by reading the machine's user manual. Clinical uses and what specific effects are attributed to the anode or cathode of a monophasic waveform are presented in Chapter 14.

HVPC is typically administered using one of three modes: continuous, reciprocating, or surge. *Continuous mode* refers to the continuous and uninterrupted flow of pulsatile current for the entire treatment session. This is not to be confused with direct current, as

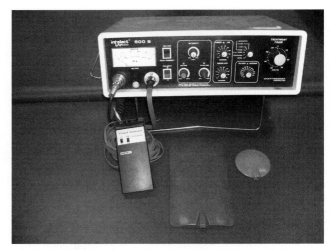

Fig 9•27 An identifying characteristic of many high-volt pulsed current devices is a large dispersive electrode.

HVPC is the flow of monophasic pulsed current not DC. Continuous mode does not have on and off times, as would be used in activating skeletal muscle, but rather remains on until the current is turned off. With continuous mode, the amplitude of each pulse remains constant throughout the duration of the session.

Reciprocating mode delivers current first to one of the active electrodes, then to the other active electrode (assuming more than two active electrodes) in an alternating or reciprocating manner. This mode does not alter the flow of current to the dispersive pad but simply reciprocates the flow between the two active electrodes. If only one active electrode is used, reciprocating mode is not chosen. Clinicians select the time that current flows at each electrode before switching. With reciprocating mode, the amplitude of each pulse remains constant throughout the duration of the session unless the clinician adjusts it; this is called *balancing*. Balancing allows the peak intensity of the current at one or both active electrodes to be decreased by a selected percentage. For example, the current in one active electrode may be dampened by 25% to accommodate a sensitive placement site.

Finally, *surge mode* modulates the amplitude of the pulse train so that the amplitude of each successive pulse progressively increases to a peak over the duration of the on-time. This is similar to the ramp-up function of other pulsatile currents.

The specific waveform characteristics of HVPC (amplitude, frequency, and pulse duration) make it possible to stimulate both sensory and motor nerves, so HVPC is used for a variety of clinical purposes. Pain modulation, activation of skeletal muscle, and tissue healing are the most common uses. Because HVPC has a true anode and cathode, it has become a widely used and evidenced waveform for tissue repair and wound healing.[23,24] Tissue repair and wound healing are undoubtedly the areas of use that have the greatest degree of support for HVPC. (More information on use of electrical stimulation for tissue healing appears in Chapter 14.) Modifying the pulse duration and frequency of HVPC can yield a waveform similar to conventional TENS for electroanalgesia, making HVPC useful in managing pain.

Because HVPC can stimulate skeletal muscle, it has also been used for muscle reeducation. Keeping in mind the strength-duration relationship of a stimulus, the very short pulse duration of HVPC necessarily requires a high-intensity stimulus, and this is often perceived as painful by the patient. In contrast to the 400-μsec pulse duration and 50% relative duty cycle of Russian current, the 100-μsec duration and 1% relative duty cycle of HVPC is considerably less. To date, there is no sufficient evidence to support using HVPC to strengthen muscle despite its ability to stimulate skeletal muscle. The bottom line for using HVPC to strengthen muscle is this: Simply because HVPC can elicit a motor response does not make it suitable—or, more importantly, effective—for that purpose. Other waveforms more suitable to muscle activation and strengthening are available and are addressed in Chapter 11.

KEY POINT! Occasionally, therapeutic currents will be referred to "high volt" or "low volt"—terms that refer to the magnitude of the voltage used to drive the current. Conventional use of these terms has led to the designation that *high volt* refers to a current with a voltage in excess of 150 V and typically up to 500 V. In contrast, the term *low volt* is given to a current with a voltage less than 150 V.

Interferential Current

In the early to mid-2000s, interferential current (IFC) was reported to be the most popular and commonly used form of electrotherapy in Europe and Australia.[25] Although no such data is available for use in the United States, IFC remains a popular waveform here. IFC is derived from the interference or superimposition of two symmetrical but asynchronous, kilohertz frequency, sinusoidal alternating currents resulting in a single treatment, or interference, current with properties uniquely different than the original input currents.[26] The premise of IFC is that when two asynchronous kilohertz frequency (1 to 10 KHz) sinusoidal currents are directed to intersect or interfere, the waves are periodically in synch or in phase with each other, and the amplitudes of the two currents will sum together[27,28] (Fig. 9-28). This is termed *constructive interference*. Equally periodic, the currents will be out of phase, resulting in destructive interference, and the amplitudes will negate each other.[26] As the two currents go in and out of synch, the amplitude of the interference current gradually increases and decreases. Because of the modulation of amplitude, IFC is referred to as *amplitude modulated AC*.

The currents are maximally in or out of phase at a rate equal to the difference between frequencies of the currents interfered. For example, interference of a 4,000 Hz and a 4,100 Hz current, the lesser of which is termed the *carrier frequency*, results in an interference current of 100 Hz. This frequency is termed the *beat frequency* and typically ranges from 1 to 200 Hz. The amplitude of the IFC will peak and fall at a frequency equal to the beat frequency. The beat frequency reflects the therapeutic frequency—that is, the frequency that elicits the therapeutic effect. Most devices on the market today allow the clinician to select a specific beat frequency. A specific beat frequency can be obtained from a number of possible interference currents as long as the difference between the currents is the same. The physiological effects elicited by IFC are based on the beat frequency, not the frequencies of the input currents. For example, to elicit a tetanic muscle contraction, a beat frequency consistent with a tetanic response is used (e.g., 50 Hz). On most contemporary devices, the clinician selects the beat frequency while the carrier frequency is prefixed at 4,000 Hz. Still other devices permit the clinician to adjust the carrier frequency within 1,000 to 5,000 Hz. The effect of a lesser carrier frequency is a longer pulse duration; however, there remains no evidence to support the selection of one carrier frequency over another.

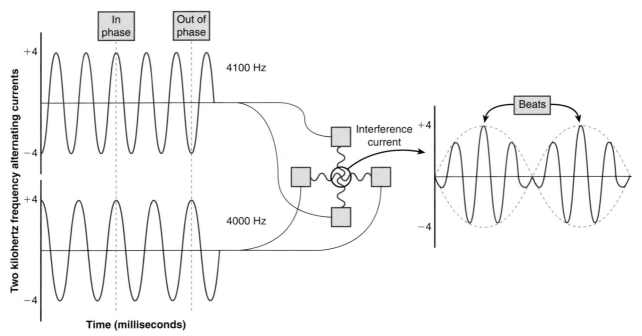

Fig 9•28 Interferential current is the interference of 2 asynchronous kilohertz frequency currents to form a current with amplitude modulation.

KEY POINT! ▶ A 100-Hz beat frequency is obtained from each of these input currents: 4,000 and 4,100 Hz; 2,500 and 2,600 Hz; 4,900 and 5,000 Hz; or any combination differing by 100 Hz.

Some IFC devices allow the frequencies of the input currents to be modulated, resulting in a modulated beat frequency (Fig. 9-29). This effect is termed *sweep* but is not available on all devices. Sweep is either a linear or peak-to-peak sweep. With linear sweep, the beat frequency is modulated continuously from a maximum to a minimum frequency, whereas a peak-to-peak sweep results in the alteration of the beat frequency between only the maximum and minimum[29] (Table 9-2). *Swing* is used to denote the temporal characteristics of the sweep pattern with "∧" used to denote a linear or continuous sweep and "∫" used to denote peak-to-peak sweep.[29] For example, a 2∧2 sweep from 100 to 10 Hz will decrease continuously from 100 Hz to 10 Hz over 2 seconds and then increase continuously and linearly over the next 2 seconds. In contrast, a 2∫2 sweep from 100 to 10 Hz denotes that the beat frequency remained at 100 Hz for 2 seconds before switching to 10 Hz for 2 seconds. The proposed benefits of sweep are a modulated rather than fixed beat frequency, thus avoiding accommodation, and the ability to use both high- and low-frequency stimulation within the same treatment, although these have not been substantiated.

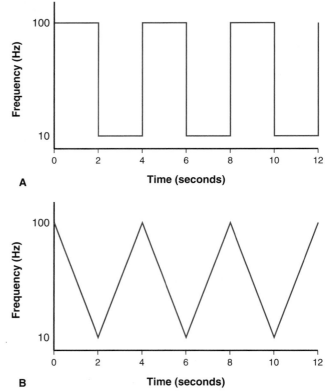

Fig 9•29 Sweep is modulation of the beat frequency of IFC and is either peak-to-peak or continuous. Swing represents the temporal characteristics of the sweep or the timing of the sweep. (A) A peak-to-peak sweep, denoted by "∫", alternates the beat frequency between only the lowest and highest beat frequency selected. (B) A continuous sweep, denoted by "∧", results in a beat frequency that progressively increases and decreases between the lowest to highest beat frequency selected.

Table 9•2 Language of Interferential Current

Parameter Frequency	Definition	Effect	Use
Carrier frequency	Lesser frequency of the two currents interfered		
Beat frequency	Frequency the interfered currents are maximally in and out of synch	Resultant frequency from interference of two KHz currents	The beat frequency determines the physiological effect
Sweep	Modulation of the beat frequency	Varies the beat frequency of the interference wave	To provide low and high frequency stimulation within the same treatment
Swing			
"∫"	Temporal characteristics of sweep	Alters the beat frequency from minimum to maximum	To use only the minimum and maximum beat frequencies
"∧"		Linear and continuous sweep between the minimum and maximum beat frequency	To use a continuously changing beat frequency from minimum to maximum
Vector scan	Amplitude modulation of the input currents	Increases the area of the interference pattern	To provide stimulation to a larger tissue area

KEY POINT! The increase and decrease in amplitude created by asynchronous currents going in and out of phase is similar to the effect of jumping on a trampoline with another person. When two jumpers are in synch, the height of the jump is increased, but when out of synch, the jumpers can cancel out each other's bounce.

IFC is administered using four electrodes positioned so that the two currents intersect each other perpendicularly. This is known as *quadripolar IFC* (Fig. 9-30). The point of intersection and site of the new interference current is assumed to be in the geometric center of the electrodes. However, this cannot be accurately determined because of nonhomogenous tissue resistances. Current will take the path of least resistance, so the path of one or both currents will probably be altered, resulting in interference at some point other than the one assumed.

The perpendicular interference of two currents results in a pattern that looks like a clover leaf electrical field (Fig. 9-31). To increase the area of the interference and stimulate greater tissue area, modulation to the interfered currents can be used. *Vector scan,* offered on some devices, is the modulation of the amplitude of one or both of the input currents, resulting in a rhythmic change in position of the interference pattern.[26] This is depicted as an oscillating clover-leaf shape,

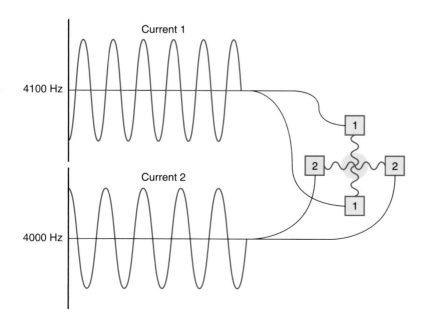

Fig 9•30 Quadripolar interferential current.

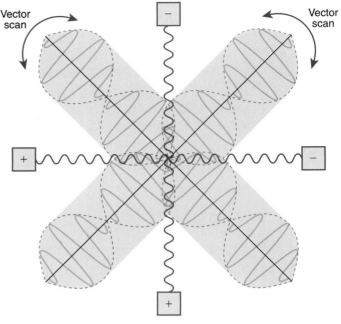

Fig 9•31 With the perpendicular interference of currents, a clover-leaf-shaped field of current is created. Vector scan is amplitude modulation resulting in expansion of the clover-leaf field.

much like the motion of the agitator of a washing machine rotating back and forth.

There are three proposed and theoretical advantages of IFC compared to other waveforms: (1) alternating sinusoidal currents with frequencies exceeding 1 KHz are hypothesized to more easily penetrate the skin due to reduced skin impedance; (2) the amplitudes of the two currents summate in the deeper tissues, thereby passing the more superficial sensory afferent nerves; and (3) a beat frequency of the interference current can be selected that is similar to other waveforms used for muscle stimulation and pain modulation.[5,25–27]

More recently, however, the proposed benefits of IFC have been questioned.[13] The proposed decrease in skin impedance noted with kilohertz frequency current is not specific to the frequency but rather to the short pulse duration necessarily associated with kilohertz frequencies. Skin impedance is directly related to pulse duration, not frequency, so that at very short pulse durations, impedance is reduced. If a pulsed current has a similar pulse duration as the kilohertz frequency current, the impedance across the skin is similarly low.[13] Furthermore, the interference pattern that characterizes IFC is not simply in the region geometrically predicted by electrode applications; rather, it is much more diffuse based on the nonhomogeneity of resistance in various tissues in the path of the current (Box 9-9).

Clinical Principles in Practice: Clinical Use of Interferential Current

A patient is referred for acute low back pain secondary to a lifting injury. Pain is local to the lumbar paraspinals, and active contraction of the muscles increases the pain. The clinician chooses interferential current to provide electroanalgesia. A treatment, or beat, frequency of 100 Hz is desired, so the clinician selects a carrier frequency of 4,000 Hz from one channel and 4,100 Hz for the second channel. The four electrodes of the two currents are applied paraspinally, such that the currents are directed to intersect perpendicularly. The stimulus intensity is increased until the patient reports a sensory level sensation.

Low-Intensity Direct Current (Microcurrent)

Technically speaking, microcurrent is any current with an amplitude less than 1 mA (10^{-3}A).[1] The microcurrent waveforms offered on electrotherapy devices are either

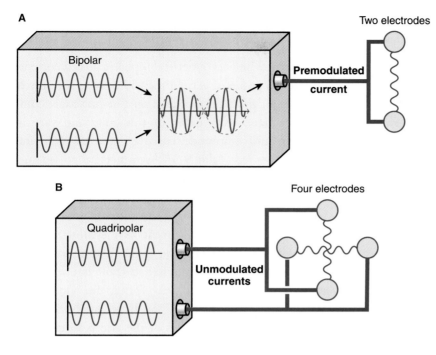

A

Bipolar

Premodulated current

Two electrodes

B

Quadripolar

Unmodulated currents

Four electrodes

Fig 9•32 (A) Premodulated (bipolar) IFC is created in the stimulator, resulting in a single current delivered by two electrodes. (B) Quadripolar IFC is created by two currents crossing in the tissues and is delivered by four electrodes.

DC or monophasic pulsed current. While *microcurrent* is the name by which this waveform is offered on many multiwaveform devices, it has also been called *low-volt pulsed current* (LVPC), *microelectrical neuromuscular stimulator* (MENS), or *microelectrical stimulation* (MES). A current of microamperage amplitude is insufficient to excite sensory or motor nerves. Thus, names implying stimulation of nerve or muscle are deceiving. Any notion of therapeutic benefit derived from activation of sensory or motor nerves is physiologically implausible.[20] The APTA recommends use of the term *low-intensity direct current* (LIDC) for this microamperage current.[1]

LIDC is typically DC or monophasic pulsed current with a peak current amplitude in the microamperage range. If the waveform is monophasic pulsed current, the pulse duration is dependent on the frequency. A typical pulse duration is 500 msec (0.5 sec)—much longer than most other pulsed currents. Frequency on most LIDC stimulators varies from 1 to 1,000 Hz. Because LIDC is either DC or monophasic, one electrode will remain the anode and the other the cathode. Unique behaviors or characteristics demonstrated by particular cell populations in response to anodal or cathodal stimulation have been reported.[30,31] A more specific discussion of cell and tissue responses to electrical stimulation appears in Chapter 14.

LIDC originated after observations of microamperage DC flowing out of injured tissue.[24,31,32] The outward flow of current indicated the presence of an electrical potential across the skin—termed the transepithelial potential (TEP). Different from the resting membrane potential of single cells, the TEP is created by the separation of ions across sheets of epithelial cells (i.e., skin; Fig. 9-33). This separation of ions across the skin leaves the external skin surface with a net negative charge, known as the *skin battery*.[24,32] When the skin is injured, a pathway is created that allows flow of positively charged ions from the deeper tissues to the skin surface.[32] As positive charges leave the injured tissue, the wound loses it positivity and becomes negative relative to the flow of positive ions to the surface. Because of this, the wound becomes the cathode of the current. In tissues lateral to the site of injury where the TEP is maintained, the concentration of positive ions now

Transepithelial Potential

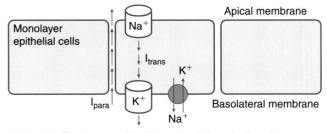

Monolayer epithelial cells

Apical membrane

Na^+

I_{trans}

K^+

I_{para}

K^+

Na^+

Basolateral membrane

Fig 9•33 The transepithelial potential underlies the "current of injury."

flows toward the wound cathode, creating what is termed *lateral currents of injury*. The outward flow of current and the lateral currents have been termed the *currents of injury*. Clinical use of LIDC is based on these endogenously produced currents and is intended to augment the current of injury.

KEY POINT! At low pulse durations and frequency, HVPC can result in current with microamperage intensity despite its name. If the frequency or pulse duration of HVPC is increased, the total current amplitude delivered is likely to exceed microamperage levels, resulting in milliamperage intensity.[20]

Clinical Principles in Practice: Clinical Use of Microcurrent

A patient is referred for treatment of a skin wound that has failed to close following an open reduction and internal fixation of the left distal radius 4 weeks ago. The clinician wants to facilitate tissue healing and chooses to use LIDC to stimulate epithelialization of the tissues. A device offering LIDC is chosen, and the anode of the current is placed over the wound site with the cathode placed adjacent to the wound.

Symmetrical and Asymmetrical Biphasic Pulsed Currents

Symmetrical and asymmetrical biphasic pulsed currents represent a group of waveforms widely used for muscle stimulation and pain modulation. The pulses are commonly square, rectangular, or triangular and vary in duration and amplitude based on the physiological response desired (Table 9-3). Asymmetrical pulsed currents are often included along with symmetrical biphasic pulsed currents on many clinical and handheld stimulators, yet there is little data to support or refute use of asymmetrical pulsed current over symmetrical for purposes of activating muscle or modulating pain.

Symmetrical biphasic pulsed current is one of the most commonly used waveforms for activating skeletal muscle along with the burst modulated AC (i.e., Russian). Most studies of the effects of electrical stimulation on skeletal muscle have used symmetrical biphasic pulsed or Russian current. Examination of the ability of each current to generate muscular torque has suggested that either there is little to no difference in the peak torque elicited[11] or that torque was greater using the biphasic pulsed current.[10]

Table 9•3 Waveforms, Uses, and Common Parameters

Type	Use	Waveform	Parameters	Settings
Russian	Activation of skeletal muscle for strengthening and endurance (NMES)	Burst modulated AC	Pulse duration:	200–600 μsec
			Frequency:	30–100 Hz
			Amplitude:	To maximal contraction for strengthening/endurance (NMES)
			Treatment Time:	10 sec on/50 sec off x ≥ 10 reps
			Ramp-up:	1–2 sec
			Ramp-down:	1–2 sec
High volt	Pain modulation	Twin-peak monophasic pulsed	Pulse duration:	50–100 μsec
			Frequency:	1–100 Hz
			Amplitude:	Sensory level: to perceivable level:
			Duration:	10–30 min
			Amplitude:	Motor level: to visible motor response:
			Duration:	1–30 min
	Wound/tissue healing		Pulse duration:	50–100 μsec
			Frequency:	100 Hz
			Amplitude:	Below sensory threshold
			Duration:	Several minutes

Russian waveform labels: 10 msec segments; High volt: 100 μsec

Table 9•3 Waveforms, Uses, and Common Parameters—cont'd

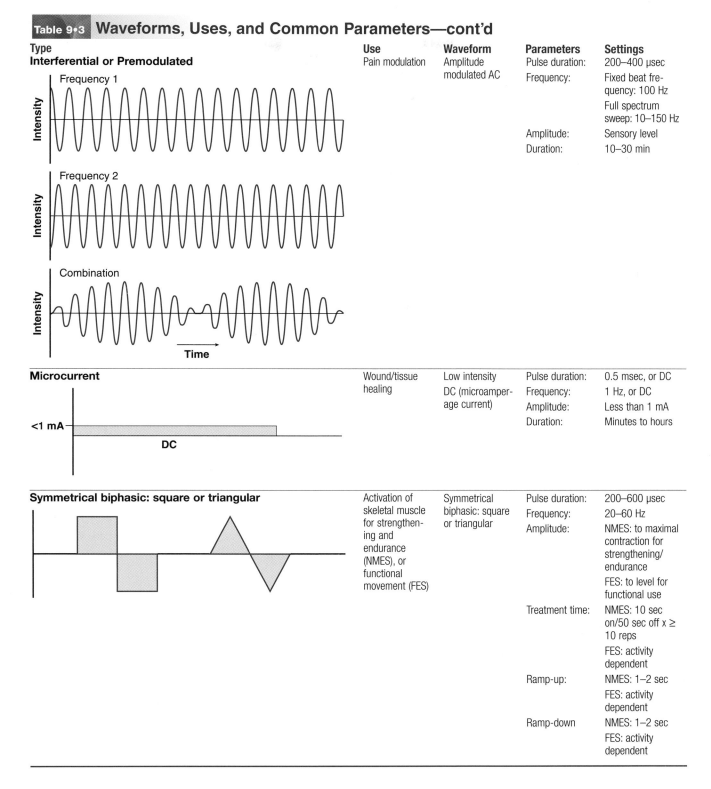

Type	Use	Waveform	Parameters	Settings
Interferential or Premodulated	Pain modulation	Amplitude modulated AC	Pulse duration:	200–400 µsec
			Frequency:	Fixed beat frequency: 100 Hz
				Full spectrum sweep: 10–150 Hz
			Amplitude:	Sensory level
			Duration:	10–30 min
Microcurrent	Wound/tissue healing	Low intensity DC (microamperage current)	Pulse duration:	0.5 msec, or DC
			Frequency:	1 Hz, or DC
			Amplitude:	Less than 1 mA
			Duration:	Minutes to hours
Symmetrical biphasic: square or triangular	Activation of skeletal muscle for strengthening and endurance (NMES), or functional movement (FES)	Symmetrical biphasic: square or triangular	Pulse duration:	200–600 µsec
			Frequency:	20–60 Hz
			Amplitude:	NMES: to maximal contraction for strengthening/ endurance
				FES: to level for functional use
			Treatment time:	NMES: 10 sec on/50 sec off x ≥ 10 reps
				FES: activity dependent
			Ramp-up:	NMES: 1–2 sec
				FES: activity dependent
			Ramp-down	NMES: 1–2 sec
				FES: activity dependent

A newer variation of symmetrical biphasic pulsed current is a burst modulated form in which three symmetrical square or rectangular biphasic pulses are delivered consecutively in each burst. It may be easier to think of this waveform as a burst modulated polyphasic waveform containing six phases with 100-µsec interphase intervals per burst (Fig. 9-34). The VMS™ Burst waveform is similar to burst modulated AC (i.e., Russian or Aussie currents), in that a kilohertz frequency carrier current can be delivered in a burst format with burst durations in the millisecond range. The burst duration is dependent on the phase duration selected. With typical phase durations

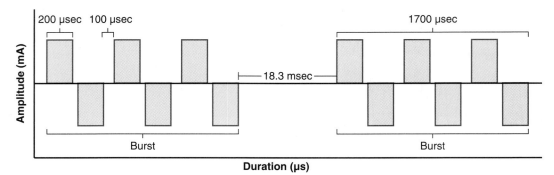

Fig 9•34 Burst modulated pulsed current. With six phase durations of 200 μsec and five interphase intervals of 100 μsec, the burst duration is 1.7 msec. Six phases (three biphasic pulses) in 1.7 msec equates to a carrier frequency of 1,675 Hz. At a burst frequency of 50 bps, the interburst interval is 18.3 msec, equating to a duty relative cycle of 9%.

of a few hundred microseconds, as is common for activating muscle, the burst duration and effective carrier frequency of this waveform are consistent with those examined by Ward and colleagues, [13,17] who suggested greater torque is elicited with burst durations of 2 to 5 msec and carrier frequencies less than 2,500 Hz. This burst modulated polyphasic current appears to be a viable waveform for activating skeletal muscle.

KEY POINT! When using the VMS™ Burst, it is critical to note that the phase duration, not pulse duration, is selected. Selecting a 200-μsec phase duration, and accounting for the five 100-μsec interphase intervals, the total burst duration is 1,700 μsec, or 1.7 msec (see Fig. 9-34). When the six phases (three biphasic pulses) in 1.7 msec bursts are compared to 50 phases (25 sinusoidal cycles) of AC in 10-msec bursts of Russian current, the effective carrier frequency of the VMS™ Burst waveform is easily calculated as 1,765 Hz (but only when the phase duration is 200 μsec). If the phase duration is increased to 400 μsec, the burst duration increases to 2,900 μsec, or 2.9 msec, and equates to a carrier frequency of 1,034 Hz.

The Bottom Line for Electrotherapy

Competent, safe, and effective use of electrical stimulation requires that the clinician understand the basics of electrotherapeutic currents and waveforms. Use of electrotherapy offers a variety of physiological effects that can be used to provide substantial therapeutic benefits to patients. While many variations of electrical waveforms have emerged over time, the electrophysiological effects remain relatively well understood. Recognizing the role of clinical electrotherapy in patient management and its potential offerings is a starting point.

Documentation Tips

Appropriate documentation of the application of electrical stimulation should include the following:

- Waveform:
  - Symmetrical biphasic square, twin-peak monophasic, Russian, interferential, etc.
- Waveform parameters (these will depend on the waveform used)
  - Pulse duration and frequency, amplitude, on and off time, ramp-up and ramp-down, burst duration, beat frequency, sweep, scan, swing
- Electrode
  - Type, shape, and size
  - Placement location
  - Integrity of skin before and after treatment
- Patient position
- Dosage
  - For NMES: the amplitude required to achieve the desired response
  - For iontophoresis: the product of current amplitude x treatment duration (e.g., 80 mA × min)
- Treatment duration

REFERENCES

1. APTA. *Electrotherapeutic Terminology in Physical Therapy.* Alexandria, VA: American Physical Therapy Association; 1990:39.
2. Giancoli D. *Physics: Principles and Applications.* 6th ed. Upper Saddle River, NJ: Pearson-Prentice Hall; 2009:1040.
3. Sherwood L. *Human Physiology: From Cells to Systems.* 7th ed. Belmont, CA: Brooks/Cole; 2010:78–83.

4. Robinson A. *Clinical Electrophysiology: Electrotherapy and Electrophysiologic Testing.* Baltimore, MD: Lippincott, Williams, and Wilkins; 2008.

5. Palmer S, Martin D. *Interferential Current.* London, England: Churchill Livingstone; 2008:297–315.

6. Ward A, Oliver W, Buccella D. Wrist extensor torque production and discomfort associated with low frequency and burst modulated kilohertz-frequency currents. *Phys Ther.* 2006;86: 1360–1367.

7. Ciccone C. Electrical stimulation for delivery of medications: Iontophoresis: In: *Clinical Electrophysiology.* 3rd ed. Baltimore: Williams and Wilkins; 2008:351–388.

8. Lundy-Ekman L. *Neuroscience: Fundamentals for Rehabilitation.* 3rd ed. St. Louis, MO: Saunders-Elsevier; 2007.

9. Ward A, Shkuratova N. Russian electrical stimulation: the early experiments. *Phys Ther.* 2002;82(10):1019–1030.

10. Laufer Y, Ries J, Leininger P, Alon G. Quadriceps femoris muscle torques produced and fatigue generated by neuromuscular electrical stimulation with three different waveforms. *Phys Ther.* 2001;81:1307–1316.

11. Snyder-Mackler L, Garrett M, Roberts M. A comparison of torque generating capabilities of three electrical stimulating currents. *J Orthop Sports Phys Ther.* 1989;11:297–301.

12. Walmsley R, Letts G, Vooys J. A comparison of torque generated by knee extension with a maximal voluntary contraction vis-à-vis electrical stimulation. *J Orthop Sports Phys Ther.* 1984;6:10–17.

13. Ward A. Electrical stimulation using kilohertz frequency alternating current. *Phys Ther.* 2009;89(2):181–190.

14. Delitto A, Brown M, Strube M, et al. Electrical stimulation of quadriceps femoris in an elite weight lifter: a single-subject experiment. *Int J Sports Med.* 1989;10:187–191.

15. St. Pierre D, Taylor A, Lavoie M, et al. Effects of 2500 Hz sinusoidal current on fibre area and strength of the quadriceps femoris. *J Sports Med Phys Fitness.* 1986;26:60–66.

16. Ward A, Robertson V. The variation in torque production with frequency using medium frequency alternating current. *Arch Phys Med Rehabil.* 1998;79:1399–1404.

17. Ward A, Robertson V, Ioannou H. The effect of duty cycle and frequency on muscle torque production using KHz frequency range alternating current. *Med Eng Phys.* 2004;26:569–579.

18. Laufer Y, Elboim M. Effect of burst frequency and duration of kilohertz-frequency alternating currents and of low-frequency pulsed currents on strength of contraction, muscle fatigue, and perceived discomfort. *Phys Ther.* 2008;88:1167–1176.

19. Newton R. High Voltage Pulsed Galvanic Stimulation: Theoretical Bases and Clinical Application. East Norwalk, CT: Appleton Century Crofts; 1987.

20. Picker R. Low volt pulsed microamp stimulation. *Clinical Management.* 1989;9(2):10–14.

21. Alon G. *Principles of Electrical Stimulation.* Stamford, CT: Appleton Lange; 1999:64.

22. Gersh M. Microcurrent electrical stimulation: putting it in perspective. *Clinical Management.* 1989;9(4):51–54.

23. Kloth L. *Electrical Stimulation for Wound Healing.* Philadelphia: FA Davis; 2002:302–303.

24. McCaig C, Rajnicek A, Song B, Zhao M. Controlling cell behavior electrically: current views and future potential. *Physiol Rev.* 2005;85:943–978.

25. Robertson V, Ward A, Low J, Reed A. *Electrotherapy Explained: Principles and Practice.* 4th ed. Oxford, United Kingdom: Butterworth Heinemann; 2006.

26. Goats G. Interferential current therapy. *Br Med J.* 1990; 24(2):87–92.

27. Draper D, Knight K. Interferential current therapy: often used but misunderstood. *Athl Ther Today.* 2006;11(4):29–31.

28. Ganne J. Interferential therapy. *Aust J Physiother.* 1976;22(3): 101–110.

29. Johnson M, Wilson H. The analgesic effects of different swing patterns of interferential currents on cold-induced pain. *Physiotherapy.* 1997;83(9):461–468.

30. Raja K, Garcia M, Isseroff R. Wound re-epithelialization: modulating keratinocyte migration in wound healing. *Front Biosci.* 2007;12:2849–2868.

31. Zhao M, Song B, Pu J, et al. Electrical signals control wound healing through phoshatidylinositol-3-OH kinase-y and PTEN. *Nature.* 2006;442:457–460.

32. Nuccitelli R. A role for endogenous electric fields in wound healing. *Curr Top Dev Biol.* 2003;58:1–26.

chapter 10

Clinical Electrical Stimulation: Application and Techniques

James W. Bellew, PT, EdD

Considering the many waveform parameters presented in Chapter 9, it should not be surprising that many clinicians feel intimidated or confused by clinical electrotherapy. However, this is entirely unnecessary, as a competent and clinically effective knowledge of electrotherapeutics can easily be obtained by understanding how parameters result in the many effects produced with electrotherapy. Unfortunately, intimidation and confusion are perpetuated by commercial hype, poorly informed clinicians, complex-appearing instrumentation, and sometimes misleading user's manuals. Waveforms vary in so many ways, and these variations are even more obvious when looking at the variety of dials, knobs, switches, and lights that are found on electrotherapeutic devices.

Instrumentation for Electrotherapy

Classifying Electrotherapeutic Devices

Electrotherapeutic devices can be described by the type of current generated and the power sources. Common clinical names used to describe devices include *Russian, high-volt, microcurrent,* and *interferential.* While these names are common, use of more specific descriptors of the individual waveforms is encouraged. When classifying by power source, devices are either line-powered or

241

battery-powered. Line-powered devices are powered by wall current (110 volt, 60 Hz in North America) and are plugged into a wall outlet for use. These devices are sometimes referred to as *clinical devices* because their portability is limited. Battery-powered devices obtain their power from a variety of different battery sources, including the common AA, AAA, and 9-volt batteries, as well as rechargeable batteries. The major advantage of battery-powered devices is their portability, allowing them to be used outside the clinic and while the patient is engaged in activity.

Line-powered devices have traditionally been capable of delivering greater current intensities than battery-powered devices. This was particularly true with stimulators delivering large amplitude currents for muscle strengthening. For many years, evidence suggested that battery-powered stimulators used for muscle strengthening were insufficient in their ability to activate skeletal muscle when compared to line-powered devices. Recent evidence has altered this opinion. In studies of healthy, strong adults, Laufer and colleagues[1] and Lyons and associates[2] reported evidence that newer battery-powered devices can stimulate skeletal muscle to levels once considered achievable only by line-powered devices.

Clinical Controversies

A common misconception is that because batteries provide DC, battery-powered devices must deliver DC to the patient. This is for the most part inaccurate, the exception being devices used for iontophoresis. While DC is provided by a battery, electrotherapeutic devices may provide a variety of other waveforms, none or only one of which may be DC. Likewise, line-powered devices receiving AC current from the wall outlet do not deliver true 60 Hz AC to the patient. Rather, the alteration of battery-provided DC and household AC to other therapeutic waveforms occurs through the use of rectifiers, transformers, filters, and regulators within electrical devices. These take an input current and modify the current into a waveform to be used for therapeutic purposes.

Therapeutic electrical devices generally consist of two primary components—a signal generator and modulator circuits for modulating the source current into the output current. For the majority of applications, this rectified current is pulsed. For most line-powered electrotherapeutic devices in clinical use today, several waveform options are available, whereas battery-powered devices tend to have only one type of current or a limited few (Fig. 10-1). Because electrotherapeutic devices generate an output current, they are sometimes referred to as generators, although this is not as common as it once was.

Control of Electrical Stimulation: The Dials and Buttons

Various waveform parameters, such as amplitude, frequency, pulse duration, and ramp, are often at the practitioner's control. The many dials, buttons, and switches on most devices are controlled by some form of oscillator circuitry. An output amplifier helps modify the intensity of the current delivered to the patient by controlling either the voltage or the current. Some devices available today allow the clinician to choose between a current output with constant voltage (CV) or constant current (CC). Voltage and current are directly proportional. Thus, a change in one necessitates a change in the other based on the resistance of the circuit. With CV devices, the voltage force driving the current will remain constant. As a result of the varying biological

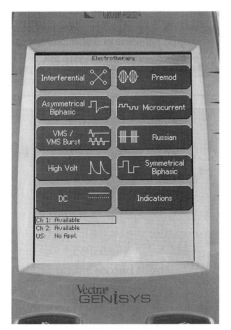

Fig 10•1 Most line-powered units offer a variety of electrotherapy waveforms.

resistances encountered by current as it passes through the body, such as bone and fat, the current will increase or decrease while the voltage remains constant. If a patients sweats while receiving stimulation from a CV device, resistance decreases and current may increase to unsafe levels. This should always be considered when using heating packs with stimulation.

A constant current (CC) device maintains a constant flow of current, despite varying biological resistances, by adjusting the voltage force pushing the current. Regarding which is better for clinical use, it is helpful to keep in mind that without the flow of current, none of the electrophysiological responses elicited by electrotherapy would be possible. With constant voltage, the current may decrease to an ineffective intensity, whereas with CC, the intensity is maintained closer to the level required for the desired therapeutic effect (Fig. 10-2).

Controls for pulse duration and frequency are also common to many devices. Pulse duration may often be labeled *pulse width*, although this is not preferred terminology, because *pulse duration* implies a chronological unit (i.e., milliseconds) whereas *width* implies linear measurement. Pulse frequency is often labeled as *rate*, *pps* (pulses per second), or *frequency*, and the clinician can select the number of pulses per second of pulsatile current. For waveforms using bursts (e.g., Russian), the burst frequency is either fixed or controlled by an altogether different mechanism. Keep in mind that devices

offering control for pulse width generate pulsatile current, because neither DC nor AC has pulse duration.

KEY POINT! Pulse duration is the total time elapsed from beginning to end of all phases, including the interphase interval within a pulse.

To understand what a device can be used for, simply look at what parameters the dials and buttons control. For example, if a device has controls for on-time and off-time as well as ramp-up and ramp-down, it is probably designed to activate skeletal muscle for strengthening or functional activity. If a device offers control of frequency and pulse duration but lacks on- and off-time controls, it is probably used for electroanalgesia and not strengthening (Fig. 10-3).

It cannot be assumed with accuracy that a numerical change on the control, whether the display is analog or digital, will result in the same change in parameter output. For example, many analog or digital controls allow linear increments from 0 to 10, or something similar. One cannot assume that with a 0-to-10 range, the increase from 1 to 2 will result in a 10% change in parameter output, nor can one assume that a single unit increase from 5 to 6 or from 7 to 8 and so on will result in equal change. In addition, it cannot be assumed that a half turn of a dial will result in a 50% change in that parameter. While most handheld and many line-powered units have amplitude dials that go from zero to maximum amplitude in one 360-degree turn, some

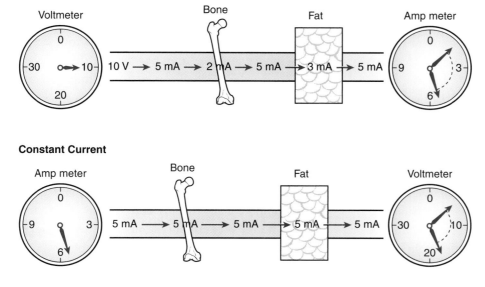

Constant Voltage

Constant Current

Fig 10•2 Constant voltage devices maintain the voltage, but current flow will vary through tissues with different resistance. Constant current devices maintain current flow by modulating the voltage through tissues with varying resistance.

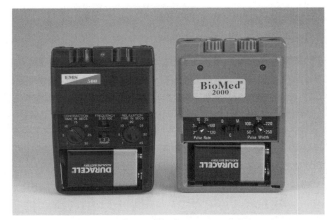

Fig 10•3 A look at the controls will likely indicate what a device can do. A muscle stimulator allows control of the on- and off-time, ramp, and frequency. TENS units often have controls for pulse duration, frequency, and modulation.

line-powered devices have rotary dials that are not fixed to one complete turn and must be rotated several times to increase or decrease the current output.

KEY POINT! To understand the linearity of the output controls, clinicians should familiarize themselves with each device and observe the electrophysiological effect on tissue when changing parameters. It is prudent to never deliver to a patient a current that you have not first tried yourself. Only through personal experience and familiarity can one truly understand and describe the feeling of the current to the patient.

Two noticeable changes in electrotherapeutic devices have evolved due to advances in technology. The first is the transition from analog controls (often dials) to digital controls (often buttons). While the progression from analog to digital control may seem like technological progression, there are limitations to the use of digitally controlled parameters. For example, some devices used for activation of skeletal muscle only allow the practitioner the option of selecting 30, 50, or 100 pps. These may be suitable for many applications, but the use of any other frequencies is not possible. The second noticeable technological change is the advent and inclusion of preprogrammed clinical treatment protocols. While these are designed to assist the practitioner in clinical decision-making and parameter selection, choosing parameters based on patient-specific needs and desired electrotherapeutic effects is encouraged. One of the main reasons

modern electrotherapeutic devices are made with less manual control is because clinical competency in using these parameters has declined. A well-educated clinician should strive to select specific waveform parameters rather than opt for preprogrammed settings.

Electrodes: Types and Choices

An *electrode* is defined as the device that serves as the interface relaying current between an electrical stimulation device and the patient. Often, little consideration is given to the choice of electrodes, preparation for electrode placement, placement sites, and care of electrodes. This is ironic because electrodes can be considered the most important link between the device and the patient. Successful use of electrotherapy depends on correct selection of electrodes so the appropriate tissues are stimulated.

There are two classes of electrodes: (1) surface or transcutaneous electrodes and (2) invasive or indwelling electrodes. Most clinical applications of electrotherapy use surface electrodes to deliver current transcutaneously from the device to the patient. Surface electrodes can be used in reverse fashion to relay electrical signals from the patient to a device during electromyographic biofeedback. The most common use of invasive electrodes is for recording the electrical activity of subjects during electrodiagnostic examinations. Invasive or indwelling electrodes may also be used to deliver therapeutic stimulation, but this is much less common and typically used for kinesiologic examination where fine-wired electrodes are inserted into muscle.

Electrodes vary in many ways, such as shape, dimensions, flexibility, method of adherence to the skin, cost, and material (Fig. 10-4). Electrodes must conduct current well, be flexible enough to conform to varying body surfaces, and be durable. Metal electrodes are usually made of tin, steel, or aluminum and require a wet sponge as an interface between the metal and the tissue. Electrodes made from metal are excellent conductors and are usually durable, but they often lack the flexibility to allow them to conform over body contours. Use of metal electrodes is associated with increased risk of electrical burns and has largely given way to commercially manufactured disposable electrodes. The most common use of metal electrodes is seen in handheld applicators and stimulating probes.

Flexible electrodes are usually made of carbonized silicon rubber, having the advantage of pliability while maintaining good conductivity. Flexible electrodes may be designed for long-term repeated use, short-term use (several days to weeks), or one-time use. Short-term or one-time-use electrodes are intended for single-patient use and are disposable. They are often coated with a conductive coupling agent, such as karaya gum (an organic extract of sterculia trees), whereas reusable clinical electrodes may not have a conductive agent and, therefore, require the addition of electroconductive gel before use.

Disposable electrodes come in many different sizes and shapes, including those designed for small sites, such as the fingers, to much larger sites, such as the lumbosacral region. One disadvantage of disposable electrodes is that they need to be replaced often, yet the number of times that reusable electrodes can be safely and effectively used varies greatly. Disposable electrodes used for strengthening typically have a life of 18 to 20 applications before patients notice a change in tolerance to the stimulus or a greater intensity stimulus is needed to achieve the same effect.[3] The number of uses of each electrode should be recorded. A subjective and more obvious indication that electrodes need to be replaced is when the perceived quality of the stimulus changes as in a prickling sensation or a decreased feeling of current (assuming the parameters are the same as in previous applications). For sanitary reasons, each patient should be issued a set of electrodes that are not to be shared with others; these can be kept in their chart.

The interface where the pin lead from the electrical stimulation (ES) device joins the electrode should be examined. The pin may enter directly into the electrode or may connect to a small lead wire connected to the electrode. This junction is clinically referred to as a *pigtail*. This pigtail junction is a common site of breakdown in the machine-to-electrode interface. A compromise of this interface can lead to current leakage and the potential for electrical burn. The conductive surface of the electrodes should be checked before and after use. The surface should appear uniform and without pitting, pocking, tears, or other areas of compromised integrity (Fig. 10-5). All of these increase the risk for adverse events and, at the very least, reduce the effectiveness of the application (e.g., current delivered to the patient).

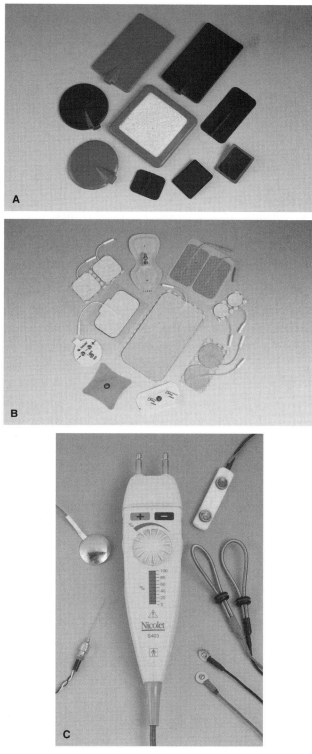

Fig 10•4 Electrodes come in many shapes and sizes, indicating a variety of uses, including (A) carbon and sponge reusable electrodes; (B) adhesive disposable electrodes; and (C) needle, bar, disk, ring, and probe electrodes used for diagnostic studies.

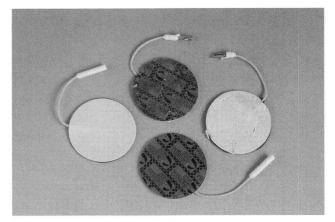

Fig 10•5 Visual inspection of electrodes prior to and after use is recommended. Breakdown of the connector and conductive surface is common after several uses.

Applying Electrodes

Before applying electrodes, the skin surface must be evaluated and prepared to ensure optimal conductance and to limit impedance. A thorough cleansing of the skin with soap and water is recommended to remove oils, dirt, and lotions, which act as resistance to current. Preparing the skin with alcohol-based cleaners is common, but this should be used with caution, as the drying and desiccating effect on the skin can lead to increased resistance to current. It is recommended to shave hair at the electrode placement site to improve adherence of the electrodes, but shaving should occur the day prior to application of electrotherapy, because scraping of the skin acts to acutely denude the stratum corneum, reducing overall skin impedance; this can result in uncomfortable stimulation. More aggressive preparation of the skin by abrasive scrubbing, often with alcohol wipes, is not necessary, again considering the acute effect of reducing skin impedance to current and exposing the more sensitive layers of the dermis.

Electrodes using sponges for interfaces must be wet with a conductive liquid. Tap water is commonly used because it is a good conductor; distilled water will not conduct as well because the natural impurities that act as conductive ions have been removed. Saline is a good conductor and is often used, but it is more costly than tap water. Flexible carbonized silicon rubber electrodes that are not manufactured with a coupling agent require the addition of a hypoallergenic aqueous gel ("electrode" or ultrasonic gel). Most flexible adhesive electrodes are manufactured with a self-adhesive conductive polymer that serves as both the conductive medium and the adhesive. Electrode adhesiveness can be improved by applying a drop or two of water. This is especially true after repeated applications, but with too many uses, conductivity will be reduced. Following treatment, sponges used must be sanitized with soap or bleach solutions between patient use. It may be prudent for each patient to have sponges issued that are not shared with others. Even flexible carbonized silicon rubber electrodes deteriorate over repeated use and need to be replaced. If the patient reports a decrease in the tolerance to the current or noticeably more current is required to elicit the same effect, the electrodes likely need to be replaced.

Short-use disposable electrodes also begin to deteriorate, with erosion of the coupling agent occurring after repeated use. Often the patient will report a burning sensation under an electrode. These "hot spots" are often due to a compromise or erosion of the conductive medium. To prolong the life of short-use disposable electrodes, care should be given to keeping the conductive surface from drying out. Electrodes should be stored on the plastic sheet from the package. Most of these plastic sheets are marked "NO" on one side and "ON" on the other side. The "ON" side is covered with a special polymer to prolong the life of the electrode, so electrodes should be placed on the "ON" side.

The choice of electrode size should be made with two things in mind: the goal of the treatment and the size of the area to be stimulated. Usually, the larger the area to be stimulated, the larger the electrodes need to be. For example, electrodes used to stimulate the quadriceps muscles should be larger than those for the forearm muscles. Electrode size and the amount of current it conducts determine current density. *Current density* is the current per unit area of the electrode (mA/cm^2 or mm^2). This assumes that there is uniform conduction of current across the electroconductive surface of the electrode, that the electrode surface is in full contact with the skin, and that no hot spots are present. Current density is inversely proportional to electrode size. For the same amount of current, the current density in a smaller electrode will be greater than that in a larger electrode (Fig. 10-6).

High levels of stimulation are generally not used with small electrodes, because the greater current density may

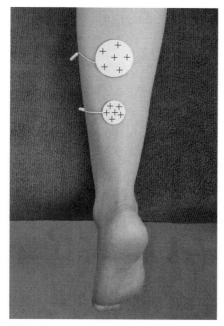

Fig 10•6 With the same amount of current delivered to electrodes of differing size, the current density will be greater under the smaller electrode.

result in uncomfortable burning sensations. If electrodes of different shapes are used at the same time, the current density across the smaller electrode will be greater, resulting in the perception of a stronger stimulus under the smaller electrode. Some electrode configurations will take advantage of this, as we will see shortly. It is more common that the electrode size is equal for most clinical applications. Electrode size should reflect the size of the area that is to be stimulated. Although larger electrodes will have less current density than smaller electrodes (assuming like current amplitude) and will be more comfortable for the patient, use of larger than necessary electrodes can lead to stimulation of tissues that are not necessary and even counter to the purpose of the stimulation. Take, for example, using electrical stimulation to activate the anterior tibialis with the goal of dorsiflexing the ankle to clear the toes during swing phase of gait. Electrodes that are larger than necessary may likely stimulate the peroneus longus and introduce a plantarflexion and eversion component, which opposes the desired effect of the anterior tibialis.

Attaching electrodes to the skin also requires some consideration. While self-adhesive electrodes usually require no additional adhesive or means of fixing the electrodes to the skin, other electrodes will. The primary consideration when attaching electrodes is to make sure

the conductive surface is over the tissue to be treated and that the full surface remains in contact with the skin. Use of adhesive tapes and elastic bands are an effective way to keep electrodes in place. Sometimes, small weights are placed atop the electrode to keep them in position, but this method and the use of tape or elastic bands must be used with attention. It is not uncommon to see flexible electrodes bend or curl under the pressure of weights or excessively tight tape or elastic bands (Fig. 10-7). This can result in a lack of contact of the outer edges of some electrodes and increased current density, impedance, discomfort, and risk of electrical burn under the compressed area of the electrode.

Insecure or loose attachment of electrodes can result in their movement and in changes of the electrode-to-skin contact. Loose contact is usually an early sign that self-adhesive electrodes need to be replaced. Special attention needs to be given to electrodes specifically designed for iontophoresis, which use DC current. These should not be attached with additional tape, bands, or weights because these may greatly increase the current density with DC and result in skin irritation, discomfort, or electrical burn. Sleeping with active electrodes could also be dangerous because the electrode may peel and lose full contact with the skin, increasing the current density to a dangerous level.

Placement of Electrodes

Where electrodes are placed is determined by the goal electrotherapy is trying to accomplish and what tissues need to be stimulated to achieve that goal.

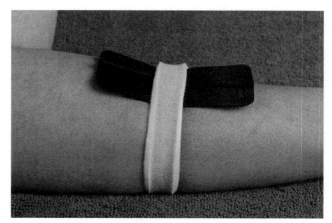

Fig 10•7 When using elastic or tape to place electrodes, avoid curling or bending of the electrode. Curling will reduce the conductive area of the electrode, increase the charge density, and increase the risk of burn.

Dermatomal, sclerotomal, or myotomal sensory distributions can be used. If, for example, stimulation of sensory nerves is desired, electrodes need to be placed over the relevant sensory nerves. If motor stimulation is desired, the stimulus needs to be placed over the motor nerve innervating the muscle to be activated. In normally innervated patients, the neurolemma (nerve membrane) of a motor nerve has a lower threshold for activation than the sarcolemma (muscle membrane); therefore, ES will depolarize the motor nerve, not the muscle directly. Motor nerves are traditionally stimulated over the motor point, which is the region where the motor nerve is most easily excited and thus accessible to stimulation. It is typically found in the muscle belly or proximal third of the muscle. In electrophysiological terms, the motor point is the place where the greatest motor response is found for a given amount of stimulus, or in other words, the place where resistance to the current is least. While motor point charts have traditionally been used and are still widely available and distributed by manufacturers as clinical guides to electrode placement, variability does exist between individuals.

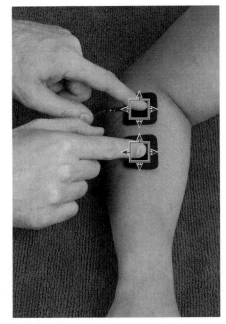

Fig 10•8 Moving or gliding small, gelled electrodes over the muscle belly while providing stimulation will assist in locating the motor point. The area with the greatest motor response to the stimulation is the motor point.

Clinical Application

It is relatively easy to find the motor point of a muscle in most patients. Using a stimulator capable of eliciting a motor response, place two small, gelled electrodes (versus adhesive) on the muscle to be stimulated. Set the parameters to produce a motor response and increase the amplitude. Slowly move or glide the electrodes on the surface of the muscle belly while observing for the greatest muscle response. The area demonstrating the greatest response is likely the motor point and the area where electrodes should be placed during muscle stimulation (Fig. 10-8).

Another technique used to identify the location for electrode placement uses direct palpation by the clinician.[99,100] To do this, the clinician applies one electrode to his or her forearm, palm, or dorsum of the hand while placing the other electrode on the patient (Fig. 10-9).

The clinician then applies conductive gel to three or four fingers of the hand used to palpate and places the fingers on the patient in the intended area of stimulation. (The current density through the therapist's fingers will be higher if only one or two fingers are used, so use three or four fingers.) Finger contact with the patient creates a circuit between the patient and the subject. In this manner, the clinician's fingers become an electrode, which will be used to explore and locate the region of least resistance. After increasing the intensity of the stimulus, the clinician simply moves his or her fingers around the intended area of stimulation, looking for the site that elicits the greatest motor response. Electrodes are then applied to this area for stimulation in the customary manner.

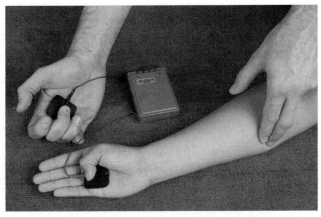

Fig 10•9 Creating a circuit between the patient and clinician allows for a moving palpation to identify the motor point. One electrode is in the hand of the clinician and the other is on the patient. Finger contact with the patient completes the circuit.

When placing electrodes for motor stimulation, a very common mistake occurs when one electrode is placed over the motor point and the other over a more distal site. The problem with this can be twofold: (1) the distal electrode is often placed away from the region of the motor nerve where the optimal response is obtained, rendering the stimulus less effective, and (2) the distal electrode is often placed in a region where there is significantly less or no depolarizable muscle tissue (Fig. 10-10). Thus, when the clinician increases the intensity, the patient is more likely to report a strong sensation of the stimulus but with little to no motor activity. This problem seems to be very common in motor stimulation of the muscles of the forearm and lower leg, where the majority of the muscle mass lies in the upper one-half of the limb segment. An electrode is commonly placed over the proximal muscle mass and one placed distally near the wrist or ankle. While the proximal one is likely near to the motor point, the distal electrode is not over the muscle group but rather a large tendon area. Besides not achieving the motor response desired, stimulation of nonmotor tissues with motor-level stimulation can cause discomfort and will likely require a decrease in the stimulus amplitude, thus diminishing the effect of the treatment.

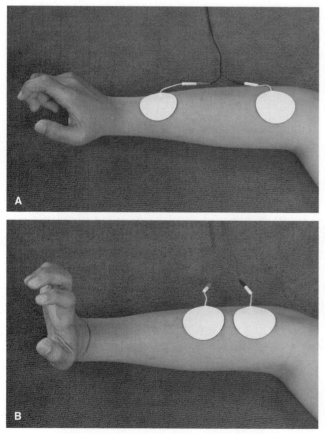

Fig 10•10 Electrodes should be positioned over the muscle tissue to be stimulated. Placement of electrodes distal to the muscle fibers (A) results in stimulation over areas without muscle tissue and may be uncomfortable or result in lesser response from the muscle. Placement over more muscular tissue (B) results in a more robust response.

Clinical Application

Recall from Chapter 9 that the normal order of response to ES is a sensory followed by motor and then noxious (e.g., painful) response. During stimulation of muscle, if the patient's sensation goes straight from a sensory to a noxious response, it is probably because one or more of the electrodes is not over an area of muscle tissue. A relocation of electrodes closer to the motor point will result in the appropriate order of response.

The distance between electrodes is termed *interelectrode distance.* Considering that current will take the path of least resistance, the clinician must ensure that the stimulus current has the best chance of reaching the desired tissue. Electrodes should not be so close together that they may come in contact with each other. This may result in increased current density in the superficial tissue between the electrodes and increase the chance of burning the patient. Making sure the stimulus current reaches deeper tissues where motor nerves, muscles, and bone lie requires appropriate spacing of electrodes. With electrodes appropriately spaced, the current is less likely to travel in the superficial tissues between electrodes. Instead, current travels in the deeper tissues, thus increasing the likelihood that the desired tissues will be stimulated (Fig. 10-11). With wider spacing, greater current amplitude can often be used to reach the deeper tissues. Wider spacing can also lead to more motor units being activated (for an NMES application) or more sensory fibers activated (in a TENS mode).

Electrode Configurations

The placement, or configuration, of electrodes will greatly impact the effect of ES. The majority of electrotherapy techniques consist of a single circuit and two electrodes placed over the target tissue. The most common electrode configuration is a *bipolar electrode configuration,* in which all the electrodes of a single circuit are placed over the treatment area (Fig. 10-12B). A bipolar configuration is most commonly used with biphasic pulsed currents, burst modulated AC (e.g., Russian), and premodulated current during stimulation of muscle (i.e., NMES and FES) and electroanalgesia (i.e., TENS). The electrodes are usually the same size, so the current density through each electrode is equal. If the two electrodes differ in size, the smaller

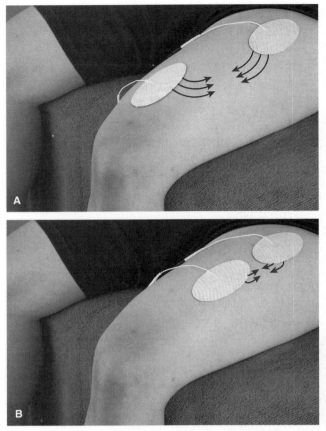

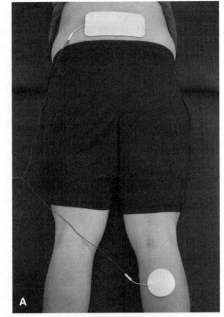

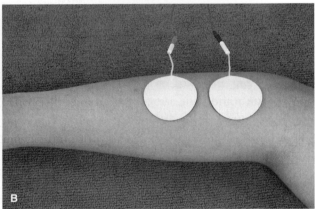

Fig 10•11 The interelectrode distance will affect the depth of penetration of current. Wider placements (A) will result in greater depth of penetration than narrower (B).

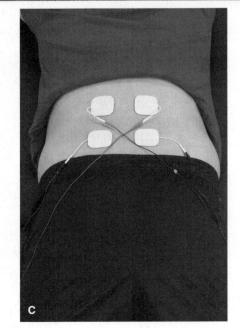

of the two will necessarily have a greater current density and impedance than the larger electrode. All the electrodes are considered treatment or active electrodes with a bipolar electrode orientation.

Sometimes it is desirable to have stimulation only under a single electrode. In this case, an electrode of a single circuit may be positioned over the treatment area while the other electrode is placed at a site where a therapeutic effect is not intended. This configuration is termed a *monopolar arrangement* (Fig. 10-12A). Monopolar electrode placement is most commonly used with DC, and monophasic pulsed currents during iontophoresis and many applications for wound or tissue healing. It is important to recognize that the lead wires from a device generating a single circuit can be split, or bifurcated, allowing two (or even more) electrodes to be used at the treatment site. If a lead wire is bifurcated to allow more than one electrode at the treatment area with a third placed over a nontreatment area, it is still considered a monopolar arrangement. With a

Fig 10•12 (A) Monopolar, (B) bipolar, and (C) quadripolar electrode placements.

monopolar electrode orientation, the electrode(s) over the target tissue is the treatment or active electrode, whereas the other electrode is termed the *reference* or *inactive* electrode.

Clinical Principles in Practice: Monopolar Electrode Configuration With One or Two Active Electrodes and a Single Inactive Electrode

The clinician treating a stage IV pressure ulcer with twin-peak monophasic current may choose to place an active electrode over the wound to deliver cathodal (negative) stimulation while placing the inactive or reference electrode adjacent to the wound. In this application, there are only two electrodes of a single circuit—one treatment and one reference. If treating acute swelling of the lateral and medial ankle secondary to sprain, the clinician may choose to bifurcate the lead wire of the active electrodes to deliver cathodal (negative) stimulation to both sides of the joint while placing the inactive electrode on the leg. In this application, there are three electrodes—two over the treatment area and one away yet still maintaining a single circuit.

As with bipolar orientation, if electrodes differ in size, the smaller electrode will have a greater current density. Because of the electrochemical effects of DC and monophasic pulsed current, asymmetrical electrode size with these currents must be considered so as to avoid adverse effects. More often than not, if one electrode of an electrotherapy device uses a much larger electrode (2 in. × 4 in. and ranging up to 8 in. × 10 in.), then the device likely provides DC, monophasic pulsed current, or unbalanced asymmetrical pulsed current. In these currents, one electrode will remain the anode and the other the cathode.

Bifurcation of lead wires can allow a greater area to be treated but decreases the current density at each individual electrode since the current is now shared between the electrodes. For example, if a monopolar electrode arrangement with a single active electrode placed over the gastrocnemius with current amplitude of 50 mA is then bifurcated to allow two electrodes over the gastrocnemius, the current density under the two electrodes is now 25 mA (assuming both electrodes are of equal size and impedance and total current output remains 50 mA). The overall effect of the change in stimulus amplitude must be considered when choosing to use more than one active electrode.

A third electrode configuration exists, which involves the application of two or more electrodes from two separate circuits. The electrodes are placed so that the currents are intentionally crossed, or interfered, as in interferential current. This configuration, using at least four electrodes, is termed a *quadripolar configuration* (Fig. 10-12C). True quadripolar interferential current is the most common application using a quadripolar electrode configuration. Table 10-1 summarizes these configurations.

KEY POINT! Simply using four electrodes does not constitute a quadripolar orientation. It is not uncommon to see four electrodes used for muscle activation or pain modulation over large areas. These uses are usually two separate circuits with bipolar electrode arrangement applied to treat the larger area.

The name *monopolar* is misleading because there are always two poles—an anode and a cathode—required to make a complete circuit. The electrode with the greater concentration of negative ions or electrons is the cathode, whereas the anode has a lesser concentration of negative ions or electrons. The greater concentration of negative ions near the cathode reduces the resting membrane potential across the cell, thereby depolarizing the nerve. In contrast, the lesser concentration of negative ions at the anode results in hyperpolarization of the cell and decreased responsiveness to stimulation. Because the cathode is the site of depolarization and the anode is the site of hyperpolarization, the cathode is termed the *active electrode* and the anode the *inactive electrode*. However, with AC and biphasic currents that regularly alternate or change direction of current flow, the electrodes also alternate from being the cathode or anode.

Whether an electrode elicits the effect of a specific pole (i.e., has a polar effect) is a matter of whether polarity is sustained under that electrode. For example,

Table 10·1	Basic Electrode Configurations and Clinical Use	
Name	**Electrode Location**	**Common Use**
Monopolar	Active electrode of single circuit over target area; inactive over nearby non-treatment area	Pain modulation, iontophoresis, tissue healing
Bipolar	Both or all electrodes of single circuit over target tissues	Muscle activation, pain modulation
Quadripolar	Four electrodes of two circuits over target tissues	Pain modulation

AC, symmetrical biphasic pulsed current, and balanced asymmetrical pulsed current result in no net charge (sometimes termed *zero net DC*); thus, the electrodes do not remain a true anode or cathode for longer than

a few hundred microseconds because the current is regularly "alternating" between positive and negative, depending on the frequency. Consider the polarity of each electrode to be constantly changing from positive to negative, never maintaining or accumulating enough charge to induce a polar effect (i.e., a cathodal or anodal effect). In contrast, three waveforms—DC, monophasic pulsed current, and unbalanced asymmetrical biphasic pulsed current—can cause true polar effects, because current either flows in only one direction (DC) or flows in one direction more than the other. This results in greater-than-zero net charge at the electrodes. A sustained anode and cathode with polar effects are present only with the latter three waveforms (Fig. 10-13). It should be noted that the pictures of waveforms in a manual depict what is happening only at one electrode.

Box 10•1	Which Color Wire Should I Use Where?

The lead wires of many electrotherapy devices are manufactured with red and black ends. Many clinicians assume this indicates the positive and negative leads, respectively. However, with currents that continually change direction, such as AC and biphasic currents, the polarity is continually changing, so the red or black lead is neither the anode or cathode for more than the duration of a single phase of a biphasic pulse (i.e., microseconds). Only when using DC, monophasic pulsed current, or unbalanced asymmetrical pulsed current would the red and black truly indicate an anode and cathode.

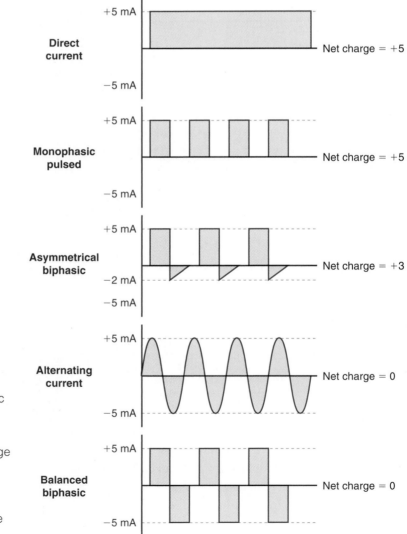

Fig 10•13 Direct current (DC), monophasic pulsed, and unbalanced asymmetrical biphasic pulsed currents will develop a net charge and thus have a sustained anode and cathode because current flows in only one direction or one direction more than the other. No net charge is accumulated with alternating current (AC), symmetrical biphasic pulsed current, and balanced biphasic currents. Note that net charge would be negative if current flowed only in the negative direction or more current flowed in the negative direction than positive.

What is happening at the other wire is a mirror image of this, reflected about the isoelectric line.

Electrotherapy Application and Techniques: Why Use Electrotherapy?

Deciphering the "Electro Lingo Code"

Clinical applications of ES are most commonly used for the following purposes: to activate skeletal muscle for improving muscle performance or strengthening, to attenuate or alleviate pain, to improve blood flow, to decrease or control edema, or to facilitate tissue healing. For various reasons, ES for these purposes has come to be known or recognized by a variety of acronyms, abbreviations, or clinical lingo. Activation of skeletal muscle for strengthening is referred to as *neuromuscular electrical stimulation* (NMES). Activation of skeletal muscle for reeducation or movement training for functional use is referred to as *functional electrical stimulation* (FES). ES for modulation of pain is called *transcutaneous electrical nerve stimulation* (TENS), despite nearly all forms of clinical electrotherapy being transcutaneous.

Use of ES to skeletal muscle below the threshold for muscle contraction has recently become known as *therapeutic* or *threshold electrical stimulation* (TES).[4-6] ES for scoliosis—*scoliotic electrical stimulation* (SES)—is not as common as it once was but nevertheless represents another use of an acronym to describe a type of application or ES.[7-8]

Other forms of ES are often recognized and referred to by the type of current used—for example, interferential current (IFC), high-volt pulsed current (HVPC), Russian current, microcurrent (low-intensity direct current), and others not listed in this chapter. Because of all the confusion in terminology, documentation of electrotherapy should more appropriately specify the type of waveform used and any pertinent parameters, particularly if the treatment is to be replicated in subsequent sessions (Box 10-2).

Electrotherapy for Activation of Skeletal Muscle: Strengthening and Reeducation

Clinical electrotherapy for muscle strengthening and reeducation is often directed toward treating or preventing muscular atrophy following disuse,

Box 10•2	Clinical Decision-Making With ES

Regardless of the purpose, when deciding to use ES, the steps in the clinical decision-making process remain the same. Questions to ask when considering use of electrotherapy include the following:

1. What is the clinical goal?
2. Is the patient appropriate for an electrotherapeutic agent?
3. Is there a type of electrotherapeutic agent that can assist in achieving this goal?
4. If there is an identifiable goal and the answers to the latter two questions are yes, then use of electrotherapy is indicated. The clinician must then continue with the following questions.
5. Is equipment with the appropriate waveform available?
6. What are the specific parameters of the selected waveform?
7. What electrodes and electrode configuration should be used?
8. What factors would necessitate a change in the treatment plan?

The clinician should always explain the procedures to the patient and interpret the effectiveness of the treatment, making appropriate accommodations as necessary. It is prudent for the clinician to apply to patients only an electrotherapeutic agent that they themselves have tried. In this manner, the clinician can offer a more factual description of the sensation and effect. This can only serve to enhance the patient-clinician relationship and trust.

immobilization, or detraining; increasing or maintaining range of motion; and reeducating, retraining, or facilitating muscle for movement and posture. Neuromuscular electrical stimulation (NMES) has generally come to imply use of ES for purposes of increasing strength in innervated muscle, whereas *electrical muscle stimulation* (EMS) implies the stimulation of denervated muscle. The fundamental difference between NMES and EMS is the tissue that is actually stimulated and depolarized to elicit the therapeutic effect. With NMES in innervated muscle, the intact peripheral nerve, which has a lower threshold for depolarization, depolarizes first and initiates contraction of the skeletal muscle—thus the name *neuromuscular electrical stimulation*. In contrast, ES in denervated muscle does not depolarize the peripheral nerve, but rather the muscle itself—thus the name electrical muscle stimulation. The term *functional electrical stimulation* (FES) has come to describe ES of innervated or denervated skeletal muscle for the purposes of facilitating or enhancing functional movement (e.g., to assist in dorsiflexion of the ankle or wrist extension in the paretic anterior tibial muscles or wrist extensors, respectively).

Strengthening: NMES

The effect of ES for activating skeletal muscle, whether for strengthening or for reeducation, has been studied much more than some other common physical therapy techniques. ES for strengthening in healthy, nonweak subjects has shown that (1) use of electrical stimulation for strengthening yields better results than no exercise at all,[9,10] (2) there is no difference between the strength gains resulting from voluntary exercise or the use of electrical stimulation alone,[9,11] and (3) there appears to be no benefit to the use of ES combined with exercise versus using each separately.[12,13]

Using ES for strengthening in weak but normally innervated subjects has shown that (1) in the initial periods of rehabilitation when voluntary exercise may be difficult, ES results in greater gains in strength than voluntary exercise or no exercise at all; (2) in the postrehabilitation stages, there is often little to no difference in strength between subjects who used ES and those who did not; and (3) there appears to be a significant positive relationship between the intensity of the ES and the strength gained.[14,15]

KEY POINT! Most studies examining the effect of ES on weak but innervated subjects have examined the quadriceps.[15]

The most commonly used waveforms for strengthening are burst-modulated AC current (e.g., Russian) and symmetrical biphasic waves of square, rectangular, or triangular shape (Table 10-2). Evidence suggests that the most effective waveform for eliciting muscle force varies between patients, so more than one waveform may need to be tried.[16] The typical pulse duration used to activate muscle for strengthening is 200 to 600 μsec, with frequencies ranging from 20 to 100 pps. Interestingly, abdominal stimulators commonly advertised on television do not offer pulse duration and frequency suitable for contracting skeletal muscle; these devices are merely gimmicks.

A bipolar electrode configuration is used with NMES, and the electrodes are placed directly over the muscle to be stimulated. Keep in mind that in healthy, innervated muscle, depolarization of the peripheral nerve innervating the muscle results in contraction, so the electrode placement should be consistent with the anatomic location of peripheral nerve to the muscle(s) being treated (i.e., near the motor point). Typical treatment sessions should consider the number of contractions (i.e., repetitions) rather than the duration of the treatment (e.g., 15 minutes) in the same manner a strength training program would count repetitions. A more detailed discussion of using ES for muscle strengthening and musculoskeletal applications appears in Chapter 11 (Box 10-3).

Reeducation and Retraining: FES

ES is often used in patients with paralysis or in those who have an inability to volitionally activate skeletal muscle secondary to stroke, cerebrovascular insult, head injury, spinal cord injury, peripheral nerve injury, or other neurological disorders. ES is used to facilitate and improve purposeful movement, assist with ambulation, reverse cardiopulmonary deconditioning, attenuate bone demineralization following spinal cord injury (SCI), and improve circulation. By virtue of its use for functional purposeful activity, FES is used for this application of ES and is differentiated from NMES in that the primary goal is not increased strength (Fig. 10-14).

Use of ES as a substitute for the intact nervous system was popularized in the 1960s by Liberson and colleagues,[17] who reported using ES as a means of improving gait in patients with hemiparesis and common peroneal nerve palsy. This example of nervous system plasticity underlies much of the continuing clinical

Table 10•2 **Parameters for NMES and FES**						
Indication	**Type**	**Waveform**	**Pulse Frequency**	**Pulse Duration**	**Amplitude**	**Duration**
Muscle strengthening	NMES	Biphasic PC or burst modulated AC (e.g., Russian)	20–100 pps or bursts per sec	200–600 μsec	As high as tolerated with a goal of reaching more than 60%–70% MVC	10–20 strong contractions
Muscle contraction for functional use	FES	Biphasic PC or burst modulated AC (e.g., Russian)	20–60 pps or bursts per sec	200–600 μsec	To level commensurate with functional activity	Task specific

Box 10•3 **How Long Is a Treatment of NMES?**

Many applications of ES and other modalities are applied for a fixed duration. But ES for muscle strengthening should be considered differently. Use of defined sets and repetitions are the cornerstone of strength and conditioning programs and should likewise be used when determining ES duration. For example, figure out the number of contractions, or repetitions, a patient should do and calculate the duration of the treatment from the contraction (i.e., on-time) and rest time (i.e., off-time) of the ES. If using 10-second contraction time with 50 seconds between contractions, the subject would complete one contraction with a rest period every minute. To complete 20 contractions would require a treatment duration of 20 minutes.

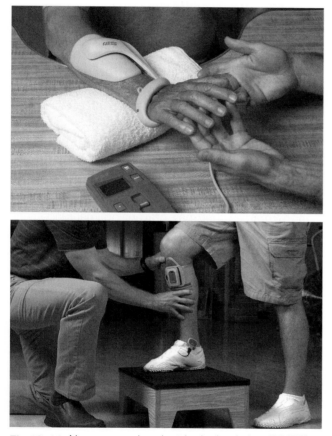

Fig 10•14 Neuromuscular electrical stimulation (NMES) and functional electrical stimulation (FES) are used in a variety of ways. (Courtesy of Bioness, Inc., Valencia, California.)

and investigative efforts given to better understanding how stimulation can be used to enhance purposeful and functional movement in patients with compromised nervous systems or difficulty voluntarily activating their muscles.

More recently, electromyographic (EMG) FES was used to trigger muscle stimulation in paretic muscles (primarily wrist and finger extensors) following neurological compromise. EMG-triggered muscle stimulation requires the patient to generate a threshold level of muscle activation from either the paretic muscle or other muscle of the same extremity in order to elicit or trigger an electrical stimulus to the paretic muscles, often the wrist and finger extensors.[18-20] This technique is held to link motor intention of the extremity with motor response.[19]

The use of contralateral controlled functional electrical stimulation (CCFES) has emerged from the EMG-triggered stimulation and uses sensors placed on the contralateral hand. Motions performed in the contralateral hand are detected and used to trigger or stimulate muscles in the contralateral side paretic hand.[19] The stimulated hand can then perform functional tasks or complete exercise retraining activities. Knutson and colleagues[19,21] have shown promising results using CCFES in patients with loss of hand function secondary to hemiplegia.

ES to facilitate functional movement is based on activation of the skeletal muscle. Thus, the stimulus parameters used will be similar to those used to strengthen muscle; however, some parameters differ, reflecting the difference in the clinical goals of each type of stimulation. Whereas ES use for strengthening requires intensities at or near those maximally tolerated, the intensity for FES should only be enough to meet the demands of the specific functional task. For example, to assist in dorsiflexion of the ankle to clear the toes during the swing phase of gait, the intensity need only be enough to move the ankle through enough range of motion so the functional task of clearing the toes is accomplished. The pulse rate or frequency of the stimulus should be considered in light of fatigue. A higher frequency will result in fatigue sooner than a lesser frequency; thus, lower frequencies are desirable with FES to avoid or delay fatigue of the activated muscle. However, keep in mind that the parameters chosen must still be capable of activating the muscle to accomplish the task.

The most common waveforms used for FES are symmetrical biphasic square and triangular waves and burst-modulated AC (e.g., Russian; see Table 10-2). The pulse duration must be capable of activating the muscle and typically will range between 200 and 600 μsec. When stimulating muscle for functional activity, pulse frequency typically ranges from 20 to 60 pps—less than NMES. Ultimately, the determination of specific stimulus parameters depends on whether the muscle activation accomplishes the functional task. In this regard, slight variations will exist within and between patients. Further description of FES for functional activity and specific treatment techniques appears in Chapter 12.

Electrical Stimulation of Denervated Muscle

The majority of evidence regarding ES for increasing strength has involved healthy, nonweak or healthy, weak subjects, but all of the subjects remained innervated.

CASE STUDY 10•1 **NMES**

A patient is referred for strengthening of the right ankle secondary to chronic lateral instability. Upon testing, the patient shows laxity in the ligaments of the lateral ankle and weakness of the peroneals.

CLINICAL DECISION-MAKING

1. Does the patient have a dysfunction, limitation, or problem that can be improved with the use of electrotherapy?
   Answer: Yes, the patient has weakness of the lateral muscles of the ankle that is associated with chronic instability.

2. Is the patient appropriate for electrotherapy (i.e., do any of the general precautions or contraindications to electrotherapy apply, or are there any specific considerations regarding application of electrotherapy to this patient)?
   Answer: The patient does not present with any contraindications or precautions.

3. What are the specific goals to be achieved with the use of electrotherapy?
   Answer: To increase strength of the lateral muscles of the ankle to reduce ankle instability.

4. Do you have the specific type of electrotherapy that is appropriate for the patient?
   Answer: NMES can be used to strengthen the lateral ankle muscles.

5. Can you select the specific parameters of electrotherapy that are appropriate for the patient?
   Answer:
   Waveform: Biphasic PC or burst-modulated AC (e.g., Russian) may be used
   Pulse duration: 200 to 600 microseconds
   Pulse frequency: 30 to 80 pps
   On:off time: 10 sec on (contraction) with 30 to 50 seconds off (rest)
   Ramps: Ramp-up 1 to 2 sec; ramp-down 1 to 2 sec

Intensity: Maximally tolerated contractions with a goal of 60% to 70% of the maximal isometric contraction of the uninvolved side
Duration: 10 to 20 strong contractions

6. What are the proper application procedures for electrotherapy?
   Answer:
   Instruct the patient: Inform the patient of the purpose and procedure. Be sure to explain the anticipated sensation and effect of the stimulation. In this case, a strong sensation of stimulation should be noted in the muscles of the lateral leg that will lead to contraction of the muscles.
   Preinspection: Clean the area to be treated and check for skin compromise. Identify any surface abnormalities that may prevent optimal placement of electrodes.
   Electrode placement: Identify the motor point for optimal electrode placement over the peroneus longus. Both electrodes should be placed over muscular tissue, avoiding placement of the distal electrode over more tendinous area. Electrodes may be adhesive-disposable or carbon-gelled but should be proportionate to the size of the area to be stimulated. Too-large electrodes may result in cross-stimulation of additional muscles, and too-small electrodes will increase current density and likely result in an uncomfortable sensation.
   Patient position: The ankle may be rested on the treatment table with the patient supine or recumbent. The patient should not be positioned so that the electrodes are compressed by body weight.
   Postinspection: Remove the electrodes and inspect the skin for any signs of skin irritation or adverse effects. If redness appears, explain that this is not uncommon and should disappear in less than 24 hours.

CASE STUDY 10•2 FES

A patient suffered a fracture of the fibular head, resulting in damage to the deep peroneal nerve, and remains unable to actively dorsiflex the ankle against gravity. The patient is referred for electrical stimulation for orthotic substitution during gait. Manual muscle testing reveals trace volitional contraction of the anterior tibialis.

CLINICAL DECISION-MAKING

1. Does the patient have a dysfunction, limitation, or problem that can be improved with the use of electrotherapy?
   Answer: Yes, the patient has decreased ability to volitionally contract the anterior tibialis and has gait impairment with decreased dorsiflexion secondary to recent nerve injury.

2. Is the patient appropriate for electrotherapy (i.e., do any of the general precautions or contraindications to electrotherapy apply, or are there any specific considerations regarding application of electrotherapy to this patient)?
   Answer: The patient does not present with any contraindications or precautions.

3. What are the specific goals to be achieved with the use of electrotherapy?
   Answer: To facilitate recruitment of the anterior tibialis to provide dorsiflexion during gait.

4. Do you have the specific type of electrotherapy that is appropriate for the patient?
   Answer: FES can be used to recruit the anterior tibialis.

5. Can you select the specific parameters of electrotherapy that are appropriate for the patient?
   Answer:
   Waveform: Biphasic PC or burst-modulated AC (e.g., Russian) may be used
   Pulse duration: 200 to 300 microseconds
   Pulse frequency: 20 to 40 pps (less than NMES so as to prevent fatigue)
   On:off time: To be set based on patient's cadence or use of heel-switch to trigger stimulation to muscle

Ramps: Ramp-up 1 sec; ramp-down 1 sec; modified to the patient's gait pattern.
Intensity: In contrast to NMES, where maximal contractions are desired, contraction intensity for FES is to a level commensurate with the desired effect. In this case, the functional goal is dorsiflexion that permits normalized gait. Therefore, the intensity should be increased to elicit contractions of this magnitude.

6. What are the proper application procedures for electrotherapy?
   Answer:
   Instruct the patient: Inform the patient of the purpose and procedure. Be sure to explain the anticipated sensation and effect of the stimulation. In this case, a sensation of stimulation should be noted in anterior tibialis with muscle contraction upon unloading and clearing the foot from the floor during gait.
   Preinspection: Because this patient will use FES often and for prolonged periods of time, it is critical to properly clean the area to be treated and check for skin compromise and to instruct the patient in these procedures for future applications.
   Electrode placement: Identify the motor point for optimal electrode placement over the anterior tibialis. Both electrodes should be placed over muscular tissue, avoiding placement of the distal electrode over more tendinous area. Electrodes may be adhesive-disposable or carbon-gelled but should be proportionate to the size of the area to be stimulated. Electrodes that are too large may result in cross-stimulation of the peroneus longus and result in unwanted ankle eversion. Electrodes that are too small will increase current density and likely result in an uncomfortable sensation.
   Postinspection: Remove the electrodes and inspect the skin for any signs of skin irritation or adverse effects. If redness appears, explain that this is not uncommon and should disappear in less than 24 hours. It is prudent to reiterate that the patient should inspect the skin if getting frequent FES treatments.

FES has likewise focused primarily on patients with intact peripheral nervous systems (i.e., intact lower motor neurons). Thus, for NMES and the majority of applications for FES, ES works via an intact peripheral nervous system supplying the muscle(s) to be activated.

The process of activating denervated muscle by ES is uniquely different from stimulating innervated muscle. In innervated muscle, the electrical stimulus depolarizes the peripheral nerve, which results in depolarization and activation of the skeletal muscle. In the case of denervation, the peripheral nerve can no longer be depolarized. Thus, activation of the muscle requires depolarization of the muscle membrane itself—the sarcolemma. This requires a stimulus of significantly greater amplitude and duration than is required for depolarizing intact peripheral nerve and thus innervated muscle (see Chapter 9). Pulse durations of 10 milliseconds or greater may be required, and the majority of electrical stimulators on the market do not offer a pulse duration of this magnitude. DC has been used with the clinician applying the electrode to the muscle for several seconds. Modern devices offering DC cannot deliver sufficient amplitude to activate denervated muscle. If the muscle has not been activated for an extensive period (e.g., several months), either by stimulation or volition or if denervation occurred some time ago, the contractile mechanisms of the muscle may have fibrosed and will no longer be able to operate.[22]

The major premise underlying use of ES in denervated muscle is that ES will maintain contractile properties of the muscle while awaiting reinnervation, but the literature remains controversial. Supporters of using stimulation to denervated muscle contend that atrophy and fibrosis can be attenuated and delayed while improving recovery;[23-25] however, opponents assert that stimulation may interfere with or interrupt endogenous mechanisms for reinnervation and collateral nerve sprouting[26-31] (Box 10-4).

Box 10•4 | **Stimulation of Denervated Muscle: Continued Controversy**

Use of ES for denervation of the muscles innervated by the facial, or seventh cranial, nerve (i.e., Bell's palsy) was once a common yet controversial use of ES. Despite recent reports of modest improvements in voluntary control of facial muscles following use of high-volt pulsed current (e.g., twin-peak monophasic) up to 6 hours per day,[98] evidence for ES of denervated muscle remains sparse and with questionable design and validity. Collectively, these factors have resulted in a declining use of ES for denervated muscle over what was once seen years ago.

Bottom line: Electrical stimulation can be used to effectively activate innervated skeletal muscle for purposes of strengthening and for participation in functional activity. Although the type of stimulus parameters used for both are similar (pulse frequency, duration, waveform, etc.), the specific determination of each parameter (i.e., frequency or intensity) can vary greatly, depending on the goals. ES for denervated muscle remains controversial and unsupported.

Electrotherapy for Modulating Pain

Using ES to modify or modulate pain may be the most common utilization of electrotherapy. Interest in the use of ES for pain modulation or electroanalgesia greatly heightened in the 1960s with Melzak and Wall's gate theory of pain control. Their theory asserted that selective stimulation of the large diameter afferent A-beta sensory fibers can result in a gating, or blocking, of noxious afferent input from smaller diameter unmyelinated nociceptive C fibers and small myelinated A-delta fibers at the level of the spinal cord.[32] Melzack and Wall's gating theory led to an increase in the production and use of handheld, battery-operated, electrical stimulators for treatment of pain via TENS. To this day, the term *transcutaneous electrical nerve stimulation* implies the use of ES for purposes of attenuating or alleviating pain.

TENS has been used for modulating pain and has been reported in a variety of patient populations. It is generally divided into applications for acute or chronic pain. The majority of studies examining the effect of TENS on pain have used portable stimulators, most of which are handheld and battery-powered despite similar waveform options on line-powered clinical units.[33] The majority of clinical applications of electrotherapy are based on pain modulation through stimulation of sensory and motor nerves. To a lesser degree is the use of ES at subsensory levels.

Sensory-level stimulation, often termed *conventional, sensory,* or *high-frequency TENS,* is characterized by a pulse frequency approximately 100 pps and a short pulse duration of 50 to 100 μsec (Table 10-3). These parameters appear well suited for selective stimulation of the large A-beta fibers for gating pain.[34] Electrodes are placed over or adjacent to the site of pain or along the dermatome or myotome, usually in a bipolar arrangement. With conventional TENS, the patient will likely describe a sensation of tingling or buzzing. Sensory-level TENS appears to be effective only during the treatment, with little evidence of benefit lasting beyond the actual application. For this reason, the gate control theory of pain is thought to underlie sensory-level TENS and acts as an ascending method of pain modulation. Sensory-level TENS is often used during activities and for prolonged periods of time, making it the most common form of TENS used.

Table 10·3 Parameters for Pain Modulation (TENS)*

Indication	Type	Waveform	Pulse Frequency	Pulse Duration	Amplitude	Duration
Acute pain: for relief during stimulation	Sensory-level stimulation	Mono- or biphasic pulsed current	High: approximately 100 pps	Short: 50–100 μsec	mA to comfortable sensory perception	20–30 min (longer if used during activity)
Acupuncture stimulation	Motor-level stimulation	Mono- or biphasic pulsed current	Short: less than 10 pps	High: greater than 150 μsec	mA to visible muscle twitches	20–45 min
Brief-intense stimulation	Motor-level stimulation	Mono- or biphasic pulsed current	High: approximately 100 pps	High: greater than 150 μsec	mA to visible strong muscle twitches	Less than 15 min
Noxious-level stimulation	Hyperstimulation (point stimulation)	DC or monophasic	High: 100 pps Low: 1–5 pps	Long: greater than 250 μsec, up to 1 second	mA to highest tolerated painful stimulus	30–60 sec to each area

*These parameters are not specific to traditional TENS units and can be repeated on many line-powered clinical stimulators.

Motor-level stimulation for electroanalgesia is based on stimulation of muscle and is commonly referred to as *low-frequency* or *acupuncture TENS*. The pulse frequency is typically 1 to 10 pps, and because a motor response is desired, a longer pulse duration of 150 μsec or greater is required (Table 10-3). The intensity should elicit a strong visible motor response, which is often seen as robust twitches corresponding to the frequency. Electrodes are placed over the affected area or in areas related to the pain, such as dermatomes or acupuncture points—thus the name *acupuncture TENS*. A bipolar electrode arrangement is most common. The patient's sensation should be of obvious muscle twitching and may be associated with prickling and stinging. In contrast to sensory-level TENS, motor-level TENS is thought to act via descending methods of pain modulation by the release of endogenous opioids (e.g., endorphins and enkephalins).[35,36]

The effects of motor-level stimulation appear to last several hours, longer than sensory-level stimulation, and appear to be more beneficial for chronic pain than acute. Because of the stronger stimulus intensity and activation of muscles, use of motor-level TENS during activity or work is not recommended. Motor-level stimulation is often used periodically throughout the day in 15- to 30-minute applications instead of continuously. Sensory-level TENS is often used in the acute stages of recovery when motor-level stimulation may not be indicated or tolerated. In later phases of rehabilitation, motor-level stimulation may be used. In this manner, a clinician may use both forms of TENS on the same patient.

A method of ES combining both sensory TENS (high frequency with short pulse duration) and motor TENS (low frequency with long pulse duration) is known as *brief-intense TENS*. The stimulus is increased to a patient's maximal tolerance, resulting in a motor response of marked fasciculations or tetanic nonrhythmic muscle contraction. Brief-intense TENS is applied similarly to motor-level TENS in periodic and brief applications but usually not greater than 15 minutes (Table 10-3). This type of stimulation is often uncomfortable for the patient and is considered a form of noxious-level stimulation thought to elicit the release of endogenous opioids.

Hyperstimulation, another form of noxious-level stimulation, is usually applied locally via probe electrodes or small electrodes and uses monophasic currents with long pulse durations approaching 1 second or direct current. Either a low pulse frequency (1 to 5 pps) or high pulse frequency (100 pps) is used. Hyperstimulation is often applied over acupuncture points or dermatomal distributions of a peripheral nerve but not over areas of motor nerve where a strong motor response would be elicited.[33] Hyperstimulation is thought to lessen pain through descending methods via release of endogenous opioids. Collectively, acupuncture (low-frequency TENS), brief-intense, and hyperstimulation TENS are considered to work via descending opiate-mediated electroanalgesia.

Current waveforms used for pain modulation differ but are generally characterized by variations in two basic parameters—pulse frequency and duration. Pulsed currents, including monophasic waveforms such as twin-peaked monophasic (e.g., high volt), symmetrical and asymmetrical, balanced and unbalanced, and biphasic currents as well as amplitude-modulated AC (e.g., interferential current) are commonly used. With TENS, there are no on-times or off-times or ramp-up or ramp-down controls, as with NMES or FES. The parameters manipulated for TENS are not specific to handheld units and are found on many line-powered clinical units, but, by convention, many clinicians would not consider these TENS units. Traditionally, a TENS unit could be identified by analog controls or dials for pulse duration and frequency with amplitude dials for each of two channels. The dial for pulse duration often ranged from 50 to 250 μsec while frequency ranged from less than 10 pps up to 200 pps. The last two decades have shown an increase in digital units with preprogrammed settings and clinical protocols designated for pain of a particular type or region (e.g., neck, shoulder, knee). Some newer handheld TENS units no longer allow the clinician to manipulate the specific parameters apart from selecting a preprogrammed protocol and the treatment intensity.

Common to many TENS units are options to select burst and modulated TENS. The burst function of most TENS units delivers the selected current in brief, intermittent periods of stimulation or packages of pulses (i.e., bursts). Modulated TENS varies per manufacturer, but in general, *modulation* implies that the specific waveform parameters (usually pulse duration and frequency) are periodically altered or modulated by the internal circuitry of the device. Modulation is used to prevent or lessen the chances of developing accommodation to the electrical stimulus, thus rendering the stimulation less effective. A patient experiencing a modulated waveform is likely to describe the sensation of the stimulus as changing, moving, waving, or increasing and decreasing (Fig. 10-15).

Electrotherapy for Preventing or Reducing Edema

Edema, or swelling, from soft tissue injury or trauma can hinder tissue repair and can lead to pain, reduced mobility, and delayed return to maximum possible function.[37–39] Edema at the knee and ankle has been clearly associated with motor inhibition and decreased excitability, which further reduces function and prolongs rehabilitation.[29,40] Increased capillary permeability and leakage of plasma proteins, leukocytes, and water into the interstitial space following soft tissue injury results in localized swelling.[37] The effects of ES on vascular permeability in rats have suggested that cathodal high-voltage pulsed current (i.e., twin-peaked monophasic current) at 120 pps frequency and 10%

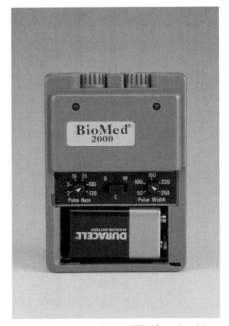

Fig 10•15 A typical handheld TENS unit with controls for pulse duration, frequency, and options for modulating the current output.

below the motor threshold may be best at limiting edema formation in the acute posttraumatic period when vessel permeability is increased.[41–49] Evidence suggests that although four 30-minute applications 30 to 60 minutes apart resulted in significant edema reduction,[45,47] continuous applications of 3 to 4 hours are more effective.[41,43,44,46,49]

What appears clear is that cathodal high-voltage electrical stimulation is an effective means of limiting the onset of swelling but only during the acute period, when vascular permeability is increased. After leakage has occurred and localized swelling has been produced, management of swelling becomes more challenging. This is frequently the case, as patients are often not seen for treatment for days or weeks after their injury.

After edema has accumulated and become chronic, management must focus on clearing the swelling, rather than preventing it. Evidence for management of chronic edema is limited to a few studies, mostly given to chronic hand edema, and all used electrically stimulated muscle contractions (e.g., NMES). It is thought that repetitive contractions of the muscles compress venous and lymphatic vessels, helping to reduce swelling while increasing venous and lymphatic return.[50,51]

The waveform most supported for edema management in the acute phase is high-volt monophasic pulsed current (e.g., twin-peak monophasic), but when using

CASE STUDY 10•3   TENS

A patient involved in a motor vehicle accident 2 days ago presents with soft tissue injury to the posterior cervical spine and the upper thoracic region on the right side. Active and resisted ROM is painful and limited. Palpation is more revealing of tenderness in the right upper trapezius.

CLINICAL DECISION-MAKING

1. Does the patient have a dysfunction, limitation, or problem that can be improved with the use of electrotherapy?
   Answer: Yes, the patient demonstrates decreased ROM, pain, and tenderness to palpation of the upper trapezius following a motor vehicle accident.

2. Is the patient appropriate for electrotherapy (i.e., do any of the general precautions or contraindications to electrotherapy apply, or are there any specific considerations regarding application of electrotherapy to this patient)?
   Answer: Given that there are no contraindications or precautions, this patient is appropriate for the use of electrical stimulation.

3. What are the specific goals to be achieved with the use of electrotherapy?
   Answer: To decrease the acute pain associated with soft tissue injury stemming from the accident.

4. Do you have the specific type of electrotherapy that is appropriate for the patient?
   Answer: TENS can be used to address acute musculoskeletal pain. Because the patient demonstrates increased pain with resisted testing of the paracervical muscles, sensory-level TENS is indicated. Keep in mind that use of TENS is not limited to handheld stimulators, as many line-powered stimulators offer the same stimulus parameters as the handheld ones.

5. Can you select the specific parameters of electrotherapy that are appropriate for the patient?
   Answer:
   Waveform: Mono- or biphasic pulsed current may be used.
   Pulse duration: 100 microseconds secondary to acute pain and pain with resisted ROM

Pulse frequency: 100 pps for acute musculoskeletal pain
Intensity: To a noticeable and comfortable sensation of tingling without visible motor response. Modulation of the stimulation may be used to minimize effects of accommodation.
Duration: 20 to 30 min or longer as needed

6. What are the proper application procedures for electrotherapy?
   Answer:
   Instruct the patient: Inform the patient of the purpose and procedure. Be sure to explain the anticipated sensation and effect of the stimulation. In this case, a perceivable yet comfortable sensation of stimulation should be noted in the muscles of the paracervical spine.
   Preinspection: Clean the area to be treated and check for skin compromise. If excessive hair is present in the area, shaving it off may enhance the delivery of the stimulation.
   Electrode placement: Two electrodes in a bipolar configuration are placed over the right upper trapezius.
   Patient position: The patient may be supine or prone with head resting on pillows or may be sitting upright.
   Postinspection: Remove the electrodes and inspect the skin for any signs of skin irritation or adverse effects. If redness appears, explain that this is not uncommon and should disappear in less than 24 hours.

Six weeks later, the patient demonstrates the ability to perform active and resisted ROM but remains symptomatic in the right upper trapezius. The clinician now opts to use motor-level or acupuncture TENS. The same waveform and device may be used, but now the pulse duration is increased to 250 μsec while the pulse frequency is reduced to 10 pps. The electrodes are placed over the muscle tissue of the right upper trapezius, and the intensity is increased to elicit visible muscle contraction of the muscle up to patient tolerance.

---

muscle activation, other waveforms suitable to motor activation can be used (Table 10-4). High-volt pulsed current is often applied with the active or treatment electrodes placed in the immediate area of injury. In many cases, this may be directly over a peripheral joint or soft tissue region, with the electrodes bracketing the joint and the dispersive pad placed nearby (a monopolar arrangement; Fig. 10-16). The size of the electrodes should reflect the size of the joint or area. Thus, larger electrodes are used at the knee than at the wrist. The clinician should designate the active electrodes placed over the swollen area as the cathode. In the acute

Table 10•4	**Parameters for Edema Management**					
Indication	**Type**	**Waveform**	**Pulse Frequency**	**Pulse Duration**	**Amplitude**	**Duration**
Acute (within 24–72 hours)	Sensory level stimulation	Monophasic pulsed (e.g., twin peak)	100–125 pps	2–100 µsec	mA to comfortable sensory perception (approximately 10% below motor threshold)	20–45 min to several hours
Existing edema (subacute or chronic)	Motor-level stimulation (e.g., NMES)	Biphasic PC or burst-modulated AC (e.g., Russian)	20–80 pps or bursts per sec	100–600 µsec if PC	mA to tetanic contraction	1:1 on:off ratio (e.g., 10–20 min of rhythmic contractions at 3 sec on–3 sec off)

stages, where motor activation is not desired, a pulse frequency of 100 to 125 pps is common, with an intensity eliciting a perceptible sensory response but below the motor threshold. If using high-volt pulsed current (e.g., twin-peak monophasic), the twin-phase pulse duration is most likely fixed at 2 to 100 µsec.

KEY POINT! There has remained some clinical opinion that changing the polarity of the active or treatment electrodes halfway through a treatment session from negative (cathodal) to positive (anodal) provides some additional benefit over continual negative stimulation. This practice has never been supported by the literature; thus, continuous use of negative stimulation over the swollen area remains recommended.

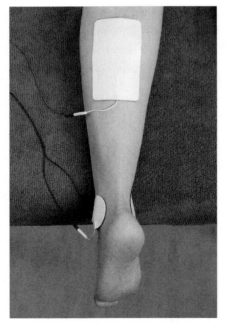

Fig 10•16 Use of electrical stimulation to reduce swelling. Cathodal stimulation with high-volt pulsed current is used in the acute stages. Muscle stimulation for pumping is used after the acute stage.

Treatment duration in the acute phase can range from several minutes to hours, but additional precaution should be taken if applying stimulation consistently for several hours secondary to the electrochemical effects that can occur at the anode and cathode when using monophasic current. When using stimulated muscle activation for reducing edema in the postacute and chronic stages, the waveform selected must be suitable for stimulating muscle. Symmetrical or asymmetrical biphasic pulsed currents (e.g., square, rectangular, or triangular waveforms) and burst-modulated AC (e.g., Russian) are commonly used. Because muscle activation is desired, electrodes must be placed over muscle tissue of the swollen joint. The bracketing of joints used in the acute stage would not allow for stimulation of muscle, since little muscle exists directly over joints. The specific parameters should allow for rhythmic contraction and relaxation of the muscle (e.g., 10-second contraction followed by 10-second rest). Pulse frequency may range from 20 to 80 pps and pulse duration from 100 to 600 µsec with an intensity capable of eliciting rhythmic tetanic contractions. Typical treatment sessions of muscle pumping last 10 to 20 minutes. Stimulation beyond 10 to 20 minutes may increase blood flow to the area and provoke further swelling.

KEY POINT! In the acute and, particularly, subacute periods following injury, the local vasculature may remain weakened and prone to further leakage. It is possible that repeated muscle contractions via NMES may result in increased local blood flow and may overload weakened local vasculature. Therefore, use of NMES for managing edema is recommended only when swelling has stabilized or does not increase following use of motor-level stimulation.

CASE STUDY 10•4 USING ELECTRICAL STIMULATION FOR MANAGEMENT OF EDEMA

Karen is a 17-year-old lacrosse player who sprained her ankle in a match yesterday afternoon. She presents to the clinic the next morning with acute swelling of the left lateral ankle and laxity in ligaments of the lateral ankle. ROM is decreased secondary to discomfort and swelling.

CLINICAL DECISION-MAKING

1. Does the patient have a dysfunction, limitation, or problem that can be improved with the use of electrotherapy?
   Answer: Yes, the patient has acute swelling, pain, and decreased ROM following musculoskeletal injury to the ankle.

2. Is the patient appropriate for electrotherapy (i.e., do any of the general precautions or contraindications to electrotherapy apply, or are there any specific considerations regarding application of electrotherapy to this patient)?
   Answer: The patient does not present with any contraindications or precautions.

3. What are the specific goals to be achieved with the use of electrotherapy?
   Answer: Reduction of acute swelling to reduce pain and permit ROM exercises as indicated in the therapy plan

4. Do you have the specific type of electrotherapy that is appropriate for the patient?
   Answer: High-volt pulsed current (i.e., twin-peak monophasic) is selected, as it may assist in reducing and preventing further swelling.

5. Can you select the specific parameters of electrotherapy that are appropriate for the patient?
   Answer:
   Pulse duration: 100 microseconds

Pulse frequency: Approximately 100 pps
Intensity: Increase intensity until a small but visible motor response is elicited and then reduce the intensity to a level approximately 10% below the motor threshold.
Duration: 15 to 30 minutes.

6. What are the proper application procedures for electrotherapy?
   Answer:
   Instruct the patient: Inform the patient of the purpose and procedure. Be sure to explain the anticipated sensation and effect of the stimulation. In this case, a sensation of buzzing or strong tingling should be noted at the ankle. Depending on the amount of swelling at each malleoli, the patient may have more or less sensation of the electrical stimulus.
   Preinspection: Clean the area to be treated and check for skin compromise. Observe any bony areas where appropriate electrode contact may be a challenge.
   Electrode placement: Electrodes are placed on the lateral and medial aspect of the ankle bracketing the joint. A dispersive pad is placed on the posterior thigh to complete the circuit. The treatment pads are designated as the cathode and the reference as the anode.
   Patient position: Because the intervention is addressing swelling, the patient should be positioned with the ankle elevated above torso. Supine positioning with the ankle elevated by pillows or a bolster is recommended.
   Postinspection: Remove the electrodes and inspect the skin for any signs of skin irritation or adverse effects. If redness appears, explain that this is not uncommon and should disappear in less than 24 hours.

Electrotherapy for Increasing Circulation

ES is often used to increase blood flow in superficial and deep tissues. This can be accomplished using various types of ES, but all generally fall into either sensory or motor-level stimulation (see Table 10-5). Local increase in skin blood flow occurs by vasodilation of cutaneous vessels;[52,53] low-frequency TENS at a sensory level (e.g., 4 pps at 250 μsec) appears to be more effective than high-frequency TENS (e.g., 100 pps at 100 μsec).[54] Deeper arterial blood flow does not appear to increase with sensory-level stimulation, but it does with motor-level stimulation using rhythmic muscle contractions.[55–58] Miller and colleagues[55] reported that the increased blood flow following motor-level electrical stimulation resulted in a longer lasting increase in flow than was measured following voluntary muscular contraction alone.

Table 10•5	**Parameters for Increasing Peripheral Blood Flow**					
Indication	**Type**	**Waveform**	**Pulse Frequency**	**Pulse Duration**	**Amplitude**	**Duration**
Vasospastic disorders	Sensory-level stimulation	Mono- or biphasic pulsed current	4–100 pps	4–600 μsec	mA to comfortable sensory perception	15–30 min
	Motor-level stimulation	Mono- or biphasic pulsed current	1–5 pps	200–600 μsec	mA to visible muscle twitches	15–30 min
Diminished arterial blood flow	Motor-level stimulation (e.g., NMES)	Biphasic pulsed current or burst-modulated AC (e.g., Russian)	20–80 pps or bursts per sec	100–600 μsec	mA to robust tetanic muscle contractions	1:1 on:off ratio (e.g., 10–15 min of rhythmic contractions)

To promote superficial local blood flow via cutaneous vasodilation, sensory-level stimulation is used with electrodes placed paraspinally, over peripheral nerves, acupuncture points, dermatomes, myotomes, or other tissue areas where increased blood flow is desired. Because low-frequency TENS appears most effective, a stimulus with a pulse frequency between 4 and 100 pps and a pulse duration of 4 to 600 μsec at a sensory-level intensity is recommended. To promote deeper blood flow via arterial or venous flow, ES capable of eliciting a motor-level response at least 10% of the maximal voluntary contraction is required. Stimulation at a frequency of 20 to 80 pps, a pulse duration of 100 to 600 μsec, and 5- to 10-second on-time and 5- to 10-second off-time is recommended. Electrodes should be placed over muscle of the area where increased blood flow is desired. Treatments for both sensory- and motor-level stimulation are recommended for 15 to 30 minutes. Because of the resistance to blood flow created by muscle contraction, sustained contractions without rest intervals are not recommended. The rhythmic effect of muscular contraction with intermittent relaxation may assist in venous blood flow and prevention of deep-vein thrombosis in the lower extremities during period of immobilization, when voluntary motor activity is impaired, or following surgery[59] (Table 10-5).

Electrotherapy for Promoting Tissue Healing

Use of ES for healing of chronic wounds is well supported in the peer-reviewed literature. In a meta-analysis of ES helping to heal chronic wounds, Gardner and associates[60] concluded that wounds treated with ES showed a 144% greater healing rate when compared to the normal rate of healing; the greatest effect was noted in pressure ulcers. Use of ES for wound healing is based on the transepithelial potential (TEP) and injury current, which is presented in Chapter 14. Wounds that fail to heal properly appear to have lost the injury current and are unable restore the TEP. The application of exogenous or clinical ES is thought to replace or augment the natural or endogenous current associated with healing.

The benefit of ES for chronic wounds appears greatest in recalcitrant stage III and IV ulcers. Reimbursement standards support use in these conditions. The Centers for Medicare and Medicaid Services (CMS) recognize ES for treating wounds only if the wound is a chronic stage III or IV ulcer and there have been no measurable signs of healing for at least 30 days of treatment with standard wound care. Therefore, documentation of the stage of the ulcer, duration of standard care, and any responses to treatment (such as wound size, presence of granulation tissue, and epithelialization) is essential for reimbursement of services.

There are a variety of cellular and tissue responses to ES. It appears that cells associated with tissue healing, such as neutrophils, macrophages, and lymphocytes, are charged and are attracted to migrate toward the opposite charge when exposed to an electrical field.[61,62] This migration of cells to a specific pole of an electrical field is termed *galvanotaxis*. Intracellular influx of calcium (Ca^{2+}) increases when cells are exposed to electrical fields, increasing activity of cytoskeletal elements, such as actin microfilaments, that underlie the galvanotaxic properties exhibited by some cells.[61,62]

CASE STUDY 10•5   INCREASING BLOOD FLOW

A patient with diabetic neuropathy and decreased sensation in the plantar aspect of both feet is referred for exercise and intervention. The clinician wants to increase arterial circulation in the feet to decrease the risk of ulceration.

CLINICAL DECISION-MAKING

1. Does the patient have a dysfunction, limitation, or problem that can be improved with the use of electrotherapy?
   Answer: Yes, the patient has diabetes-related peripheral neuropathy with decreased sensation of the plantar aspects of both feet.

2. Is the patient appropriate for electrotherapy (i.e., do any of the general precautions or contraindications to electrotherapy apply, or are there any specific considerations regarding application of electrotherapy to this patient)?
   Answer: The patient has decreased sensation in the intended treatment area. Decreased sensation is a precaution for electrotherapy, so the clinician must carefully monitor the treatment both prior to and after stimulation.

3. What are the specific goals to be achieved with the use of electrotherapy?
   Answer: To increase local blood flow in the plantar aspect of the feet to facilitate improved sensation.

4. Do you have the specific type of electrotherapy that is appropriate for the patient?
   Answer: Motor-level stimulation is indicated to increase local blood flow. Waveforms and parameters used for eliciting motor-level stimulation may be used. The stimulation should produce rhythmic muscle twitches in the plantar intrinsic muscles.

5. Can you select the specific parameters of electrotherapy that are appropriate for the patient?
   Answer:
   Waveform: Mono- or biphasic pulsed current may be used.
   Pulse duration: 300 microseconds—suitable for motor-level stimulation
   Pulse frequency: 5 pps for low-frequency motor stimulation
   Intensity: Until small but visible muscle twitches are produced in the plantar muscle region
   Duration: 15 to 30 min

6. What are the proper application procedures for electrotherapy?
   Answer:
   Instruct the patient: Inform the patient of the purpose and procedure. Be sure to explain the anticipated sensation and effect of the stimulation. Decreased sensation in the treatment area may limit the patient's perception of the stimulation. Careful monitoring by the clinician is required to ensure proper administration of the stimulation.
   Preinspection: Clean the area to be treated and check for skin compromise and possible ulceration. Excessive callus formation on the plantar areas may increase resistance to the stimulation.
   Electrode placement: Two electrodes in a bipolar configuration are placed over the plantar aspect of each foot.
   Patient position: The patient will be placed supine on a treatment table.
   Postinspection: Remove the electrodes and inspect the skin for any signs of skin irritation or adverse effects.

Other specific cell activities are noted in response to ES. The large negatively charged surface membrane proteins of the fluid-mosaic phospholipid cell wall show movement to the side of the cell facing the anode. Certain cells, such as endothelial cells, elongate and orient themselves to the field lines created by ES. Cell adhesion molecules, such as fibronectin, show increased binding of cells within the extracellular matrix. Intracellular second messenger systems, such a cyclic AMP and G-proteins, show increased activity. Additionally, protein kinase activity is increased, resulting in increased expression of epithelial and fibroblastic growth factors.[61,62]

KEY POINT! An understanding of the effects of ES on tissue healing has come from studies using calcium (Ca^{2+}) channel antagonists (e.g., lanthanum) or blockers (e.g., nitrendipine or verapamil). These drugs can slow or even stop increased cell activity observed in response to an electrical field.[61,72]

High-volt pulsed current (e.g., twin-peak monophasic) remains the most commonly used and supported current for tissue healing. The current may be applied directly into the wound or in the region around it. Prior to application, the specific polarity to be used must be determined and is termed the *active* or *treatment electrode*. In general, the cathode is used first in the early period of wound inflammation and infection. The anode is then used for debridement (e.g., phagocytosis and autolysis) and for promotion of epithelialization during the later proliferation stage of healing. The other electrode (dispersive or inactive electrode), and thus pole, is placed nearby on the skin (approximately 15 to 30 cm from the wound) in a monopolar arrangement. If stimulation is to be introduced directly into the wound, the active electrode should be placed in a saline-moistened sterile gauze and placed into or onto the wound. (Keep in mind that distilled water will not conduct, so saline is best used.) If the stimulus is to be delivered near the wound, the electrodes are placed on either side of it so current will travel through the wound (Fig. 10-17).

A pulse frequency of approximately 100 to 125 pps at a sensory-level intensity is recommended. Pulse duration is usually maintained on most high-volt pulsed devices at 2 to 100 μsec. Low-intensity direct current (e.g., microcurrent) is also used and by definition is below the sensory threshold. Like high-volt pulsed monophasic current, the anode and cathode of DC are used for their specific properties. In patients with compromised sensation in the wound area, a trial application of the stimulus over an area of intact sensation can be used to gauge patient comfort and tolerance. Daily treatments of 45 to 60 minutes are recommended

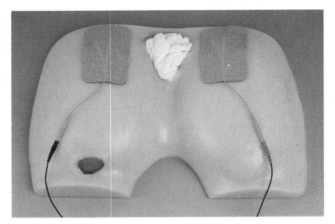

Fig 10•17 Use of electrical stimulation for wound healing. Electrodes may be placed on either side of the wound. The clinician should rotate the dispersive electrode or the pair of electrodes 30 to 90 degrees on subsequent treatments to fully expose all edges of the wound to the current.

(Table 10-6). Further discussion of ES for tissue healing is presented in Chapter 14.

KEY POINT! Because current flow will be greatest directly between the electrodes, the electrode placement sites should be rotated around the wound edge approximately 45 to 90 degrees on subsequent applications to ensure the wound is fully exposed to the stimulation. Failure to do so may result in the wound closing on only one side.

Biofeedback

Electromyographic (EMG) biofeedback differs from the previously described uses of ES in that no current is

Table 10•6 **Parameters for Enhancing Tissue Healing**						
Indication	**Type**	**Waveform**	**Pulse Frequency**	**Pulse Duration**	**Amplitude**	**Duration**
Epithelialization, autolysis, and reactivation of inflammatory process	Sensory-level stimulation; anode placed at wound	Monophasic pulsed current (e.g., twin-peak monophasic)	100 pps	4–100 μsec	mA to comfortable sensory response	60 min, 5–7 days per week
Promotion of granulation of wound	Sensory-level stimulation; cathode placed at wound	Monophasic pulsed current (e.g., twin-peak monophasic)	100 pps	4–100 μsec	mA to comfortable sensory response	60 min, 5–7 days per week
Bactericidal effect for infected wound	Sensory-level stimulation; cathode or cathode followed by anode placed at wound	Monophasic pulsed current (e.g., twin-peak monophasic)	100 pps	4–100 μsec	mA to comfortable sensory response	30–60 min of cathodal stimulation or 20 min of cathodal stimulation followed by 40 min of anodal stimulation

CASE STUDY 10•6 TISSUE HEALING

A 49-year-old man with diabetes is referred with a stage IV recalcitrant pressure ulceration at the lateral lower leg. There have been no observable signs of tissue healing for the last 30 days of standard wound care. The clinician wishes to facilitate granulation in the wound area.

CLINICAL DECISION-MAKING

1. Does the patient have a dysfunction, limitation, or problem that can be improved with the use of electrotherapy?
   Answer: Yes, the patient has a stage IV recalcitrant pressure ulceration at the posterior lower leg.

2. Is the patient appropriate for electrotherapy (i.e., do any of the general precautions or contraindications to electrotherapy apply, or are there any specific considerations regarding application of electrotherapy to this patient)?
   Answer: Diabetes may be associated with decreased sensation in the treatment area. Assessment of sensation is recommended prior to stimulation, and close monitoring of treatment is warranted if compromised sensation is noted.

3. What are the specific goals to be achieved with the use of electrotherapy?
   Answer: To promote and encourage granulation of the wound bed.

4. Do you have the specific type of electrotherapy that is appropriate for the patient?
   Answer: High-volt pulsed current (i.e., twin-peak monophasic current) may be used, as this monophasic waveform can deliver cathodal and anodal stimulation.

5. Can you select the specific parameters of electrotherapy that are appropriate for the patient?
   Answer:
   Waveform: Monophasic (high-volt) pulsed current
   Pulse duration: 100 microseconds
   Pulse frequency: 100 pps
   Intensity: To produce a mild sensory sensation
   Duration: 60 min

6. What are the proper application procedures for electrotherapy?
   Answer:
   Instruct the patient: Inform the patient of the purpose and procedure. Be sure to explain the anticipated sensation and effect of the stimulation. Decreased sensation in the treatment area may limit the patient's perception of the stimulation.
   Preinspection: The ulceration represents an area of decreased resistance to current and should be inspected prior to stimulation.
   Electrode placement: The treatment electrode is placed within a saline-moistened sterile gauze pad placed directly within the ulceration, and the reference or inactive electrode is placed adjacent to the ulceration. The treatment electrode is designated as the cathode and the reference the anode.
   Patient position: The patient will be placed supine or side-lying on the opposite side.
   Postinspection: Remove the electrodes and inspect the ulceration and adjacent skin for any signs of adverse effect.

---

actually delivered to the patient. In contrast, EMG biofeedback involves the assessment and recording of skeletal muscle activity so that the practitioner and patient can use the information to alter future muscle activity, whether that be to increase or decrease movement.[63] Improvement in function and decrease in pain are still the primary goals with EMG biofeedback, despite the differences with other forms of electrotherapy. Oftentimes, EMG biofeedback is not included in the same category as other electrotherapeutic applications where current is applied to the patient, but EMG biofeedback can be used to enhance volitional muscle activation, thereby providing therapeutic benefit. More

details and clinical applications of EMG biofeedback are presented in Chapter 11.

Iontophoresis

Iontophoresis is a technique in which current is used to induce the transcutaneous movement of ions across the skin into target tissues. Clinical use of iontophoresis is based on the fundamental concept that like charges repel and opposites attract. An ion is an atom that has lost or gained electrons and thus becomes positively or negatively charged. To mobilize or deliver negatively charged ions into the treatment area, an electrode containing the negative ions attached to the cathode of an electrical circuit is placed over the treatment area. For a positively charged ion, the anode is used. For the majority of clinical applications, iontophoresis implies the delivery of a medicinal ion for therapeutic benefit. The electrode containing the medicinal ion is termed the *treatment, active,* or *delivery electrode,* and the other electrode is termed the *inactive, reference,* or *dispersive electrode.* Note that either the anode or cathode can be used as the treatment electrode, depending on the polarity of the ions being delivered.

Current is delivered to the electrodes via a device. Most devices used for iontophoresis use DC and are small and portable and battery-operated. The DC provides a unidirectional electric current to induce ion movement. There are some devices that use alternating current, although evidence for their use is limited.[64,65] It has been proposed that the alternating nature of AC current may increase the permeability of the tissue, facilitating the passage of the ions.[66] Still, some units using AC for iontophoresis do so using AC with a "DC offset" that in essence mimics the properties of DC that induce ion movement.[67]

Iontophoresis has been used for many conditions, including soft tissue inflammatory conditions,[68,69] neuralgia,[70] edema,[71] ischemic skin ulcers,[72] hyperhidrosis,[73,74] plantar warts,[75] gouty arthritis,[76] calcific tendonitis,[77] scar tissue,[78] Peyronie's disease,[78–80] and other disorders of connective tissue. For most of these uses, the evidence is generally favorable.[81] The most studied use of iontophoresis is of corticosteroids, such as dexamethasone, which is used to reduce inflammation of local soft tissues.

Physiology of Iontophoresis

Underlying the process of iontophoresis is the electrical repulsion of ions. Using ES to move charged ions into the target tissues has long been the cornerstone explanation for iontophoresis and is termed *electromigration.* However, more recent explanations of the physiological mechanisms underlying iontophoresis have been described.[82]

Electroporation is an increase in the porosity of the superficial skin in response to ES and may facilitate movement of ions into the tissues.[82–85] Skin is naturally hydrophobic, so it presents a barrier to the transcutaneous movement of ions in a solution.[86] Following ES, a temporary increase in the skin's porosity allows ions to more easily penetrate the tissues. The exact mechanisms by which electroporation occurs are not known, but it is clear that cell organization and function of skin are altered in response to ES.[83–85]

Another mechanism that is used to explain the migration of ions into the tissues is based on "volume flow," or the bulk movement of solute in response to an electric field. Not to be confused with simple diffusion, this movement is in response to an applied electrical field and not concentration gradients.[82] When electrodes are applied to the skin, ions of positive charge within the extracellular fluid—that is, sodium (Na^+)—are attracted to the cathode, whereas negatively charged ions such as chloride (Cl^-) are attracted to the anode. The bulk movement of solute such as Na^+ and Cl^- in response to the electrical field is thought to provide a mechanism by which ions are moved into the tissues. This process is termed *electroosmosis,* or *ionohydrokinesis*[82,87] (Fig. 10-18).

Electroosmotic flow occurs in the same direction as flow of counterions (ions of charge opposite the skin). Because human skin maintains a net negative charge, the direction of electroosmotic flow is from the anode to the cathode.[82] For positively charged ions delivered from the anode, electroosmotic flow may assist in transdermal delivery, but in contrast, electroosmotic flow may hinder delivery of negatively charged ions from the cathode.[82] This opposition to delivery of

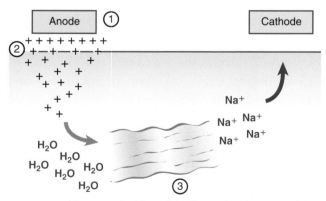

Fig 10•18 Movement of ions into tissue by three mechanisms: (1) electrical repulsion of like charges; (2) electroporation, increasing openings in the skin surface for ions; and (3) electroosmosis or movement of water and sodium (Na^+) toward the cathode, creating a stream by which ions are moved.

negative ions from the cathode is increased only when using larger current amplitudes, as the increased force of the electrical field will necessarily increase the ionic movement.

When considering the collective effects of electromigration, electroporation, and electroosmosis, there is reason to consider use of smaller amplitude current for delivery of negative ions to minimize the counterflowing electroosmosis. The "wear-home" iontophoresis systems with self-contained electrocircuitry use this principle by delivering a smaller amplitude current over a longer period of time versus in-clinic systems. Likewise, the effect of electroosmosis and counterion flow makes anodal delivery of negatively charged ions or neutral drug molecules such as glucose a future consideration. This use of anodal delivery for negatively charged ions has been termed *wrong-way iontophoresis* but reflects the idea that delivery of larger, negatively charged ions may be more effective when delivered secondary to properties of electroporation and electroosmosis.[82]

Application of Iontophoresis

There are two important aspects of iontophoresis: (1) knowing the polarity of the ion or drug to be used and (2) having good conductivity so there is not a chemical burn under the electrodes. If the incorrect pole is used during the procedure, there is little to no chance the ions will make it into the desired tissue.

KEY POINT! Selecting an ion with a known polarity may seem obvious, but at one time there was considerable controversy over the polarity of dexamethasone, the most commonly used drug for iontophoresis. Dexamethasone was once considered to be positively charged, and many textbooks and guidelines for iontophoresis instructed in using the anode to deliver dexamethasone. It was not until 1992 that dexamethasone was shown to be best phoresed from the cathode. This is now the standard procedure for using dexamethasone.[88]

Selecting an Ion

The primary determinant in selecting an ion or drug for iontophoresis is whether the ion has a therapeutic effect on the condition being treated. For example, if treating an inflamed tendon with the goal of reducing

inflammation and pain, an ion with anti-inflammatory capability is recommended. Because iontophoresis is a procedure in which ions are transferred across the skin, it is critical to specify what specific ion or medicine is to be phoresed. A number of both pharmacological and nonpharmacological ions are used in therapeutic iontophoresis (Table 10-7). The most common of these is dexamethasone sodium phosphate. Because of the widespread use of this drug, the term *iontophoresis* has conventionally come to imply the use of dexamethasone, although this does not accurately reflect the procedure of iontophoresis. Therefore, it is recommended that use of the term *iontophoresis* be clarified by specifying what type of ion or medication was used. In summary, when performing iontophoresis, you should always answer the question, "Phoresis of what?"

KEY POINT! Effective iontophoresis is predicated on several factors, one of which is the concentration of the ion or drug used. It is advised that drugs for iontophoresis be obtained from a licensed pharmacist to ensure proper concentrations and storage.

Electrode Selection and Placement

Current density is the amount of current per unit of the electrode's conductive surface area and is calculated as:

$$\text{Current density (CD)} = \frac{\text{current amplitude (mA)}}{\substack{\text{conductive surface area} \\ \text{of the electrode (cm}^2)}}$$

It is critical to note that an electrode's size and its conductive surface area are not the same. Most commercially manufactured electrodes for iontophoresis have a region of adhesive material extending beyond the edges of the conductive surface area (Fig. 10-19). This renders the conductive surface area smaller than the apparent electrode size. A maximal current density of 0.5 mA/cm² (3.3 mA/in.²) at the cathode and 1 mA/cm² (6.6 mA/in.²) at the anode have been recommended as safe.[87,89,90] Caustic damage to the tissue at the cathode caused by formation of sodium hydroxide is of great concern. Therefore, it is recommended that the cathode's electroconductive surface area exceed that of the anode, even up to twice the area.

When using cathodal stimulation to the smaller active electrode, it is recommended that the current amplitude be monitored to minimize risk of tissue damage. Most commercially manufactured iontophoresis

Table 10•7 Indications and Drugs Commonly Used With Iontophoresis

Indication	Drug	Solution	Delivery Electrode Polarity	Effect
Inflammation	Dexamethasone	4 mg/mL in aqueous solution	Negative	Anti-inflammatory
Calcific tendonitis, myositis ossificans	Acetic acid	2–5% aqueous solution	Negative	Believed to increase solubility of calcium deposits
Adhesive capsulitis and other soft tissue adhesions	Iodine	5–10% solution or ointment	Negative	Sclerolytic effects
Soft tissue pain and inflammation	Lidocaine	4–5% solution or ointment	Positive	Local anesthetic effects
Muscle and joint pain	Salicylates	10% trolamine salicylate ointment or 2–3% sodium salicylate solution	Negative	Analgesic and anti-inflammatory
Local subacute or chronic edema	Hyaluronidase	Reconstitute with 0.9% sodium chloride to provide a 150 mg/ml solution	Positive	Dispersion of local edema
Skeletal muscle spasms	Calcium chloride	2% aqueous solution	Positive	Decreased excitability of peripheral nerves and skeletal muscle
Skeletal muscle spasms, myositis	Magnesium sulfate	2% aqueous solution or ointment	Positive	Muscle relaxant
Skin ulcers	Zinc oxide	20% ointment	Positive	Acts as a general antiseptic and may increase tissue healing
Hyperhidrosis	Tap water	N/A	Alternating polarity	Decreased sweating of palms, feet, or axillae

Source: Ciccone, CD: Pharmacology in Rehabilitation, ed. 3. FA Davis, Philadelphia, 2002, p 651.

electrodes have a conductive surface area that allows a current density within acceptable ranges for most iontophoresis devices, with a maximal current output of 4 to 5 mA. Many of the commercially prepared electrodes include chemical buffers within the electrode to minimize the chance of electrical burn. Although the process of iontophoresis can theoretically be administered using any type of electrode placed over a porous material containing the ions (e.g., a sponge or towel), for reasons of safety, commercially prepared electrodes should be used.

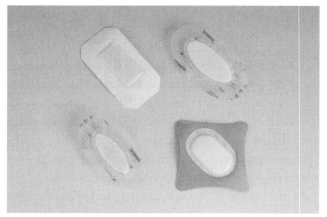

Fig 10•19 The electroconductive surface of most electrodes used for iontophoresis is less than the apparent size of the electrode.

The placement of electrodes for iontophoresis is directly dependent on the site being treated. The active electrode delivering the therapeutic ion is placed over the desired treatment area. In many cases, palpation to identify the most painful area will reveal the local area best suited for application. Prior to application, inspect the skin for color and integrity and record this in the patient's treatment record. Repeat this upon removing the electrodes to determine the skin's tolerance of the current. The inactive electrode is placed at a site distant from the treatment electrode, but some consideration should be given to the distance between electrodes (i.e., the interelectrode distance). The closer the electrodes, the more superficial will be the current and potential movement of ions. A greater interelectrode distance will facilitate greater depth of current penetration and potentially ion delivery.

Dosage and the Iontophoretic Equation

Because iontophoresis usually involves delivery of a drug, it is necessary to specify the dose that is delivered. The iontophoretic equation is used to calculate the dose and is based on the current amplitude of the DC current and the duration the current is delivered:

$$\text{Dosage (mA·min)} = \text{Current (mA)} \times \text{Duration (min)}$$

Typical clinical dosages range from 20 to 80 mA·min with maximal dosages reaching 160 mA·min. As of yet, there has been no clearly defined dosage that is more effective than another and, in many cases, is decided upon by patient response and tolerance.[64] Current amplitude with clinical iontophoresis at dosages of 20 to 80 mA·min typically range from 0.1 to 4 mA, depending on patient tolerance and the duration current flows to obtain the desired dose. Duration is variable and has been a source of discussion. There remains disagreement as to the optimal dose and specific parameters used to obtain it. Some evidence has suggested that longer duration with lower amplitude facilitates greater depth of delivery.[91]

KEY POINT! To date, there remains no universal agreement as to whether the process of iontophoresis is specific to the administration of a medicinal ion or simply implies the use of current to mobilize ions. Thus, it is suggested that when performing iontophoresis, the clinician should clearly state what ion was "phoresed."

Adverse Effects: Current not Drugs

There is a greater risk of skin irritation and redness when using DC than with other currents. This is why it is critical to inspect the skin both before and after treatment. The tingling, itching, and redness that can occur with iontophoresis have inaccurately been attributed to the drug(s) used when actually it is the DC current that causes these effects. Cations such as Na^+ that form sodium hydroxide (NaOH) are attracted to the cathode. The formation of NaOH creates an alkaline reaction, and the movement of water with sodium via osmosis results in a decrease in protein density (sclerolysis) in the tissues under the cathode, which softens the tissue. This increases the risk of tissue breakdown or electrical burn. At the anode, an acidic reaction is created as anions such as Cl^- are attracted to it, reducing the local pH in the tissues near the anode. Likewise, as water moves away from the anode with Na^+, protein density increases (sclerosis) and tissue hardens. These factors must be considered even after a single treatment but certainly when iontophoresis is applied multiple times per week. In some patients showing skin compromise, it may be necessary to skip a treatment to allow the skin to heal. A summary of these reactions is presented in Table 10-8.

Table 10•8 **Associated Reactions at Each Electrode During Iontophoresis**

	Anode	Cathode
Attracts	Cl^-	Na^+
Forms	HCl	NaOH
Process	Sclerotic	Sclerolytic
Effect	Skin hardens	Skin softens*

* Increases risk of electrical burn and tissue damage to DC

Recent Advances in Iontophoresis

If using typical peak current amplitudes of 4 mA, typical clinical treatments of 20 to 80 mA·min require a 5- to 20-minute duration. At peak amplitude, patients may report stinging, tingling, or itching and mild reversible irritation.[92] Because maximal amplitude can be uncomfortable and patients are required to remain in the clinic, manufacturers designed wireless, disposable, battery-operated electrodes. These electrodes can be worn home by the patient, eliminating the need to remain in the clinic for the treatment, and they can deliver a low amplitude current for a longer duration, even up to 24 hours.[93] Newer iontophoresis electrodes consist of a single adhesive "patch" containing a complete microcircuit. A small button-sized battery delivers DC from 0.1 to 4 mA to an embedded anode and cathode to which the ionized drug and saline have been added (Fig. 10-20).

These newer iontophoresis electrodes may be initially charged while the patient is in the clinic. This charging provides an initial voltage that overcomes the skin's initial resistance to the current. After a few minutes of charging and a reduction in skin resistance, the wear-home disposable electrode then delivers a lower intensity current to phorese the drug. The electroconductive surface area is generally 6 to 9 cm², keeping the current density well within a safe range. Protocols for these electrode systems provide dosages similar to in-clinic procedures but seem to be gaining popularity for their ability to provide the same dose but at a lower (i.e., more comfortable) amplitude.

At the time of this writing, the literature is void of studies examining efficacy for these new wireless iontophoresis systems, but studies are under way. Positive evidence does seem to exist for the iontophoretic delivery of fentanyl, a rapid-acting opioid, for management of acute pain.[94,95]

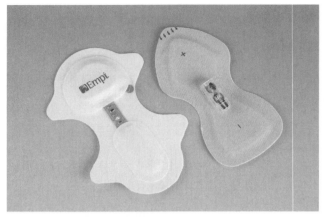

Fig 10•20 Wireless disposable electrode systems for iontophoresis.

Iontophoresis Versus Tap Water Galvanism

Although iontophoresis is the movement of ions in response to ES, conventional clinical use of the term has led the process to be associated with delivery of a pharmacological ion. Tap water galvanism (TWG) is the use of DC in tap water to create a constant, unidirectional electrostatic field.[74] The naturally occurring impurities found in tap water, such as magnesium, calcium, and chloride ions, are sufficient enough to conduct electrical current. TWG has long been shown to help reduce the symptoms of hyperhidrosis, a condition of excessive sweat production from the eccrine

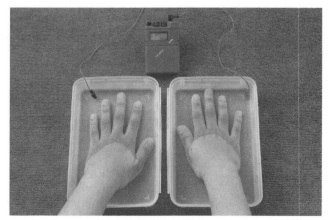

Fig 10•21 Most devices used for iontophoresis deliver direct current which can be used to treat hyperhidrosis. Placement of the hands in a water bath with an electrical field created by direct current can be used to address palmar hyperhidrosis.

sweat glands, typically of the hands and feet.[74,96] The hands or feet are placed within water, becoming part of the electrical field as a low-amplitude DC current is applied (Fig. 10-21).

TWG's mechanism of action remains unclear, but two mechanisms have been proposed: (1) DC current encourages hyperkeratinization in which waxy, keratinous plugs form and act to obstruct the sweat glands, and (2) DC may induce a functional disturbance that interferes with the stimulus-secretion coupling, impairing the electrochemical gradient of sweat output and thus decreasing sweat production.[97] Evidence for the use of TWG in the management of hyperhidrosis has existed for decades,[74,96] with the most recent evidence showing therapeutic benefit using a commercial iontophoresis device delivering DC current[73] (Box 10-5).

Precautions and Contraindications

Effective use of ES is founded on two primary factors: (1) careful differentiation of patients who stand to benefit from the intervention from those for whom electrotherapy is not appropriate and (2) careful, knowledgeable, and safe application of the intervention. Thus, precautions and contraindications to application of electrotherapy must be considered during treatment selection (Box 10-6 and 10-7).

CASE STUDY 10•7   IONTOPHORESIS

The patient is a 28-year-old female recreational tennis player who developed right lateral elbow pain 6 weeks ago. She presents to the clinic with a chief complaint of right elbow pain during tennis and when grasping with her hand. Palpation reveals tenderness and elicits pain over the lateral epicondyle and common extensor tendon of the right elbow. Wishing to address the acute soft tissue inflammation of the extensor tendon, the practitioner chooses to use iontophoresis and selects dexamethasone for its anti-inflammatory properties. After choosing an electrode with a 3 × 3 cm conductive surface area, the dexamethasone is applied to the electrode, and the electrode is placed over the lateral epicondyle and extensor soft tissue. Because dexamethasone is a negatively charged ion, the cathode of the DC current will be delivered to the electrode containing the dexamethasone. To complete a circuit, saline is placed on the inactive electrode, which is placed at a distance not less than twice the diameter of the smallest electrode. The amplitude of the current is increased to 4 mA, creating a current density of 0.44 mA/cm^2 (4 mA/9 cm^2). A 40 mA·min dosage is selected, so at 4 mA, the duration of the treatment will be 10 minutes. To complete the treatment, the clinician removed the electrodes and inspected the tissue for signs of adverse effect of the current.

CLINICAL DECISION-MAKING

1. Does the patient have a dysfunction, limitation, or problem that can be improved with the use of electrotherapy?
   Answer: Yes, the patient exam reveals relatively acute and localized tenderness to the extensor tendon of the lateral epicondyle.

2. Is the patient appropriate for electrotherapy (i.e., do any of the general precautions or contraindications to electrotherapy apply, or are there any specific considerations regarding application of electrotherapy to this patient)?
   Answer: The patient is a 28-year-old female and of reproductive age. Pregnancy is contraindicated with iontophoresis, so the practitioner should explain this concern and ask the patient if she is pregnant.

3. What are the specific goals to be achieved with the use of electrotherapy?
   Answer: To decrease local tissue inflammation and damage.

4. Do you have the specific type of electrotherapy that is appropriate for the patient?
   Answer: Iontophoresis offers a method for delivering dexamethasone sodium phosphate transcutaneously to a localized soft tissue area.

5. Can you select the specific parameters of electrotherapy that are appropriate for the patient?
   Answer:
   Waveform: DC
   Dosage: 40 to 80 mA·min
   Intensity: Up to 4 to 5 mA
   Duration: 10 to 20 min, depending on dosage and intensity

6. What are the proper application procedures for electrotherapy?
   Answer:
   Instruct the patient: Inform the patient of the purpose and procedure. Be sure to explain the anticipated sensation and effect of the stimulation.
   Preinspection: Inspect the skin in the area to be treated as well as the area where the reference, or inactive, electrode will be placed.
   Electrode placement: The appropriate volume of dexamethasone is applied to a commercially manufactured electrode and placed over the lateral epicondyle. The volume of medication is dependent on the electrode size and is often marked on the electrode. The reference electrode is placed on the triceps of the same arm away from the treatment electrode. Because dexamethasone is a negatively charged ion, the treatment electrode is designated as the cathode and the reference electrode as the anode.
   Patient position: The patient may be placed sitting with the arm resting on the treatment table.
   Postinspection: Remove the electrodes and inspect the skin beneath the treatment and reference electrode for any signs of adverse effect. The practitioner must be aware that frequent treatments may result in tissue breakdown at the lateral epicondyle (cathode) and hardening at the triceps (anode).

| Box 10•6 | **Contraindications** |

Electrodes should not be placed over:

- The trunk or heart region in patients with demand-type pacemakers or implantable cardioverter defibrillators (ICDs)
  - In patients where use of electrotherapy is desired but contraindicated for pacemakers or ICDs, electrocardiographic examination by a cardiologist during a trial application of stimulation can determine the potential for interference with these devices.
- The pelvic, abdominal, lumbar, or hip region in pregnant women
  - Although the effects of electrical stimulation on the fetus or uterus are not clearly known, caution is recommended if using stimulation near these areas. For this reason, it is advised to ask all premenopausal women about the possibility of being pregnant prior to administering stimulation in these areas.
  - Pregnant women with known history of miscarriage may not be suitable to receive electrical stimulation, regardless of the area of application. The unknown effects of electrical stimulation on fetal health should be disclosed to the patient.
- Carotid bodies
  - Located on the anterolateral neck between the sternocleidomastoid and trachea; stimulation of these bodies may induce abnormal heart function. For this reason, proper electrode placement when treating posterior cervical musculature must ensure that carry-over of stimulation to the anterolateral neck does not occur.
- Phrenic nerve or urinary bladder stimulators
  - Interference from electrical stimulators may alter or compromise the function of these stimulators
- Areas of known peripheral vascular disease, including arterial or venous thrombosis or thrombophlebitis
  - Because stimulation may increase blood flow to the treatment area, avoid stimulating areas of compromised blood flow
- The phrenic nerve, eyes, or gonads
- Areas of active osteomyelitis
- Areas of hemorrhage

| Box 10•7 | **Precautions** |

1. Electrotherapy should be used with caution in patients:
   - Without intact sensation, as they may be unable to sense or detect and recognize abnormal sensations. An exception to this is when using low amplitude current for wound healing.
   - Who are unable to communicate, as they may be incapable of accurately providing feedback regarding the stimulation.
   - With compromised mental ability or lack of cognition, as they may be unable to understand directions.
   - With cardiac dysfunction, including uncontrolled hypertension or hypotension, or irregular heart rate or rhythm.
   - With epilepsy or other seizure disorders.
2. Over neoplasms (active or previous):
   - Use of electrotherapy in patients with active cancer should include consultation with the patient's physicians and documentation of patient consent.
   - Use of electrotherapy over sites of inactive neoplasm or elsewhere in patients with history of cancer should be done only after thorough explanation of the anticipated risks and benefits.
   - Written documentation of patient and physician consent is recommended.
3. Electrodes should not be placed over:
   - Compromised skin (except if treating for wound/tissue repair).
   - Tissues vulnerable to hemorrhage or hematoma.
   - Cervical (i.e., neck) or craniofacial regions in patients who have a history of cerebrovascular accident (CVA) or seizures.
4. Do not use electrical stimulation devices within approximately 5 yards of diathermy units or other source of electromagnetic radiation.

Safety With Electrotherapeutics: "Primum Non Nocere"

Latin for "first, do no harm," the phrase *primum non nocere* should always be considered when preparing to use an electrotherapeutic agent. The use of electrical current by nature brings with it inherent risk, danger, and potential for adverse events. However, clinicians aware of safety measures and safety practices can greatly minimize these risks and safely and effectively deliver therapeutic electrical stimulation. The primary concern with the use of electrical current is shock. While the intensity of the current flowing from the therapeutic device to the patient is often well below

harmful levels, the danger of electrical shock lies in the current flowing between the electrotherapeutic device and the wall current (household current). So while battery-powered devices may present less risk than line-powered ones, attention must nevertheless be given to ensure the safest environment for the patient and clinician. Any excess or short circuit must be terminated before it reaches a patient or the clinician.

Perhaps the most common and effective safety measures regarding electrical current from line-powered devices are the hospital-grade, three-prong plugs that have a safety ground in direct connection to the earth ground and the ground fault circuit interrupters

(GFCI). True ground returns current to the ground (i.e., earth) and does not include passage through the patient. GFCIs detect any loss or leak of current in the circuit created between the patient and the device. Most GFCIs are activated when a differential in current out versus current returned is greater than 3 to 5 mA. If a leak of this level is detected, the GFCI immediately stops flow of current within approximately 25 msec.

Although grounded plugs and GFCIs are essential safety measures, routine inspection is still important. Prior to every use, the clinician should take the time to inspect the integrity of the three-prong plug, the GFCI wall outlet, the power cord to the device, and the insulated coating on the lead wires. It is not uncommon that lead wires are run over by carts holding the devices or that the leads get caught on objects while moving the device, stretching and stressing the leads. This can damage the protective rubber or plastic coating and present a potential pathway for current to leak; this creates a risk to the patient or clinician. Likewise, the power cord from the wall to the device can be run over, pinched, or pulled loose. Thus, careful inspection of these components is critical.

More extensive inspections performed by trained personnel are also recommended and required by many standards. While there is presently no stipulation as to the frequency of formal inspection, an annual inspection should be done at the minimum, and more frequent inspections should be directly related to the frequency the device is used. Careful attention should also be given to the position of the patient and the placement of the electrodes so that electrodes do not come in contact with conductive surfaces that may lead to current leak. Some examples include metals from treatment tables and chairs, including bed rails and armrests, and other equipment that may be nearby such as orthotic equipment or a variety of hospital equipment containing metal. Likewise, lead wires can easily become caught or snagged on beds, tables, and chairs, so a watchful eye for these potential situations can lead to greater safety with electrotherapeutic stimulators.

Documentation Tips

Follow the documentation guidelines explained in Chapter 9.

REFERENCES

1. Laufer Y, Ries J, Leininger P, Alon G. Quadriceps femoris muscle torques produced and fatigue generated by neuromuscular electrical stimulation with three different waveforms. *Phys Ther.* 2001;81:1307–1316.
2. Lyons C, Robb J, Irrgang J, et al. Differences in quadriceps femoris muscle torque when using a clinical electrical stimulator versus a portable electrical stimulator. *Phys Ther.* 2005;85:44–51.
3. Manal T. Unpublished data: personal communication; 2009.
4. Dali C, Hansen F, Pedersen S, et al. Threshold electrical stimulation (TES) in ambulant children with CP: a randomized double-blind placebo controlled clinical trial. *Dev Med Child Neurol.* 2002;44:364–369.
5. Pape K. Therapeutic electrical stimulation for the treatment of disuse muscle atrophy in cerebral palsy. *Pediatr Phys Ther.* 1997;9:110–112.
6. Sommerfelt K, Markestad T, Berg K, Saetesdal I. Therapeutic electrical stimulation in cerebral palsy: a randomized, controlled, cross-over trial. *Dev Med Child Neurol.* 2001;43:609–613.
7. Axelgaard J, Brown J. Lateral electrical surface stimulation for treatment of progressive idiopathic scoliosis. *Spine.* 1983;8:242–260.
8. Eckerson L, Axelgaard J. Lateral electrical surface stimulation as an alternative to bracing in the treatment of idiopathic scoliosis. *Phys Ther.* 1984;64:483–490.
9. Currier D, Mann R. Muscular strength development by electrical stimulation in healthy individuals. *Phys Ther.* 1983;63:915–921.
10. Massey B, Nelson R, Sharkey B, et al. Effects of high frequency electrical stimulation on the size and strength of skeletal muscle. *J Sports Med Phys Fitness.* 1965;5:136–144.
11. Swearingen J. *Electrical Stimulation for Improving Muscle Performance.* Stamford, CT: Appleton and Lange; 1999:143–182.
12. Kramer J, Semple J. Comparison of selected strengthening techniques for normal quadriceps. *Physiother Can.* 1983;35:300–304.
13. Wolf S, Ariel G, Saar D, et al. The effect of muscle stimulation during resistive training on performance parameters. *Am J Sports Med.* 1986;14:18–23.
14. Delitto A, McKowen J, McCarthy J, et al. Electrically elicited co-contraction of the thigh musculature after anterior cruciate ligament surgery. A description and single-case experiment. *Phys Ther.* 1988;68:45–50.
15. Gremeaux V, Renault J, Pardon L, Deley G, Lepers R, Casillas J. Low frequency electrical stimulation combined with physical therapy after total hip arthroplasty for hip osteoarthritis in elderly patients: a randomized controlled trial. *Arch Phys Med Rehabil.* 2008;89:2265–2273.
16. Delitto A, Rose S. Comparative comfort of three waveforms used in electrically eliciting quadriceps femoris muscle contractions. *Phys Ther.* 1986;66(11):1704–1707.
17. Liberson W, Holmquest H, Scott M. Functional electrotherapy: stimulation of the common peroneal nerve synchronized with the swing phase of gait in hemiplegic patients. *Arch Phys Med Rehabil.* 1961;42:202–205.
18. Alon G, Levitt A, McCarthy P. Functional electrical stimulation enhancement of upper extremity functional recovery during stroke rehabilitation: a pilot study. *Neurorehabil Neural Repair.* 2007;21:207–215.
19. Knutson J, Hisel T, Harley M, Chae J. A novel functional electrical stimulation treatment for recovery of hand function in hemiplegia: a 12 week pilot study. *Neurorehabil Neural Repair.* 2009;23(1):17–25.

20. Kowalczewski J, Gritsenko V, Ashworth N, Ellaway P, Prochazka A. Upper-extremity functional electrical stimulation-assisted exercises on a workstation in the subacute phase of stroke recovery. *Arch Phys Med Rehabil.* 2007;88:833–839.

21. Knutson J, Harley M, Hisel T, Chae J. Improving hand function in stroke survivors: a pilot study of contralaterally controlled functional electrical stimulation in chronic hemiplegia. *Arch Phys Med Rehabil.* 2007;88:513–520.

22. Eberstein A, Eberstein S. Electrical stimulation of denervated muscle: is it worthwhile? *Med Sci Sports Exerc.* 1996; 28(12):1463–1469.

23. Kern H, Salmons S, Maryr W, et al. Recovery of long-term denervated human muscles induced by electrical stimulation. *Muscle Nerve.* 2005;31:98–101.

24. Pachter B, Eberstein A, Goodgold J. Electrical stimulation effect on denervated skeletal myofibers in rats: a light and electron microscopic study. *Arch Phys Med Rehabil.* 1982;63:427–430.

25. Schmitt LC, Schmitt LA, Rudolph K. Management of a patient with a forearm fracture and median nerve injury. *J Orthop Sports Phys Ther.* 2004;34:47–56.

26. Davis H. Is electrostimulation beneficial to denervated muscle? A review of results from basic research. *Physiother Can.* 1983;35:306–310.

27. Hayes K. Electrical stimulation and denervation: proposed program and equipment limitations. *Top Acute Care Trauma Rehabil.* 1988;3:27–37.

28. Hennig R. Late reinnervation of the rat soleus muscle is differentially suppressed by chronic stimulation and by ectopic innervation. *Acta Physiol Scand.* 1987;130(1):153–160.

29. Hennig R, Lomo T. Effects of chronic stimulation on the size and speed of long-term denervated and innervated rat fast and slow skeletal muscles. *Acta Physiol Scand.* 1987;130: 115–131.

30. Merletti R, Pinelli P. A critical appraisal of neuromuscular stimulation and electrotherapy in neurorehabilitation. *Eur Neurol.* 1980;19:30–32.

31. Schimrigk K, McLaughjlin J, Gruninger W. The effect of electrical stimulation on the experimentally denervated rat muscle. *Scand J Rehabil Med.* 1977;9:55–60.

32. Melzack R, Wall P. Pain mechanisms: a new theory. *Science.* 1965;150:971–978.

33. Manal T, Snyder-Mackler L. *Electrical Stimulation for Pain Modulation.* Baltimore, MD: Lippincott, Williams, and Wilkins; 2008;167.

34. Levin M, Hui-Chan C. Conventional and acupuncture-like transcutaneous electrical nerve stimulation excite similar afferent fibers. *Arch Phys Med Rehabil.* 1993;74:54–60.

35. Low J, Reed A. *Electrotherapy Explained: Principles and Practice.* 3rd ed. Oxford, UK: Butterworth-Heinemann; 2000: 94–95.

36. Sjolund B, Terenius L, Eriksson M. Increased cerebrospinal fluid levels of endorphins after electroacupuncture. *Acta Physiol Scand.* 1977;100:382–384.

37. Dolan M, Mendel F. Clinical application of electrotherapy. *Athl Ther Today.* 2004;9(5):11–16.

38. Man I, Morrisey M, Cywinski J. Effect of neuromuscular electrical stimulation on ankle swelling in the early period after ankle sprain. *Phys Ther.* 2007;87:53–65.

39. Wilkerson G, Horn-Kingery H. Treatment of the inversion ankle sprain: comparison of different modes of compression and cryotherapy. *J Orthop Sports Phys Ther.* 1993;17:240–246.

40. Hall R, Nyland J, Nitz A, et al. Relationship between ankle invertor H-reflexes and acute swelling induced by inversion ankle sprain. *J Orthop Sports Phys Ther.* 1999;29:339–344.

41. Bettany J, Fish D, Mendel F. Influence of high voltage pulsed direct current on edema formation following injury. *Phys Ther.* 1990;70:219–224.

42. Dolan M, Graves P, Nakazawa C, Delano T, Hutson A, Mendel F. Effects of ibuprofen and high-voltage electric stimulation on acute edema formation after blunt trauma to limbs of rats. *J Athl Train.* 2005;40(2):111–115.

43. Dolan M, Mychaskiw A, Mattacola C, Mendel F. Effects of cool water immersion and high-voltage electric stimulation for 3 continuous hours on acute edema in rats. *J Athl Train.* 2003;38:325–329.

44. Dolan M, Mychaskiw A, Mendel F. Cool-water immersions and high-voltage electric stimulation curb edema formation in rats. *J Athl Train.* 2003;38:225–230.

45. Mendel F, Fish D. New perspectives in edema control via electrical stimulation. *J Athl Train.* 1993;28:63–74.

46. Mendel F, Wylegala JA, Fish D. Influence of high-voltage pulsed current on edema formation following impact injury in rats. *Phys Ther.* 1992;72:668–673.

47. Reed B. Effect of high voltage pulsed electrical stimulation on microvascular permeability to plasma proteins. *Phys Ther.* 1988;68:491–495.

48. Taylor K, Mendel F, Fish D, Hard R, Burton H. Effects of high-voltage pulsed current and alternating current on macromolecular leakage in hamster cheek pouch microcirculation. *Phys Ther.* 1997;77:1729–1740.

49. Thornton R, Mendel F, Fish D. Effects of electrical stimulation on edema formation in different strains of rats. *Phys Ther.* 1998;78:386–394.

50. Bettany J, Fish D, Mendel F. High voltage pulsed direct current: effect on edema formation after hyperflexion injury. *Arch Phys Med Rehabil.* 1990;71:677–681.

51. Goddard A, Pierce C, McLeod K. Reversal of lower limb pump edema by calf muscle pump stimulation. *J Cardiopulm Rehabil Prev.* 2008;28:174–179.

52. Al Malty A, Petrofsky J, Akhavan S. Aging in women: the effect of menopause on skin blood flow and the response to electrical stimulation. *Phys Occup Ther Geriatr.* 2008;27(2):139–159.

53. Kaada B. Vasodilation induced by transcutaneous nerve stimulation in peripheral ischemia (Raynaud's phenomenon and diabetic polyneuropathy). *Eur Heart J.* 1982;3:303–314.

54. Scudds R, Helewa A, Scudds R. The effects of transcutaneous electrical nerve stimulation on skin temperature in asymptomatic subjects. *Phys Ther.* 1995;75:621–628.

55. Miller B, Gruben K, Morgan B. Circulatory responses to voluntary and electrically induced muscle contractions in humans. *Phys Ther.* 2000;80:53–60.

56. Scremin O, Cuevas-Trisan R, Scremin A, Brown C, Mandelkern M. Functional electrical stimulation effect on skeletal muscle blood flow measured with H2150 positron emission tomography. *Arch Phys Med.* 1998;79(6):641–646.

57. Sherry J, Oehrlein K, Hegge K, Morgan B. Effect of burst-mode transcutaneous electrical nerve stimulation on peripheral vascular resistance. *Phys Ther.* 2001;81:1183–1191.

58. Tracy J, Currier D, Threlkeld A. Comparison of selected pulse frequencies from two different electrical stimulators on blood flow in healthy subjects. *Phys Ther.* 1988;68:1526–1532.

59. Kloth L. *Electrical Stimulation for Wound Healing.* Philadelphia: FA Davis; 2002:302–303.

60. Gardner S, Frantz R, Schmid F. Effect of electrical stimulation on chronic wound healing: a meta-analysis. *Wound Repair Regen.* 1999;7:495–503.

61. McCaig C, Rajnicek A, Song B, Zhao M. Controlling cell behavior electrically: current views and future potential. *Physiol Rev.* 2005;85:943–978.

62. Nuccitelli R. A role for endogenous electrical fields in wound healing. *Curr Top Dev Biol.* 2003;58:1–27.
63. Basmajian J. Introduction. Principles and background. In: *Biofeedback: Principles and Practices for Clinicians.* 3rd ed. Baltimore: Williams & Wilkins; 1989.
64. Banga A, Panus P. Clinical applications of iontophoretic devices in rehabilitation medicine. *Crit Rev Phys Rehabil Med.* 1998;10(2):147–179.
65. Howard J, Drake T, Kellogg D. Effects of alternating current iontophoresis on drug delivery. *Arch Phys Med Rehabil.* 1995;76(5):463–466.
66. Shibaji T, Yasuhara Y, Oda N, et al. A mechanism of the high frequency AC iontophoresis. *J Control Release.* 2001;73: 37–47.
67. Banga A, Bose S, BGhosh T. Iontophoresis and electroporation: comparisons and contrasts. *Int J Pharm.* 1999;179:1–19.
68. Chandler T. Iontophoresis of 0.4% dexamethasone for plantar fasciitis. *Clin J Sport Med.* 1998;8:68.
69. Gudeman S, Eisele S, Heidt R, et al. Treatment of plantar fasciitis by iontophoresis of 0.4% dexamethasone. A randomized, double-blinded, placebo-controlled study. *Am J Sports Med.* 1997;25:312–316.
70. Ozawa A, Haruki Y, Iwashita K, et al. Follow-up of clinical efficacy of iontophoresis therapy for postherpetic neuralgia. *J Dermatol* 1999;26:1–10.
71. Magistro C. Hyaluronidase by iontophoresis in the treatment of edema: a preliminary clinical report. *Phys Ther.* 1964;44: 169–175.
72. Cornwall M. Zinc iontophoresis to treat ischemic skin ulcers. *Phys Ther.* 1981;61:359–360.
73. Bellew J, Baker R, Williams J. A novel method of delivering tap water galvanism for management of hyperhidrosis: a case report. *Br J Med.* 2008;13(2):40–44.
74. Gillick B, Kloth L, Starsky A, Cincinelli-Walker L. Management of post surgical hyperhidrosis with direct current and tap water. *Phys Ther.* 2004;84:262–267.
75. Gordon A, Weistein M. Sodium salicylate iontophoresis in the treatment of plantar warts: case report. *Phys Ther.* 1969; 49:869–870.
76. Kahn J. A case report: lithium iontophoresis for gouty arthritis. *J Orthop Sports Phys Ther.* 1982;4:113–114.
77. Psaki C, Carol L. Acetic acid ionization: a study to determine the absorptive effects upon calcified tendinitis of the shoulder. *Phys Ther.* 1955;35:84–87.
78. Tannenbaum M. Iodine iontophoresis in reduction of scar tissue. *Phys Ther.* 1980;60:792.
79. Montorsi F, Salonia A, Guazzoni G, et al. Transdermal electromotive multi-drug administration for Peyronie's disease: preliminary results. *J Androl.* 2000;21:85–90.
80. Reidl C, Plas E, Engelhardt P, Daha P, Pfluger H. Iontophoresis for treatment of Peyronie's disease. *J Urology.* 2000;163: 95–99.
81. Belanger A. *Evidenced Based Guide to Therapeutic Physical Agents.* Philadelphia, PA: Lippincott, Williams, and Wilkins; 2002.
82. Pikal M. The role of electroosmotic flow in transdermal iontophoresis. *Adv Drug Deliv Rev.* 2001;46:281–305.
83. Banga A. New technologies to allow transdermal delivery of therapeutic proteins and small water-soluble drugs. *Am J Drug Deliv.* 2006;4(4):221–230.
84. Fang J, Sung K, Wang JJ, Chu C, Chen K. The effects of iontophoresis and electroporation on transdermal delivery of buprenorphine from solutions and hydrogels. *J Pharm Pharmacol.* 2002;54:1329–1337.
85. Zhu H, Li S, Peck K, Miller D, Higuchi W. Improvement on conventional constant current DC iontophoresis: a study using constant conductance AC iontophoresis. *J Control Release.* 2002;82:249–261.
86. Viscusi E. Emerging treatment modalities: balancing efficacy and safety. *Am J Health Syst Pharm.* 2007;64(15):S6–11.
87. Ciccone C. Electrical stimulation for delivery of medications: Iontophoresis: In: *Clinical Electrophysiology.* 3rd ed. Baltimore: Williams and Wilkins; 2008:351–388.
88. Petelenz T, Buttke J, Bonds C. Iontophoresis of dexamethasone: laboratory studies. *J Control Release.* 1992;20:55–66.
89. Cummings J. *Iontophoresis.* Norwalk, CT: Appleton and Lange; 1991:317–329.
90. Henley E. Transcutaneous drug delivery: iontophoresis and phonophoresis. *Crit Rev Phys Med Rehabil Med.* 1991;2: 139–151.
91. Anderson C, Morris R, Boeh S, Panus P. Effects of iontophoresis current magnitude and duration on dexamethasone deposition and localized drug retention. *Phys Ther.* 2003; 83(2):161–170.
92. Li G, Van Steeg T, Putter H, et al. Cutaneous side-effects of transdermal iontophoresis with and without surfactant pretreatment: a single blinded randomized controlled trial. *Br J Dermatol.* 2005;153(2):404–412.
93. Yarrobino T, Kalbfleisch J, Ferslew K, Panus P. Lidocaine iontophoresis mediates analgesia in lateral epicondylalgia treatment. *Physiother Res Int.* 2006;11(3):152–160.
94. Layzel M. Current interventions and approaches to postoperative pain management. *Br J Nurs.* 2008;17(7):414–419.
95. Momeni M, Crucitti M, De Kock M. Patient-controlled analgesia in the management of postoperative pain. *Drugs.* 2006;66(18):2321–2337.
96. Bouman H, Lentzer E. The treatment of hyperhidrosis of hands and feet with constant current. *Am J Phys Med.* 1952;31:158–162.
97. Stolman L. Treatment of hyperhidrosis. *Dermatol Clin.* 1998;16(4):863–867.
98. Hyvärinen A, Tarkka I, Mervaala E, Pääkkönen A, Valtonen H, Nuutinen J. Cutaneous electrical stimulation treatment in unresolved facial nerve paralysis: an exploratory study. *Am J Phys Med Rehabil.* 2008;87:992–997.
99. Berlant S. Method of determining optimal stimulation sites for transcutaneous electrical nerve stimulation. *Phys Ther.* 1984;64:924–928.
100. Kahn J. *Principles and Practice of Clinical Electrotherapy.* 4th ed. Philadelphia, PA: Churchill Livingstone; 2000.

Clinical Applications of Modalities

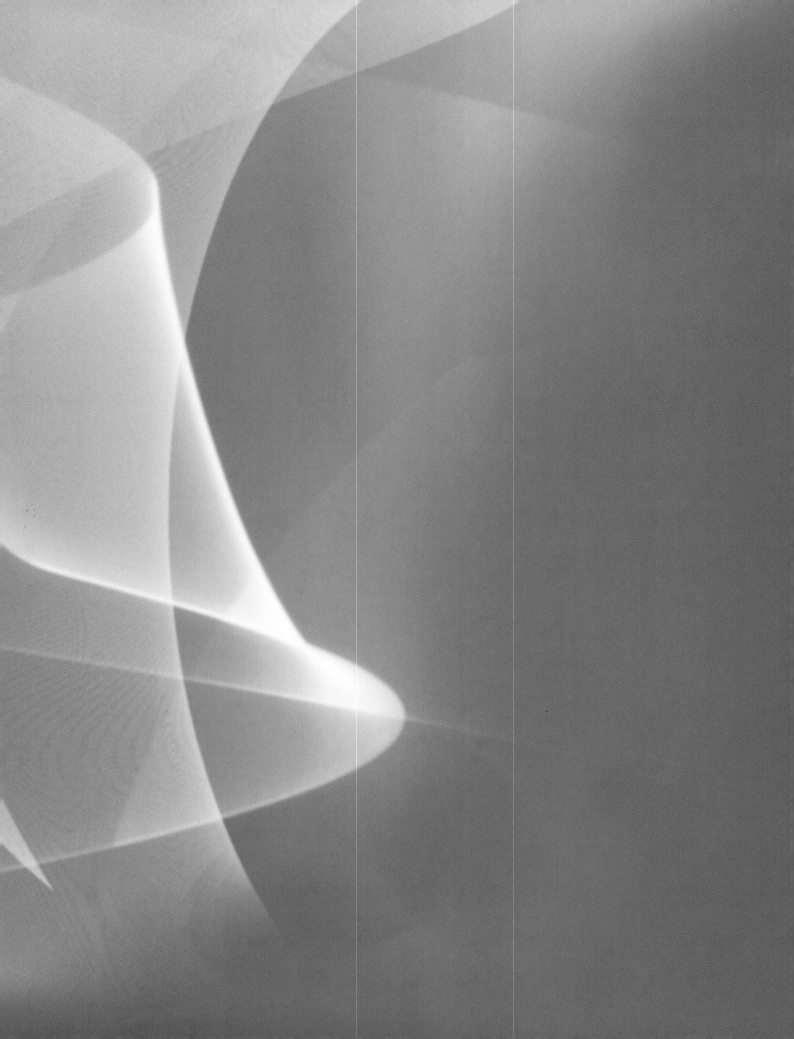

chapter 11

Electrotherapy for Musculoskeletal Disorders

C. Scott Bickel, PT, PhD | Chris M. Gregory, PT, PhD |
James W. Bellew, PT, EdD

Neuromuscular electrical stimulation (NMES) is commonly used in a variety of clinical settings to mimic or augment voluntary contractions and to enhance the rehabilitation of human skeletal muscles.[1–3] This chapter will (1) review early training studies that incorporated NMES training of skeletal muscle, (2) provide data to support the idea that properly designed NMES training protocols can result in improved neuromuscular performance, (3) provide guidelines for the implementation of NMES training for individuals with musculoskeletal disorders, (4) provide an overview of NMES-induced muscle recruitment, and (5) outline some of the drawbacks associated with NMES training. This information is intended to help practitioners provide evidence-based treatment when utilizing NMES to improve muscle size and strength.

Rationale for NMES

The common goal of using NMES is to mimic voluntary contractions to obtain the physiological improvements that result from training. NMES is a widely accepted modality that is used to treat atrophic muscle after injury or disease, although a consensus on specific programs and parameters to improve neuromuscular performance has yet to be reached. Early studies targeting increases in muscle mass were not consistently successful. However, recent studies have demonstrated the potential of NMES training protocols to elicit a hypertrophic response in skeletal muscle; this suggests that this training modality has the potential to be a valuable tool for rehabilitation if utilized in an appropriate manner.

The neuromuscular system is perhaps the most highly plastic system in the human body, showing dramatic adaptations in response to changes in activity. Skeletal muscle can adapt by increasing or decreasing the amount of contractile proteins, by changing its fiber type composition, or by altering its metabolic profile to sustain force production.[4,5] Adaptations resulting from activity are not limited to peripheral skeletal muscle, with concurrent adaptations occurring in neural systems in response to activity.[6,7] Specifically, enhanced recruitment of motor units (an alpha motor neuron and all the muscle fibers innervated by it) is accomplished through improved central control of firing frequency or synchronization of motor units—that is, by activating motor units more frequently and in unison, muscle force can be increased. These factors underlie the use of NMES.

NMES for Muscle Strengthening

NMES is used as a method to strengthen weakened muscle in persons with musculoskeletal disorders and is supported by evidence in the scientific literature. Muscle strengthening is thought to result from two primary mechanisms: increased muscle size or improved motor unit recruitment (nonmuscle mass adaptations).[8] Increasing muscle mass usually takes several weeks to occur, while nonmuscle mass adaptations occur more rapidly. The nonmuscle mass adaptations are typically due to increased motor unit recruitment, which is caused by increasing the frequency that motor units are recruited and recruiting motor units in a more synchronized manner (i.e., at that same time) (Fig. 11-1).[7,9] The manner in which NMES-induced motor unit recruitment increases muscle force is similar to the game of tug-of-war. If the team pulls more frequently and at the same time, the result is a more forceful pull or tug.

KEY POINT! Improved muscle size is an adaptation that occurs with repeated muscle overload and is consistent with the principles of voluntary muscle strengthening. Increases in muscle mass typically take several weeks to occur; this may not be a reasonable expectation during rehabilitation programs in the

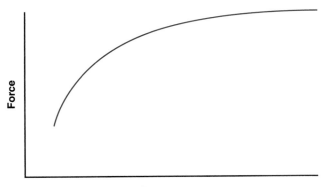

Fig 11•1 Force-frequency relationship. Note that as frequency of activation is increased, force is progressively increased until tetany is reached (the point where further increases in frequency do not produce increases in force production). *(Adapted with permission from Gregory CM, Dixon W, Bickel CS. Impact of varying pulse frequency and duration on muscle torque production and fatigue.* **Muscle Nerve.** *2007;35(4):504–509.)*

current health-care environment, where shorter supervised training and reduced visits are typical. Increases in strength observed in the initial weeks of training are due to changes in motor unit recruitment.

Previous studies have investigated the effects of NMES on muscle strength in participants without disability. These studies often compared the effects of NMES, voluntary isometric exercise, and no exercise on strength of the quadriceps femoris.[10–13] Results generally showed that both the NMES and exercise groups displayed increased strength, but there were no differences between these two groups. As expected, strength in the no-exercise control group was unchanged. One criticism of these studies is that NMES and voluntary exercise may not have produced equivalent forces during treatment, leading to inequality in training doses. Many early NMES studies did not in fact try to maximize the amount of stimulation delivered. Therefore, activated motor units were not necessarily being exercised to the same degree in both the voluntary and NMES groups, which potentially impacted results. Despite this potential, studies have shown gains in strength following NMES training to be similar to voluntary exercise.

KEY POINT! Similar gains in strength have been observed in studies comparing voluntary exercise and NMES. However, voluntary exercise often used maximal contractions, whereas less-than-maximal contractions were used with NMES.

A few studies have investigated changes in muscle size after NMES training in healthy, nonweak individuals; the results provided a foundational basis for understanding the effects of NMES on muscle. These studies have reported increases in voluntary strength after NMES training; however, this finding alone does not imply a resultant hypertrophy, because factors other than increases in muscle size can account for improved voluntary force generation after training (i.e., nonmuscle mass adaptations). For example, in a single subject design, Delitto and colleagues[14] reported impressive strength gains despite average fiber size decreasing by approximately 16% following NMES training. Although a reduction in fiber size is surprising, strength gains were realized without remarkable muscle fiber hypertrophy. These findings confirm that improvements in strength and size after NMES are not necessarily related.

There is evidence that NMES can prevent atrophy and induce hypertrophy in individuals with weakness caused from neurological disorders[15,16] or from orthopedic injury,[3,17] but clear, foundational data on the effects of NMES on muscle size are limited. However, there are studies demonstrating that NMES can elicit muscle hypertrophy in skeletal muscle when utilized appropriately (i.e., suitable mode, dosage). For example, the triceps brachii in primates was trained using NMES, and skeletal muscle biopsies were obtained pre- and post-training.[18] NMES was used to cause contraction of the elbow extensors (60 Hz, 5 sec on/10 sec off × 60 min) 5 days per week for 3 weeks at the maximum contraction intensity tolerated "without causing discomfort to the animals." The results showed that average size of all muscle fiber types increased between 13% and 45%. It should be noted that these gains were realized over an extremely short training period. In another study, the triceps surae was stimulated for 21 consecutive days with 15 to 20 contractions per session at an amplitude of 40 to 45 mA. Skeletal muscle biopsy analyses revealed that muscle fiber size increased approximately 16% after 21 days of stimulation.[19] The fact that such increases in fiber size can be realized in such short training programs illustrates the potential impact of NMES.

Additional data examining the effects of NMES training on muscle size have also shown promise.[20,21] These studies have incorporated the use of dynamic contractions with high training loads (about 70% to 80% of maximal voluntary isometric contraction) in an effort to mimic voluntary training studies that are known to result in muscle hypertrophy (i.e., progressive resistance training). Ruther and associates[20] studied subjects who trained 2 days per week for 9 weeks with either voluntary or NMES-induced isokinetic exercise. Stimulation intensity was set to elicit 70% of maximal voluntary isometric torque. The results indicated a 10% and 4% increase in quadriceps femoris muscle size in NMES and in voluntary training groups, respectively, suggesting that resistance training with NMES may be superior to voluntary training—at least during the early phase of a resistance-training program. These findings are consistent with data showing that early strength gains are not typically due to muscle fiber hypertrophy.[22] Stevenson and Dudley[21] used a similar protocol in subjects who reported active participation in a voluntary resistance-training program at least 2 days per week. One leg received NMES training at approximately 70% of maximal voluntary isometric torque. Stimulation intensity was progressively increased, and by the end of 8 weeks of training, muscle size increased by about 10% in the NMES-trained leg. Table 11-1 summarizes the results of these studies and others for NMES for muscle strengthening or hypertrophy.

For several decades, neuromuscular electrical stimulation has been used after various surgical procedures for the knee. This probably stems from the fact that quadriceps force is reduced with knee effusion due to neural inhibition (i.e., arthrogenic muscle inhibition).[23,24] Because the quadriceps femoris is an important muscle to focus on during rehabilitation of the knee, practitioners will often turn to NMES for assistance if the patient is unable to volitionally activate the quadriceps. Studies using NMES following knee surgery have shown positive changes in muscle performance. Several reports in the literature address the use of NMES in patients following anterior cruciate ligament (ACL) reconstruction surgeries (Tables 11-2 and 11-3).

Several studies have examined the effect of NMES on the quadriceps femoris muscles after ACL reconstruction,[2,25–28] and some suggest that early intervention with intense NMES enhances recovery of strength and function.[26,27] Early studies compared the use of NMES-evoked contractions to voluntary exercise during the

Table 11•1 NMES for Muscle Strengthening or Hypertrophy

Author	Training	NMES Parameters	Outcome
Cabric et al.[19]	Isometric 15–20 contractions 1 time/day 21 days	PC Group 1: 50 Hz Group 2: 2,000 Hz	Increased type I muscle fiber area
Caggiano et al.[12]	Isometric 10 contractions 3 days/week 4 weeks	PC: biphasic symmetrical 200 µsec 25 pps 36% MVIC	Increased strength
Currier et al.[10]	Isometric 10 contractions of 15 sec with 15 sec of rest 3 days/week 5 weeks	Burst-modulated AC (Russian) 2,500 Hz 50 bps > 60% MVIC	Increased strength
Delitto et al.[14]	Isometric 10 contractions/ session 3 days/week 4 weeks	Burst-modulated AC (Russian) 2,500 Hz 75 bps Max tolerable current (95%–126% MVIC)	Increased strength Increased type I fiber area Reduced type II fiber area
Iwasaki et al.[63]	Isokinetic 10 sets of 10 3 days/week 6 weeks	Burst-modulated AC (Russian) 5,000 Hz 20 bps Max tolerable current	Increased strength
Laughman et al.[11]	Isometric 10 reps 5 days/week 5 weeks	Burst-modulated AC (Russian) 2,500Hz 50 bps 33% MVIC	Increased strength
McMiken et al.[13]	Isometric 10 contractions 4 days/week 3 weeks	PC 100 µsec 75 pps Max tolerable current	Increased strength
Mohr et al.[64]	Isometric 10 contractions 3 days/week 5 weeks	PC: twin-peak monophasic pulses 45 µsec 50 pps Max tolerable	Increased strength in voluntary exercise only
Ruther et al.[20]	Isokinetic 3 to 5 sets of 10 2 days/week 9 weeks	PC: symmetrical biphasic pulses 500 µsec 50 pps 70% MVC	Increased muscle cross-sectional area with NMES (10%)
Stevenson et al.[21]	Isokinetic 3 to 5 sets of 10 2 days/week 8 weeks	PC: symmetrical biphasic pulses 450 us 70 pps 70% MVC	Increased muscle cross-sectional area (11%)

PC = Pulsed current

early phase of rehabilitation (first 6 weeks)[25] or compared the addition of NMES to the rehabilitation programs.[27] These studies utilized burst-modulated AC (Russian current) at intensities that were "maximally tolerated"; a greater increase in quadriceps muscle strength was seen in those subjects in the NMES groups.[25,27] One study randomly assigned participants who were 1 week post-ACL reconstruction into four isometric strengthening treatment groups: high-intensity NMES, high-intensity voluntary exercise, low-intensity NMES, and a combination of high- and low-intensity NMES.[26] The groups that trained with high-intensity NMES and the combination of low- and high-intensity NMES showed significant improvements in strength and knee flexion/extension during gait when compared to the other two groups.[26] The intensity of stimulation used

Table 11•2 NMES for Anterior Cruciate Ligament Reconstruction

Author	Training	NMES Parameters	Outcome
Delitto et al.[25]	Isometric 15 contractions 5 days/week 3 weeks	Burst-modulated AC (Russian) 2,500 Hz 50 bps Max tolerable current	Increased strength
Fitzgerald et al.[2]	Isometric 10 contractions 2 days/week 11 weeks	Burst-modulated AC (Russian) 2,500 Hz 75 bps Max tolerable current	Increased strength
Paternostro-Sluga et al.[28]	Isometric 48 5-sec and 24 10-sec contractions 7 days/week 6 weeks	PC: biphasic symmetrical 220 μsec 100 pps Tolerable, strong visible contraction	Increased strength (no difference between groups)
Snyder-Mackler et al.[26]	Isometric 15 contractions 3 days/week 6 weeks	Burst-modulated AC (Russian) 2,500 Hz 75 bps Max tolerable current	Increased strength
Snyder-Mackler et al.[27]	Isometric 15 contractions 3 days/week 3 weeks	Burst-modulated AC (Russian) 2,500 Hz 75 bps Max tolerable current	Increased strength Improved gait pattern

Table 11•3 NMES for Total Knee Arthroplasty

Author	Training	NMES Parameters	Outcome
Lewek et al.[31]	Isometric 10 contractions 11 sessions	Burst-modulated AC (Russian) 2,500 Hz 40–75 bps Max tolerable current (35%–50%)	Single case study, patient showed improvements in strength and met goals
Petterson et al.[32]	Isometric 10 contractions 2–3 days/week 6 weeks	Burst-modulated AC (Russian) 2,500 Hz 50 bps Max tolerable current (min level = 30% MVIC)	Improvements in strength and function (no differences between groups that did not receive NMES)
Stevens et al.[3]	Isometric 10 contractions 3 days/week 6 weeks	Burst-modulated AC (Russian) 2,500 Hz 50 bps Max tolerable current	Increased strength

was the "maximum tolerated" by each participant, suggesting the training was intense enough to evoke neuromuscular adaptations. It should be noted that not all studies that have utilized NMES in the treatment of patients following ACL reconstruction have shown significantly better results with NMES[28] (see Table 11-2).

NMES is also commonly used in patients following total knee arthroplasty (see Table 11-3). Individuals in this population have considerable knee effusion, pain, and impaired ability to voluntarily activate their quadriceps femoris similar to that seen following ACL reconstruction.[29] Data have shown that 1 year after TKA, muscle atrophy, weakness, and functional limitations persist.[30] Case studies done on patients post-TKA surgery found promising results using burst-modulated AC (Russian current) delivered to evoke 10-second contractions for a total of 10 repetitions at "maximally tolerated" intensity.[3,31] The case studies suggested that after 6 weeks of training, some subjects showed greater strength in the surgical leg at 6 months post-TKA than the limb that was not surgically repaired. A randomized controlled trial has been published that investigated how a progressive strengthening program with or without NMES influenced function after TKA and compared them to a group that received conventional rehabilitation with perhaps a less intense training protocol.[32] Their results indicated that as long as the individuals were participating in a structured progressive strengthening program (with or without NMES), they made significantly greater improvements than those who were undergoing standard rehabilitation. This study highlights the importance of training intensity, and in this case, function was apparently achieved regardless of whether NMES was used. In some cases, NMES may be required to achieve sufficient intensity during rehabilitation due to impairments with voluntary muscle activation.

Examination, Evaluation, and Prognosis

The initial examination should evaluate the patient's medical history, paying specific attention to possible precautions and contraindications for the use of NMES. Individuals with musculoskeletal disorders will typically have some degree of impairment with voluntary muscle activation, but they may still benefit from neuromuscular electrical stimulation. The practitioner should assess the muscle innervation status of patients who have a possible neurological injury, such as peripheral nerve injuries (e.g., nerve compression, crush, or laceration), or who have a history of neurological disorders (e.g., multiple sclerosis, stroke, spinal cord injury). It is important to note whether the patient has an upper or lower motor neuron injury, because lower motor neuron injuries do not respond to NMES. (See the "EMS Applied to Denervated Muscle" section.)

If innervation status is unknown, the practitioner can test for this by applying NMES to the involved muscle and observing its response. Electrodes should be applied so that the motor nerves of the weak muscles are within the area where current will flow. Ask the patient to report the first sensation of electrical stimulation, noting the milliamps when this occurs and understanding that if sensation is compromised, the patient may not feel anything. Continue to increase the current until you see a motor response. If the patient reports sensation and there is an observed motor response, then the muscle is innervated and able to respond to NMES. Should there be no

sensation of electrical stimulation and a lack of motor response, further neurophysiological testing may be indicated (see Chapter 16). If this is the case, the practitioner may need to refer to another health-care provider who can conduct electromyography tests to evaluate the degree of injury. Additional tests for strength, ROM, pain, and functional status are indicated to evaluate the appropriateness of NMES compared to other interventions (Table 11-4).

KEY POINT! Stimulation of denervated muscle requires long pulse durations (greater than 1 millisecond), which most stimulators are unable to deliver.

Intervention

Patients with decreased muscle strength caused by musculoskeletal dysfunction can benefit from NMES, especially those with muscle atrophy. However, it should be noted that the *intensity of training* is a key factor in the efficacy of NMES strengthening protocols. Most studies that have shown effectiveness have used intensities or dosages that were "maximally tolerated" and resulted in approximately 70% of maximum voluntary contractions (see Tables 11-1 through 11-3). It is important to realize that prescription of NMES exercise should be done in a similar fashion as voluntary training programs. Thus, the sets and reps performed as well as the load (i.e., % MVC [maximal voluntary contraction]) used should be carefully prescribed and monitored in NMES training programs.

Practitioners need to consider several factors when applying NMES: electrode placement, on- and off-times, number of repetitions, frequency, and duration of treatment, and it's important to choose the appropriate muscle stimulator, based upon the desired stimulation parameters to achieve the neuromuscular response. NMES is utilized in an effort to facilitate the contraction of skeletal muscle when there is sufficient need to do so. Understanding the differences between voluntary and artificial activation of skeletal muscle is necessary to determine whether NMES is indicated (Box 11-1).

Voluntary Versus NMES Exercise: Differences in Muscle Recruitment

Recruitment of skeletal muscle during voluntary contractions (i.e., without NMES) follows a predictable and orderly pattern—starting with smaller and progressing to larger motor units as increasing forces are required. It

Table 11•4 **Examination for NMES for Strengthening**

Tests of	Question	Reason
Muscle innervation	Has innervation status been compromised?	NMES for strengthening typically requires innervation of the muscle.
Strength	What is current voluntary strength (manual muscle test or muscle dynamometry)?	To determine effect of treatment.
Range of motion	Are there any ROM limitations present?	Decreased ROM may impact functional outcomes.
Sensation	Is sensation present, absent, or diminished?	More frequent monitoring of skin integrity is needed with reduced sensation.
Pain	Is there pain at rest or with activity? How severe?	Pain could be a limiting factor for the strength-training program.
Spasticity	Is spasticity present?	Antagonist spasticity may affect ability to accurately assess strength.
Function	What functional limitations are present?	To determine effect of treatment on function.
Cognitive status	Is cognitive status sufficient to provide feedback?	To ensure safety of use.

should also be noted that the number of motor units and the firing frequency can be altered during voluntary activities. In contrast, artificial activation (e.g., during NMES) does not follow these same principles and results in a more random pattern of activation of motor units (e.g., small and large motor units will be recruited even when low forces are produced). Additionally, alterations in the number of motor units or firing frequency are typically not available with clinical stimulators without stopping and starting the treatment multiple times. Consequently, all activated motor units have the same firing rate and will produce relatively similar forces, which could be 100% of their force-producing capacity at higher frequencies of stimulation. When the decision is made to utilize NMES, the practitioner should apply the basic principles of muscle conditioning to the design of the protocol (i.e., current intensity, repetitions, sets, and frequency of treatment) while considering the differences in motor unit activation. It is also important to monitor the patient's initial response to treatment and all subsequent contractions.

Selecting a Stimulator

The electrical stimulation device should be able to deliver parameters that are capable of maximizing force

---

Box 11•1 **Factors to Consider When Applying NMES**

- Line or battery-powered stimulator
- Stimulation parameters
- Electrode placement
- On- and off-times
- Dosage (intensity)
- Number of repetitions/sets
- Frequency of application

---

development of muscle and activating a large percentage of the muscle fibers in an effort to provide muscle overload. Studies have examined the use of small portable stimulators versus larger line-powered devices with mixed results (Fig. 11-2). Snyder-Mackler et al.[17] initially reported that significantly greater forces were created using a line-powered stimulator as compared to a portable one in participants who had had ACL reconstruction. However, they also acknowledged that there might be other portable stimulators available that may create more force.

More recently, Laufer and colleagues[33] compared two portable stimulators and one line-powered device and reported that when stimulation parameters were kept constant across stimulators, the portable stimulators created more force. Other reports have also indicated that portable stimulators can evoke similar torque outputs as line-powered stimulators.[34] Based upon these studies, practitioners should realize the importance of understanding the capabilities of their available stimulators and choose one appropriate for the intervention desired (Table 11-5).

Clinical Controversies

Until recently, most battery-powered, handheld NMES stimulators were incapable of delivering current intensities sufficient to elicit muscle contractions to improve strength. More modern battery-powered devices have shown the ability to elicit contractions similar to those evoked by line-powered clinical stimulators.

Stimulation Parameters

When selecting the parameters, there are several options from which the practitioner can choose to achieve the desired response. If the goal of NMES is to enhance muscle strength, the highest pulse duration

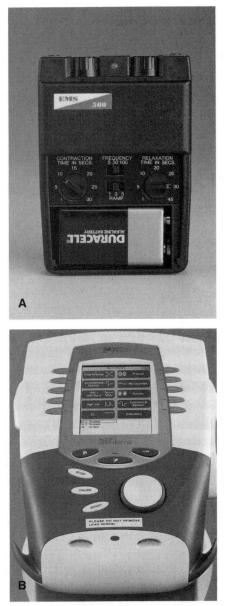

Fig 11•2 Examples of (A) portable and (B) clinical plug-in stimulators.

Table 11•5	NMES Parameters Typically Used for Muscle Strengthening[2,3,20,21,26,31,36]
Waveform	Symmetrical or asymmetrical biphasic pulsed current, burst-modulated alternating current (e.g., Russian current)
Pulse duration	200–600 μsec
Frequency	20–100 pps (bursts per second)
Amplitude	To obtain strong muscle contraction (maximum tolerated or current necessary to achieve $\geq$ 50% of MVC)
Ramp-up time	1–5 seconds
Ramp-down time	1–2 seconds
Duty cycle	1:3 to 1:5 with on-time up to 10 seconds and off-time up to 50 seconds
Treatment time and duration	At least 10 contractions or up to 1 hour/day 3–5 times/week 4–8 weeks
Carrier frequency*	1,000–2,500 Hz
Burst duration*	2–10 msec
Relative duty cycle*	10%–50%

*Specific to burst-modulated AC (BMAC)

and amplitude tolerated by the patient should be used.[35] The frequency should be adjusted to achieve a smooth, forceful contraction, generally achieved with greater than 30 pps (see Fig. 11-1). If one chooses to use burst-modulated AC (BMAC), then we recommend a burst frequency of 50 bursts per second. Although Russian current may be the most recognized form of BMAC, other variations are available that may be more effective at eliciting muscle torque.[36] Therefore, when using BMAC for muscle strengthening, the following parameters are recommended: a burst duration of 2 to10 msec, a relative duty cycle of 10% to 50%, a carrier frequency of 1,000 to 2,500 Hz, and the highest amplitude tolerated.[36]

It is important to understand that higher stimulation frequencies (pps or bursts per second) will also lead to greater muscle fatigue. Therefore, choose an on-time to off-time ratio that allows for sufficient muscle recovery between repetitions. Support for this is provided by a study that investigated the effects of duty cycle on metabolic changes within the calf musculature; there was a significantly greater force decline during contraction and a significantly decreased muscle pH with a 10-sec on/10-sec off on:off time ratio as compared to 10 sec on/50 sec off.[37] If muscle fatigue is an ongoing problem, the practitioner can reduce frequency and increase the rest time between contractions, so each stimulated contraction is evoking maximum force.

KEY POINT! To decrease the effect of fatigue and ensure that NMES is eliciting as much muscle force as possible, it may be necessary to increase the rest period between maximally tolerated contractions.

Ramp time is often used for patient comfort during electrical stimulation, allowing time for the current to increase and decrease slowly rather than abruptly. However, a longer ramp-up time is not always the most comfortable for each patient and will reduce the amount of time that all motor units are activated. It is recommended to have shorter ramp times so the muscle can be activated for sufficient periods of time. It is prudent to be mindful that the patient's feedback and muscle response are critical to assist with guiding these decisions.

Electrode Placement

Electrode placements for NMES applications depend on the size and location of the targeted muscle (Box 11-2). If the goal is to optimize muscle strength by facilitating the contractions, the electrode placement should be arranged to recruit as many motor units as possible. Electrode configurations may be monopolar, bipolar, or quadripolar, depending on the size of electrodes and the size of the target muscle. Figure 11-3 shows examples of different electrode configurations. The practitioner should recognize that current density is inversely proportional to electrode area and should select electrodes of an appropriate size for the targeted muscle. A photo image of electrode placement can be taken to record treatment and make it easier to reproduce a successful stimulation session.

Intensity or Dosage

The appropriate intensity or amplitude of the electrical stimulation is perhaps the most important

---

| **Box 11•2** | **Tips for Electrode Placement** |

- If electrodes are too small for the targeted muscle, increased current density may lead to discomfort.
- If large electrodes are not available, splitting or bifurcating the two electrodes into four or using two channels will increase the target area.
- It may take several attempts to optimize the electrode placement to get the desired response.

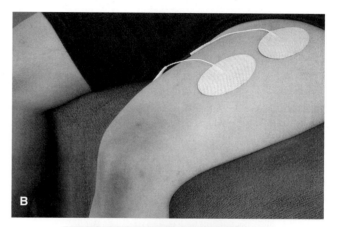

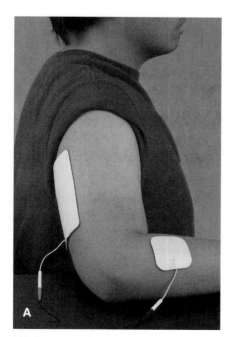

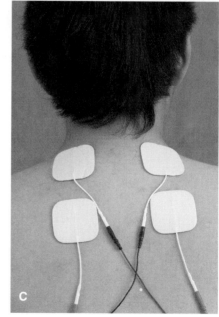

Fig 11•3 (A) A monopolar arrangement involves placing one electrode over the target muscle(s), such as the wrist extensors pictured here, and a larger electrode in another area where muscle activation is not desired, such as the triceps. Two different sizes of electrodes are used because the current density needs to be greater over the targeted muscle. (B) A bipolar arrangement places two electrodes over the targeted muscle(s) pictured here for the quadriceps femoris. (C) Another example of a bipolar arrangement splits or bifurcates the lead wires from the single circuit to use four electrodes over the target area. Two separate circuits in bipolar arrangement can also be used.

parameter of NMES and the one most often underused by practitioners. The "overload" principles of strength training and prior studies of NMES clearly show that contractions near maximal tolerance are required for increasing strength. Contractions near 70% of the MVC of the opposite limb are common in studies reporting increased strength following NMES. Many practitioners do not deliver an appropriate intensity to elicit contractions of this level; thus, patients are less likely to realize the benefits of NMES.

Determining or quantifying the appropriate stimulus intensity for NMES is easy and should be performed prior to the first session. To ascertain an appropriate treatment intensity or dosage, the maximal isometric strength of the patient's uninvolved side should be measured first. This can be completed with an isokinetic dynamometer, a standard pulley-style weight stack, or a handheld dynamometer. The patient is then positioned on the same device to test the involved side. Following appropriate setup of the NMES, the intensity of the electrical stimulation is increased as muscle force is measured. The stimulus intensity required to reach a

specific submaximal percentage of the opposite side is recorded and used as the dosage for subsequent applications of NMES. The patient can then be moved to a treatment table or area using the newly quantified intensity or dosage. Typical target percentages for NMES training sessions may be 50% or greater, although initial applications may need to be closer to 30%. This process of quantifying the dosage of stimulus intensity should be repeated at regular intervals throughout rehabilitation as strength improves so as to optimize the effects of the treatment (see Figs. 11-3 and 11-4).

KEY POINT! The amplitude required to elicit a specific level of muscle force can be measured and is termed *dosage*. A dosage eliciting greater than 50% of the MVC is recommended for strengthening.

Monitoring Treatment

Similar to voluntary exercise, treatment with NMES may lead to delayed-onset muscle soreness (DOMS). Consequently, the practitioner needs to educate the patient regarding the possible effects of muscle soreness as would be done following volitional exercise.

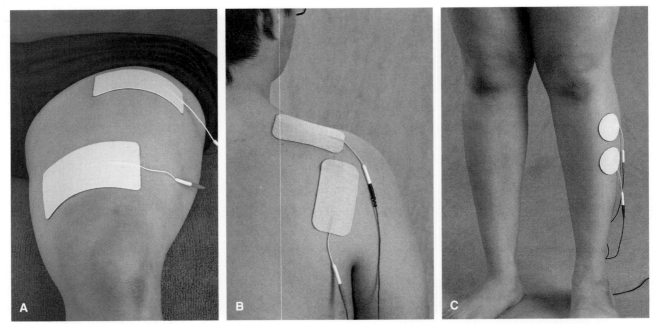

Fig 11•4 (A) This picture demonstrates one possible placement of electrodes to stimulate the quadriceps femoris muscle. To cause this large muscle group to contract, the practitioner should use appropriately sized electrodes, which may vary between patients. (B) Electrodes to posterior rotator cuff muscles; the exact location to optimize the response will vary among patients. The goal is to move the humerus superiorly into the glenoid fossa without creating abduction. (C) This picture demonstrates one possible placement of electrodes to obtain balanced dorsiflexion. This placement will vary among patients, and the practitioner may need to try several different placements before obtaining the desired response.

It is normal for the skin under the electrodes to feel warm and appear pink after treatment due to the electrothermal effects of the stimulus. However, skin should be checked for any excessive redness or irritation. As with any exercise program, adjustments may need to be made to the NMES regimen based upon individual patient responses. For example, it may not be possible to achieve the targeted intensities on the first day of treatment, as the patient may be a little apprehensive with the new program. Treatments from day to day may change. It is recommended that each time that electrical stimulation is utilized, practitioners proceed with caution, being aware of the patient's response (both verbal and nonverbal).

CASE STUDY 11•1 NMES FOR MUSCLE STRENGTHENING

A 42-year-old police officer presents with a chief complaint of decreased strength of the knee extensors following left ACL reconstruction 4 weeks ago. The ACL rupture occurred 6 months prior while playing basketball.

CLINICAL DECISION-MAKING

1. Does the patient have a dysfunction, limitation, or problem that can be improved with the use of neuromuscular electrical stimulation (NMES)?
   Answer: Yes, decreased strength secondary to orthopedic injury can be improved with NMES.

2. Is the patient appropriate for NMES (i.e., do any of the general precautions or contraindications to NMES apply to the patient, or are there any specific considerations regarding application of NMES to this patient)?
   Answer: If the patient has been screened to ensure general precautions or contraindications do not apply, then it is appropriate to use NMES.

3. What are the specific goals to be achieved with the use of NMES?
   Answer: Increase strength of the quadriceps femoris muscle by using NMES to evoke strong contractions in accordance with principles of muscle strengthening. A functional goal would be a return to full duty at work.

4. What specific form of electrical stimulation would be appropriate for the patient?
   Answer: A waveform that evokes muscle contractions. This would be either biphasic pulsed current or burst-modulated AC (i.e., Russian).

5. What specific parameters of NMES are appropriate for the patient?
   Answer:
   Current: Biphasic pulsed current (or burst-modulated AC)
   Pulse duration: 400 to 500 μsec
   Frequency: 50 Hz (or 50 bursts per second)

   Amplitude: A dosage set to obtain as strong of a contraction as tolerated or according to specific percentage of MVC
   Ramp time: 1 to 2 seconds
   Duration: Select 1:5 ratio of 10 seconds on, 50 seconds off. Perform at least 10 contractions, 3 days per week.

6. What are the proper (i.e., effective and safe) application procedures for NMES related to this case example?
   Answer:
   Instruct the patient: Inform the patient of the purpose and procedure and explain the anticipated sensation and effect of the stimulation. The goal of treatment is a motor response, so explain to the patient how much contraction is expected and required for the treatment to be effective. Initially, it may be necessary to offer the patient a familiarization session to become accustomed to the sensation of electrical stimulation.
   Preinspection: Generally observe the area to be treated for skin integrity.
   Electrode application: Two electrodes in a bipolar arrangement using a single channel, one proximally and laterally over the vastus lateralis and rectus femoris and one distally and medially over the vastus medialis. Application of the electrodes may take several attempts to optimize the response.
   Patient position: Patient is positioned on an isokinetic dynamometer or table with the knee flexed 45° to 90°. The distal extremity should be securely fixed to ensure isometric contraction.
   Treatment monitoring: Observe the muscle response and the reaction of the patient to NMES. The amplitude may need to be increased during the session to achieve the effect, if tolerated.
   Postinspection: Remove the electrodes and inspect the skin for any signs of skin irritation or adverse effects. If redness occurs, explain to the patient that this is not uncommon and should disappear in less than 24 hours.

CASE STUDY 11•2 **NMES FOR DECREASING SHOULDER SUBLUXATION**

A 16-year-old female gymnast has chronic posterior-lateral glenohumeral joint instability that increases toward the end of practice sessions.

CLINICAL DECISION-MAKING

1. Does the patient have a dysfunction, limitation, or problem that can be improved with the use of NMES?

   Answer: Yes, assuming there are no structural problems that require surgery, it appears that muscles involved in shoulder stability are susceptible to muscle fatigue, and NMES-induced exercise can improve neuromuscular performance.

2. Is the patient appropriate for NMES (i.e., do any of the general precautions or contraindications to NMES apply to the patient, or are there any specific considerations regarding application of NMES to this patient)?

   Answer: If the patient has been screened to ensure general precautions or contraindications do not apply, then it is appropriate to use NMES. She may have even experienced NMES during her knee rehabilitation.

3. What are the specific goals to be achieved with the use of NMES?

   Answer: Improve neuromuscular performance of specific muscles that contribute to stabilizing the shoulder during activity. A functional goal would be a return to full workouts without pain.

4. What specific form of electrical stimulation would be appropriate for the patient?

   Answer: A waveform that is appropriate for evoking muscle contractions. This would be either biphasic pulsed current or burst-modulated AC (i.e., Russian).

5. What specific parameters of NMES are appropriate for the patient?

   Answer:

   Type of stimulator: A portable stimulator that can meet desired parameters is preferable so treatment can be done outside of the clinic.

   Current: Biphasic pulsed current (or burst-modulated AC)

   Pulse duration: 400 to 500 μsec

   Frequency: 50 Hz (or 50 bursts per second)

   Amplitude: A dosage set to obtain as strong of a contraction as tolerated.

   Ramp time: 1 to 2 seconds

   Duration: Select 1:2 ratio of 10 seconds on, 20 seconds off. Perform at least 15 contractions, 3 to 5 days per week. As treatment progresses, gradually decrease the off-time and increase the on-time to improve fatigue resistance and increase the number of contractions.

6. What are the proper (i.e., effective and safe) application procedures for NMES related to this case example?

   Answer:

   Preinspection: Generally observe the area to be treated for skin integrity.

   Electrode application: Two electrodes in a bipolar arrangement—one over the supraspinatus and one over the posterior deltoid. Additional electrodes may be added to scapular stabilizers, if necessary. Application of the electrodes may take several attempts to optimize the response.

NMES and Motor Unit Recruitment

The ability to discriminately select and properly implement NMES requires an awareness of the physiological and functional differences that exist between electrically elicited and voluntary contractions. Specifically, it is important to understand potential differences with respect to temporal (i.e., firing pattern of recruited motor units/fibers) and spatial characteristics (i.e., location of recruited fibers within the muscle) of motor unit recruitment as well as the amount of fatigue realized when using NMES versus voluntary contractions. These issues are the subject of some debate,[38] and their impact on skeletal muscle function must be considered in the design of appropriate training paradigms when using this modality.

The Henneman size principle of voluntary motor unit recruitment describes the progressive recruitment of alpha-motorneuron cell bodies in order of increasing size from small to large.[39] Although this principle describes the activation of motor units based on their size rather than their type, it is often associated with the progressive recruitment of slow, typically small, motor units followed by the fast, typically large, motor units. Some have suggested that the use of NMES results in a reversal of the size principle, therefore recruiting fast motor units prior to slow.[40,41] This rationale is based on the fact that larger cell bodies are more easily depolarized due to less impedance to current flow, and their axons have faster conduction velocities than their smaller counterparts.[42,43] Although the premise of a reversal in the size principle may hold true during direct nerve stimulation, evidence surrounding transcutaneous application of NMES suggests that muscle fiber recruitment during electrical stimulation occurs in a nonselective, spatially fixed, and temporally synchronous pattern rather than a reversal of the physiological voluntary recruitment order.[38,44,45]

KEY POINT! There is a fundamental difference between activating motor units voluntarily versus passively via electrical stimulation. Voluntary activation results in a predictable order of recruitment, resulting in activation of fast, fatigable fibers typically at high relative intensities, whereas with electrical stimulation there is no predictable order of recruitment—thus the potential to activate fast fibers at lower contraction intensities.

In addition to recruitment order, differences exist in the amount of muscle fatigue when voluntary and NMES activities are compared. A functional consequence of NMES is an increased fatigability relative to voluntary activation, which is independent of stimulation intensity.[46,47] Reasons other than recruitment order (i.e., recruiting fast, fatigable fibers) can account for this outcome. One explanation for this phenomenon is that during voluntary actions, asynchronous motor unit recruitment patterns allow for additional motor units to be activated when muscle fibers that were initially recruited become fatigued.[48] As previously mentioned, NMES recruitment is not based on motor unit characteristics, such as size or fiber type, and is not spatially fixed. Thus, NMES recruitment does not allow for alterations in recruitment between repeated contractions during treatment and therefore contributes to increased fatigability.

An additional mechanism explaining increased fatigability during NMES is that during voluntary actions, muscle force can be maintained by modulating the firing frequency of active motor units. However, during NMES, firing frequency is fixed based on the selected frequency of the current used.[48] Thus, the ability to counter fatigue (i.e., maintain external force production) in voluntary efforts can be accomplished by one or both of the following: (1) recruiting additional motor units as those initially recruited become fatigued (i.e., asynchronous recruitment) or (2) activating more motor units at lower (i.e., subtetanic) firing frequencies. Neither of these recruitment strategies is available during NMES-induced muscle contractions. Therefore, recruitment of muscle fibers using NMES is spatially and temporally fixed and results in a subsequent drop in force whenever any of the fibers being activated becomes fatigued. This increased fatigability is a fundamental problem when using NMES for functional activities and could potentially limit training responses.

A common misconception associated with motor unit recruitment through NMES is that only motor units near the skin's surface can be activated. Patterns of activation after NMES of the quadriceps femoris have been mapped using magnetic resonance imaging (MRI).[46] MRI is a valid and reliable method of quantifying the amount of muscle utilized during both voluntary and electrically stimulated activities.[49] Images reveal that even during lower levels of stimulation intensity (about 25% of maximum voluntary isometric contraction), skeletal muscle fibers near the femur are activated. Even if the electrical current activates only the most superficial nerves, the muscle fibers innervated by these nerves are seemingly spread throughout the muscle; this results in the recruitment of muscle fibers located deep within the muscle (Fig. 11-5).

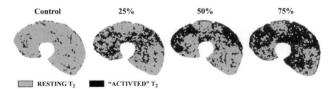

Fig 11•5 Representative single slice T2 maps of the quadriceps femoris from one subject at rest (control) and after NMES at a level that elicited an initial torque equal to 25%, 50%, or 75% of MVIT. Dark regions represent "activated" skeletal muscle. *(Adapted with permission from Adams GR, Harris RT, Woodard D, Dudley GA. Mapping of electrical muscle stimulation using MRI. J Appl Physiol. 1993;74(2):532–537.)*

KEY POINT! Because of differences in the way motor units are activated during voluntary activity versus during electrical stimulation, repeated contractions with electrical stimulation will result in greater and earlier muscle fatigue than with voluntary actions.

Limitations of NMES

Although there are some distinct advantages for using NMES-evoked contractions to activate skeletal muscles, these same factors can be used to suggest limitations of its use. For example, consideration should be given to the fact that synchronous or fixed recruitment of motor units may not be advantageous from a metabolic perspective. Needle EMG has been utilized to measure the frequency of activation of human skeletal muscles during voluntary activation and has shown that slow and fast skeletal muscles have in vivo firing frequencies of approximately 10 and 30 Hz, respectively, during MVC.[47] These

frequencies are lower than what is typically applied during clinical NMES. Oftentimes, practitioners utilize frequencies of 50 Hz or more to ensure tetanic contractions that produce large amounts of force.

KEY POINT! The indiscriminate activation of fast and slow motor units at firing frequencies that are higher than typically achieved voluntarily may contribute to increased fatigue and may potentially limit the amount of training that can be completed. This can be addressed to some degree by providing sufficient rest periods between contractions or by lowering the activation frequency. Previous studies have had success by using 10-second contractions with 50-second rest intervals.

Clinical Controversies

Because commonly used stimulation frequencies of NMES can exceed in vivo firing frequencies of some motor units, fatigue may happen sooner and may limit

---

CASE STUDY 11•3 **NMES FOR ENDURANCE**

A 38-year-old postal carrier is being treated for chronic mechanical low back pain aggravated by prolonged walking while carrying his mailbag. He has decreased endurance of the lumbar paraspinals.

CLINICAL DECISION-MAKING

1. Does the patient have a dysfunction, limitation, or problem that can be improved with the use of NMES?
   Answer: Yes, conditioning of the lumbar paraspinals is a key component to many rehabilitation programs for low back pain. Electrical stimulation can be used to address both gross strength and endurance for his occupational demands.

2. Is the patient appropriate for NMES (i.e., do any of the general precautions or contraindications to NMES apply to the patient, or are there any specific considerations regarding application of NMES to this patient)?
   Answer: Yes, the patient is appropriate with no precautions or contraindications noted.

3. What are the specific goals to be achieved with the use of NMES?
   Answer: To increase the endurance of the patient's lumbar paraspinals with consideration of his prolonged walking while carrying the mailbag.

4. What specific form of electrical stimulation would be appropriate for the patient?
   Answer: NMES with emphasis on parameters for increasing endurance. Biphasic pulsed current or burst-modulated AC (i.e., Russian) can be used.

5. What specific parameters of NMES are appropriate for the patient?
   Answer:
   Pulse duration: 400 to 600 usec
   Frequency: 60 to 80 pps; higher frequency will train the muscle for endurance
   Amplitude: Maximally tolerated contractions are not necessary since we are addressing endurance of the muscles.
   Ramp time: 1- to 2-sec ramp-up
   Duration: At least 10-sec contractions and up to 20 sec with progressively decreasing off-time.

6. What are the proper (i.e., effective and safe) application procedures for NMES related to this case example?
   Answer:
   Electrode application: Bipolar electrode placement using two channels, one for each of the left and right lumbar paraspinals. One electrode placed paraspinally just proximal to L5 with the other on the ipsilateral side placed just above.

the extent of training that can be completed with NMES. Longer rest periods between contractions are recommended to limit the potential for this fatigue.

Contraction-induced muscle injury and the resultant DOMS is typically associated with eccentric muscle actions.[50,51] While this phenomenon is common to most resistance-training paradigms, the magnitude of this response may be exaggerated using NMES and could potentially limit training volume and subsequent adaptations. For example, in a traditional resistance-training program, eccentric and concentric forces are dictated by the external load applied. In addition, the amount of muscle recruited to accomplish these actions is less during the eccentric phase of the contraction. However, programs that incorporate electrically evoked actions may be performed on an isokinetic dynamometer where external loads are not predetermined or limited. The spatially fixed recruitment strategies previously discussed keep the amount of activation constant during NMES, thus resulting in eccentric forces well above those measured concentrically.[52] Thus, the use of high-intensity eccentric contractions during NMES could potentially induce greater muscle damage than a voluntary training program. These are limiting factors because practitioners often see the need to reduce eccentric loading with electrical stimulation. However, it has been reported that eccentric contractions are necessary to obtain sufficient degrees of skeletal muscle hypertrophy.[53]

A final limitation to NMES training is the limited number of muscle groups that can be trained. As previously mentioned, high-intensity NMES is facilitated by the use of an isokinetic dynamometer or a similar piece of equipment that can safely secure the limb and control joint motion during training. While traditional resistance-training programs favor large-muscle group, multijoint exercises (i.e., dead lift, squat, bench press), it is difficult to incorporate NMES with these activities. NMES training is limited to muscle groups using isolated joints and within a given plane of motion. Examples of potential muscle groups to be trained include those that elicit flexion and extension about the ankle (triceps surae and tibialis anterior), knee (quadriceps femoris and hamstrings), and elbow (biceps and triceps brachii). Thus, although the benefits of NMES training are potentially great, significant limitations do exist to its use and resultant application to training.

NMES is often criticized because it does not involve muscle activation during multijoint activities, as traditional resistance-training programs can. However, NMES can be used during rehabilitation to retard loss of and increase strength when multijoint activities cannot be performed.

Electrical Muscle Stimulation (EMS) Applied to Denervated Muscle

The efficacy of electrical stimulation with muscles that have been denervated is controversial and has been questioned in the scientific literature.[54] It should be noted that when referring to the use of electrical stimulation with denervated muscle, the term *NMES* is no longer appropriate, because this assumes the peripheral nervous system is intact and the muscle is being activated through stimulation of the peripheral nerve. When using ES for denervated muscle, the practitioner is attempting to directly activate the muscle through depolarization of the sarcolemma. This act requires different stimulation parameters than standard NMES. Differences include utilizing longer pulse durations, greater amplitude of stimulation, and often a different waveform (direct current). Many commercially available stimulators may not allow modulation of these parameters to accomplish direct stimulation of muscle. In addition, using direct current increases the risk of electrode-related burns, especially when using higher amplitudes of stimulation.

The literature on stimulating denervated muscle generally reports mixed results regarding its effect on preserving muscle and its potential effect on reinnervation.[54–58] Previously published studies have utilized a variety of stimulation parameters, because most practitioners and researchers do not agree on the optimal method to stimulate denervated muscle. Some have suggested that a low-frequency current (2 to 4 pps) preserves denervated muscle tissue better while others argue that a higher-frequency current (20 to 40 pps) is optimal. However, most would agree that the pulse duration should be greater than or equal to 1 millisecond (msec). In fact, many studies have greatly exceeded this value.[54]

There is some controversy as to whether nerve growth is suppressed when electrical stimulation is used or if reinnervation is suppressed due to the activity at the motor end plate with electrical stimulation. A review of relevant studies using electrical stimulation for denervated muscle suggests several conflicting conclusions.[54]

Clinically, electrical stimulation for denervated muscles has most commonly been applied to facial muscles after facial nerve palsy (i.e., Bell's palsy) to preserve the muscle while reinnervation occurs. Some studies suggest using stimulation could be beneficial[55] and some claim it could be harmful.[59] In cases of lower motor neuron injury at the cauda equina, it has been reported that the affected muscle can be trained with a long pulse duration (30 to 50 ms), moderate frequency (16 to 25 pps), and high amplitude (250 mA).[56] However, it took these researchers 1 to 4 years to induce significant muscle hypertrophy. More research is needed to determine whether EMS for denervated muscle shows any future promise as a clinical intervention. There is a renewed interest in this topic for using functional electrical stimulation (FES) to provide function or to preserve muscle to allow for future regenerative techniques. However, this requires specialized equipment, and results are inconclusive thus far.[56,60,61]

Examination, Evaluation, and Prognosis

If ES for denervated muscles is to be considered, tests of strength, ROM, sensation, and function are important—just as with applying NMES for innervated muscle. A review of the patient's medical history should include the cause and length of time of denervation. Electromyography tests should be conducted by a trained electromyographer to evaluate the degree of denervation (see Chapter 16). Patient prognosis for improvement with EMS appears to depend upon length of time since denervation and the number of remaining motor units. Overall, the prognosis for strengthening denervated muscle with EMS is not as good as it is for innervated muscle.

Intervention

Because of the high variability between studies, parameters are more difficult to select in trying to stimulate denervated muscle. Table 11-6 provides the range of parameters used by the majority of studies reviewed. As shown in the table, very long pulse durations (ms as

Table 11•6 EMS Parameters Typically Used for Stimulating Denervated Muscle[54,56]	
Waveform	Monophasic or DC
Pulse duration	1–450 ms (long)
Frequency	1–500 pps
Amplitude	To obtain contraction but low to prevent burns
Ramp-up time	Not identified
Ramp-down time	Not identified
Duty cycle	Highly variable
	30 minutes, 8 hours per day
Treatment time and duration	5–7 days per week
	4 days to 4 years

opposed to μs) are required to stimulate denervated muscle. One potential risk associated with this is burning the patient. Careful attention must be given to the skin during treatment, especially since these patients are likely to also have impairments in sensation.

Electrodes used for denervated muscles tend to be either very large to cover the entire bulk of the muscle or very small to attempt to isolate the motor end plate. A probe type of electrode is often used for stimulating small muscles (Fig. 11-6).

KEY POINT! The stimulation of denervated muscles is not widely endorsed but is often done despite questionable efficacy. We suggest practitioners proceed with caution.

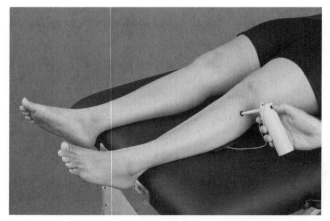

Fig 11•6 An example of a stimulator designed to stimulate denervated muscle. The small tip is placed over the muscle. With denervation, the practitioner needs to move the point of the stimulator along the muscle to attempt to activate any intact motor units. The long pulse duration with this stimulator allows muscle fibers to be stimulated directly.

CASE STUDY 11•4   ELECTRICAL STIMULATION FOR DENERVATED MUSCLE

A 43-year-old female awoke 10 days ago with insidious onset of right-sided facial paralysis with inability to fully close her lips and eye on the right side following a recent sinus infection. Examination shows only trace contraction of the right-sided facial muscles.

CLINICAL DECISION-MAKING

1. Does the patient have a dysfunction, limitation, or problem that can be improved with the use of NMES?
   Answer: Yes, the patient has loss of volitional muscle control of the right-sided facial muscles. Electrical stimulation may be used to activate these muscles.

2. Is the patient appropriate for NMES (i.e., do any of the general precautions or contraindications to NMES apply to the patient, or are there any specific considerations regarding application of NMES to this patient)?
   Answer: No specific contraindications or precautions are present.

3. What are the specific goals to be achieved with the use of ES?
   Answer: To stimulate the involved muscles in order to facilitate restoration of volitional control of the right-sided facial muscles.

4. What specific form of electrical stimulation would be appropriate for the patient?
   Answer: Based on the strength-duration relationship discussed in Chapter 9, activation of muscles demonstrating denervation requires a pulse duration and amplitude greater than that required for innervated muscle.

5. What specific parameters of ES are appropriate for the patient?
   Answer:
   Pulse duration: At least 1 msec or greater. Since many clinical stimulators do not offer pulse durations greater than 1 msec, practitioners should use the longest pulse duration possible. DC or monophasic currents are often used with a probe electrode and manual trigger controls to administer stimulation (see Fig. 11-6).
   Frequency: Low frequency (1 to 4 pps) or higher frequency (20 to 40 pps)
   Amplitude: A dosage set to elicit as much muscle contraction as tolerated by the patient
   Ramp time: 1 to 2 seconds for comfort
   Duration: Contractions should be sustained for several seconds as tolerated; on-times of 3 to 10 sec with off-times of 30 to 50 sec between contractions.

6. What are the proper (i.e., effective and safe) application procedures for NMES related to this case example?
   Answer:
   Electrode application: Because of the smaller facial muscles, electrodes should be appropriately small for the area to be stimulated. Practitioners should be aware of the increase in current density when using smaller electrodes. A probe electrode should be appropriately small and allow for more localized stimulation of specific facial muscles. Practitioners should also be aware that there is an increased risk of burning the patient, so close monitoring of the skin is essential.

Biofeedback

Electromyographic (EMG) biofeedback is the monitoring, detection, or assessment of skeletal muscle activity so that the information gained can be used by the patient and clinician to influence future activity of skeletal muscle, whether for increasing or decreasing activity.[62] Biofeedback shares the same purpose as other forms of electrotherapy—to improve function and decrease pain. Where biofeedback differs is that none of the currents or waveforms previously described is actually delivered to the patient. Instead, the electrical activity generated by contraction of skeletal muscle is detected and used for therapeutic purpose. Because current never reaches the patient, biofeedback is not generally considered an electrotherapeutic agent; however, because the electrical activity is still part of the therapeutic process, biofeedback is discussed with other forms of electrotherapy used for therapeutic purpose.

KEY POINT! Biofeedback does not involve the delivery of electrical current. It can be offered as an option in the initial therapy sessions when patients are apprehensive about electrical stimulation or when the clinician wants to provide kinesthetic awareness of motion. After a trial or two of biofeedback, many patients feel more comfortable receiving electrical stimulation for muscle activation.

Clinically, EMG biofeedback is generally used to either increase or decrease activity of skeletal muscle. Techniques in which increased volitional activity of muscle is desired are considered facilitatory; techniques in which decreased activity is desired are considered inhibitory. Examples of facilitatory and inhibitory EMG biofeedback are listed in Table 11-7.

Recording and Displaying the EMG Signal

EMG biofeedback requires specialized equipment to detect and record the electrical activity associated with muscle recruitment (Fig. 11-7). A device for detecting and transducing the electrical activity of muscle contraction into visual or audio feedback to the patient is required. Most biofeedback devices offer both visual and audio feedback and are portable.

Electrical activity associated with skeletal muscle depolarization is measured in units of microvolts (1,000,000 uV = 1 V) and is then amplified to millivolts for transduction to audio or visual feedback. The degree to which these electrical signals are amplified reflects "sensitivity," which refers to the ability to detect an event. In terms of biofeedback, *sensitivity* refers to the ability to detect the electrical activity associated with muscle contraction. Typical devices used for EMG biofeedback offer sensitivity settings (sometimes called *gain*) of 1, 10, 100, or 1,000 microvolts (uV). This means the smallest level of muscle activity that can be detected is 1 uV. Sensitivity and gain are inversely related, although the terms are often used synonymously,

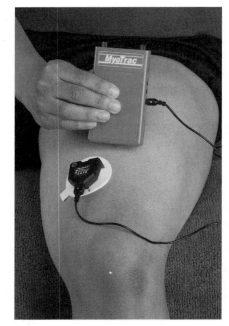

Fig 11•7 An example of biofeedback device and electrode placement.

such that at the highest sensitivity, the gain setting is lowest. For example, at the lowest gain setting of 1 uV, the sensitivity is greatest, capable of detecting as little as one microvolt (uV) of change in muscle activity. In contrast, a high gain setting of 1,000 uV is much less sensitive, only capable of detecting change of 1,000 uV. As the need for sensitivity decreases, the gain setting will be increased accordingly. The sensitivity of a biofeedback device is set depending on the need for amplification and the clinical goals. Less sensitivity is needed when muscle activity is very high. More sensitivity is needed when volitional muscle activity is low.

Electrode Type and Electrode Placement Considerations for EMG Biofeedback

The electrodes used for biofeedback are often specifically made for detecting electrical activity of muscle, but some devices that serve as electrical stimulators also offer EMG biofeedback and use conventional disposable adhesive electrodes similar to those used with other forms of electrotherapy. Placement of electrodes should consider the intent of the biofeedback (i.e., facilitatory or inhibitory) and whether the muscles are demonstrating high or low activity. The muscle fibers most likely to be detected are those closest to the electrodes, if, in fact, these are activated. A wider electrode placement will detect electrical activity from a larger volume of muscle than will a

Table 11•7	**Clinical Examples of Facilitatory and Inhibitory Biofeedback**
Facilitatory	• To increase muscle activity following surgery or injury when volitional recruitment is impaired
	• To normalize the balance of muscles acting at a joint where one muscle group may be insufficient
	• To improve volitional motor control following dysfunction of the central nervous system
	• To increase volitional control of pelvic floor muscles for rehabilitation of urinary incontinence
Inhibitory	• To help decrease activity in muscles demonstrating spasticity caused by dysfunction of the central nervous system
	• To help decrease activity in muscles demonstrating increased activity caused by postural stress or anxiety
	• To help decrease muscle activity associated with chronic pain

narrower electrode placement. When trying to assess "very active" muscles, closer electrode placements are recommended. In contrast, when the volitional activity of muscle is decreased, there is a greater need to assess or monitor a larger muscle volume. In this case, a greater sensitivity and wider electrode placement is recommended to detect activity over more muscle volume. Electrode size does not increase the amplitude of the activity detected but rather simply detects more area of muscle fiber.

Patient Training Strategies With EMG Biofeedback

A requirement for the use of clinical EMG biofeedback is that the muscle be at least partially innervated, and the patient must be able to somewhat activate the muscle. The level of muscle activity the patient is able to reach, whether it be increased or decreased activity, is termed the *threshold*. If the clinical goal is to increase volitional activation of a muscle, then a facilitatory threshold is set so that when the patient increases the muscular activity to a threshold target, audio or video feedback is provided. If the clinical goal is to decrease volitional activity of muscle, then an inhibitory threshold may be set so that when the patient decreases the muscular activity to a threshold target, audio or video feedback is likewise provided.

As a patient is able to increase volitional activity, the sensitivity can be decreased and the electrode placement can be narrowed to focus on more specific areas that may need additional facilitation. As a patient is able to relax or quiet a highly active muscle, the sensitivity may need to be increased and electrode placement widened in order to continue assessing muscle activity.

EMG biofeedback provides a clinically useful and indirect intervention to increase or decrease volitional muscle control by recording muscle activity and using this information to allow the patient to alter future muscle activity. Because no electrical stimulus is applied to the patient, there are no contraindications to using EMG biofeedback, assuming volitional activation of the muscles to be examined is appropriate (Box 11-3).

Box 11•3	**Six Questions to Answer When Considering Use of Biofeedback**

1. Is the patient appropriate for use of biofeedback?
2. What are the muscles to be monitored?
3. Is the intent to facilitate or inhibit muscle activity?
4. How sensitive must the assessment be?
5. Should the electrodes be placed close together or wider apart?
6. How will these factors change as the patient improves?

CASE STUDY 11•5   BIOFEEDBACK FOR FACILITATING MUSCLE ACTIVATION

A 76-year-old female with right total knee arthroplasty completed 4 weeks ago is referred for strengthening of the knee extensors. She is unable to tolerate NMES at a dosage intensity sufficient for increasing strength. Biofeedback is chosen to assist her in activating her quadriceps.

CLINICAL DECISION-MAKING

1. Does the patient have a dysfunction, limitation, or problem that can be improved with the use of NMES?
   Answer: Yes, the patient has postoperative weakness and dysfunction with contracting her quadriceps.

2. Is the patient appropriate for NMES (i.e., do any of the general precautions or contraindications to NMES apply to the patient, or are there any specific considerations regarding application of NMES to this patient)?
   Answer: Yes, given that biofeedback only records electrical activity from the patient rather than delivering it, EMG biofeedback is appropriate.

3. What are the specific goals to be achieved with the use of NMES?
   Answer: To enhance the patient's ability to volitionally recruit her muscle for purposes of increasing strength.

4. What specific form of electrical stimulation would be appropriate for the patient?
   Answer: EMG biofeedback for facilitation.

5. What specific parameters of EMG biofeedback are appropriate for the patient?
   Answer: Initially, the clinician chooses a higher sensitivity setting (gain of 1uV) and wider electrode placement over the proximal muscle belly and the distal vastus medialis, because the patient demonstrates decreased volitional activity of the quadriceps. Two weeks later, the patient's right knee extensor strength is measured at 60% of the left. Because the patient is demonstrating increased ability to volitionally activate the quadriceps, the clinician chooses to decrease the sensitivity (gain increased to 100 uV) and place the electrodes closer together over the vastus medialis.

Documentation Tips

Appropriate documentation of NMES application should include the following:

- Waveform type
  - Russian, biphasic pulsed, etc.
- Waveform parameters
  - Pulse duration and frequency, contraction and rest time, ramp-up and ramp-down
- Electrode
  - Type, shape, and size
  - Placement or location
  - Integrity of skin before and after treatment
- Patient position
- Treatment duration
  - Number of contractions or duration of treatment

REFERENCES

1. Carmick J. Managing equinus in children with cerebral palsy: electrical stimulation to strengthen the triceps surae muscle. *Dev Med Child Neurol.* 1995;37(11):965–975.
2. Fitzgerald GK, Piva SR, Irrgang JJ. A modified neuromuscular electrical stimulation protocol for quadriceps strength training following anterior cruciate ligament reconstruction. *J Orthop Sports Phys Ther.* 2003;33(9):492–501.
3. Stevens JE, Mizner RL, Snyder-Mackler L. Neuromuscular electrical stimulation for quadriceps muscle strengthening after bilateral total knee arthroplasty: a case series. *J Orthop Sports Phys Ther.* 2004;34(1):21–29.
4. Baldwin KM, Haddad F. Skeletal muscle plasticity: cellular and molecular responses to altered physical activity paradigms. *Am J Phys Med Rehabil.* 2002;81(11 Suppl):S40–S51.
5. Pette D. Historical perspectives: plasticity of mammalian skeletal muscle. *J Appl Physiol.* 2001;90(3):1119–1124.
6. Semmler JG, Nordstrom MA. Motor unit discharge and force tremor in skill- and strength-trained individuals. *Exp Brain Res.* 1998;119(1):27–38.
7. Milner-Brown HS, Stein RB, Lee RG. Synchronization of human motor units: possible roles of exercise and supraspinal reflexes. *Electroencephalogr Clin Neurophysiol.* 1975;38(3):245–254.
8. Kraemer WJ, Adams K, Cafarelli E, et al. American College of Sports Medicine position stand. Progression models in resistance training for healthy adults. *Med Sci Sports Exerc.* 2002;34(2):364–380.
9. Leong B, Kamen G, Patten C, Burke JR. Maximal motor unit discharge rates in the quadriceps muscles of older weight lifters. *Med Sci Sports Exerc.* 1999;31(11):1638–1644.
10. Currier DP, Mann R. Muscular strength development by electrical stimulation in healthy individuals. *Phys Ther.* 1983;63(6):915–921.
11. Laughman RK, Youdas JW, Garrett TR, Chao EY. Strength changes in the normal quadriceps femoris muscle as a result of electrical stimulation. *Phys Ther.* 1983;63(4):494–499.
12. Caggiano E, Emrey T, Shirley S, Craik RL. Effects of electrical stimulation or voluntary contraction for strengthening the quadriceps femoris muscles in an aged male population. *J Orthop Sports Phys Ther.* 1994;20(1):22–28.
13. McMiken DF, Todd-Smith M, Thompson C. Strengthening of human quadriceps muscles by cutaneous electrical stimulation. *Scand J Rehabil Med.* 1983;15(1):25–28.
14. Delitto A, Brown M, Strube MJ, Rose SJ, Lehman RC. Electrical stimulation of quadriceps femoris in an elite weight lifter: a single subject experiment. *Int J Sports Med.* 1989;10(3):187–191.
15. Mahoney ET, Bickel CS, Elder C, et al. Changes in skeletal muscle size and glucose tolerance with electrically stimulated resistance training in subjects with chronic spinal cord injury. *Arch Phys Med Rehabil.* 2005;86(7):1502–1504.
16. Dudley GA, Castro MJ, Rogers S, Apple DF Jr. A simple means of increasing muscle size after spinal cord injury: a pilot study. *Eur J Appl Physiol Occup Physiol.* 1999;80(4):394–396.
17. Snyder-Mackler L, Delitto A, Stralka SW, Bailey SL. Use of electrical stimulation to enhance recovery of quadriceps femoris muscle force production in patients following anterior cruciate ligament reconstruction. *Phys Ther.* 1994;74(10):901–907.
18. Bigard AX, Lienhard F, Merino D, Serrurier B, Guezennec CY. Effects of surface electrostimulation on the structure and metabolic properties in monkey skeletal muscle. *Med Sci Sports Exerc.* 1993;25(3):355–362.
19. Cabric M, Appell HJ, Resic A. Effects of electrical stimulation of different frequencies on the myonuclei and fiber size in human muscle. *Int J Sports Med.* 1987;8(5):323–326.
20. Ruther CL, Golden CL, Harris RT, Dudley GA. Hypertrophy, resistance training, and the nature of skeletal muscle activation. *J Strength Cond Res.* 1995;9(3):155–159.
21. Stevenson SW, Dudley GA. Dietary creatine supplementation and muscular adaptation to resistive overload. *Med Sci Sports Exerc.* 2001;33(8):1304–1310.
22. Staron RS, Karapondo DL, Kraemer WJ, et al. Skeletal muscle adaptations during early phase of heavy-resistance training in men and women. *J Appl Physiol.* 1994;76(3):1247–1255.
23. Jensen K, Graf BK. The effects of knee effusion on quadriceps strength and knee intraarticular pressure. *Arthroscopy.* 1993;9(1):52–56.
24. Hopkins JT, Ingersoll CD, Krause BA, Edwards JE, Cordova ML. Effect of knee joint effusion on quadriceps and soleus motoneuron pool excitability. *Med Sci Sports Exerc.* 2001;33(1):123–126.
25. Delitto A, Rose SJ, McKowen JM, Lehman RC, Thomas JA, Shively RA. Electrical stimulation versus voluntary exercise in strengthening thigh musculature after anterior cruciate ligament surgery. *Phys Ther.* 1988;68(5):660–663.
26. Snyder-Mackler L, Delitto A, Bailey SL, Stralka SW. Strength of the quadriceps femoris muscle and functional recovery after reconstruction of the anterior cruciate ligament. A prospective, randomized clinical trial of electrical stimulation. *J Bone Joint Surg Am.* 1995;77(8):1166–1173.
27. Snyder-Mackler L, Ladin Z, Schepsis AA, Young JC. Electrical stimulation of the thigh muscles after reconstruction of the anterior cruciate ligament. Effects of electrically elicited contraction of the quadriceps femoris and hamstring muscles on gait and on strength of the thigh muscles. *J Bone Joint Surg Am.* 1991;73(7):1025–1036.
28. Paternostro-Sluga T, Fialka C, Alacamlioglu Y, Saradeth T, Fialka-Moser V. Neuromuscular electrical stimulation after anterior cruciate ligament surgery. *Clin Orthop Relat Res.* 1999;(368):166–175.
29. Mizner RL, Petterson SC, Stevens JE, Vandenborne K, Snyder-Mackler L. Early quadriceps strength loss after total knee arthroplasty. The contributions of muscle atrophy and failure of voluntary muscle activation. *J Bone Joint Surg Am.* 2005;87(5):1047–1053.

30. Walsh M, Woodhouse LJ, Thomas SG, Finch E. Physical impairments and functional limitations: a comparison of individuals 1 year after total knee arthroplasty with control subjects. *Phys Ther.* 1998;78(3):248–258.

31. Lewek M, Stevens J, Snyder-Mackler L. The use of electrical stimulation to increase quadriceps femoris muscle force in an elderly patient following a total knee arthroplasty. *Phys Ther.* 2001;81(9):1565–1571.

32. Petterson SC, Mizner RL, Stevens JE, et al. Improved function from progressive strengthening interventions after total knee arthroplasty: a randomized clinical trial with an imbedded prospective cohort. *Arthritis Rheum.* 2009;61(2):174–183.

33. Laufer Y, Ries JD, Leininger PM, Alon G. Quadriceps femoris muscle torques and fatigue generated by neuromuscular electrical stimulation with three different waveforms. *Phys Ther.* 2001;81(7):1307–1316.

34. Lyons CL, Robb JB, Irrgang JJ, Fitzgerald GK. Differences in quadriceps femoris muscle torque when using a clinical electrical stimulator versus a portable electrical stimulator. *Phys Ther.* 2005;85(1):44–51.

35. Gregory CM, Dixon W, Bickel CS. Impact of varying pulse frequency and duration on muscle torque production and fatigue. *Muscle Nerve.* 2007;35(4):504–509.

36. Ward AR. Electrical stimulation using kilohertz-frequency alternating current. *Phys Ther.* 2009;89(2):181–190.

37. Matheson GO, Dunlop RJ, McKenzie DC, Smith CF, Allen PS. Force output and energy metabolism during neuromuscular electrical stimulation: a 31P-NMR study. *Scand J Rehabil Med.* 1997;29(3):175–180.

38. Gregory CM, Bickel CS. Recruitment patterns in human skeletal muscle during electrical stimulation. *Phys Ther.* 2005;85(4):358–364.

39. Henneman E, Somjen G, Carpenter DO. Functional significance of cell size in spinal motoneurons. *J Neurophysiol.* 1965;28:560–580.

40. Kubiak RJ, Whitman KM, Johnston RM. Changes in quadriceps femoris muscle strength using isometric exercise versus electrical stimulation. *J Orthop Sports Phys Ther.* 1987;8(11):537–541.

41. Sinacore DR, Delitto A, King DS, Rose SJ. Type II fiber activation with electrical stimulation: a preliminary report. *Phys Ther.* 1990;70(7):416–422.

42. Solomonow M. External control of the neuromuscular system. *IEEE Trans Biomed Eng.* 1984;31(12):752–763.

43. Blair E, Erlanger J. A comparison of the characteristics of axons through their individual electrical responses. *Am J Physiol.* 1933;106:524–564.

44. Binder-Macleod SA, Halden EE, Jungles KA. Effects of stimulation intensity on the physiological responses of human motor units. *Med Sci Sports Exerc.* 1995;27(4):556–565.

45. Knaflitz M, Merletti R, De Luca CJ. Inference of motor unit recruitment order in voluntary and electrically elicited contractions. *J Appl Physiol.* 1990;68(4):1657–1667.

46. Adams GR, Harris RT, Woodard D, Dudley GA. Mapping of electrical muscle stimulation using MRI. *J Appl Physiol.* 1993;74(2):532–537.

47. Bellemare F, Woods JJ, Johansson R, Bigland-Ritchie B. Motor-unit discharge rates in maximal voluntary contractions of three human muscles. *J Neurophysiol.* 1983;50(6):1380–1392.

48. Carpentier A, Duchateau J, Hainaut K. Motor unit behaviour and contractile changes during fatigue in the human first dorsal interosseus. *J Physiol.* 2001;534(Pt 3):903–912.

49. Meyer RA, Prior BM. Functional magnetic resonance imaging of muscle. *Exerc Sport Sci Rev.* 2000;28(2):89–92.

50. Bowers EJ, Morgan DL, Proske U. Damage to the human quadriceps muscle from eccentric exercise and the training effect. *J Sports Sci.* 2004;22(11-12):1005–1014.

51. Lu SS, Wu SK, Chen JJ. The effects of heavy eccentric contractions on serum creatine kinase levels. *Chin J Physiol.* 1992;35(1):35–44.

52. Dudley GA, Harris RT, Duvoisin MR, Hather BM, Buchanan P. Effect of voluntary vs. artificial activation on the relationship of muscle torque to speed. *J Appl Physiol.* 1990;69(6):2215–2221.

53. Hather BM, Tesch PA, Buchanan P, Dudley GA. Influence of eccentric actions on skeletal muscle adaptations to resistance training. *Acta Physiol Scand.* 1991;143(2):177–185.

54. Eberstein A, Eberstein S. Electrical stimulation of denervated muscle: is it worthwhile? *Med Sci Sports Exerc.* 1996;28(12):1463–1469.

55. Hyvarinen A, Tarkka IM, Mervaala E, Paakkonen A, Valtonen H, Nuutinen J. Cutaneous electrical stimulation treatment in unresolved facial nerve paralysis: an exploratory study. *Am J Phys Med Rehabil.* 2008;87(12):992–997.

56. Kern H, Hofer C, Modlin M, et al. Denervated muscles in humans: limitations and problems of currently used functional electrical stimulation training protocols. *Artif Organs.* 2002;26(3):216–218.

57. Kern H, Hofer C, Strohhofer M, Mayr W, Richter W, Stohr H. Standing up with denervated muscles in humans using functional electrical stimulation. *Artif Organs.* 1999;23(5):447–452.

58. Lindsay RW, Robinson M, Hadlock TA. Comprehensive facial rehabilitation improves function in people with facial paralysis: a 5-year experience at the Massachusetts eye and ear infirmary. *Phys Ther.* 2010;90(3):391–397.

59. Diels HJ. Facial paralysis: is there a role for a therapist? *Facial Plast Surg.* 2000;16(4):361–364.

60. Mandl T, Meyerspeer M, Reichel M, et al. Functional electrical stimulation of long-term denervated, degenerated human skeletal muscle: estimating activation using T2-parameter magnetic resonance imaging methods. *Artif Organs.* 2008;32(8):604–608.

61. Modlin M, Forstner C, Hofer C, et al. Electrical stimulation of denervated muscles: first results of a clinical study. *Artif Organs.* 2005;29(3):203–206.

62. Basmajian JV. Introduction. In: *Principles and Background. Biofeedback: Principles and Practices for Clinicians.* 3rd ed. Baltimore: Williams & Wilkins; 1989.

63. Iwasaki T, Shiba N, Matsuse H, et al. Improvement in knee extension strength through training by means of combined electrical stimulation and voluntary muscle contraction. *Tohoku J Exp Med.* 2006;209(1):33–40.

64. Mohr T, Carlson B, Sulentic C, Landry R. Comparison of isometric exercise and high volt galvanic stimulation on quadriceps femoris muscle strength. *Phys Ther.* 1985;65(5):606–612.

chapter 12

NMES and FES in Patients with Neurological Diagnoses

Therese E. Johnston, PT, PhD, MBA

Patients with neurological conditions have specific impairments and functional limitations that may be addressed through the use of electrical stimulation. For example, a person who has sustained a stroke may have multiple impairments, such as decreases in strength, motor control, and passive ROM; compromised balance; and spasticity. These impairments contribute to the functional limitations and disability that often result from a stroke. Mobility is compromised, so an important component of rehabilitation is to improve mobility to allow for greater independence. Neuromuscular electrical stimulation (NMES) and functional electrical stimulation (FES) may be used clinically to address some of these areas. NMES is defined as the use of electrical stimulation (ES) to activate muscles through stimulation of intact peripheral motor nerves. FES is the use of NMES to promote functional activities.[1]

Examination Needs

A thorough examination must be performed to determine the patient's appropriateness for receiving ES (Box 12-1). Table 12-1 identifies items that should be considered when determining if a patient with a neurological condition is suitable for ES. This table is not all-inclusive. Other pertinent examination items specific to the patient should be included.

One of the examination items is testing muscle innervation, which is critical to deciding appropriateness

Box 12•1	**Concerns Specific to Diagnosis**

Stroke
- Cognitive status
- Preexisting medical issues
- Spasticity
- Blood pressure

Spinal Cord Injury
- History of spontaneous fractures (osteoporosis)
- History of autonomic dysreflexia
- Sensation
- Orthopedic concerns
- Respiratory demands
- Spasticity
- Pressure sores
- Preexisting medical issues

Cerebral Palsy
- Orthopedic issues
- History of seizures
- Implanted devices
- Cognitive status

Multiple Sclerosis
- Spasticity
- Fatigue
- Cognitive status
- Preexisting medical issues

Pediatric Onset Conditions
- Scoliosis
- Hip subluxation
- Torsional deformities of bones
- Osteoporosis

Table 12•1	**Examination and Rationale for the Use of Electrical Stimulation in Populations With Neurological Conditions**

Tests of	Question	Reason
Muscle innervation	If a neurological condition is present, are muscles capable of being stimulated?	Electrical stimulation applications typically require innervation of the muscle (an upper motor neuron injury).
Strength	What is current strength (manual muscle test or muscle torque)?	To determine muscles to treat and effect of treatment.
Range of motion	Are any ROM limitations present?	Decreased ROM may impact functional outcomes. Electrical stimulation may increase ROM.
Sensation	Is sensation present, absent, diminished?	More frequent monitoring is needed with insensate skin.
Pain	Is pain present at rest or with activity? How severe?	To determine any positive or negative effects on pain.
Spasticity	Is spasticity present?	Spasticity can impact the choice of stimulation parameters. Spasticity may be positively or negatively impacted by electrical stimulation.
Function	Are any functional limitations present?	To determine effect of treatment on function.
Cognitive status	Is cognitive status sufficient to provide feedback?	Safety of use.
Caregiver assistance	Does patient require caregiver assistance to use electrical stimulation at home if needed?	Determine availability of assistance.
Other treatments	Are any other treatments being used or modified that may impact the intervention with electrical stimulation?	May impact ability to assess effects of intervention.

for ES. The patient must have an upper motor neuron injury to the targeted muscles in order to obtain a muscle response with standard clinical stimulation. A quick test for gross innervation is to apply electrical stimulation and observe if the muscle achieves a fused contraction. However, a more in-depth evaluation may be needed if sensation or spasticity prevents a visible response. An examination of the signs of an upper motor neuron lesion (i.e., presence or absence of spasticity) should also be performed. If denervation is suspected, nerve conduction velocity or electromyography tests can be conducted by a trained electroneuromyographer to evaluate the degree of denervation and appropriateness for electrical stimulation.

Neuromuscular Electrical Stimulation (NMES)

NMES for Muscle Strengthening

NMES has been applied to patients with neurological conditions to enhance strength in a variety of affected muscles groups (Table 12-2). Primary diagnoses studied include stroke, cerebral palsy (CP), spinal cord injury

Table 12•2 **Summary of Studies Using NMES for Strengthening**

Authors	Population	Method	Results
Powell et al.[3]	Acute stroke	Rehab + NMES to wrist extensors 3×/wk, 8 wks vs. rehab alone	Increased isometric strength and hand function
Kimberley et al.[4]	Chronic stroke	NMES to wrist and finger extensors vs. sham treatment	Increased finger extensor strength, grasp and release ability, and cortical activity
Knutson et al.[5]	Chronic stroke	NMES for hand opening (on/off times started in cycles of 5/20 sec with on-times increasing and off-times decreasing over the 12-week intervention	Increased finger extension AROM, torque production, and upper extremity function
de Kroon and IJzerman[6]		EMG triggered NMES to the wrist extensors vs. cyclical NMES	Improvements in grip strength and function with no differences between groups
Wright and Granat[7]	Hemiplegic CP	35-day program of NMES 30 min/day to wrist extensors	Increase wrist extension strength and hand function
Kamper et al.[8]	Hemiplegic CP	NMES to wrist extensors and flexors (15 min, 6 days/wk, for 3 months)	Improved wrist extension torque and muscle coactivation with movement
Vaz et al.[9]	Hemiplegic CP	NMES to wrist extensors (3×/wk for 8 wks)	Increase in wrist strength without functional change
Ozer et al.[10]	Hemiplegic CP	NMES to wrist extensors and dynamic bracing vs. dynamic bracing alone	Increased grip strength and ROM
Hazlewood et al.[11]	Hemiplegic CP	NMES to dorsiflexors 1 hour a day for 35 consecutive days vs. matched controls	Increase dorsiflexion strength and PROM
van der Linden et al.[12]	Diplegic, hemiplegic, quadriplegic CP	NMES to gluteus maximus for 1 hour/day, 6 days/wk for 8 weeks	No effects on strength, gait, or PROM
Stackhouse et al.[13]	Diplegic CP	Intensity of isometric quadriceps and plantar flexor stimulation based on ≥ 50% of maximal voluntary contraction (percutaneous electrodes)	Larger strength and walking speed gains compared to volitional exercise group
Bélanger et al.[18]	SCI	NMES to quadriceps 5 days/wk, for 24 wks, one leg given resistance, the other no resistance	Greater rate of increase seen on the resisted side. Both sides increased distal femur and proximal tibia bone density
Livesly et al.[22]	MS	NMES to quadriceps and hamstrings, 12 min, 5 days/wk, for 6 wks vs. sham	No to small effect on strength

(SCI), and multiple sclerosis (MS). In the neurological population, studies have examined NMES using a strengthening paradigm and have shown that patients who display decreased muscle strength due to a neurological problem may benefit from the use of NMES, especially when muscle atrophy is present. However, a recent systematic review[2] concluded that NMES primarily has modest support in the stroke population and that it is difficult to make conclusions for other neurological populations because of the small number of low-quality studies.

NMES can lead to improvements in strength and other impairments in those with neurological conditions, so the practitioner may have combined goals of enhancing strength, ROM, and functional outcomes in these patients. Overall, studies are very difficult to compare due to the different outcome measures, stimulation parameters, and treatment durations. Table 12-3 identifies the ranges of parameters used.

This section will focus on NMES applications. However, many studies have used FES to improve function yet reported a strengthening effect of the treated muscles. FES studies are described in the FES section of this chapter, because these two techniques in theory use a different approach.

KEY POINT! It is important to keep in mind that traditional strengthening protocols require overload for strengthening to occur. Although this principle also applies to NMES for strengthening, many studies investigating NMES involving those with neurological conditions do not overload the muscle to the extent used for treating musculoskeletal diagnoses without neurological injury.

Stroke

Research has shown improvements in upper extremity strength and function following an NMES strengthening program. Improvements have been reported in isometric strength of the wrist[3] and finger extensors,[4,5] grip strength,[6] hand function,[3,5] grasp and release ability,[4] and cortical activity (seen via functional MRI).[4]

Table 12•3	Parameters Typically Seen for Muscle Strengthening[3,5,6,9,11,18,23,113,116–121]	
Waveform	Symmetrical or asymmetrical biphasic, burst-modulated AC (i.e., Russian current)
Pulse duration	100–700 µsec
Frequency	30–85 pps
Amplitude	To obtain strong contraction (may be related to a percentage of maximum voluntary isometric contraction)
Ramp-up time	1–5 seconds
Ramp-down time	1–2 seconds
Duty cycle	1:3 to 1:5 with on-times up to 10 seconds
Treatment time and duration	At least 10 contractions or up to 1 hour/day, three to five times per week, for 4 to 8 weeks

Cerebral Palsy

Improvements have been reported following both upper and lower extremity NMES applications in children with CP. Upper extremity changes have included improved wrist extension strength,[7–9] hand function,[7] muscle coactivation with movement,[8] grip strength,[10] and ROM.[10] NMES to the dorsiflexor muscles has led to gains in dorsiflexion strength and passive ROM,[11] while NMES to the gluteus maximus resulted in no gains.[12] The quadriceps and plantar flexor muscles were stimulated in another study using percutaneous electrodes (electrodes implanted into the muscle but exiting the skin), resulting in larger strength and walking speed gains compared to volitional exercise.[13]

For children with CP, a technique that gained popularity in the 1990s and early 2000s is threshold electrical stimulation (TES). This technique involves low-level (sensory only) stimulation delivered overnight with the theory that muscle strength would result from an increase in blood flow. Even though an earlier report showed some benefits of this approach,[14] more recent randomized control trials (RCTs) have shown it to have no impact on motor or walking function,[15] spasticity,[16] ROM,[16] or muscle growth.[16]

Spinal Cord Injury

For patients with a diagnosis of complete SCI (no motor function below level of injury), electrical stimulation has been studied to increase muscle mass and stimulated muscle strength, often with goals of decreasing secondary complications of SCI. However, most of these studies have used FES rather than NMES to achieve outcomes (see the "Functional Electrical Stimulation" section). Two studies have looked specifically at NMES for strength and

reported increases in strength,[17,18] self-care,[18] and mobility.[18] Another application of NMES for SCI involves stimulation to the gluteal muscles to improve seated pressure for skin protection and prevention of pressure ulcers. Studies have reported decreased seating interface pressures,[19,20] decreased pain,[21] increased skin pliability,[21] and increased muscle bulk[21] using NMES.

Multiple Sclerosis

One study (NMES vs. sham treatment) has examined NMES strengthening for people with MS[22] and showed no to small effects on quadriceps and hamstrings muscle strength following a 12-minute, 5 times weekly, 6-week NMES program (3, 10, or 35 pps; 200 ms).

Examination for Muscle Strengthening

Specific examination items for strengthening are listed in Table 12-4.

Intervention for Muscle Strengthening

The practitioner needs to make many decisions to determine the optimal means of applying NMES. The appropriate muscle stimulator must be chosen based upon the desired stimulation parameters to achieve a strong muscle response. Electrode placement, on- and off-times, number of repetitions, and frequency and duration of treatment are all important considerations. The practitioner should apply the basic principles of muscle strengthening in designing the intervention, always monitoring the patient's response to treatment. However, there are some differences between voluntary exercise and exercise with NMES in terms of muscle fiber type recruitment that should be kept in mind.

Table 12•4 **Examination and Rationale for NMES for Strengthening**

Tests of	Question	Reason
Muscle innervation	Are muscles capable of being stimulated?	NMES for strengthening typically requires innervation of the muscle.
Strength	What is current strength (manual muscle test or muscle torque)?	To determine effect of treatment.
Range of motion	Are any ROM limitations present?	Decreased ROM may impact functional outcomes.
Sensation	Is sensation present, absent, diminished?	More frequent monitoring needed with insensate skin.
Pain	Is pain present at rest or with activity? How severe?	To determine effect of strengthening on pain.
Spasticity	Is spasticity present?	Antagonist spasticity may affect ability to accurately assess strength.
Function	Are any functional limitations present?	To determine effect of treatment on function.
Cognitive status	Is cognitive status sufficient to provide feedback?	Safety of use.

Stimulation Parameters

See Table 12-3 for typical strengthening parameters. The practitioner does have options in selecting these parameters in order to achieve the desired response, and as with any intervention, patient response will guide the practitioner in determining stimulation parameters. If the goal of NMES is to enhance muscle strength, the highest pulse duration, amplitude, and frequency tolerated by the patient should be used.[23] It is important to realize, however, that maximizing stimulation parameters will also lead to greater muscle fatigue. Therefore, it is critical to choose an appropriate duty cycle to allow for muscle recovery between repetitions (Box 12-2).

KEY POINT! Ramp-up and ramp-down times are often selected for patient comfort. However, it is important to remember that a longer ramp-up time will lead to a slower generation of force and is not always the most comfortable for the patient. The patient's feedback and muscle response will help guide decision-making. In patients with neurological conditions who have spasticity, a longer ramp-up time is often required when stimulating the antagonist muscle to avoid a quick stretch of the spastic muscle.

Electrode Placement

Electrode placement for NMES applications depends primarily on the size of the targeted muscle. Because the goal is to optimize muscle strength, the electrode should be of sufficient size to recruit as many motor units as possible.

Monitoring Treatment

Patients with neurological conditions have impairments that require close monitoring during electrical

Box 12•2 **Critical Considerations for Strengthening With NMES**

- Overload of muscle is important.
- Longer ramp-up times may be uncomfortable when trying to get a maximal contraction.
- There is some evidence for the use of NMES in neurological populations, but stronger research is needed.
- A wide range of stimulation parameters are reported, making it difficult to determine optimal parameters and dosing.

stimulation. For example, sensation may be decreased over the targeted area, hypersensitivity may be present, or spasticity may be triggered by NMES. As with any exercise program, adjustments may need to be made to the NMES program based upon patient response. A patient should not be sent home with a home-based NMES program until the practitioner is confident that it can be properly carried out at home (Box 12-3).

NMES for Increasing Range of Motion

NMES has been applied as an alternate method to increase tissue extensibility or ROM. Chapter 13 discusses the principles behind the use of modalities to address decreased ROM. NMES is potentially advantageous for increasing ROM, as it can provide repetitive motion of the shortened musculotendinous complex and surrounding tissues over a period of time by stimulating the antagonist muscle. NMES used in this manner may be an efficient way for a practitioner to increase ROM, as the patient or family can often be taught to perform this technique safely at home, increasing the amount of time that the tissues are exposed to stretch.

Box 12•3	General Application and Monitoring Information for NMES and FES

- Instruct the patient: Inform the patient of the purpose and procedure. Be sure to explain the anticipated sensation and effect of the stimulation. Since you want a motor response, explain to the patient how strong of a contraction is expected and required for the treatment to be effective. Initially, it may be necessary to offer the patient a familiarization session to become accustomed to the sensation of electrical stimulation. With a child, make a game of it or distract the child with a video or other activity.
- Preinspection: Inspect the area to be treated for skin compromise and assess for intact sensation over the area to be treated.

- Treatment monitoring: Monitor the patient's response to treatment by observing the muscle response and his reaction to it. The amplitude may need to be increased during the session to achieve the effect if tolerated. If the patient has cognitive deficits, ask the patient for feedback about how the electrical stimulation feels. If the patient is unable to respond, stop the treatment after several minutes, remove the electrodes, and check the skin. If there are no skin issues, the treatment can resume.
- Postinspection: Remove the electrodes and inspect the skin for any signs of skin irritation or adverse effects. If redness occurs, explain to the patient that this is not uncommon and should disappear in less than 24 hours.

Studies have reported that NMES helped prevent wrist flexion contractures following acute stroke,[24] increase wrist extension passive ROM (PROM) following stroke,[25] increase wrist flexion PROM and improvability to manipulate objects for children with CP,[7] and increase ankle dorsiflexion PROM for children with CP.[26] Other studies have reported increases in passive ROM when NMES has been applied for a variety of reasons,[27–29] including strengthening, reducing spasticity, and increasing function.

ROM improvements have been seen with NMES either used directly to increase ROM or as a result of NMES applied for another application. Due to these findings, more controlled research is needed to identify the best method to apply when using NMES to increase tissue extensibility and to predict anticipated outcomes.

Examination, Evaluation, and Prognosis

Table 12-5 indicates some important aspects of an examination when considering using NMES to increase tissue extensibility. The general precautions and contraindications for using NMES mentioned in Chapter 10 are still applicable and should be included in the examination.

Intervention

Electrodes should be selected based upon the size of the antagonist muscle. Table 12-6 identifies commonly used stimulation parameters to improve tissue extensibility.

KEY POINT! A critical factor when using NMES for tissue extensibility is to minimize fatigue so the patient can then increase treatment time. Fatigue can be minimized by using the lowest frequency and highest amplitude that creates the needed force.[23]

Amplitude should be set to achieve a 3+/5 contraction that will stretch the tightened muscle. A contraction stronger than this may cause discomfort, because the

Table 12•5	Examination and Rationale for NMES for Tissue Extensibility	
Tests of	Question	Reason
History	Is there a history of bony injury or deformity?	NMES will address only soft tissue impairment.
Strength	Is voluntary movement present in agonist or antagonist?	Potential for strength improvement using NMES.
Range of motion	What is available ROM? How long has decreased ROM been present?	Significantly decreased ROM and chronic contracture have poorer prognosis.
Sensation	Is sensation present, absent, diminished?	More frequent monitoring needed with insensate skin.
Pain	Is pain present at rest? With activity? How severe?	To determine effect of increasing ROM on pain.
Spasticity	Is spasticity present?	Strong spasticity may impact outcomes if not addressed.
Function	What are the functional limitations due to decreased ROM?	To determine effect of treatment on function.
Cognitive status	Is cognitive status sufficient to provide feedback?	Safety of use.
Caregiver assistance	Does patient require caregiver assistance to use NMES at home?	Determine availability of assistance.

CASE STUDY 12•1 NMES TO IMPROVE STRENGTH

An 8-year-old boy with mild spastic diplegic cerebral palsy is experiencing an increase in his crouched gait pattern (increased hip and knee flexion during stance) that you feel is due to decreased quadriceps muscle strength.

CLINICAL DECISION-MAKING

1. Does the patient have a problem that can be improved with the use of NMES?
   Answer: This patient may benefit from quadriceps strengthening with NMES.

2. Is the patient appropriate for application of NMES (i.e., do any of the general precautions or contraindications to NMES apply, or are there any specific considerations regarding application of NMES to this patient)?
   Answer: Considerations include orthopedic concerns, cognitive status and ability to understand treatment, seizure history, ROM limitations, and spasticity.

3. What are the specific goals to be achieved with the use of NMES?
   Answer: Increased strength of the quadriceps muscles and decreased knee flexion during stance. A functional goal could be to have him play soccer with his friends.

4. What specific parameters of NMES would be appropriate for the patient?
   Answer: Pulse duration: 200–400 μsec
   Frequency: 50+ pps
   Amplitude: To obtain a strong contraction as tolerated
   Ramp time: 1–2 seconds
   Duration: Start low to get him used to the stimulation (5 seconds on, 25 seconds off) and work up to 10 seconds on, 30 seconds off. Perform at least 10 contractions, 3 days per week.

5. What are the proper (i.e., effective and safe) application procedures for NMES related to this case example?
   Answer:
   Electrode application: Two electrodes, one proximally and laterally over the vastus lateralis and

rectus femoris and one distally and medially over the vastus medialis and the rectus femoris (Fig. 12-1).
Patient position: The exercise can be done a few different ways and may require some creativity of the physical therapist. The child can work with the stimulation, or you can have the child try to relax and let the stimulation turn on the muscle.
- The child can sit in a comfortable chair with the leg moving against gravity. Weights can be added if more of an effect is needed.
- The child can sit on a computerized dynamometer with the knee fixed at 60° of flexion. An isometric contraction can then be performed.
- The activity can be turned into a functional activity (as FES) by having the child do step-ups, squats, or other closed-chain quadriceps exercises. The physical therapist can trigger the FES through a remote switch to time the stimulation with the activity.

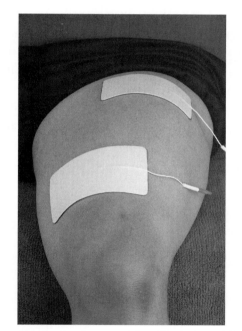

Fig 12•1 Electrode placement for stimulation of the quadriceps femoris muscle.

joint will be more forcefully moved to its limits in ROM. As maximal stimulation parameters aren't used, a portable stimulator may be sufficient for this application, making home treatment more feasible. The greatest variation in treatment recommendations involves the treatment times and duration. Therefore, the practitioner should base the treatment times first on patient tolerance (monitoring for muscle soreness) and then on clinical judgment based upon the goals of the treatment and the patient's current status (i.e., acute versus chronic stroke).

Table 12•6	Parameters Typically Seen for Enhancing Tissue Extensibility[26–29,31,32,122]
Waveform	Symmetrical or asymmetrical biphasic
Pulse duration	200–300 μsec
Frequency	12–33 pps
Amplitude	To obtain 3+/5 contraction
Ramp-up time	3 seconds (for comfort)
Ramp-down time	1–2 seconds
Duty cycle	1:1 (typically 10 seconds on, 10 seconds off)
Treatment time and duration	15 minutes to 6 hours per day, 1 to 4 times/day, for 2 weeks to 6 months

In starting a program using NMES, the practitioner may begin with a longer off-time and a shorter treatment time and advance quickly to a 1:1 duty cycle and longer treatment times in order for the patient to develop tolerance and muscle endurance for the length of the treatment (Box 12-4).

NMES for Decreasing Spasticity

Spasticity is defined as a velocity-dependent increase in tone that is frequently assessed by moving the limb quickly and observing the response.[30] Clinically, spasticity can interfere with function. Three theories have been proposed for the mechanisms for decreasing spasticity using NMES. The first theory states that NMES applied to the antagonist muscle decreases spasticity through reciprocal inhibition of the spastic

Box 12•4	Critical Considerations for Using NMES to Increase ROM

- Parameters should be set so that stretching principles are followed (low load, prolonged application).
- Stimulation parameters should be set to minimize fatigue (low frequency and amplitude), since goal is longer treatment time.
- A wide range of stimulation parameters are reported, making it difficult to determine optimal parameters and dosing.
- Stronger research is needed.

agonist muscle.[31] Reciprocal inhibition occurs through inhibitory interneurons within the spinal cord.[32] The second theory proposes that NMES applied to the spastic agonist muscle works by fatiguing the muscle or by providing recurrent inhibition via Renshaw cells.[31] Stimulating the motor units of the spastic agonist muscle excites the Renshaw cells, which then inhibit the same spastic motor units.[32] The third theory states that electrical stimulation that delivers only sensory stimuli (doesn't create a muscle contraction) leads to sensory habituation that then leads to a decrease in spasticity.[31]

Clinically, NMES has been used to address spasticity in many patients who have neurological conditions with or without voluntary movement. Table 12-7 reviews studies that address spasticity in different populations. Several problems exist with much of the literature. Few studies include a control or comparison group, and inconsistencies exist in regard to

Table 12•7 Literature on NMES for Decreasing Spasticity

Authors	Population	Method	Results
Kamper et al.[8]	CP	NMES to wrist flexors and extensors	No change in spasticity
King[123]	Stroke	NMES to wrist extensors: passive stretch and NMES groups	NMES group had greater decrease in spasticity of wrist flexors as measured by torque meter.
Miller et al.[124]	MS	TENS to quadriceps muscles	Decreased spasticity per Global Spasticity Scale after 2 weeks for group using TENS 8 hrs/day but not for group using 1hr/day.
Potisk et al.[125]	Stroke	Sensory stimulation over sural nerve	Decreased plantar flexor spasticity as measured by an electrohydraulic brace.
Robinson et al.[126]	SCI	NMES to quadriceps femoris	Decreased quadriceps spasticity immediately after treatment only.
Scheker et al.[127]	CP	NMES to wrist and finger extensors while wearing a wrist splint	Decreased wrist flexor spasticity as measured by a compliance scale. Increased upper extremity function.
Seib et al.[128]	SCI, TBI	NMES to anterior tibialis: sham and treatment groups	Treatment group had subjective decrease in plantar flexor spasticity lasting 24 hours after treatment.
Wang et al.[31]	Stroke	Sensory stimulation to T12 and L1 paravertebral areas to decrease plantar flexor spasticity	Decreased passive resistance of plantar flexors as measured by dynamometer.
Weingarden et al.[28]	Stroke, TBI	NMES to wrist and finger extensors	Decreased wrist flexor spasticity

CP, cerebral palsy; *MS*, multiple sclerosis; *SCI*, spinal cord injury; *TBI*, traumatic brain injury.

Table 12•8	Examination and Rationale for NMES for Spasticity Management	
Tests of	**Question**	**Reason**
Strength	Is voluntary movement present in agonist or antagonist?	Potential for strength improvement using NMES and for decreased antagonist spasticity to allow weak agonist to move.
Range of motion	Is a fixed contracture present?	A decrease in spasticity may have limited results if significant ROM deficits are present.
Sensation	Is sensation present, absent, diminished?	More frequent monitoring needed with insensate skin.
Pain	Is pain present? How severe?	To determine effect of decreased spasticity on pain.
Spasticity	How significant is the spasticity?	To determine effect of intervention.
Function	Does spasticity affect functional abilities?	To determine effect of treatment on function.
Cognitive status	Is cognitive status sufficient to provide feedback?	Safety of use.
Caregiver assistance	Does patient require caregiver assistance to use NMES at home?	Determine availability of assistance.
Other treatments	Are antispasticity medications or other treatments being used or modified?	May impact ability to assess effects of intervention.

treatment duration, length of time of effect, and how spasticity is measured.

Examination, Evaluation, and Prognosis

Table 12-8 provides some important aspects of the patient examination when considering using NMES to decrease spasticity. Based upon the literature, the treatment needs to be provided on an ongoing basis to maintain the effect and a longer treatment time may be necessary.

Intervention

Table 12-9 identifies parameters reported in the literature for decreasing spasticity by creating a muscle contraction with NMES. One important parameter when treating patients with spasticity is the ramp-up time. When stimulating the antagonist to the spastic muscle, a short ramp-up time may create a spastic response of the agonist due to the quick stretch. The practitioner should monitor the patient for this response and adjust the ramp-up time accordingly.

Studies using sensory-level electrical stimulation use similar parameters except that the amplitude is kept low to avoid a muscle contraction. Another difference is that the stimulation typically is delivered continuously for the treatment time, rather than using a duty cycle. A higher frequency (up to 100 pps) is often used.

As with other NMES applications, electrode size must be relative to the muscle size. A small, portable stimulator may be sufficient for using NMES to reduce spasticity, because the goal is not to maximize force production. A portable stimulator also offers the advantage of being easily used at home after patient/caregiver training has occurred (Box 12-5).

NMES for Decreasing Urinary Incontinence

NMES has mainly been used to decrease incontinence for people without neurological conditions;

Table 12•9	Parameters Typically Seen for Decreasing Muscle Spasticity Using NMES[8,28,31,123–128]
Waveform	Symmetrical or asymmetrical biphasic, burst-modulated AC (i.e., Russian current)
Pulse duration	250–500 µsec
Frequency	20–60 pps
Amplitude	To obtain a contraction (at least a grade 3+/5)
Ramp-up time	0.5–3 seconds
Ramp-down time	0–3 seconds
Duty cycle	Variable (1:1, 3:4, 10:7) but typically larger ratio than for muscle strengthening
Treatment time and duration	10–60 minutes per day except one study treated for 8 hrs. Treatment typically needs to continue for effect to remain, unless recovery of movement is occurring.

CASE STUDY 12•2 NMES FOR INCREASING TISSUE EXTENSIBILITY AND DECREASING SPASTICITY

A 71-year-old woman presents with complaints of tightness and spasticity in her left hand and wrist and the inability to use the hand functionally. She holds her hand and wrist in flexion. Her past medical history reveals a right cerebral vascular accident 1 month prior, hypertension, and coronary artery disease. She currently lives with her daughter. Her goals are to become independent with several activities of daily living.

CLINICAL DECISION-MAKING

1. Does the patient have a problem that can be improved with the use of NMES?
   Answer: Yes, she has decreased ROM, spasticity, and likely has decreased strength.

2. Is the patient appropriate for application of NMES (i.e., do any of the general precautions or contraindications to NMES apply, or are there any specific considerations regarding application of NMES to this patient)?
   Answer: This patient may have decreased cognition and sensory awareness that may impact safety of using NMES. Her PROM needs to be assessed. If her contracture is significant (little motion), the issue may involve more than just soft tissue, and NMES would not be appropriate. However, since her stroke was 1 month ago, she likely has primarily a soft tissue limitation.

3. What are the specific goals to be achieved with the use of NMES?
   Answer: Your immediate goals can be to increase ROM and decrease spasticity. If successful, later goals can focus on strength and functional outcomes. A functional goal could be for her to hold a fork in that hand or to use that hand as an assist for bimanual activities.

4. What is an appropriate electrode placement for this patient to address both immediate goals?
   Answer: Place electrodes on the wrist extensor muscles to provide a stretch to the wrist flexors (Fig. 12-2). Spasticity reduction will be targeted based on the principle of reciprocal inhibition using this approach. If your clinic has access to a NESS H200 (see "Functional Electrical Stimulation" section), this device may be assessed with this patient to also meet her goals. The device would then allow the advancement to functional use once sufficient passive ROM is gained.

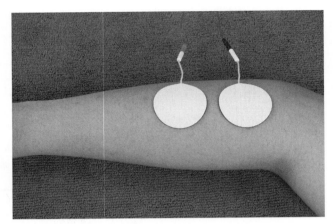

Fig 12•2 Electrode placement for stimulation of the wrist extensors.

5. What specific parameters of NMES would be appropriate for the patient?
   Answer:
   Pulse duration: 200–300 μsec
   Frequency: 20–30 pps
   Amplitude: To obtain a 3+ contraction
   Ramp-up time: Up to 3 seconds (watch for spastic response)
   On/off time: Start with 10:30 and change to 10:10 as endurance improves
   Duration: 15-minute sessions to start, working up to several hours

6. What are the proper (i.e., effective and safe) application procedures for NMES related to this case example?
   Answer:
   Electrode application: Electrodes should be placed in a bipolar arrangement using a single channel to the wrist and finger extensor muscles on the forearm. The best response will allow her wrist and fingers to move through their full available passive ROM.
   Patient position: With her seated comfortably with good posture, place her forearm on a towel or other soft surface on a table. Position her forearm in neutral pronation/supination to allow the wrist to extend in a gravity-eliminated position. If her hand quickly returns to a fully flexed position after each muscle contraction, place a soft roll in her hand to maintain a better position.

however, some studies have addressed its use for patients with neurological conditions. An RCT with subjects with MS showed a greater reduction in incontinence episodes when intravaginal NMES was added to a program of pelvic floor training and biofeedback (85% reduction compared to 47% reduction with sham NMES).[33]

Implanted sacral nerve stimulators have been approved by the FDA for patients with urinary retention or with urge incontinence who have failed all conservative therapies. The device stimulates the third or fourth sacral nerve root through a quadripolar electrode placed in the sacral foramen and an implanted stimulator placed in the upper buttock[34] (Fig. 12-3). Reduction in symptoms has been sufficient for Medicare to provide coverage for the device beginning June 2001.[35,36] In addition to reducing symptoms for patients without neurological

conditions, success has been shown with patients with multiple sclerosis.[34]

Examination, Evaluation, and Prognosis

Precautions and contraindications for NMES for urinary incontinence include decreased sensation, pregnancy or plans to become pregnant, recurrent vaginal or urinary infections, vaginal lesions or fistulas, anal fissures, prolapsed uterus, atrophic vaginitis, recent pelvic surgery, pelvic irradiation, and neurological conditions.[37,38] Examination may include an assessment of strength of the pelvic floor muscles using an intravaginal probe that measures intravaginal pressure. A patient diary is recommended before and after treatment to document changes in incontinence (Box 12-6).

Intervention

Intervention strategies have varied in terms of electrodes, waveforms, and parameters used. Table 12-10 provides the range of parameters typically used. The frequency is important based on different physiological mechanisms. Lower frequencies are used to create inhibition (primarily for urge incontinence), and the higher

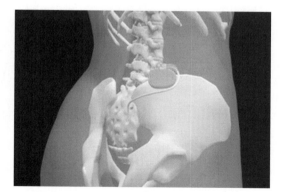

Fig 12•3 An electrode is surgically passed through the skin and placed immediately adjacent to the S3 nerve root within the sacral foramen. The implanted stimulator is placed subcutaneously in the buttock. This completely implanted system allows a signal to be delivered to the S3 nerve root to control incontinence. *(Reprinted with the permission of Medtronic, Inc. © 2004.)*

Table 12•10	Parameters Used for Decreasing Incontinence[33–35,37,39–41,115]	
Waveform	Symmetrical or asymmetrical biphasic, amplitude-modulated AC (i.e., interferential current)	
Pulse duration	250–1,000 µsec	
Frequency	Urge incontinence: 5–20 pps (12 pps common)	
	Stress incontinence: 20–50 pps (50 pps common)	
Amplitude	To maximum tolerable levels (max 100 mA)	
Ramp-up time	2 seconds	
Ramp-down time	2 seconds	
Duty cycle	1:3, 1:2, 1:1 (typically 5 seconds on time)	
Treatment time and duration	15–30 minutes, 1–3 times/day, 4–12 weeks	

frequencies are used to activate motor units (primarily for stress incontinence). Typically a vaginal electrode is used for women (Fig. 12- 4) and a rectal electrode for men. Studies have also used surface electrodes applied to the anus or pubic symphysis[39,40] or to the posterior tibial nerve.[41] Several companies manufacture stimulators specific for treating urinary incontinence, including the typically used parameters and vaginal/rectal electrodes.

Functional Electrical Stimulation

FES is the use of NMES within a functional activity. There are many activities in which FES can be incorporated, and the practitioner can be creative in how it is applied. There are some more common uses of FES, such as for reducing shoulder subluxation, improving hand function, decreasing foot drop

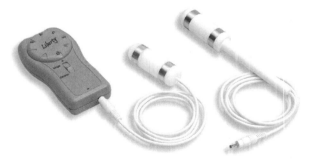

Fig 12•4 Examples of incontinence electrodes. A vaginal electrode is typically inserted to stimulate the pelvic floor muscles to decrease incontinence. This figure shows a stimulator and two types of vaginal electrodes. *(Courtesy of Utah Medical Products, Inc., Midvale, UT.)*

during gait, and exercise to maintain joint mobility, cardiovascular function, and lean mass, among other things.

As mentioned earlier, patients with neurological conditions and spasticity usually require a longer ramp-up time when stimulating the antagonist muscle to avoid a quick stretch of the spastic muscle. However, with FES applications, ramp time needs to be considered in relation to the length of the contraction required for the activity. For example, dorsiflexion to clear the foot occurs quickly during gait. If using electrical stimulation to create dorsiflexion while walking, a long ramp time would be inappropriate and may delay the onset of the contraction or extend the length of the contraction beyond the needs of the activity (the muscle would be on too long).

FES for Shoulder Subluxation

Subluxation of the shoulder is a common problem after an acute stroke, occurring in up to 80% of patients within the first few weeks following stroke. This problem results from the lack of musculature support around the flaccid shoulder girdle, creating stress on the supporting ligaments and joint capsule as gravity creates a traction-type force. As a result, the humerus subluxes inferiorly[42] (Fig. 12-5). Subluxation is usually

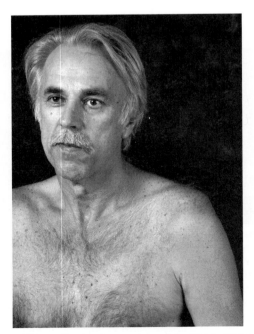

Fig 12•5 This patient, who sustained a stroke, presents with a resulting shoulder subluxation.

painful and can limit the patient's ability to participate in rehabilitation of the upper extremity. Subluxation is typically treated with a supportive sling. However, the use of a sling does not address the flaccid muscles that caused the subluxation and can interfere with rehabilitation of the rest of the upper extremity.

FES using electrodes on the skin surface was introduced in the 1980s as a potential way to decrease shoulder subluxation by stimulating muscles around the shoulder girdle, most commonly to the posterior deltoid and supraspinatus muscles. This orthotic assist can help to provide more normal glenohumeral alignment and create stability for distal movement during rehabilitation.[43]

Several studies, with a meta-analysis,[44] have reported on the benefits of FES for shoulder subluxation; findings indicated that FES was successful for subluxation in the acute stage following stroke but not the chronic stage (Table 12-11). Across the studies reviewed, a subluxation on average of 6.5 mm was reduced by an average of 1.9 mm with the use of FES as compared to conventional treatment alone.

An alternative method for providing FES for shoulder subluxation is the use of percutaneous electrodes as opposed to electrodes applied to the skin surface. Percutaneous electrodes are thin wires implanted near the motor point of a muscle. The electrode exits the skin to allow connection of the cables that attach to a stimulator (Fig. 12-6). Some potential advantages of this type of electrode are decreased discomfort, ease of use because electrodes do not need to be reapplied for each treatment session, and repeatability of muscle responses.[45] Similar outcomes have been reported with the use of percutaneous electrodes as compared to electrodes applied to

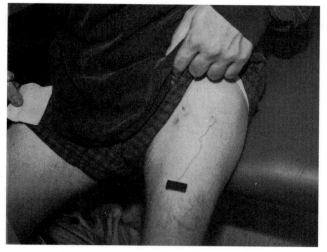

Fig 12•6 Percutaneous electrodes are implanted near the nerve or the motor point. In this picture, an electrode was implanted to the quadriceps femoris via the femoral nerve. To protect the electrode throughout the day, an occlusive bandage is placed over the electrode and connector block. Percutaneous electrodes can be tunneled underneath the skin to exit in any location. When more than one percutaneous electrode is implanted, they typically all exit in the same location.

the skin surface.[29,46] Yu and colleagues[46] reported that 9 out of 10 patients perceived less discomfort with percutaneous electrodes.

Examination, Evaluation, and Prognosis

When determining if a patient is suitable for receiving FES for shoulder subluxation, the examination should include tests of upper extremity strength, ROM, spasticity, the degree of shoulder subluxation, and function (Table 12-12). Ratings of pain should be obtained, and medical history should be reviewed to determine time since stroke and any medical contraindications for use of FES.

Table 12•11	Studies Using FES to Decrease Shoulder Subluxation		
Authors	**Population**	**Method**	**Results**
Faghri et al.[42]	Acute stroke	FES for 6 weeks vs. conventional physical therapy	Decreased shoulder subluxation, spasticity, and pain.
Linn et al.[129]	Acute stroke	FES vs. conventional physical therapy	Decreased shoulder subluxation and pain after 4 weeks. No difference between groups after 12 weeks.
Chantraine et al.[130]	Acute stroke	FES vs. conventional physical therapy	Increased motor scores and decreased pain and subluxation in the FES group after 5 weeks.
Chae et al.[131]	Acute stroke	Percutaneous FES vs. sling (6-week program)	Greater decreases in pain than subjects treated with a sling. Effects lasted for 12 months.

Table 12•12 Examination and Rationale for FES for Shoulder Subluxation

Tests of	Question	Reason
History	Onset of stroke?	Greatest effect seen with acute stroke
Strength	Is voluntary movement present in involved upper extremity?	Potential for improvement
Range of motion	What is upper extremity ROM?	Potential for improvement
Sensation	Is sensation present, absent, diminished?	More frequent monitoring needed with insensate skin
Pain	Is pain present at rest or with activity? How severe?	To determine effect on pain
Spasticity	Is spasticity present?	Potential for improvement
Function	What are the functional limitations?	To determine effect of treatment on function
Pain	Is shoulder or upper extremity pain present?	Potential for improvement
Cognitive status	Is cognitive status sufficient to provide feedback?	Safety of use
Caregiver assistance	Does patient require caregiver assistance to use NMES at home?	Determine availability of assistance

Intervention

Electrodes are typically applied to the posterior deltoid and the supraspinatus muscles. The middle deltoid may be used if there is difficulty isolating the posterior deltoid. The practitioner may find a better response by placing a smaller electrode on the posterior deltoid to increase the current density and a larger one on the supraspinatus in order to create the feeling of the humerus being pulled superiorly without creating significant abduction of the upper extremity. Activation of the upper trapezius muscle should be avoided. Table 12-13 provides typical parameters used for FES for shoulder subluxation.

FES for Upper Extremity Function

FES has been applied to improve hand and upper extremity function in patients following stroke, traumatic brain injury (TBI), CP, and SCI. Some studies conducted in the 1970s demonstrated the feasibility of using FES in patients following stroke.[43] Using commercial devices such as the NESS H200, FES has been more recently applied for hand function in patients who have had a stroke as well as for TBI. The NESS H200 is a forearm- and hand-molded orthosis with five electrodes to stimulate the extensor digitorum, the extensor pollicis brevis, the flexor digitorum superficialis, the flexor pollicis longus, and the thenar muscles. The wrist is held in approximately 10° to 20° of extension within the orthosis (Fig. 12-7). The H200 can provide both exercise and functional grasping abilities. Studies have reported effects on spasticity,[28,47] range of motion,[28] motor function,[47,48] and functional abilities[48–50] with the use of the NESS

Table 12•13 Parameters Typically Seen for FES for Shoulder Subluxation[42,129,130,132]

Waveform	Symmetrical or asymmetrical biphasic
Pulse duration	200–350 μsec
Frequency	30–40 pps
Amplitude	To achieve effect without abduction or shoulder elevation
Ramp-up time	3 seconds
Ramp-down time	3 seconds
Duty cycle	Range 1:5 to 15:1. Typically start with a 1:5, 1:3, or 1:1 but goal is to quickly increase on-time and decrease off-time as muscle endurance improves. On-times up to 30 seconds can be used if tolerated by muscles.
Treatment time and duration	30 minutes to 6 hours (start low and increase as endurance improves), 5–7 days per week, for 4–6 weeks

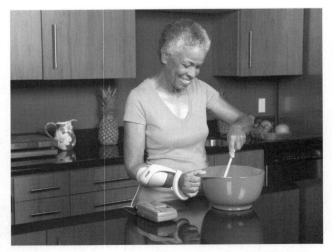

Fig 12•7 Patient following a CVA using the NESS H200 for upper extremity functional activity. *(Courtesy © 2009 Bioness, Inc., Valencia, CA.)*

CASE STUDY 12•3 **FES FOR DECREASING SHOULDER SUBLUXATION**

A 65-year-old man sustained a left CVA 2 weeks ago. He has been complaining of right shoulder pain in the past week and is hesitant about attempting to use the right upper extremity for function. A radiograph showed the presence of a 7 mm inferior subluxation of the humerus from the glenoid fossa. He has been wearing a sling during the past week. His medical history reveals hypertension. His goal is to decrease the pain.

CLINICAL DECISION-MAKING

1. Does the patient have a problem that can be improved with the use of FES?
   Answer: Yes, FES can help to decrease the shoulder subluxation and pain.

2. Is the patient appropriate for application of FES (i.e., do any of the general precautions or contraindications to FES apply, or are there any specific considerations regarding application of FES to this patient)?
   Answer: FES is appropriate for this patient. Special considerations include any possible cognitive and sensory deficits that may limit safety.

3. What are the specific goals to be achieved with the use of FES?
   Answer: The goals are to decrease the degree of subluxation and reduce pain so that he can participate in functional upper extremity training.

4. What specific parameters of FES would be appropriate for the patient?
   Answer:
   Stimulator: Portable stimulator preferred so treatment can continue outside of therapy.
   Pulse duration: 200–350 µsec
   Frequency: 30–40 pps
   Amplitude: Enough to achieve effect of seeing visible reduction in subluxation (elevation of head of humerus). If shoulder abduction is seen, amplitude is too high.
   Ramp time: 3 seconds
   Treatment: You decide to start with on-times of 10 seconds and off-times of 30 seconds, providing treatment for 30 minutes, three times per day. If tolerated, increase on-times and total treatment time with goals of reaching up to 30-second on-times and 2-second off-times for up to 6 hours. Progression should be made as quickly as possible.

5. What are the proper (i.e., effective and safe) application procedures for FES related to this case example?
   Answer:
   Electrode application: Two electrodes, one over the posterior deltoid and one over the supraspinatus (Fig. 12-8). Goal is to move the humerus superiorly into the glenoid fossa without creating abduction. The middle deltoid can also be tried instead of the posterior deltoid if needed.

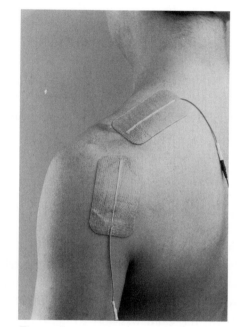

Fig 12•8 Electrodes to reduce a shoulder subluxation are typically placed over the posterior deltoid and the supraspinatus. The exact location to optimize the response will vary between patients. The goal is to move the humerus superiorly into the glenoid fossa without creating abduction.

Patient position: To start, the patient's arm needs to be supported on a table or with a sling. As subluxation and pain reduce, the support may be removed.
Treatment monitoring: Monitor his response to the treatment by observing the decrease in subluxation and asking about pain.

H200 (and its earlier counterpart, the Handmaster) in patients following TBI and stroke. Two of these studies were RCTs[48,50] that compared traditional therapy and traditional therapy plus FES. Both studies included subjects with acute stroke, but Thrasher et al.[48] also included those with chronic effects of stroke and reported that the effects were only significant when applied after an acute stroke.

Other studies have used different devices to apply FES for hand function, using a variety of techniques, including EMG control[6,51] or intensity control using the other hand,[5] bilateral hand activities,[52] percutaneous electrodes,[51] and clinically available stimulators.[53] These studies have reported similar effects on decreasing spasticity, increasing motor ability, and increasing function. However, one study that provided the intervention for only 4 weeks concluded that more sessions would be needed to have a significant effect compared to a control group.[53]

More limited research has been done on FES for upper extremity function in children with CP. Several case studies have looked at FES for hand function. Carmick[54] applied FES for finger and wrist extension and finger flexion in a child with hemiplegic CP. The child initially wore a splint to control wrist position while using FES. The therapist or the parents triggered the FES to create flexion or extension while the child attempted to use the hand functionally. After 9 months of treatment, the child was able to perform activities such as tying his shoes without the splint or FES. In another report, Carmick[55] indicated increased awareness of the involved upper extremity after treatment with FES in one child with hemiplegic CP and increased bilateral hand use in another child, also with hemiplegic CP. Although these are all case studies, they do suggest that FES can impact functional hand use in these populations.

More research effort has been directed toward providing hand function for patients with complete tetraplegia at the fifth and sixth cervical levels. Studies have reported improved function with the use of the Handmaster®[53] and with implanted FES systems.[56,57] Numerous studies of implanted FES systems have reported increased functional independence using a device (called the Freehand®) that stimulates eight upper extremity muscles and provides a control source that allows the user to activate and control the grasp and release patterns. The Freehand, which was clinically available, is no longer on the market.

Examination, Evaluation, and Prognosis

In considering the use of FES for hand function, important tests include those of strength, ROM, sensation, function, and spasticity. The diagnosis and presence of voluntary movement will help the practitioner decide if functional benefits are expected only with the stimulation turned on or if functional benefits with it off are anticipated due to muscle reeducation. For example, a patient following stroke may gain enough muscle strength and motor control to be able to function without the FES. However, another patient may not make these same gains and thus want to use the device throughout the day to provide the ability to grasp. Another important consideration is that if FES is to be used for the hand or forearm only, the patient needs to have sufficient shoulder and elbow strength and ROM to operate the device functionally.

Intervention

In a clinical environment, FES for upper extremity applications can be applied using a surface stimulator. If the practitioner wants to control the stimulation during functional activities, remote switches are available for some stimulators. The practitioner then needs to trigger the FES when appropriate for the activity. For example, grasp can be triggered during a functional reaching activity and then turned off when the patient is ready to release the item. It is important that the practitioner be creative in selecting activities that may be aided by FES in an attempt to provide a new functional movement or to enhance one already present (Box 12-7). Table 12-14 identifies typically used stimulation parameters.

FES for Ambulation

Much focus with FES has centered on ambulation—either in enhancing it for those with some voluntary muscle movement or in creating it for those with no voluntary lower extremity movement. It is common for practitioners to use FES as a dorsiflexion assist for patients who present with decreased foot clearance (foot drop) during the swing phase of gate (Fig. 12-9). This technique has been applied to patients with stroke,

Key Points for Using FES to Increase Upper Extremity Function

- Patients with an acute stroke can increase their functional abilities following combined programs of traditional therapy and FES. The intervention may need to last longer than 4 weeks for an effect.
- FES can be delivered through commercially available systems specifically designed for the forearm/hand or other types of stimulators.
- More research is needed on FES for upper extremity function in children with CP.
- Patients with tetraplegia at C5 or C6 levels can improve hand function with an implanted FES system.

Table 12•14 **Parameters Typically Seen for Hand Function**[28,47–51,53,55–57,133]

Waveform	Symmetrical or asymmetrical biphasic
Pulse duration	200–350 µsec
Frequency	12–40 pps
Amplitude	To achieve desired movement for function. Keep as low as is feasible.
Ramp-up time	Very short to achieve effect
Ramp-down time	Very short to achieve effect
Duty cycle	N/A. Stimulation is timed with demand of functional activity.
Treatment time and duration	30–45 minutes once or twice per day, 3–6 times per week, 6–16 weeks

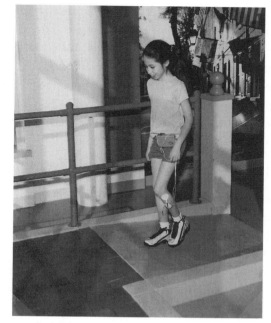

Fig 12•9 A child with hemiplegic cerebral palsy using FES to assist with clearance during the swing phase of gait.

TBI, CP, and incomplete SCI, but is not limited to these populations.

KEY POINT! The most common clinical application of FES for ambulation involves using it as a dorsiflexion assist for decreased foot clearance during swing. FES applied in this manner may replace the use of an ankle foot orthosis, and functional ambulation has been shown to be comparable with an ankle foot orthosis versus FES following stroke.[58]

Timing of the stimulation is controlled with a remote switch or a foot switch placed in the shoe, typically underneath the patient's heel. When pressure is removed from the foot switch, as in the initiation of swing, stimulation will begin. It will end when pressure is again placed onto the foot switch. If a patient does not achieve heel contact during gait, alternate positions for the foot switch can be investigated.

Other means for triggering FES for foot drop are incorporated into devices made specifically for this application. Two systems are currently on the market in the United States: the WalkAide and the NESS L300. Both systems involve placing a cuff containing the electrodes around the upper calf to deliver the stimulation (Fig. 12-10). The WalkAide uses a tilt sensor that detects the leg's position in order to trigger the FES. The NESS L300 uses a sensor mounted on the shoe and computer-based algorithms to control the timing of the simulation (Fig. 12-11). For both devices, the

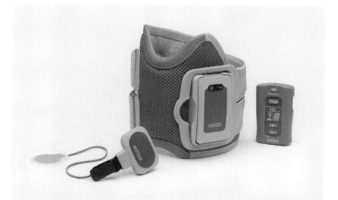

Fig 12•10 This figure shows, from left to right, the sensor that detects pressure increasing and decreasing beneath the heel, the cuff that contains the electrodes that is wrapped around the patient's proximal tibia/fibula to stimulate dorsiflexion during swing, and the FES controller. *(Courtesy © 2009 Bioness, Inc., Valencia, CA.)*

practitioner determines the specific needs of each patient during the initial training phase. The stimulation levels provided by the WalkAide are 50 to 250 μsec, 16.7 to 33 pps, and up to 200 mA. Those for the NESS L300 are 200 μsec, 30 pps, and approximately 30 to 35 mA. As of January 2009, Medicare approved coverage for the WalkAide and the NESS L300 for people with incomplete SCI.

Stroke and Multiple Sclerosis

Early studies showed effects of FES for foot drop following stroke with improvements reported in dorsiflexion during swing,[59] spontaneous recovery,[59] recovery in muscle force three times greater than controls,[60] and walking speed.[61] A more recent study reported improvements in function, social integration, and walking speed for subjects following stroke who had used the NESS L300 for 1 year.[62] Other studies have examined the outcomes with implanted electrodes for FES for foot drop. Implanted electrodes have the advantage of being in a consistent place, so the muscle response should be more consistent. Reported findings include increased walking speed[61,63,64] and distance.[61]

Improvements in walking speed and energy expenditure have been seen with FES applied to the peroneal

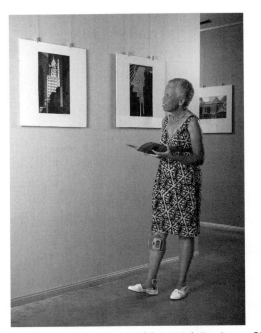

Fig 12•11 Patient using the NESS L300 following a CVA. *(Courtesy © 2009 Bioness, Inc., Valencia, CA.)*

nerve in patients with MS or following stroke.[65] However, another study that involved subjects with MS found increased walking speed and decreased physiological cost of walking when subjects walked with or without FES (which was applied for foot drop).[66]

Cerebral Palsy

Research on FES for gait has received less attention in children with CP. Of the work that has been done, outcomes have included increases in ROM and improvements during ambulation with the FES turned off.[67] Other studies have reported improved ambulation and other functional improvements with FES applied to both the gastrocnemius and peroneal nerve or to just the gastrocnemius muscle in this population.[68,69] One study examined the immediate effects of percutaneous FES on the anterior tibialis and gastrocnemius muscles during gait; findings showed improvements in dorsiflexion during gait whenever the anterior tibialis was stimulated in swing either by itself or in combination with the gastrocnemius (stimulated during terminal stance).[70] Another study applied FES to the gastrocnemius during gait and reported an increase in force production during walking.[71]

Spinal Cord Injury

FES for walking in those with SCI has received considerable focus. FES for dorsiflexion assist alone or in combination with FES to other muscles has augmented swing, increased walking speed, and increased strength for patients with incomplete SCI.[72–74]

Much focus has also been directed to providing ambulation for patients with complete thoracic SCI using surface or percutaneous electrodes or implanted systems.[75–79] The Parastep® is an FDA-approved device for ambulation that stimulates the peroneal nerve to create a flexor withdrawal response for stepping and stimulates the gluteal and quadriceps muscles for stance. It is controlled through push buttons on a walker (Fig. 12-12). The Parastep has been reported to improve lower extremity blood flow,[80] cardiovascular status,[81] muscle size,[82] and lean tissue;[82] however, it had no effect on bone density.[83] In July 2002, a Medicare review panel concluded that FES is at least comparable to interventions currently covered, such as orthoses, so Medicare approved the use of FES for standing and

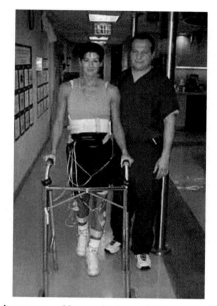

Fig 12•12 A woman with a spinal cord injury uses the Parastep system to ambulate down a hallway at the Miami Project. The push buttons are located on the walker handles, enabling this woman to initiate steps as desired. *(Reprinted with the permission of Sigmedics, Inc.)*

walking for individuals with SCI. Coverage is limited to those individuals who continue to use FES following a trial period, and the goal must be ambulation.[84]

Other methods for standing and walking involve percutaneous or implanted electrodes to create stepping or a swing-through gait pattern (advancing both limbs simultaneously).[77,78,85–88] These other methods all involve research devices. Long-term benefits of these devices have not yet been established. Other research designs combine FES with orthoses, such as reciprocating gait orthoses.[89]

FES Gait Combined With Treadmill Training

The combination of FES for gait and treadmill training has received some recent attention in people who have had a stroke or who have incomplete SCI. These studies range from stimulating for dorsiflexion and stepping only[90] or for multiple muscles.[91] A study with incomplete SCI showed that dorsiflexion for walking on the treadmill led to an increase in overground walking speed and in muscle strength.[90] A pilot study for one subject following stroke used FES to the dorsiflexors and plantar flexors while walking on the treadmill with the assistance of a robotic device. Improvements were reported in the Timed Up and Go test, walking speed, and gait.[92] Although these applications on the treadmill

are newer and less common, these combined techniques show promise.

Examination, Evaluation, and Prognosis

Clinically, the main application of FES for ambulation is to assist dorsiflexion. Because this technique is typically applied to those with neurological conditions, the practitioner must know if the targeted muscles are innervated. As with other applications, tests of strength, ROM, sensation, function, and spasticity are important. Walking speed is an additional test that may be helpful in evaluating results of the treatment and describing the gait pattern before treatment. The diagnosis and presence of voluntary movement will help the practitioner to decide if functional benefits are expected with the stimulation turned on or if functional benefits with it off are anticipated due to muscle reeducation.

Intervention

In applying FES for dorsiflexion assist, two electrodes are applied to create balanced dorsiflexion—meaning the foot is balanced between inversion and eversion. A small amount of eversion is acceptable. However, excessive inversion places the patient at risk of an inversion ankle sprain. Electrodes are typically applied to stimulate the anterior tibialis and the peroneal muscles. Some portable stimulators can be equipped with a remote switch that the therapist will control or a foot switch that will react to the patient's movement. A foot switch is placed into the shoe on the patient's affected side. When weight is removed from the switch to initiate swing, stimulation will be triggered. When weight is reapplied at initial contact, stimulation stops. This method is the ideal way to create a dorsiflexion assist in the clinic, as the therapist can focus on the patient's response rather than the timing with the remote switch.

Again the practitioner should be creative in other ideas for enhancing ambulation using FES or using FES as a tool for muscle reeducation (Box 12-8). Table 12-15 identifies typically used stimulation parameters for dorsiflexion assist.

FES for Exercise

FES Cycling

FES has also been applied as a form of exercise, mainly for patients with diagnoses of SCI. One method for this

Table 12•15 Parameters Typically Seen for Dorsiflexion Assist[62,65,67–69,72,73,134,135]

Waveform	Symmetrical or asymmetrical biphasic
Pulse duration	200–350 μsec
Frequency	30–40 pps
Amplitude	To achieve 3+/5 contraction
Ramp-up time	0–1 second
Ramp-down time	0–1 second
Duty cycle	N/A. Stimulation is timed with demand of functional activity.
Treatment time and duration	Determined by muscle fatigue

is FES cycling. A specially designed bicycle that provides cyclical stimulation to the quadriceps, gluteal, and hamstring muscles is used. Treatment, as described in the literature, is typically provided for 30 minutes, three times per week. However, a recent study applied FES cycling five times per week for 60 minutes—a protocol that is being adopted by more people who use the device at home. Studies of FES cycling have reported improvements in muscle volume and fiber size, fat-free tissue, bone density, cardiovascular fitness, and lower extremity circulation.[93] Numerous studies have examined the effects of FES cycling on the cardiovascular system of adults with SCI.[93] Studies involving cycling training 2 to 3 days per week for 12 to 16 weeks have shown increases in peak oxygen uptake,[94,95] cardiac output,[94,96] stroke volume,[96] and pulmonary ventilation.[94] Overall, these results indicate that FES cycling has a positive effect on individuals with SCI. People undergoing this exercise regimen were able to expend additional calories to improve overall fitness and showed a pronounced effect on cardiovascular health.

Another technique for FES cycling is to add volitional arm exercise at the same time. A study by Raymond et al.[97] showed that subjects could obtain higher oxygen uptake and power output, which may lead to better cardiovascular benefits.

Although FES cycling has primarily been used by patients with complete SCI, this technique is now being used for patients following stroke and for those with MS or incomplete SCI. In the past, these populations were typically excluded due to concerns with the inability to tolerate the sensation of FES. However, many patients can tolerate levels that are sufficient for making gains. Studies have shown a reduction in spasticity[98,99] and improved cycling smoothness[99] for people with MS. For patients who had had a stroke, a small RCT[100] with chronic stroke experienced gains in aerobic capacity in a 6-minute walk test and in the Berg Balance Scale after a 6-week program of FES cycling two times per week. However, these gains were not different from the subjects cycling without FES.

FES cycling is usually done on a stationary cycle, either one that the user transfers onto or one that allows the user to stay in his or her wheelchair (Fig. 12-13). However, cycling with FES overground is another

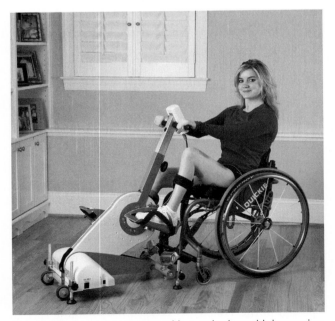

Fig 12•13 A young woman with a spinal cord injury using the RT300 FES cycle. *(Courtesy of Restorative Therapies, Inc., Baltimore, MD.)*

CASE STUDY 12•4 FES TO IMPROVE FOOT DROP

A 16-year-old female with an acute C8 incomplete spinal cord injury is experiencing recovery in both lower extremities and has started gait training with a walker. However, recovery for her left ankle muscles is slower, and she is unable to clear her left foot while walking.

CLINICAL DECISION-MAKING

1. Does the patient have a problem that can be improved with the use of FES?

   Answer: This patient may benefit from FES to achieve dorsiflexion during gait.

2. Is the patient appropriate for application of FES (i.e., do any of the general precautions or contraindications to FES apply, or are there any specific considerations regarding application of FES to this patient)?

   Answer: This patient is appropriate for FES. Since her spinal cord injury was at C8, she should have an upper motor neuron lesion to her dorsiflexors. This can be tested by applying NMES and looking at the response. Other considerations for this patient include possible autonomic dysreflexia, decreased sensation (including proprioception), ROM of her ankle, and plantar flexor spasticity.

3. What are the specific goals to be achieved with the use of FES?

   Answer: The immediate goal is to eliminate the foot drop so that she can obtain sufficient foot clearance during gait.

4. What specific parameters of FES would be appropriate for the patient?

   Answer: There are a couple of options for a stimulator. A portable stimulator with a foot switch can be used. The foot switch is placed in the shoe under the patient's heel. With the switch in place, the FES will be activated when pressure is removed from it during terminal stance/preswing. Another option is to use one of the commercially available devices designed specifically for foot drop (WalkAide or NESS L300).

   Pulse duration: 200–350 μsec
   Frequency: 30–40 pps
   Amplitude: Enough to achieve sufficient dorsiflexion for foot clearance.
   Ramp time: None, since contraction needs to occur quickly.
   Duration: Timed with gait. Monitor patient for fatigue of dorsiflexors.

5. What are the proper (i.e., effective and safe) application procedures for FES related to this case example?

   Answer:

   Electrode application: Two electrodes, one over the anterior tibialis and one over the peroneal nerve (or muscles; Fig. 12-14). The peroneal nerve electrode (for eversion) may be placed proximally near the fibular head or posterior to the lateral malleolus. The goal is to achieve dorsiflexion without inversion. Inversion is never acceptable due to the risk of an inversion sprain.

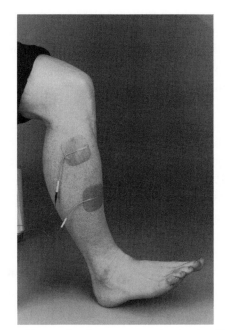

Fig 12•14 Electrode placement to obtain dorsiflexion. Placement will vary between patients, and the clinician may need to try several different placements before obtaining the desired response.

Patient position: If possible, position the knee in a position that mimics terminal stance, since that is when the FES needs to be activated. The orientation of the skin to the peroneal nerve can change with the position of the knee. You may need to readjust the electrode position once the patient is standing.

Treatment monitoring: Monitor response to the treatment by observing her gait.

option and is more widely used in Europe. Due to the power output required to cycle outdoors and muscle fatigue, cycling distance is limited. Nevertheless, one study added a motor to a cycle in order to provide power from the legs through FES and through the motor.[101]

Upper extremity cycling is another technique that has recently been used for people with tetraplegia. Using the RT300 FES Cycle, an arm attachment can be added to provide unilateral FES to up to six muscles around the shoulder, elbow, and wrist, or it can provide bilateral FES to three muscles per upper extremity. There is no research with this specific device; however, one study[102] with a different device reported gains in oxygen uptake and power output for one subject with C6 tetraplegia, and power output only for another subject, also with C6 tetraplegia. In that study, only the bilateral biceps and triceps were stimulated.

When initiating an FES exercise program, there are several decisions to be made in regard to stimulation levels, which muscle to stimulate, and treatment dosage. Typically there is a preset limit on the current level, and the cycle will adjust the amplitude delivered based upon the cadence (speed) that the user is trying to maintain. For example, the patient may have a target cadence of 50 rpm and a maximum amplitude of 140 mA. If the patient can cycle at 50 rpm with only 80 mA, the cycle won't increase the amplitude. However, if the legs start to slow down, the amplitude will increase to keep the legs cycling at 50 rpm (Box 12-9).

FES Rowing

A newer FES exercise technique is FES-assisted rowing for people with SCI. It is currently not available in the United States, but hopefully it will be in the future. This technique starts with a standard rowing ergometer and makes modifications to the seating to accommodate the needs of people with SCI. The user pulls back on the rowing handle and activates a button on the handle to turn on the stimulation to the quadriceps. The amount of pressure through the button determines the amount of stimulation delivered. The user then slowly releases the button to return to the flexed position. One study[103] showed gains in oxygen uptake and distance rowed after a program of FES rowing sessions performed for 30 minutes, three times per week for 12 weeks. The increases were reported to

Box 12•9	**Critical Considerations for Using FES Cycling in the Clinic**

- Set initial stimulation levels lower for patients with remaining sensation.
- Encourage volitional movement if present as long as it doesn't interfere with the cycling motion (i.e., if volitional movement causes significant spasticity during cycling).
- Typical muscles are quadriceps, hamstrings, and gluteal muscles, but others may be possible, depending on patient needs and the cycle being used.
- Cycling for 30 to 60 minutes, three times per week is supported by the literature for patients with SCI. Cycling five times a week is reported but may be overly fatiguing.
- Typical cycling cadence (speed) is 40 to 50 rpm with resistance increasing as the patient is able.
- Read the precautions and contraindications for the FES cycle that is being used.

be comparable to those achieved with combined FES cycling/upper extremity exercise and upper extremity exercise alone.

Biofeedback

Biofeedback (Fig. 12-15) is another option for improving function in patients with neurological conditions, and it can be combined with FES. For this technique,

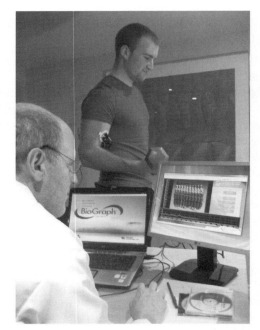

Fig 12•15 This figure displays biofeedback to the biceps and triceps muscles. This technique could be used to teach a patient to contract the biceps while relaxing the triceps. *(Courtesy © 2010 Thought Technology.com.)*

CASE STUDY 12•5 FES FOR EXERCISE

A 45-year-old man with a T8 complete spinal cord injury is concerned about his health and fitness. He has gained 10 pounds in the past year and feels that he has become more sedentary. He also complains about increased fatigue with pushing his wheelchair.

CLINICAL DECISION-MAKING

1. Does the patient have a problem that can be improved with the use of FES?
   Answer: This patient may benefit from FES cycling to improve his fitness level.

2. Is the patient appropriate for application of FES (i.e., do any of the general precautions or contraindications to FES apply, or are there any specific considerations regarding application of FES to this patient)?
   Answer: Considerations for FES cycling include osteoporosis, decreased sensation, spasticity, respiratory status, skin integrity, and any preexisting medical issues.

3. What are the specific goals to be achieved with the use of FES?
   Answer: Improvements in fitness levels (i.e., oxygen uptake, resting heart rate), bone density, and muscle volume. A functional goal could be to improve his endurance for functional tasks (i.e., wheelchair propulsion).

4. What specific parameters of FES would be appropriate for the patient?
   Answer:
   Pulse duration: 150–400 µsec
   Frequency: 30–40 pps
   Amplitude: Enough to achieve the cycling motion. FES cycles usually have a limit that can be set, and the stimulation will adjust to keep the legs cycling at a preset speed (usually 40 to 50 revolutions per minute). A common maximum amplitude is 140 mA for each muscle.
   Ramp time: None, since contraction needs to occur quickly.
   Duration: Goal is to improve endurance to achieve 30 to 60 minutes of cycling, 3 days per week.

5. What are the proper (i.e., effective and safe) application procedures for FES related to this case example?
   Answer:
   Electrode application: Electrodes are placed bilaterally on the quadriceps, hamstrings, and gluteal muscles. Attach the stimulation cables correctly, as the cycle turns the proper muscles off and on through the cable. If connected incorrectly, the wrong pattern will occur.
   Patient position: If the patient is using a cycle without a seat (e.g., RT300), the patient will remain seated in his wheelchair for cycling. It is recommended that his knees have a minimum flexion angle of 30° to 45° while cycling. Place his feet on the pedals and secure them with the straps over the foot and the calf.
   Treatment monitoring: Monitor his response to the treatment by watching blood pressure and heart rate. Suspend treatment if he exceeds safe changes in these responses to the exercise and decrease the stimulation intensity.
   Postinspection: Inspect the skin under the straps and any bony prominence that was in contact with the wheelchair while cycling (i.e., low back, ischial tuberosities). Extra care needs to be taken with his skin due to his lack of sensation.

---

the patient can volitionally activate a muscle by trying to reach a target EMG amplitude. The FES can then complete any remainder of the motion that the patient is unable to finish. This combined technique allows the patient to obtain feedback about the level of volitional activation and do as much as possible, but still have sufficient force generation to perform the functional task.

Biofeedback has been used as a tool to aid recovery following stroke, teach new movement patterns, and decrease bladder dysfunction. Current evidence does not show support for the technique when used in patients who have had a stroke;[104] however, the studies to date are small, not well designed, and report varying outcomes, which makes comparisons difficult. A few studies have reported clinical changes after stroke patients followed a program of EMG biofeedback. One study[105] reported greater improvements in upper extremity ROM and function for subjects at least 6 months after their stroke who had biofeedback added to a 1-year program of occupational therapy (OT) and FES. Subjects receiving only OT and FES also made gains, but not as much as those receiving OT, FES, and biofeedback.

Other studies have examined biofeedback for other populations. In ambulatory subjects with incomplete SCI, biofeedback training for the gluteus medius muscle during gait led to significant reductions in their Trendelenburg gait pattern. The biofeedback device in this study gave the subjects feedback if they were insufficiently activating the gluteus medius muscle while walking.[106] For children with CP, a program of biofeedback to increase activity (excitation) of the anterior tibialis muscles and to decrease the activity (inhibition) of the gastrocnemius muscles was added to a more traditional strengthening and functional program. Children who had the added biofeedback training showed reductions in gastrocnemius spasticity and increases in active ROM at the ankle. Biofeedback combined with traditional training did not provide greater improvements in gait over the traditional program alone.[107] However, biofeedback was not used during gait, suggesting specificity of treatment.

These few studies show that biofeedback may be a useful tool in the clinic with patients with neurological conditions. The same principles for use with any population can be applied, either for trying to facilitate desired motion, to inhibit unwanted motion, or to improve a functional task.

CASE STUDY 12•6   **BIOFEEDBACK TO IMPROVE ACTIVATION AND INHIBITION**

A 35-year-old woman with MS wants to work on walking without her ankle foot orthosis. She can inconsistently activate her dorsiflexors while walking and while seated, but she often coactivates both the dorsiflexors and the plantar flexors when she tries to dorsiflex her ankle. Her goal is to gain enough control of her ankle muscles so that she can walk around her home without her ankle-foot orthosis.

CLINICAL DECISION-MAKING

1. Does the patient have a problem that can be improved with the use of biofeedback?
   Answer: This patient may benefit from biofeedback to increase the activity of her dorsiflexors and decrease the unwanted activation of her plantar flexors.

2. Is the patient appropriate for application of biofeedback (i.e., do any of the general precautions or contraindications to biofeedback apply, or are there any specific considerations regarding application of biofeedback to this patient)?
   Answer: Considerations include the amount of volitional activity that she has in the muscles and her innervation status.

3. What are the specific goals to be achieved with the use of biofeedback?
   Answer: Improved control of her ankle muscles and the ability to walk at home without an ankle-foot orthosis.

4. What specific parameters of biofeedback would be appropriate for the patient?
   Answer: An assessment needs to be done as to her ability to activate the dorsiflexors and to relax the plantar flexors in order to set the targets for the EMG activity level. Since she is weak, sensitivity of the signal from the dorsiflexors should be high to start (low gain) so that you can detect muscular contractions. Sensitivity to the plantar flexors will likely need to be set lower, as this muscle is very active. However, the sensitivity may need to be increased if her attempts to decrease the activity are not being detected. Auditory and visual feedback may both be used. Visual alone may not be sufficient if she has visual disturbances related to MS.

5. What are the proper (i.e., effective and safe) application procedures for biofeedback related to this case example?
   Answer:
   Electrode application: Dorsiflexors: Two electrodes over the muscle belly of the anterior tibialis. The electrodes should be placed far apart, as the muscle is weak and you want to detect electrical activity from a greater volume of the muscle. Plantar flexors: Two electrodes placed closer together over the gastrocnemius muscle. The close placement is needed, as the muscle is likely very active; you want her to focus on a small area of the muscle at a time.
   Patient position: If her proprioception is impaired, she may need to be able to see her ankle, so the sitting position will likely be the best choice to start. Once she gains control, biofeedback can be attempted in standing.
   Treatment monitoring: Monitor her response to the treatment and adjust the sensitivity as needed to obtain the best signal.

Documentation Tips

- Muscles stimulated
- Stimulation settings
- Treatment type (NMES or FES) and purpose (e.g., spasticity reduction)
- Patient position
- Type and duration of activity for FES
- Treatment intensity and duration for NMES
- Response to treatment (e.g., improved gait for FES)
- Any skin irritation post-treatment

REFERENCES

1. Section on clinical electrophysiology. Electrotherapeutic terminology in physical therapy. Alexandria, VA: American Physical Therapy Association; 2001.
2. Glinsky J, Harvey L, Van Es P. Efficacy of electrical stimulation to increase muscle strength in people with neurological conditions: a systematic review. *Physiother Res Int.* 2007;12:175–194.
3. Powell J, Pandyan AD, Granat M, et al. Electrical stimulation of wrist extensors in poststroke hemiplegia. *Stroke.* 1999;30:1384–1389.
4. Kimberley TJ, Lewis SM, Auerbach EJ, et al. Electrical stimulation driving functional improvements and cortical changes in subjects with stroke. *Exp Brain Res.* 2004;154:450–460.
5. Knutson JS, Hisel TZ, Harley MY, Chae J. A novel functional electrical stimulation treatment for recovery of hand function in hemiplegia: 12-week pilot study. *Neurorehabil Neural Repair.* 2009;23:17–25.
6. de Kroon JR, IJzerman MJ. Electrical stimulation of the upper extremity in stroke: cyclic versus EMG-triggered stimulation. *Clin Rehabil.* 2008;22:690–697.
7. Wright PA, Granat MH. Therapeutic effects of functional electrical stimulation of the upper limb of eight children with cerebral palsy. *Dev Med Child Neurol.* 2000;42:724–727.
8. Kamper DG, Yasukawa AM, Barrett KM, Gaebler-Spira DJ. Effects of neuromuscular electrical stimulation treatment of cerebral palsy on potential impairment mechanisms: a pilot study. *Pediatr Phys Ther.* 2006;18:31–38.
9. Vaz DV, Mancini MC, da Fonseca ST, et al. Effects of strength training aided by electrical stimulation on wrist muscle characteristics and hand function of children with hemiplegic cerebral palsy. *Phys Occup Ther Pediatr.* 2008;28:309–325.
10. Ozer K, Chesher SP, Scheker LR. Neuromuscular electrical stimulation and dynamic bracing for the management of upper-extremity spasticity in children with cerebral palsy. *Dev Med Child Neurol.* 2006;48:559–563.
11. Hazlewood ME, Brown JK, Rowe PJ, Salter PM. The use of therapeutic electrical stimulation in the treatment of hemiplegic cerebral palsy. *Dev Med Child Neurol.* 1994;36:661–673.
12. van der Linden ML, Hazlewood ME, Aitchison AM, et al. Electrical stimulation of gluteus maximus in children with cerebral palsy: effects on gait characteristics and muscle strength. *Dev Med Child Neurol.* 2003;45:385–390.
13. Stackhouse SK, Binder-Macleod SA, Stackhouse CA, et al. Neuromuscular electrical stimulation versus volitional isometric strength training in children with spastic diplegic cerebral palsy: a preliminary study. *Neurorehabil Neural Repair.* 2007;21:475–485.
14. Steinbok P, Reiner A, Kestle JR. Therapeutic electrical stimulation following selective posterior rhizotomy in children with spastic diplegic cerebral palsy: a randomized clinical trial. *Dev Med Child Neurol.* 1997;39:515–520.
15. Sommerfelt K, Markestad T, Berg K, Saetesdal I. Therapeutic electrical stimulation in cerebral palsy: a randomized, controlled, crossover trial. *Dev Med Child Neurol.* 2001;43:609–613.
16. Dali C, Hansen FJ, Pedersen SA, et al. Threshold electrical stimulation (TES) in ambulant children with CP: a randomized double-blind placebo-controlled clinical trial. *Dev Med Child Neurol.* 2002;44:364–369.
17. Klose KJ, Schmidt DL, Needham BM, et al. Rehabilitation therapy for patients with long-term spinal cord injuries. *Arch Phys Med Rehabil.* 1990;71:659–662.
18. Bélanger M, Stein RB, Wheeler GD, et al. Electrical stimulation: can it increase muscle strength and reverse osteopenia in spinal cord injured individuals? *Arch Phys Med Rehabil.* 2000;81:1090–1098.
19. van Londen A, Herwegh M, van der Zee CH, et al. The effect of surface electric stimulation of the gluteal muscles on the interface pressure in seated people with spinal cord injury. *Arch Phys Med Rehabil.* 2008;89:1724–1732.
20. Liu LQ, Nicholson GP, Knight SL, et al. Pressure changes under the ischial tuberosities of seated individuals during sacral nerve root stimulation. *J Rehabil Res Dev.* 2006;43:209–218.
21. Rischbieth H, Jelbart M, Marshall R. Neuromuscular electrical stimulation keeps a tetraplegic subject in his chair: a case study. *Spinal Cord.* 1998;36:443–445.
22. Livesley E. Electrical neuromuscular stimulation on functional performance in patients with multiple sclerosis. *Physiotherapy.* 1992;78:914–917.
23. Binder-Macleod SA, Snyder-Mackler L. Muscle fatigue: clinical implications for fatigue assessment and neuromuscular electrical stimulation. *Phys Ther.* 1993;73:902–910.
24. Baker LL, Yeh C, Wilson D, Waters RL. Electrical stimulation of wrist and fingers for hemiplegic patients. *Phys Ther.* 1979;59:1495–1499.
25. Pandyan AD, Granat MH, Stott DJ. Effects of electrical stimulation on flexion contractures in the hemiplegic wrist. *Clin Rehabil.* 1997;11:123–130.
26. Maenpaa H, Jaakkola R, Sandstrom M, von Wendt L. Does microcurrent stimulation increase the range of movement of ankle dorsiflexion in children with cerebral palsy? *Disabil Rehabil.* 2004;26:669–677.
27. Bertoti BD, Stanger M, Betz RR. Percutaneous intramuscular functional electrical stimulation as an intervention choice for children with cerebral palsy. *Pediatr Phys Ther.* 1997;9:123–127.
28. Weingarden HP, Zeilig G, Heruti R, et al. Hybrid functional electrical stimulation orthosis system for the upper limb: effects on spasticity in chronic stable hemiplegia. *Am J Phys Med Rehabil.* 1998;77:276–281.
29. Chae J, Yu D, Walker M. Percutaneous, intramuscular neuromuscular electrical stimulation for the treatment of shoulder subluxation and pain in chronic hemiplegia: a case report. *Am J Phys Med Rehabil.* 2001;80:296–301.
30. Ghez C. Posture. In: Kandel ER, Schwartz JH, Jessell TM, eds. *Principles of Neural Science.* Norwalk, CT: Appleton and Lange; 1991:596–608.

31. Wang RY, Tsai MW, Chan RC. Effects of surface spinal cord stimulation on spasticity and quantitative assessment of muscle tone in hemiplegic patients. *Am J Phys Med Rehabil.* 1998;77:282–287.

32. Gordon J. Spinal mechanisms of motor coordination. In: Kandel ER, Schwartz JH, Jessell TM, eds. *Principles of Neural Science.* Norwalk, CT: Appleton and Lange; 1991:581–595.

33. McClurg D, Ashe RG, Lowe-Strong AS. Neuromuscular electrical stimulation and the treatment of lower urinary tract dysfunction in multiple sclerosis—a double blind, placebo controlled, randomised clinical trial. *Neurourol Urodyn.* 2008;27:231–237.

34. Brubaker L, Benson JT, Bent A, et al. Transvaginal electrical stimulation for female urinary incontinence. *Am J Obstet Gynecol.* 1997;177:536–540.

35. Dumoulin C, Seaborne DE, Quirion-DeGirardi C, Sullivan SJ. Pelvic-floor rehabilitation, part 1: Comparison of two surface electrode placements during stimulation of the pelvic-floor musculature in women who are continent using bipolar interferential currents. *Phys Ther.* 1995;75:1067–1074.

36. Centers for Medicare and Medicaid Services. Sacral nerve stimulation for urge urinary incontinence: decision memorandum. Available at http://www.cms.hhs.gov/coverage/8b3-v3.asp. Accessed June 29, 2001.

37. Dumoulin C, Seaborne DE, Quirion-DeGirardi C, Sullivan SJ. Pelvic-floor rehabilitation, part 2: Pelvic-floor reeducation with interferential currents and exercise in the treatment of genuine stress incontinence in postpartum women—a cohort study. *Phys Ther.* 1995;75:1075–1081.

38. Sand PK, Richardson DA, Staskin DR, et al. Pelvic floor electrical stimulation in the treatment of genuine stress incontinence: a multicenter, placebo-controlled trial. *Am J Obstet Gynecol.* 1995;173:72–79.

39. Das AK, White MD, Longhurst PA. Sacral nerve stimulation for the management of voiding dysfunction. *Rev Urol.* 2000;2:43–60.

40. Fall M, Lindstrom S. Electrical stimulation. A physiologic approach to the treatment of urinary incontinence. *Urol Clin North Am.* 1991;18:393–407.

41. Kabay SC, Yucel M, Kabay S. Acute effect of posterior tibial nerve stimulation on neurogenic detrusor overactivity in patients with multiple sclerosis: urodynamic study. *Urology.* 2008;71:641–645.

42. Faghri PD, Rodgers MM, Glaser RM, et al. The effects of functional electrical stimulation on shoulder subluxation, arm function recovery, and shoulder pain in hemiplegic stroke patients. *Arch Phys Med Rehabil.* 1994;75:73–79.

43. Binder-Macleod SA, Lee SCK. Assessment of the efficacy of functional electrical stimulation in patients with hemiplegia. *Top Stroke Rehabil.* 1997;3:88–98.

44. Ada L, Foongchomcheay A. Efficacy of electrical stimulation in preventing or reducing subluxation of the shoulder after stroke: a meta-analysis. *Aust J Physiother.* 2002;48:257–267.

45. Chae J, Hart R. Comparison of discomfort associated with surface and percutaneous intramuscular electrical stimulation for persons with chronic hemiplegia. *Am J Phys Med Rehabil.* 1998;77:516–522.

46. Yu DT, Chae J, Walker ME, et al. Comparing stimulation-induced pain during percutaneous (intramuscular) and transcutaneous neuromuscular electric stimulation for treating shoulder subluxation in hemiplegia. *Arch Phys Med Rehabil.* 2001;82:756–760.

47. Hendricks HT, IJzerman MJ, de Kroon JR, et al. Functional electrical stimulation by means of the Ness Handmaster Orthosis in chronic stroke patients: an exploratory study. *Clin Rehabil.* 2001;15:217–220.

48. Thrasher TA, Zivanovic V, McIlroy W, Popovic MR. Rehabilitation of reaching and grasping function in severe hemiplegic patients using functional electrical stimulation therapy. *Neurorehabil Neural Repair.* 2008;22:706–714.

49. Alon G, Ring H. Gait and hand function enhancement following training with a multi-segment hybrid-orthosis stimulation system in stroke patients. *J Stroke Cerebrovasc Dis.* 2003;12:209–216.

50. Alon G, Levitt AF, McCarthy PA. Functional electrical stimulation enhancement of upper extremity functional recovery during stroke rehabilitation: a pilot study. *Neurorehabil Neural Repair.* 2007;21:207–215.

51. Chae J, Harley MY, Hisel TZ, et al. Intramuscular electrical stimulation for upper limb recovery in chronic hemiparesis: an exploratory randomized clinical trial. *Neurorehabil Neural Repair.* 2009;23:569–578.

52. Chan MK, Tong RK, Chung KY. Bilateral upper limb training with functional electric stimulation in patients with chronic stroke. *Neurorehabil Neural Repair.* 2009;23:357–365.

53. Mangold S, Schuster C, Keller T, et al. Motor training of upper extremity with functional electrical stimulation in early stroke rehabilitation. *Neurorehabil Neural Repair.* 2009;23:184–190.

54. Carmick J. Use of neuromuscular electrical stimulation and [corrected] dorsal wrist splint to improve the hand function of a child with spastic hemiparesis. *Phys Ther.* 1997;77:661–671.

55. Carmick J. Clinical use of neuromuscular electrical stimulation for children with cerebral palsy, part 2: upper extremity. *Phys Ther.* 1993;73:514–522.

56. Peckham PH, Keith MW, Kilgore KL, et al. Efficacy of an implanted neuroprosthesis for restoring hand grasp in tetraplegia: a multicenter study. *Arch Phys Med Rehabil.* 2001;82:1380–1388.

57. Mulcahey MJ, Betz RR, Smith BT, et al. Implanted functional electrical stimulation hand system in adolescents with spinal injuries: an evaluation. *Arch Phys Med Rehabil.* 1997;78:597–607.

58. Sheffler LR, Hennessey MT, Naples GG, Chae J. Peroneal nerve stimulation versus an ankle foot orthosis for correction of footdrop in stroke: impact on functional ambulation. *Neurorehabil Neural Repair.* 2006;20:355–360.

59. Liberson WT, Holmquest HJ, Scot D, Dow M. Functional electrotherapy: stimulation of the peroneal nerve synchronized with the swing phase of the gait of hemiplegic patients. *Arch Phys Med Rehabil.* 1961;42:101–105.

60. Merletti R, Zelaschi F, Latella D, et al. A control study of muscle force recovery in hemiparetic patients during treatment with functional electrical stimulation. *Scand J Rehabil Med.* 1978;10:147–154.

61. Burridge JH, Taylor PN, Hagan SA, et al. The effects of common peroneal stimulation on the effort and speed of walking: a randomized controlled trial with chronic hemiplegic patients. *Clin Rehabil.* 1997;11:201–210.

62. Laufer Y, Hausdorff JM, Ring H. Effects of a foot drop neuroprosthesis on functional abilities, social participation, and gait velocity. *Am J Phys Med Rehabil.* 2009;88:14–20.

63. Kottink AI, Hermens HJ, Nene AV, et al. A randomized controlled trial of an implantable 2-channel peroneal nerve stimulator on walking speed and activity in poststroke hemiplegia. *Arch Phys Med Rehabil.* 2007;88:971–978.

64. Weber DJ, Stein RB, Chan KM, et al. Functional electrical stimulation using microstimulators to correct foot drop: a case study. *Can J Physiol Pharmacol.* 2004;82:784–792.

65. Taylor PN, Burridge JH, Dunkerley AL, et al. Clinical use of the Odstock dropped foot stimulator: its effect on the speed and effort of walking. *Arch Phys Med Rehabil.* 1999;80: 1577–1583.

66. Paul L, Rafferty D, Young S, et al. The effect of functional electrical stimulation on the physiological cost of gait in people with multiple sclerosis. *Mult Scler.* 2008;14:954–961.

67. Comeaux P, Patterson N, Rubin M, Meiner R. Effect of neuromuscular electrical stimulation during gait in children with cerebral palsy. *Pediatr Phys Ther.* 1997;9:10–19.

68. Carmick J. Clinical use of neuromuscular electrical stimulation for children with cerebral palsy, part 1: lower extremity. *Phys Ther.* 1993;73:505–513.

69. Carmick J. Managing equinus in a child with cerebral palsy: merits of hinged ankle-foot orthoses. *Dev Med Child Neurol.* 1995;37:1006–1010.

70. Orlin MN, Pierce SR, Stackhouse CL, et al. Immediate effect of percutaneous intramuscular stimulation during gait in children with cerebral palsy: a feasibility study. *Dev Med Child Neurol.* 2005;47:684–690.

71. Ho CL, Holt KG, Saltzman E, Wagenaar RC. Functional electrical stimulation changes dynamic resources in children with spastic cerebral palsy. *Phys Ther.* 2006;86:987–1000.

72. Bajd T, Kralj A, Stefancic M, Lavrac N. Use of functional electrical stimulation in the lower extremities of incomplete spinal cord injured patients. *Artif Organs.* 1999;23: 403–409.

73. Granat MH, Ferguson AC, Andrews BJ, Delargy M. The role of functional electrical stimulation in the rehabilitation of patients with incomplete spinal cord injury—observed benefits during gait studies. *Paraplegia.* 1993;31:207–215.

74. Johnston TE, Finson RL, Smith BT, et al. Functional electrical stimulation for augmented walking in adolescents with incomplete spinal cord injury. *J Spinal Cord Med.* 2003;26: 390–400.

75. Brissot R, Gallien P, Le Bot MP, et al. Clinical experience with functional electrical stimulation-assisted gait with Parastep in spinal cord-injured patients. *Spine.* 2000;25:501–508.

76. Davis R, Houdayer T, Andrews B, Barriskill A. Paraplegia: prolonged standing using closed-loop functional electrical stimulation and Andrews ankle-foot orthosis. *Artif Organs.* 1999;23: 418–420.

77. Johnston TE, Betz RR, Smith BT, Mulcahey MJ. Implanted functional electrical stimulation: an alternative for standing and walking in pediatric spinal cord injury. *Spinal Cord.* 2003; 41:144–152.

78. Kobetic R, Triolo RJ, Uhlir JP, et al. Implanted functional electrical stimulation system for mobility in paraplegia: a follow-up case report. *IEEE Trans Rehabil Eng.* 1999;7:390–398.

79. Shimada Y, Sato K, Kagaya H, et al. Clinical use of percutaneous intramuscular electrodes for functional electrical stimulation. *Arch Phys Med Rehabil.* 1996;77:1014–1018.

80. Nash MS, Jacobs PL, Montalvo BM, et al. Evaluation of a training program for persons with SCI paraplegia using the Parastep 1 ambulation system: part 5. Lower extremity blood flow and hyperemic responses to occlusion are augmented by ambulation training. *Arch Phys Med Rehabil.* 1997;78: 808–814.

81. Jacobs PL, Nash MS, Klose KJ, et al. Evaluation of a training program for persons with SCI paraplegia using the Parastep 1 ambulation system: part 2. Effects on physiological responses to peak arm ergometry. *Arch Phys Med Rehabil.* 1997;78: 794–798.

82. Klose KJ, Jacobs PL, Broton JG, et al. Evaluation of a training program for persons with SCI paraplegia using the Parastep 1 ambulation system: part 1. Ambulation performance and anthropometric measures. *Arch Phys Med Rehabil.* 1997;78: 789–793.

83. Needham-Shropshire BM, Broton JG, Klose KJ, et al. Evaluation of a training program for persons with SCI paraplegia using the Parastep 1 ambulation system: part 3. Lack of effect on bone mineral density. *Arch Phys Med Rehabil.* 1997;78:799–803.

84. Centers for Medicare and Medicaid Services. Neuromuscular electrical stimulation (NMES) for spinal cord injury: decision memorandum. Available at: http://www.cms.hhs.gov/ coverage/8b3-aaa2.asp. Accessed July 22, 2009.

85. Shimada Y, Sato K, Abe E, et al. Clinical experience of functional electrical stimulation in complete paraplegia. *Spinal Cord.* 1996;34:615–619.

86. Agarwal S, Triolo RJ, Kobetic R, et al. Long-term user perceptions of an implanted neuroprosthesis for exercise, standing, and transfers after spinal cord injury. *J Rehabil Res Dev.* 2003;40:241–252.

87. Mushahwar VK, Jacobs PL, Normann RA, et al. New functional electrical stimulation approaches to standing and walking. *J Neural Eng.* 2007;4:S181–S197.

88. Johnston TE, Betz RR, Smith BT, et al. Implantable FES system for upright mobility and bladder and bowel function for individuals with spinal cord injury. *Spinal Cord.* 2005;43: 713–723.

89. Kobetic R, Marsolais EB, Triolo RJ, et al. Development of a hybrid gait orthosis: a case report. *J Spinal Cord Med.* 2003; 26:254–258.

90. Field-Fote EC. Combined use of body weight support, functional electric stimulation, and treadmill training to improve walking ability in individuals with chronic incomplete spinal cord injury. *Arch Phys Med Rehabil.* 2001;82:818–824.

91. Postans NJ, Hasler JP, Granat MH, Maxwell DJ. Functional electric stimulation to augment partial weight-bearing supported treadmill training for patients with acute incomplete spinal cord injury: A pilot study. *Arch Phys Med Rehabil.* 2004;85:604–610.

92. Krishnamoorthy V, Hsu WL, Kesar TM, et al. Gait training after stroke: a pilot study combining a gravity-balanced orthosis, functional electrical stimulation, and visual feedback. *J Neurol Phys Ther.* 2008;32:192–202.

93. Davis GM, Hamzaid NA, Fornusek C. Cardiorespiratory, metabolic, and biomechanical responses during functional electrical stimulation leg exercise: health and fitness benefits. *Artif Organs.* 2008;32:625–629.

94. Hooker SP, Figoni SF, Rodgers MM, et al. Physiologic effects of electrical stimulation leg cycle exercise training in spinal cord injured persons. *Arch Phys Med Rehabil.* 1992;73: 470–476.

95. Ragnarsson KT. Physiologic effects of functional electrical stimulation-induced exercises in spinal cord-injured individuals. *Clin Orthop Relat Res.* 1988;53–63.

96. Faghri PD, Glaser RM, Figoni SF. Functional electrical stimulation leg cycle ergometer exercise: training effects on cardiorespiratory responses of spinal cord injured subjects at rest and during submaximal exercise. *Arch Phys Med Rehabil.* 1992;73:1085–1093.

97. Raymond J, Davis GM, Climstein M, Sutton JR. Cardiorespiratory responses to arm cranking and electrical

stimulation leg cycling in people with paraplegia. *Med Sci Sports Exerc.* 1999;31:822–828.

98. Krause P, Szecsi J, Straube A. FES cycling reduces spastic muscle tone in a patient with multiple sclerosis. *NeuroRehabilitation.* 2007;22:335–337.

99. Szecsi J, Schlick C, Schiller M, et al. Functional electrical stimulation-assisted cycling of patients with multiple sclerosis: biomechanical and functional outcome—a pilot study. *J Rehabil Med.* 2009;41:674–680.

100. Janssen TW, Beltman JM, Elich P, et al. Effects of electric stimulation-assisted cycling training in people with chronic stroke. *Arch Phys Med Rehabil.* 2008;89:463–469.

101. Hunt KJ, Stone B, Negard NO, et al. Control strategies for integration of electric motor assist and functional electrical stimulation in paraplegic cycling: utility for exercise testing and mobile cycling. *IEEE Trans Neural Syst Rehabil Eng.* 2004;12:89–101.

102. Coupaud S, Gollee H, Hunt KJ, et al. Arm-cranking exercise assisted by functional electrical stimulation in C6 tetraplegia: a pilot study. *Technol Health Care.* 2008;16:415–427.

103. Wheeler GD, Andrews B, Lederer R, et al. Functional electric stimulation-assisted rowing: increasing cardiovascular fitness through functional electric stimulation rowing training in persons with spinal cord injury. *Arch Phys Med Rehabil.* 2002;83:1093–1099.

104. Woodford H, Price C. EMG biofeedback for the recovery of motor function after stroke. *Cochrane Database Syst Rev.* 2007;CD004585.

105. Lourencao MI, Battistella LR, de Brito CM, et al. Effect of biofeedback accompanying occupational therapy and functional electrical stimulation in hemiplegic patients. *Int J Rehabil Res.* 2008;31:33–41.

106. Petrofsky JS. The use of electromyogram biofeedback to reduce Trendelenburg gait. *Eur J Appl Physiol.* 2001;85:491–495.

107. Dursun E, Dursun N, Alican D. Effects of biofeedback treatment on gait in children with cerebral palsy. *Disabil Rehabil.* 2004;26:116–120.

108. Centers for Medicare and Medicaid Services. Pelvic floor electrical stimulation for urinary incontinence: decision memorandum. Available at: http://www.cms.hhs.gov/coverage/8b3-w4.asp. Accessed October 5, 2000.

109. McIntosh LJ, Frahm JD, Mallett VT, Richardson DA. Pelvic floor rehabilitation in the treatment of incontinence. *J Reprod Med.* 1993;38:662–666.

110. Dougherty MC. Current status of research on pelvic muscle strengthening techniques. *J Wound Ostomy Continence Nurs.* 1998;25:75–83.

111. Yamanishi T, Kamai T, Yoshida K. Neuromodulation for the treatment of urinary incontinence. *Int J Urol.* 2008;15:665–672.

112. Yamanishi T, Yasuda K, Sakakibara R, et al. Pelvic floor electrical stimulation in the treatment of stress incontinence: an investigational study and a placebo controlled double-blind trial. *J Urol.* 1997;158:2127–2131.

113. Lewek M, Stevens J, Snyder-Mackler L. The use of electrical stimulation to increase quadriceps femoris muscle force in an elderly patient following a total knee arthroplasty. *Phys Ther.* 2001;81:1565–1571.

114. Luber KM, Wolde-Tsadik G. Efficacy of functional electrical stimulation in treating genuine stress incontinence: a randomized clinical trial. *Neurourol Urodyn.* 1997;16:543–551.

115. Laycock J, Jerwood D. Does pre-modulated interferential therapy curb genuine stress incontinence? *Physiotherapy.* 1993;79:553–560.

116. Delitto A, Rose SJ, McKowen JM, et al. Electrical stimulation versus voluntary exercise in strengthening thigh musculature after anterior cruciate ligament surgery. *Phys Ther.* 1988;68:660–663.

117. Paternostro-Sluga T, Fialka C, Alacamlioglu Y, et al. Neuromuscular electrical stimulation after anterior cruciate ligament surgery. *Clin Orthop Relat Res.* 1999;166–175.

118. Snyder-Mackler L, Delitto A, Bailey SL, Stralka SW. Strength of the quadriceps femoris muscle and functional recovery after reconstruction of the anterior cruciate ligament. A prospective, randomized clinical trial of electrical stimulation. *J Bone Joint Surg Am.* 1995;77:1166–1173.

119. Snyder-Mackler L, Ladin Z, Schepsis AA, Young JC. Electrical stimulation of the thigh muscles after reconstruction of the anterior cruciate ligament. Effects of electrically elicited contraction of the quadriceps femoris and hamstring muscles on gait and on strength of the thigh muscles. *J Bone Joint Surg Am.* 1991;73:1025–1036.

120. Laughman RK, Youdas JW, Garrett TR, Chao EY. Strength changes in the normal quadriceps femoris muscle as a result of electrical stimulation. *Phys Ther.* 1983;63:494–499.

121. Caggiano E, Emrey T, Shirley S, Craik RL. Effects of electrical stimulation or voluntary contraction for strengthening the quadriceps femoris muscles in an aged male population. *J Orthop Sports Phys Ther.* 1994;20:22–28.

122. Laufer Y, Ries JD, Leininger PM, Alon G. Quadriceps femoris muscle torques and fatigue generated by neuromuscular electrical stimulation with three different waveforms. *Phys Ther.* 2001;81:1307–1316.

123. King TI, II. The effect of neuromuscular electrical stimulation in reducing tone. *Am J Occup Ther.* 1996;50:62–64.

124. Miller L, Mattison P, Paul L, Wood L. The effects of transcutaneous electrical nerve stimulation (TENS) on spasticity in multiple sclerosis. *Mult Scler.* 2007;13:527–533.

125. Potisk KP, Gregoric M, Vodovnik L. Effects of transcutaneous electrical nerve stimulation (TENS) on spasticity in patients with hemiplegia. *Scand J Rehabil Med.* 1995;27:169–174.

126. Robinson CJ, Kett NA, Bolam JM. Spasticity in spinal cord injured patients: 1. short-term effects of surface electrical stimulation. *Arch Phys Med Rehabil.* 1988;69:598–604.

127. Scheker LR, Chesher SP, Ramirez S. Neuromuscular electrical stimulation and dynamic bracing as a treatment for upper-extremity spasticity in children with cerebral palsy. *J Hand Surg Br.* 1999;24:226–232.

128. Seib TP, Price R, Reyes MR, Lehmann JF. The quantitative measurement of spasticity: effect of cutaneous electrical stimulation. *Arch Phys Med Rehabil.* 1994;75:746–750.

129. Linn SL, Granat MH, Lees KR. Prevention of shoulder subluxation after stroke with electrical stimulation. *Stroke.* 1999;30:963–968.

130. Chantraine A, Baribeault A, Uebelhart D, Gremion G. Shoulder pain and dysfunction in hemiplegia: effects of functional electrical stimulation. *Arch Phys Med Rehabil.* 1999;80:328–331.

131. Chae J, Yu DT, Walker ME, et al. Intramuscular electrical stimulation for hemiplegic shoulder pain: a 12-month follow-up of a multiple-center, randomized clinical trial. *Am J Phys Med Rehabil.* 2005;84:832–842.

132. Wang RY, Chan RC, Tsai MW. Functional electrical stimulation on chronic and acute hemiplegic shoulder subluxation. *Am J Phys Med Rehabil.* 2000;79:385–390.

133. Snoek GJ, IJzerman MJ, in 't Groen FA, Stoffers TS, Zilvold G. Use of the NESS Handmaster to restore hand function in tetraplegia: clinical experiences in ten patients. *Spinal Cord.* 2000;38:244–249.

134. Stein RB, Chong S, Everaert DG, et al. A multicenter trial of a footdrop stimulator controlled by a tilt sensor. *Neurorehabil Neural Repair.* 2006;20:371–379.

135. Malezic M, Hesse S, Schewe H, Mauritz KH. Restoration of standing, weight-shift and gait by multichannel electrical stimulation in hemiparetic patients. *Int J Rehabil Res.* 1994; 17:169–179.

chapter 13

Pain and Limited Motion

Stephanie C. Petterson, PT, MPT, PhD |
Susan L. Michlovitz, PT, PhD, CHT

Pain and loss of motion, whether from disease or injury, are two of the most common impairments treated by rehabilitation practitioners. The causes of pain and loss of motion are multifaceted and need to be considered in selecting modalities to address these impairments. This chapter will discuss the use of modalities in intervention plans that are designed for pain control and for increasing motion due to reduced joint mobility and range of motion (ROM).

Clinical Reasoning

Pain is considered one of the most challenging impairments to remediate because of the complex physiological mechanisms involved in the normal response to pain as well as maladaptive pain states that frequently occur in persistent or chronic pain conditions. The variable nature of the pain associated with musculoskeletal injuries, disease processes, and medical conditions of other body systems contributes to the challenge of measuring and evaluating pain. A comprehensive assessment of pain and motion will enhance the development of an appropriate plan of care, including the judicious use of modalities. Consequences of injury, immobilization, and arthritis include loss of joint mobility and range of motion. Intervention strategies are based upon examination findings and knowledge of the course of recovery from injury.

Sources of Pain Mediation

During the examination, the practitioner will develop a hypothesis about the primary source and nature of the patient's pain impairment. Frequently this is easily determined by the referral diagnosis or history of present illness. It may be more difficult to determine the primary source of pain mediation in patients with long-standing pain complaints. The International Association for the Study of Pain (IASP) has developed a classification system for pain that includes definitions for pain terms and descriptions of pain syndromes.[1] This established taxonomy enhances communication in the scientific literature and clinical practice. Gifford and Butler[2] have used the components of the IASP classification system to promote clinical reasoning among practitioners about the primary source of pain mediation in patients whose chief complaint is pain. This is presented as one way to organize thoughts about examination and intervention strategies for pain management. Determining the source of the pain mediation allows practitioners to develop an effective plan of care to manage pain symptoms. Table 13-1 outlines these concepts.

Peripheral Nociceptive

This source of pain lies with injured musculoskeletal tissues.[1,2] Nociceptors located in the injured tissue are stimulated by noxious chemical, mechanical, or thermal stimuli associated with inflammation and tissue healing. Peripheral nociceptive fibers (A delta and C fibers) transmit this noxious stimulation to the dorsal horn, and these impulses are cortically interpreted as pain. This type of pain mediation is sharp and well localized to the area of tissue damage. Because this

source of pain mediation is most commonly associated with acute inflammation and tissue damage, pain is expected to subside as healing occurs. Failure to heal may lead to the development of chronic or persistent pain. Pain following surgery is a specific type of nociceptive pain. Common therapy interventions used to modulate pain, such as rest, modalities, and therapeutic exercise, are usually effective in reducing pain.

KEY POINT! Nociceptive pain is regarded as acute somatic pain that serves as a warning signal of tissue injury.

Peripheral Neurogenic

This source of pain is an injury or dysfunction in the peripheral nervous system.[1,2] Lesions or areas of dysfunction are referred to as *abnormal impulse generator sites* (AIGS). Pain is mediated by mechanical or chemical stimulation of injured neural tissue. Examples of this source of pain mediation are radicular pain associated with spinal dysfunction and pain associated with peripheral nerve entrapment, such as with carpal tunnel syndrome. The nature of the pain is localized to the nerve root or peripheral nerve sensory distribution and is usually accompanied by other sensory abnormalities such as paresthesia. The quality of the pain is often described as "sharp" and "shooting." Common therapy interventions used to modulate pain, such as rest, modalities, and therapeutic exercise, should be effective

Table 13•1 Sources of Pain Mediation and Suggested Interventions

Primary Pain Source	Location(s) of Lesion(s)	Nature of Pain	Suggested Intervention
Peripheral nociceptive	• Injury to musculoskeletal or skin/subcutaneous tissue • Acute inflammation due to tissue damage • Postoperative pain	• Sharp, well localized • Subsides as healing occurs	• Rest • Modalities • Therapeutic exercise
Peripheral neurogenic	• Radicular pain from spinal dysfunction • Entrapment neuropathy, such as carpal tunnel syndrome	• Paresthesia and pain • Localized to sensory distribution • Sharp, shooting	• Rest • Modalities • Therapeutic exercise
Central pain	• Central nervous system lesion	• Inconsistent • Often little correlation between stimulus and response	• Pharmacological agents • Behavior modification • Modalities not likely helpful
Pain related to sympathetic nervous system	• Sympathetic nervous system	• Intense burning • Out of proportion to expectations following injury • Vasomotor instability	• Modalities • Pharmacological agents • Therapeutic exercise • Functional activities
Affective pain	• Limbic system	• Pain behaviors linked to pain tolerance	• Patient education • Modalities not likely helpful

if the pain is treated early after onset. Long-standing nerve injury may require surgical decompression or may result in a chronic pain condition.

Central Pain

This pain is mediated by a lesion or dysfunction within the central nervous system (CNS).[1,2] It is theorized that there is an abnormal sensitivity or discharge of CNS neurons or synapses.[3] The nature of these pain symptoms is inconsistent; pain differs in characteristics from the peripheral sources of pain. There is usually little or no correlation between stimulus and response. Sudden incidences of unprovoked pain may occur due to abnormal CNS nociceptor activity. Abnormal pain states, such as allodynia and hyperalgesia, are centrally mediated.[1,3] Common therapy interventions, such as modalities, are usually ineffective. Medical management, such as pharmacological agents and behavior modification, are key components of a structured and monitored plan of care that includes therapeutic intervention.

KEY POINT! *Allodynia* refers to pain provoked by a mechanical or static stimulus that does not typically cause pain. Pain may occur at a site away from the stimulated area. *Hyperalgesia* refers to a heightened response to a painful stimulus.

Pain Related to Sympathetic Nervous System

The primary source of this type of pain is thought to be a function of the sympathetic nervous system. Both types of complex regional pain syndrome (CRPS) are linked to this source of pain mediation (Box 13-1):[1,2]

- CRPS type I (reflex sympathetic dystrophy, or RSD)
- CRPS type II (causalgia)

Affective Pain

This source of pain is within the CNS and is primarily related to neurons or pathways concerned with affect or emotion.[1] The limbic system is likely to be involved in this source of pain mediation. Other sources of pain mediation can be influenced by changes in the patient's emotional state or cognition. The pain behaviors displayed are related to the concept of pain tolerance. *Tolerance* implies a question about how much pain an

| Box 13•1 | **Complex Regional Pain Syndrome** |

Complex regional pain syndrome (CRPS) is a chronic pain condition that most commonly affects upper or lower extremities. It is characterized by severe pain, changes in skin, and sweating. There is no obvious nerve damage in type I CRPS or RSD, whereas nerve damage is present in type II CRPS or causalgia.

The primary symptom of CRPS is intense burning pain associated with vasomotor instability.[1] Causalgia is identified when this type of pain occurs with a known peripheral nerve injury. The pain is usually localized to the sensory distribution of the peripheral nerve. The diagnosis of RSD is given when it is unknown if there is any peripheral nerve involvement. Although this type of pain mediation may be seen in any body region, it is more common in the distal extremities. Complex regional pain syndromes identified early respond best to medical and therapeutic management. Pain is primarily modulated by pharmaceuticals, and modalities may be used as an adjuvant intervention to facilitate patient participation in therapeutic exercise and functional activity. Additional information on therapeutic intervention of CRPS is available.[4,5]

individual can take. Variables that affect pain tolerance include fatigue, lack of control, stress, and anxiety.[6] Practitioners should determine if any of the factors that modulate pain tolerance are present during the examination. Therapy interventions, such as patient education about the rehabilitation process and positioning during hours of sleep, may be extremely helpful in reducing some of the variables associated with pain tolerance and affective pain. Modalities are not likely to be as effective in pain modulation as addressing the factors that influence pain tolerance.

Sources of Loss of Mobility and Range of Motion

Patients referred for therapy with musculoskeletal and neuromuscular problems often have a loss of active or passive ROM. Chapter 1 provided an overview of the principles of injury and tissue repair; this should serve as a foundation for understanding tissue changes that can lead to limited ROM. This section of the chapter discusses the sources of loss of motion; later sections discuss the assessment of loss of motion and intervention strategies.

Edema and Pain Following Injury

Swelling and pain following injury indicate an inflammatory process. Both can limit motion. Edema fluid within the interstitium of an arm or a leg can increase the volume of an extremity enough to mechanically limit motion. In addition, prolonged fluid can lead to fibrosis of tissue, which in turn leads to motion losses.

Joint Stiffness Associated With Arthritis

Arthritis causes degenerative changes to joints and contracture of the periarticular joint structures.[7] Osteoarthritis, the "wear and tear" kind of arthritis, is the most common and is often associated with aging. Traumatic arthritis can occur as a result of prolonged impact to joints (e.g., as a result of prolonged heavy labor jobs) or as a long-term consequence to joint

trauma. In both of these forms of arthritis, osteophytes (e.g., bony outgrowths) and loss of joint space will also impinge on motion. Severe joint degeneration can lead to joint instability. Rheumatoid arthritis is a systemic disorder associated with changes in the joint capsule's synovial lining and the lining of tendon sheaths. Other systemic changes can occur. Table 13-2 outlines characteristics of osteoarthritis and rheumatoid arthritis. Modalities may be used to increase ROM if joint space is not reduced, if osteophytes are not impinging on motion, and if there is no subluxation and instability (as in the case of rheumatoid arthritis). Intervention goals for patients with arthritis are outlined in Box 13-2.

Table 13·2 **Features of Rheumatoid Arthritis and Osteoarthritis**

Findings	Osteoarthritis	Rheumatoid Arthritis
Joints Commonly Involved		

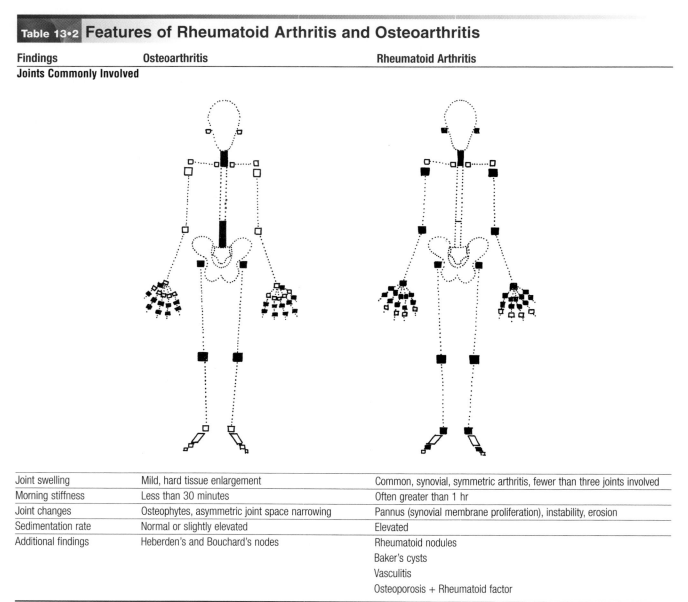

Findings	Osteoarthritis	Rheumatoid Arthritis
Joint swelling	Mild, hard tissue enlargement	Common, synovial, symmetric arthritis, fewer than three joints involved
Morning stiffness	Less than 30 minutes	Often greater than 1 hr
Joint changes	Osteophytes, asymmetric joint space narrowing	Pannus (synovial membrane proliferation), instability, erosion
Sedimentation rate	Normal or slightly elevated	Elevated
Additional findings	Heberden's and Bouchard's nodes	Rheumatoid nodules
		Baker's cysts
		Vasculitis
		Osteoporosis + Rheumatoid factor

Source: Adapted from Fields et al.[6]

Box 13•2	Potential Intervention Goals for Patient With Arthritis

- Decrease joint swelling*
- Decrease pain*
- Decrease stiffness*
- Increase cardiovascular endurance
- Increase functional mobility
- Increase muscle strength*
- Increase ROM*
- Promote weight loss

*Indicates goal where modality intervention may be appropriate.

Joint Contracture Following Injury and Immobilization

A variety of injuries and conditions can lead to joint contracture and soft tissue adhesions (Box 13-3). Following joint surgery for reconstructing ligament injuries and other soft tissue problems, joint motion will often be limited and contracture can occur. The effects of injury and immobilization on soft tissue involve structural changes in length of collagen fibers, random reorganization of collagen fibers, and biochemical changes leading to reduction of water content and glycosaminoglycans.[8] In an ideal situation, contracture will be minimized; if not, interventions need to be employed to restore motion.

Assessment of Pain and Loss of Motion

Tests and measurements have been developed to quantify pain and to attempt to objectify the pain experience and to quantify loss of motion. First, we will discuss pain assessment and then continue with examination strategies for joint stiffness and contractures. The emphasis for this chapter is on pain assessment; there is abundant information in physical therapy texts on motion assessment.

Box 13•3	Conditions Associated With Joint Contracture

- Burns
- Fractures
- Osteoarthritis and rheumatoid arthritis
- Prolonged inactivity or immobilization
- Scarring following injury
- Spasticity
- Tenosynovitis (inflammation of a tendon and its sheath)

Pain Assessment

Pain assessment is an integral part of a thorough clinical examination. The most basic assessment is to have the patient describe their pain. However, many assessment tools have been designed to quantify and qualify the pain experience and to determine the impact of pain on functional capacity. Several factors should be considered when reporting and interpreting pain information. These include the patient's age, ethnicity, cognitive status, and reading ability. Specific tools to measure pain in infants, children, and adolescents have been developed. A child's stage of development and ability to self-report pain complaints are significant considerations when selecting appropriate pain assessment measures.[9] Ethnicity can also play a role in the pain experience, influencing reports of perceived pain and the utilization of pain interventions.[10] Cognitive level and emotional status likewise affect the reliability of the pain assessment. Information provided by numeric scales may be more reliable in patients who are illiterate or who have poor cognition than information provided from multidimensional or functional pain assessment questionnaires.[11]

The selection of the appropriate measure is also dependent on the dimension of pain you are trying to capture. Table 13-3 identifies common pain instruments with the appropriate dimension of pain. Most of the measures described in this section assess only one dimension of pain. These measures usually work well in clinical practice when the patient's pain complaint is relatively straightforward, such as in postoperative pain or peripheral nociceptive pain associated with a recent ankle sprain. For complex or chronic pain cases, multidimensional measures, such as region- or condition-specific self-report questionnaires, are more beneficial. Frequently, these types of outcome measures integrate an intensity pain measure with certain functional activities at specific points in time. One limitation to the region- or condition-specific questionnaire is that it still limits the scope of pain assessment to a particular body part and does not consider the impact of the pain experience on the whole person. Additional questionnaires that expand the scope of pain intensity and the impact on physical function should also be considered with complex or chronic pain patients. These questionnaires may provide information about the impact of the pain

Table 13•3	Pain Dimension in Relation to Assessment Measures	
Dimension of Pain Assessed	**Pain Measure Used**
Spatial (location)	Body diagram
Intensity (how much)	Rating scale
	Patient interview
Quality or nature	Patient interview
Temporal	Patient interview
	Pain diary
	Repeated rating scales
	Repeated pain drawings
Impairments or disability	Patient interview
	Self-report questionnaires
Multidimensional	Patient interview
	McGill Pain Questionnaire
	Self-report questionnaires

on the patient's emotional, psychological, and social adaptations to persistent pain.[12] Several resources are available for obtaining additional information on multidimensional pain measures and self-report questionnaires related to pain, functional limitations, and disability.[13–15]

KEY POINT! Region- or condition-specific assessment scales are limited to evaluating a particular body part. Information regarding the impact on the social and mental components of health is often lacking.

Pain Interview

A key element of the clinical examination is a series of questions regarding the patient's perception of pain.[15] Questions should elicit information regarding the intensity, quality, temporal aspects, and physical characteristics of pain. Intensity is usually described in terms of the severity of the pain. The quality of the pain may include such descriptions as *burning, sharp,* and *stabbing.* The temporal aspects of pain include whether the pain is constant or intermittent. They may also include the time of day the pain is better or worse and what activities seem to exacerbate it. The physical characteristics of pain refer to the location of the pain and whether it is radiating, localized, or diffuse. When conducting the interview, the practitioner needs to be careful not to ask leading questions. Broad-based questions (e.g., Do you have pain at all times?) should also be avoided.

Pain Rating Scales

Many rating scales have been suggested in the literature as a way to measure the intensity of the patient's pain.[11,15–17] These pain-rating scales are relatively quick and easy to administer. They can be presented in a verbal or visual format. Rating scales can be used as part of the initial assessment of pain as well as before, during, or after therapy interventions. The information gained from the rating scales is momentary and may therefore provide the practitioner with only limited information regarding the effectiveness of a particular intervention in providing overall pain relief.

To administer a verbal numeric rating scale, the practitioner generally asks the patient to rate his pain on a scale of 0 to 10, with 0 referring to no pain and 10 being the worst pain that the patient has ever experienced. This 11-point scale is commonly used in clinical practice. A 101-point scale[16] that assesses pain intensity on a scale from 0 (no pain) to 100 (pain as bad as it could be) may be more responsive to change, but it may be more difficult for patients to select a number.[17] Spadoni and colleagues[11] developed an 11-point numeric pain intensity measure, the P4, which has the patient rate pain intensity at four different time points over a 2-day period: morning, afternoon, evening, and with activity. The P4 demonstrated better ability to assess change in pain intensity than a single-item, 11-point numeric rating scale.

There are several versions of the visual analog scale (VAS). Commonly, there is a 10-cm horizontal or vertical line that represents a range of levels of pain.[15–17] The line may have no marks or descriptive words except at the ends of the line, which represent no pain or the worst pain possible. The patient places a mark on the line, and the "intensity" is measured by the distance that the point is placed from 0 in either centimeters or millimeters. Other visual scales may place more word descriptors along the continuum. The patient places a mark on the line. In pediatrics, the use of facial expressions that vary from happy to sad instead of descriptor words or numbers is frequently used.

A problem that may occur when using the rating scales is that the patient may initially start marking near or at the top end of the scale, indicating the worst pain, and then the patient's pain experience becomes worse during subsequent examinations. In this situation, there is no way to indicate the increased severity of pain, unless other measures of pain as related to function are used in addition.

Body Diagrams or Pain Drawings

The patient or the practitioner can fill out a diagram of the human body with both front and back views.[15] An enlarged diagram of a specific body part may be an appropriate alternative to a full-body diagram. This would allow more detailed information regarding the location, intensity, and quality of the pain to be illustrated. However, when examining a patient with complex or persistent pain, some practitioners prefer to use a full-body diagram to determine all potential pain complaints. Colored pencils, degrees of shading, or symbols can be used to represent the intensity and the quality of the pain. (If notes must be sent for reimbursement purposes, remember to photocopy on a color printer.) Numbness and paresthesia associated with pain can be included in this format by using different identification markings, such as dotted areas for paresthesia and crosshatches for areas of numbness. Letters, such as *E* and *I*, may be used to indicate whether pain is located externally (superficial) or internally (deep). Numbers that indicate the intensity dimension of pain may be used to give a numeric rating to the different areas of pain located on the diagram.

The McGill Pain Questionnaire

This specific pain questionnaire (Fig. 13-1) provides a comprehensive look at the multidimensional aspects of pain.[18] One part of the questionnaire involves word descriptors for pain that are categorized and ranked in regard to quality and intensity. The patient selects only one word from each group of words. A particular group of words may be omitted if it does not match the patient's perception of pain. The selection of the word descriptors provides information about the affective, cognitive, and sensory components of pain. Unfortunately, some of the words are complex and are not well understood by patients.[17] Another part of the questionnaire includes a rating scale that could be a modified visual analog scale or a present pain index (PPI). This consists of a numeric value assigned to a descriptive word. The remaining parts include a body diagram and a questionnaire regarding the temporal aspects of pain.

Reduction in Pain Medications

Usage of pain medications is another important component of assessing pain characteristics. Physicians, nurses, and practitioners will monitor pain medication consumption when modalities are used to remediate pain, especially in postoperative cases. Although there is no formal instrument for this dimension of pain assessment, observations of decreased use of pain medications have been correlated with modality effectiveness.[19–25] Consumption of pain medications should be documented, including the type of pain medication, dosage, frequency of administration, and time of intake.

Mobility and Range of Motion Assessment

Assessing the patient's loss of motion due to tissue changes may be more obvious than assessing pain. Through a structured examination, taking into account patient history and present condition, it may be determined that a modality can be beneficial and can be incorporated into an intervention for enhancing motion. The assessment of motion will lay the foundation for determining whether a modality can be used to facilitate an increase in ROM and which would be most effective. There are numerous sources available to the practitioner on how to administer these tests and measures; therefore, they will not be reiterated in this chapter.[26,27]

Scar tissue, particularly when crossing over a joint surface, can limit motion (Fig. 13-2). Recently, a self-rated score for scarring following surgery has been developed.[28] The scale includes items to rate:

- Presence of symptoms (e.g., itch, red, painful)
- Concern for each symptom (e.g., bothered by itch, tightness, pain, redness, height of scar)
- Pain at rest and during (hand) use
- Color
- Scar compliance

Suggested clinical tests and measures for motion are outlined in Table 13-4.

Modality Interventions: Use of Modalities for Pain Modulation

The rationale for the use of heat and cold for pain control is largely based on clinical observation. These modalities are known to alleviate pain and inflammation; however, the specific underlying mechanisms are not well understood. The concept of counterirritation is probably similar to the gate control theory.[29] The increased firing rate of thermoreceptors within the

1. Where is your pain?

   Please mark, on the drawings below, the areas where you feel pain.
   Put E if external, or I if internal, near the areas which you mark.
   Put EI if both external and internal.

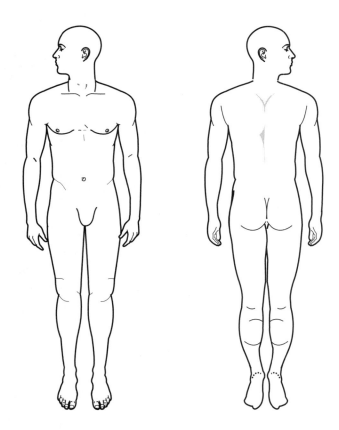

2. Please mark on the scale how much pain you have.

VISUAL ANALOGUE SCALE

PAIN AS
BAD AS IT ——————————————————— NO PAIN
COULD BE

Fig 13•1 Adapted from 1, 2, and 3 of the McGill Pain Questionnaire. Included are (1) a body diagram to be marked by the patient and (2) a visual analogue scale to quantify pain. Word descriptors that provide a quantitative description of pain are included in (3) the Pain Rating Index.

Fig 13•1 Cont'd

3. Pain Rating Index

There are many words that describe pain. From the list below, select only those words that describe your pain as it feels right now. Only select one word in each column, and only if it applies to your pain. YOU DO NOT NEED TO MARK A WORD IN EVERY COLUMN—ONLY MARK THOSE WORDS THAT DESCRIBE YOUR PAIN!

1.	2.	3.	4.
Flickering	Jumping	Pricking	Sharp
Quivering	Flashing	Boring	Cutting
Pulsing	Shooting	Drilling	Lacerating
Throbbing		Stabbing	
Beating			
Pounding			

5.	6.	7.	8.
Pinching	Tugging	Hot	Tingling
Pressing	Pulling	Burning	Itchy
Gnawing	Wrenching	Scalding	Smarting
Cramping		Searing	Stinging
Crushing			

9.	10.	11.	12.
Dull	Tender	Tiring	Sickening
Sore	Taut	Exhausting	Suffocating
Hurting	Rasping		
Aching	Splitting		
Heavy			

13.	14.	15.	16.
Fearful	Punishing	Wretched	Annoying
Frightful	Grueling	Blinding	Troublesome
Terrifying	Cruel		Miserable
	Vicious		Intense
	Killing		Unbearable

17.	18.	19.	20.
Spreading	Tight	Cool	Nagging
Radiating	Numb	Cold	Nauseating
Penetrating	Drawing	Freezing	Agonizing
Piercing	Squeezing		Dreadful
	Tearing		Torturing

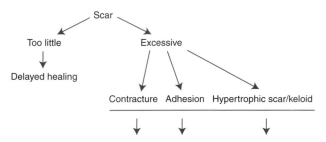

Fig 13•2 Potential consequences of scar tissue.

Table 13•4	Assessment Measures for Motion Limitation: Differentiation of Tissues Causing Limited Motion
Motion-Limiting Factor	**Technique for Assessment**
Scar	Scar assessment
	Scar self-assessment[28]
	Describe scar (keloid versus hypertrophic scar), scar color (hyperemia, pale)
Edema	Girth measurement with tape measure
	Figure-of-eight measurement (for foot and ankle, hand and wrist)
	Water displacement technique with volumeter (for foot and ankle; hand and wrist)
Muscle length	Compare joint motion with muscle slackened and muscle lengthened
Active insufficiency (e.g., muscle weakness or loss of tendon gliding)	Comparison of active and passive ROM of joint
Periarticular joint structures (joint contracture)	Comparison of active and passive ROM of joint
	Joint mobility testing: accessory motions

cutaneous tissue may block the input from the primary nociceptive afferents to the dorsal horn. Pain may be modulated by affecting the pain-muscle spasm-pain cycle. When at least one component of the cycle is removed, pain may be reduced. Reduction of muscle spasm has been described for both heat and cold.[30–33] Although this may be an effective manner for decreasing pain, the intensity of the thermal agent should be monitored to avoid dosages that cause thermal damage to the soft tissues.

According to the opinion of the Philadelphia Panel,[34] which evaluated the use of thermotherapy for spine, knee, and shoulder conditions, pain modulation via both heat and cold is short-lived. Most of the heat studies reviewed used short application heat therapy.

Cryotherapy

Cryotherapy—the use of modalities to lower tissue temperatures—can be used for pain management and treatment (Fig. 13-3). Cold may reduce the painful response to injury by reducing blood flow and preventing the excessive release of chemical mediators associated with inflammation. A variety of cold modalities can be used, including ice packs, ice massage, frozen gel packs, and vapor coolant sprays. (See Chapter 2 for a more detailed description of cold modalities.)

Cryotherapy can increase pain threshold and tolerance. The analgesic effect of tissue cooling may raise pain threshold and reduce muscle spasms via neuromuscular and hemodynamic mechanisms. A reduction in tissue temperature causes vasoconstriction of the surrounding vessels, reducing blood flow to the injured area and decreasing bleeding and the inflammatory response. By limiting this inflammatory response,

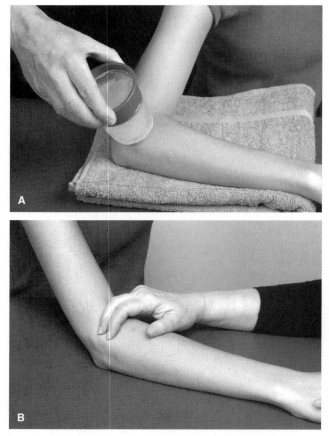

Fig 13•3 Lateral epicondylitis. (A) Ice massage to the lateral elbow. (B) Transverse friction massage to the area of lateral epicondylitis.

fewer irritants are released in the injured area, mediating the pain response. Tissue cooling also reduces nerve conduction velocity, inhibits nociceptors, and decreases muscle spasms.[35] Nerve conduction velocity has been shown to decrease by as much as 33% at tissue temperatures of 10°C (50°F).[36] By slowing the transmission of pain signals, the transmission of pain by nociceptors and pain fibers is reduced or blocked.

Cryotherapy is commonly used for pain control with acute soft tissue injuries. Ice is more effective than no ice, and it may be beneficial to apply cold before therapeutic exercises for pain control.[23] Studies have also shown a reduced consumption of analgesic medications when cryotherapy is used in acute injuries.[23] There is a paucity of evidence to support the optimal parameters for cold application (i.e., duration of application, frequency of application, mode of delivery). Therefore, clinical decisions must be made based on a case by case basis, taking into account the injury, the patient's response, and the best evidence in the literature.

The use of continuous cold application has been shown to have a positive effect in postoperative pain.[37,38] Postoperative pain may be more related to incisional pain and the surrounding superficial tissues, warranting the use of superficial cold modalities for pain management. Continuous cooling of the hip for 4 days after total hip arthroplasty at a constant cooling temperature of 5°C (41°F) immediately after surgery had a positive effect on patient-reported postoperative pain.[37] If the pain source was located in the deeper hip region, superficial cooling would not have been successful in mediating this pain. In addition, continuous cooling may improve sleep quality (i.e., less pain, more uninterrupted sleep) and improve tolerance to rehabilitation in the immediate postoperative phase.[38]

The use of controlled cooling devices for the management of postoperative pain has gained popularity in the past decade.[20–25] Table 13-5 presents an overview of the studies that discuss the use of cryotherapy after surgery and other conditions.

Thermotherapy

Thermotherapy—the use of modalities to raise tissue temperatures—can also be utilized for pain management and treatment. Heating modalities include moist hot packs, heating pads, warm whirlpools, short-wave diathermy, continuous ultrasound, and pulsed ultrasound with parameters sufficient to elevate tissue

Table 13•5	**Literature Using Cryotherapy for Pain Modulation**		
Authors	**Population**	**Method**	**Results**
Morsi, 2002[19]	Postoperative total knee arthroplasty	Staged bilateral total knee replacements. Continuous-flow cooling device applied immediately postoperatively for 6 days on one knee, but not the other knee when the same surgery was performed on the same patient weeks later.	Lower VAS score and analgesic consumption noted with cooling device.
Hochberg, 2001[20]	Postoperative carpal tunnel release	Controlled cold therapy compared with conventional ice therapy for 3 days postoperatively.	Lower VAS score and analgesic consumption noted with cooling device.
Barber , 2000[25]	Postoperative ACL reconstruction	Randomized, controlled trial comparing continuous flow cold to crushed ice. Cryotherapy was applied for 3 days, then "as needed" for an additional 4 days.	Lower pain measures (VAS, Likert scale), decreased use of analgesic medication, greater usage, greater knee flexion, and higher self-rated performance in the continuous cold group.
Fountas et al., 1999[126]	Postoperative lumbar microdiscectomy	Randomized, controlled trial comparing the use of a cold (18°C [64°F]) 5% bacitracin solution for 5 minutes followed by cooling with a microtemperature pump for 24 hours after surgery.	Significant reduction in postoperative pain, earlier ambulation, and shorter length of hospital stay.
Kullenberg et al., 2006[127]	Postoperative total knee arthroplasty	Prospective study comparing cold compression or epidural analgesia for 3 days after TKA.	Less pain, greater knee flexion ROM, and shorted hospital stay in the cold compression group.
Sellwood et al., 2007[128]	Delayed-onset muscle soreness following eccentric training	Prospective, randomized, double-blind, controlled trial comparing body submersion in ice water (5±1°C [41°F]) or tepid water (24°C [75°F])	No differences in pain, tenderness, isometric strength, swelling, hop-for-distance or serum creatine kinase.

temperature.[39] (See Chapter 3 for a more detailed description of heating agents.)

The primary mechanism of pain control through the use of heating agents is vasodilation. Increased blood flow as a result of vasodilation may facilitate healing by supplying nutrients to the wounded area and removing pain-inducing chemical mediators known to activate or sensitize nociceptors. Heating also improves soft tissue extensibility, which can reduce soft tissue tension's contribution to the pain response. Conversely, heating an area of acute inflammation may further exacerbate movement of plasma proteins and fluids into the interstitial tissue, which may facilitate activation of nociceptors by chemical mediators. Sound clinical decision-making is important to facilitate rather than impede the healing process when considering heat for pain control.

Selection of superficial versus deep heating modalities is dependent on the target tissues. Continuous-wave ultrasound (US) and short-wave diathermy are capable of affecting structures deeper than 2 centimeters under the skin and therefore may be more effective than conductive heating agents in relieving joint and muscle pain.

The ease of joint movement secondary to the increase in collagen extensibility associated with heating may add to the patient's perception of decreased pain and allow the patient to participate in therapeutic exercise. Published clinical papers on the use of hot packs for patients with adhesive capsulitis[40] and paraffin for patients with rheumatoid arthritis[41] support this phenomenon. In addition, the use of thermal agents before isokinetic exercises in women with knee osteoarthritis has been shown to have a positive effect on exercise performance, pain, and function. Hot packs used in conjunction with a transcutaneous electrical nerve stimulation or short-wave diathermy have been shown to have a more favorable outcome than ultrasound.[42]

Easing pain symptoms and raising pain threshold can be justification for giving a heat modality before exercising, posture training, or gait training if it increases patient participation. Muscle guarding spasm can perpetuate pain and limited motion. Alleviating the spasm can be accomplished by using a heat modality. Some older studies are worth reviewing, because they may spark interest in further areas of research. For example, a comparison between moist heat packs and continuous short-wave diathermy (SWD) was made for trigger-point therapy.[43] Moist heat packs or SWD were administered for 20 minutes over trigger points in the thoracic, lumbar, or gluteal region. Heat was adjusted to patient tolerance. Pain was measured at the trigger points by tolerable grams of pressure from a pressure algometer. Both moist heat packs and SWD were effective in reducing pain at the most sensitive trigger points. SWD was more effective in treating less-sensitive trigger points.

Williams and colleagues[44] compared the use of moist heat packs and exercise versus ice packs and exercise on patients with rheumatoid arthritis of the shoulder. Both the ice and heat groups demonstrated decreases in pain and increases in shoulder range of motion, and there were no significant differences between groups. These findings suggest that either heat or cold can be of benefit before exercise in this scenario or that the heat or cold provided no added benefit to exercise.

When treating a patient with pain, muscle spasm, or both, the patient's position for intervention must be carefully selected and should be as comfortable as possible, particularly considering that the patient may need to remain in this position for up to 30 minutes. If muscle spasm is present, the muscle(s) should not be in a position of "undue stretch" until some pain relief has occurred. If the patient has joint pain, the joint should be positioned in an open-packed position, with the ligaments and joint capsule in a slackened position.[26] In this position, intra-articular pressure and stress on joint structures will be lessened.[45]

Another option to reduce pain and increase flexibility is through the use of wearable heat wraps, which are designed for self-application. (The use and design of these heat wraps are discussed in Chapter 3.) A number of studies (Table 13-6) have examined the use of these wraps in managing low back pain and other conditions.[46–49]

Ultrasound

There is a lack of evidence from well-designed, controlled, randomized studies that ultrasound is effective in pain modulation for conditions other than calcific tendonitis of the shoulder, carpal tunnel syndrome, or rheumatoid arthritis. A meta-analysis by Gam and

Table 13•6 Literature Using Continuous Low-Level Heat Therapy for Pain Modulation

Authors	Population	Method	Results That Support Use
Mayer et al., 2006[129]	Subjects without low back pain who performed an eccentric exercise program to elicit low back delayed-onset muscle soreness (DOMS)	Prevention substudy: randomized to heat wrap 4 hours before and 4 hours after exercise or a control group. Treatment substudy: randomized to heat wrap or cold between 18 to 42 hours postexercise.	Prevention substudy: Heat wrap group had less pain and disability and greater self-reported physical function. Treatment substudy: Greater pain relief with the heat wrap. No significant differences in disability or self-reported function.
Michlovitz et al., 2004[46]	Wrist sprains and strains (SS), osteoarthritis (OA), carpal tunnel syndrome (CTS)	Randomized to heat wrap 8-hr wear over 3 days and placebo analgesic.	Pain relief and increased grip strength (day 3) for SS/OA heat group; pain relief, increased grip strength, decreases stiffness and CTS symptoms (Boston Carpal Tunnel Scales*) for CTS heat group.
Nadler et al., 2003[48]	Acute nonspecific low back pain (no traumatic injury within last 48 hrs)	Randomized to continuous low-level heat wrap group 8-hr wear or acetaminophen/ibuprofen group.	Self-reported pain reduction and decrease in muscle stiffness in heat wrap group. Both groups reported decreased perceived disability.
Nadler et al., 2003[49]	Acute nonspecific low back pain	Randomized to heat wrap during sleep or oral placebo for 3 consecutive nights.	Heat wrap group had pain relief throughout the next day, reduced muscle stiffness and disability, and improved trunk flexibility.

Johannsen[50] and systematic reviews by Robertson and Baker[51] and van der Windt and colleagues[52] demonstrated that randomized, controlled clinical trials generally do not support the use of ultrasound as an intervention to decrease pain in musculoskeletal disorders, such as knee osteoarthritis[53,54] and patellofemoral pain syndrome.[55] These conclusions are enlightening, particularly considering the frequency with which ultrasound is used in many outpatient facilities. The Philadelphia Panel, composed of health-care practitioners from physical therapy and medicine, concluded from their systemic reviews that ultrasound may offer some benefit in the management of shoulder pain. This group also concluded that there was either no evidence or insufficient evidence to recommend the use of ultrasound for pain management of low back, neck, or knee conditions.[34] Evidence also supports the use of ultrasound for rheumatoid arthritis with purported benefits that include a decrease in the number of swollen and painful joints, improved ROM and stiffness, and improved grip strength.[56] Table 13-7 presents a sample of the literature that supports or refutes the use of ultrasound for pain modulation in the past two decades.[57-65]

Additional research is needed with thermotherapy and ultrasound in clinical populations, controlling for placebo when possible, to determine the causal relationship between these modalities and pain modulation as well as their effect on improving functional outcome.

Electroanalgesia

Transcutaneous electrical nerve stimulation (TENS) uses externally applied electrical stimulation with surface electrodes (Fig. 13-4). TENS has been commonly used to describe pain suppression with electrotherapy since Melzack and Wall proposed the gate theory in 1965.[66] *Electroanalgesia* is a general term that describes the outcome of using electrical stimulation or TENS for pain modulation.[67]

Three modes, or levels, of stimulation have been described to promote electroanalgesia. Sensory- or motor-level stimulations are commonly used to modulate peripheral nociceptive or neurogenic mediated pain. These modes of stimulation may be produced using pulsed current generators, interferential current (IFC) devices, and high-volt pulsed current (HVPC) units. Noxious-level stimulation is recommended when other methods of pain modulation have failed or when managing CRPS or centrally mediated pain.

Overall, the evidence is inconclusive for the use of TENS for pain control. Comparison of the effects on pain is problematic, because it is difficult to categorize the different types of pain or pain syndromes. Inconsistent terminology, parameter selection, or

Table 13•7 Literature Using Ultrasound (US) for Pain Modulation

Authors	Population	Method	Results That Support or Refute Use
Dogru et al., 2008[130]	Adhesive capsulitis of the shoulder	Randomized trial of US and sham US.	No significant differences between groups at 3 months in pain or shoulder pain and disability index (SPADI) score.
Ainsworth et al., 2007[131]	Shoulder pain	Double-blind, randomized trial. Manual therapy plus US or manual therapy plus sham US in conjunction with home exercises.	No difference between groups at 6 weeks or 6 months on the Shoulder Disability Questionnaire—UK.
Giombini et al., 2006[132]	Supraspinatus tendinopathy	Randomized, controlled trial of 434 MHz hyperthermy, 1 MHz continuous ultrasound, and an exercise control.	Hyperthermy yielded greater pain relief than US or exercise on VAS score and pain reported with movement.
Almeida et al., 2003[57]	Fibromyalgia	Randomized study of two groups using combined therapy of pulsed and interferential current (CPTI) and a sham group for 12 sessions.	Quantity and intensity of painful areas measured through body diagrams and VAS score were lower following treatment before and after sleep. Touch tolerance increased.
Ebenbichler et al., 1999[133]	Calcific tendinitis in shoulder	Double-blind, randomized study of two treatment groups receiving either pulsed US or sham US over area of calcification for twenty-four 15-minute sessions.	Significant differences in pain intensity and calcium absorption noted in pulsed US group at the end of 24 treatments (6 weeks). No significant differences were found at 9-month follow-up evaluation.
Ebenbichler et al., 1998[59]	Carpal tunnel syndrome	Double-blind, randomized, controlled clinical trial consisting of two treatment groups receiving either pulsed US or sham US over the area of carpal tunnel for twenty 15-minute sessions.	VAS scores for pain complaints were significantly lower in US group at end of 20 sessions and at 6 months. Improved nerve conduction was also observed in the US group.
D'Vaz et al., 2006[134]	Lateral epicondylitis	Double-blind, randomized, controlled trial of pulsed low-intensity ultrasound therapy or placebo US daily for a 12-week period.	No significant difference between groups in VAS pain score, Patient-Related Forearm Evaluation Questionnaire (PRFEQ), and grip strength.
Gam et al., 1998[62]	Myofascial trigger points (MTrP)	Single-blind, randomized, controlled clinical trial; two treatment groups and control group, which did not receive any treatment. Difference between two treatments groups was that either US or sham US was given along with massage and exercise.	No significant differences between groups on VAS scores or analgesic medication usage. Two treatment groups had lower MTrP indices (quantity and intensity) than control group.
Ozgonenel et al., 2009[135]	Knee osteoarthritis	Double-blind, randomized controlled trial of 1 MHz continuous US at 1 W/cm^2 and sham US for 10 treatments.	Lower pain VAS pain scores, higher WOMAC scores, and faster 50-m walk time.
Falconer et al., 1992[63]	Knee osteoarthritis	Single-blind, randomized treatment groups receiving either continuous US or sham US prior to exercise for 12 treatments.	No significant differences between groups in knee AROM or VAS scores after 12 treatments or follow-up evaluation at 2 months.
Johasson et al., 2005[136]	Shoulder impingement	Single-blind, randomized controlled trial in which patients received acupuncture or US for 10 treatments in conjunction with a home-exercise program.	The acupuncture group had greater improvement at 3-, 6-, and 12-month follow-up on the Constant-Murley Shoulder Assessment, the Adolfsson-Lysholm Shoulder Score, and the University of California at Los Angeles End-Result Score.
Kurtais Gursel et al., 2004[137]	Soft tissue disorder of the shoulder	Randomized, placebo-controlled trial with patients receiving either continuous US or sham US treatment.	No difference between groups in pain, joint ROM, or Shoulder Disability Questionnaire Score.

omitted stimulation parameters contribute to the lack of comparable data. The importance of stimulation parameters has been demonstrated in producing an analgesic effect.[68,69] Some studies investigate only the effectiveness of a single treatment of electrical stimulation, while others look at multiple applications over time. This makes comparing study results difficult as well.

Transcutaneous electrical nerve stimulation using portable pulsed current generators is more commonly used in studies than are other waveforms that can produce electroanalgesia. The literature on other forms of electrotherapy, including interferential current and diadynamic currents, is less abundant.[69] Deyo and colleagues[68] concluded that there was no significant benefit to treatment with TENS or placebo TENS with or without exercise in patients with chronic low back pain. The results of this analysis demonstrate that it is difficult to control for placebo using a sham treatment and that patients with low back pain do not have the same source of pain mediation. TENS was effective in managing intractable pain of known etiology, such as musculoskeletal disorders, but patients with chronic trical stimulation and pulley traction into gleno-humeral abduction for up to 2 hours. Greater ROM gains were observed in the TENS group than the heat group. The authors concluded that TENS produced a greater analgesic response that allowed the subjects to tolerate the prolonged stretch with pulley traction. The TENS group also achieved pain-free sleep after 4 to 6 weeks compared to 4 to 5 months for the heat group.

The Philadelphia Panel's[34] conclusions support the use of TENS with therapeutic exercises for patients with osteoarthritis of the knee. Other studies on arthritis populations have also demonstrated improved joint function, theorizing that TENS allows patients with arthritis to participate in other therapy interventions, such as exercise and functional activities.[73–76] However, a 2009 Cochrane Review concluded that there was a lack of sufficient evidence to support the use of TENS in the management of arthritis-related pain.[77]

Laser Therapy

Laser therapy is the use of light radiation to alter cellular and tissue functions to promote healing. Both low-level laser therapy (LLLT) and high-level laser therapy (HLLT) can be used as an adjunct to physical therapy treatment to decrease pain and disability. The therapeutic use of laser therapy is discussed in Chapter 6.

There is conflicting evidence to support the use of LLLT in the management of soft tissue disorders of the shoulder and elbow. Several studies report successful pain reduction and reversal of weakness when LLLT was used as an adjunct to physical therapy for the management of supraspinatus tendonitis.[78–82] However, conflicting evidence suggests that LLLT is no more effective than placebo treatment.[83–85] A systematic review of LLLT in patients with rheumatoid arthritis in the hand supports its use to reduce pain and morning stiffness.[86] In addition, clinical studies in patients with lateral epicondylitis,[84,87] knee pain,[88] and myofascial pain[89] have shown positive outcomes in pain and function with LLLT.

However, LLLT does not appear to be effective in managing pain for patients with nonspecific low back pain.[90] As with other modalities, one of the major limitations of research on the use of LLLT for pain is the lack of homogeneity in treatment parameters.

Research supports the use of HLLT as a promising intervention in the management of subacromial impingement syndrome.[91] A neodymium yttrium alu-

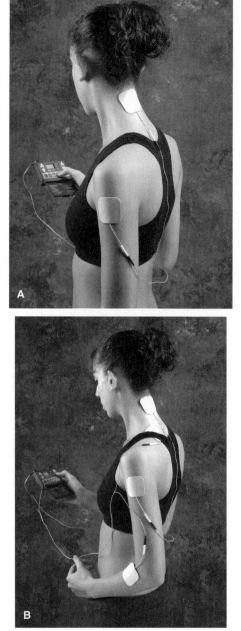

Fig 13•4 Cervical radiculopathy. (A) TENS with two electrodes. (B) TENS with four electrodes.

pain who had a strong affective pain component did not respond well to TENS.[70,71]

Rizk and colleagues[72] reported that the use of sensory-level electrical stimulation and pulley traction improved ROM and facilitated pain-free sleep in patients with adhesive capsulitis. The subjects were divided into two treatment groups. One group received heat prior to therapeutic exercises that consisted of Codman's pendulum exercises, wall climbing, and pulley exercises. The second group received sensory-level elec-

CASE STUDY 13•1 CERVICAL PAIN—SENSORY-LEVEL TENS

A 45-year-old female is referred for chronic history of upper quarter pain over the past 3 years. She has had intermittent pain in the left paracervical region from C4 to T1, the left upper trapezius and levator scapulae muscles, and the left proximal dorsal forearm and lateral elbow region pain in the C5 and C6 dermatomes for the past 4 weeks, unrelated to any specific incident or injury. Cervical flexion and right lateral rotation reproduces her pain.

CLINICAL DECISION-MAKING

1. Does the patient have a dysfunction, limitation, or problem that can be improved with the use of electrical stimulation?
   Answer: Yes, sensory-level transcutaneous electrical stimulation can be used to reduce pain.

2. Is the patient appropriate for electrical stimulation (i.e., do any of the general precautions or contraindications to electrical stimulation apply to the patient, or are there any specific considerations regarding application of electrical stimulation to this patient)?
   Answer: Yes, as long as sensation is intact and none of the generalized precautions or contraindications apply.

3. What are the specific goals to be achieved with the use of electrical stimulation?
   Answer: To decrease pain to allow patient to perform activities of daily living.

4. What specific electrical stimulation would be appropriate for the patient?
   Answer: Parameters appropriate for sensory-level stimulation.

5. Can you select the specific parameters of electrical stimulation that are appropriate for the patient?
   Answer: Sensory-level stimulation for pain control requires the following parameters:

Pulse duration: 100 μsec
Pulse frequency: 100 pps
Intensity: Strong enough to achieve perceptible tingling without muscle contraction as tolerated
Duration: 30 minutes
Type of device: A portable pulsed current stimulator (TENS unit) should be used so that the patient can use it following exacerbation of pain either at work or home.
Motor-level stimulation parameters may also be used.

6. What are the proper application procedures for sensory-level TENS?
   Answer:
   Instruct the patient: Inform the patient of the purpose and procedure, including the anticipated sensation and effect of the stimulation.
   Preinspection: Inspect the area to be treated for skin compromise and assess for intact sensation over the area to be treated.
   Electrode application: Prepare area by cleansing with soap and water or alcohol wipe. Electrodes should be placed over areas of pain in left paracervical region and along the distribution of pain. One or two channels of stimulation can be used with two or four electrodes, respectively.
   Patient position: The patient should be positioned prone or supine to take tension off antigravity cervical muscles and to avoid an upright forward head posture.
   Postinspection: Remove the electrodes and inspect the skin for any signs of skin irritation or adverse effects. If redness occurs, explain to the patient that this is not uncommon and should disappear in less than 24 hours.

---

minum garnet laser with a pulsating waveform was used to deliver a 2,050 J total dose of energy over a 10-minute treatment duration. Ten treatment sessions were provided over a period of 2 consecutive weeks. Compared to continuous US at a frequency of 1 MHz and an intensity of 2 W/cm² for 10 minutes, HLLT provided a greater reduction in pain and a greater improvement in articular movement, function, and muscle strength. Table 13-8 presents an overview of the studies that support the use of laser therapy in musculoskeletal disorders.

Transdermal Delivery of Medications or Other Substances

Iontophoresis and phonophoresis can be used to deliver analgesics and anti-inflammatory agents parenterally to resolve pain and inflammation. Iontophoresis delivers ionizable substances through the skin using electrical stimulation. Phonophoresis delivers topically applied medications using ultrasound waves. The potential benefits of transdermal delivery include direct application to the target tissue, resulting in higher concentrations

Table 13•8 **Literature Using Low-Level Laser Therapy (LLLT) for Pain Modulation**

Authors	Population	Method	Results That Support Use
Oken et al., 2008[87]	Lateral epicondylitis	Single-blind, randomized controlled trial of brace plus exercise, continuous ultrasound (1 MHz, 1.5 W/cm^2, 5 minutes) plus exercise, or LLLT (HeNe laser, wavelength 632.8 nm, output 10 mV, 10 minutes) plus exercise. US and LLLT treatments were applied 5 days per week for 2 weeks.	Pain significantly improved in all groups at the end of treatment but was only significant at 6 weeks in the US and LLLT groups. Grip strength also improved after treatment in the LLLT group.
Dincer et al., 2009[140]	Carpal tunnel syndrome	Randomized trial of splinting, splinting plus US, or splinting plus LLLT.	LLLT plus splinting was the most effective treatment for decreasing symptom severity and pain and increasing patient satisfaction.
Shirani et al., 2009[89]	Myofascial pain	Double-blind, placebo-controlled, randomized trial of laser therapy (2, 600 nm diode laser probes, 6.2 J/cm^2, 6 min, continuous wave, and 890 nm, 1 J/cm^2, 10 min, 1,500 Hz), and placebo laser 2 times per week for 3 weeks.	The laser therapy group exhibited a greater reduction in VAS pain post-treatment compared to the placebo group.
Yeldan et al., 2009[141]	Subacromial impingement syndrome	Randomized trial of laser therapy and placebo laser. Treatment was applied 5 days a week for 3 weeks in conjunction with cold therapy and a progressive exercise program.	No significant differences in pain, function, disability, and strength between groups after treatment.
Hegedus et al., 2009[88]	Mild to moderate knee osteoarthritis	Double-blind, placebo-controlled trial of LLLT (diode laser, 830 nm wavelength, continuous wave, power 50 mW, 6 J/point dose) versus a placebo control group (power 0.5 mW) 2 times per week for 4 weeks.	The LLLT showed a significant improvement in VAS pain, knee circumference, pressure sensitivity, flexion ROM, and improvement in circulation compared to the placebo laser group.

of medication to the area and elimination of gastrointestinal absorption or liver metabolism factors, which is a side effect of many oral anti-inflammatory medications. Injections are also an alternative to oral medications that may produce higher concentrations of medication to the target tissue. However, injections are an invasive procedure that poses a risk for injury and tissue damage with repeated injections, and they may be painful to the recipient.

Numerous investigations assessing the clinical effectiveness of iontophoresis and phonophoresis have been conducted in the past two decades, including case reports and clinical trials without a control group or placebo group.[92–94] Some authors have reported a decrease in pain and increased joint ROM using a combination of lidocaine and dexamethasone iontophoresis.[95–97] The technique of applying both medications is no longer popular because of the concern about competing ions within the same delivery electrode.

Iontophoresis treatment has been shown to be superior to ultrasound and muscle relaxants in alleviating myofascial shoulder girdle pain and tendonitis.[95–97] The iontophoresis groups responded more favorably to treatment than the sham-iontophoresis groups. However, more recent work by Kaya and colleagues[98] suggests that lidocaine iontophoresis was no more effective than direct current stimulation without lidocaine in the treatment of cervical and periscapular trigger points. Similar findings have also been reported in patients with temporomandibular pain[99] and plantar heel pain.[100] Other factors to consider are advancing age and degenerative changes, as these have been shown to adversely impact response to iontophoresis treatment.[95,96] Table 13-9 presents more recent studies that have evaluated the effectiveness of iontophoresis.[101–104]

There is limited evidence to support the use of phonophoresis in the management of tendinopathies.[60,105] It is difficult to interpret the results of many studies because control groups were not included in the study design; however, the evidence suggests that the use of a specific drug as the coupling medium appears to have no added benefit than continuous-wave ultrasound alone in managing upper and lower extremity tendinopathies, such as lateral epicondylitis, supraspinatus tendonitis, De Quervain tenosynovitis, biceps tendonitis, patellar tendonitis, plantar fasciitis, and Achilles tendonitis.[60]

CASE STUDY 13•2 LATERAL EPICONDYLALGIA—LOW-LEVEL LASER THERAPY (LLLT)

A 53-year-old male mechanic is referred for a diagnosis of lateral epicondylalgia. He reports difficulty using work tools and a weakening of his grip. Pain over the common extensor tendon is provoked with rested wrist and long finger extension and passive stretch of the common extensors.

CLINICAL DECISION-MAKING

1. Does the patient have a dysfunction, limitation, or problem that can be improved with the use of LLLT?
   Answer: Yes, LLLT can be used to treat soft tissue injuries.

2. Is the patient appropriate for LLLT (i.e., do any of the general precautions or contraindications to LLLT apply to the patient, or are there any specific considerations regarding application of LLLT to this patient)?
   Answer: Yes, as long as none of the generalized precautions or contraindications apply and there are no open wounds over the treatment area.

3. What are the specific goals to be achieved with the use of LLLT?
   Answer: To decrease pain and allow patient to return to work.

4. Do you have the specific type of laser that is appropriate for the patient?
   Answer: A low-level laser or cold laser is appropriate for its photochemical effects.

5. Can you select the specific parameters of LLLT that are appropriate for the patient?
   Answer: The following parameters are appropriate for LLLT:
   Laser average power: 1 to 500 mW
   Wavelength: 600 to 1,000 nm
   Pulse frequency: 2.5 Hz to 5 KHz
   Dosage: 10 to 15 J/cm^2
   Duration: Determined by painful treatment area; irradiate each area for 20 to 50 seconds.
   Optimal treatment parameters are not known.

6. What are the proper application procedures for LLLT?
   Answer:
   Instruct the patient: Inform the patient of the purpose and procedure, including the anticipated sensation.
   Preinspection: Inspect the area to be treated for skin compromise and assess for intact sensation.
   Application: The laser probe should be completely in contact with the skin, perpendicular to the treatment area.
   Patient position: The patient should be positioned in sitting or supine to allow access to the common extensor tendon.
   Postinspection: The skin should be inspected for any signs of irritation or adverse effects. A mild discomfort or ache may be felt in the treatment area and should resolve within 24 to 48 hours after treatment.

Table 13•9 Literature Using Iontophoresis for Pain Modulation

Authors	Population	Method	Results That Support Use
Nirschl et al., 2003[101]	Acute lateral epicondylitis	Double-blind, randomized, controlled study in which patients were assigned to either treatment group that received iontophoresis with dexamethasone sodium phosphate or placebo group that received iontophoresis with saline solution. Current dosage for both groups was 40 ma-min, and each subject received six treatments of iontophoresis within 13–17 days.	Dexamethasone iontophoresis group showed significantly lower VAS scores compared to saline iontophoresis group 2 days after all treatments were delivered. Pain scores at 1 month post-treatment not significantly different between groups.
Runeson et al., 2002[138]	Lateral epicondylitis	Double-blind, randomized clinical trial of corticosteroid iontophoresis (0.4% dexamethasone sodium phosphate) or placebo (saline) iontophoresis. Current dosage was 4 mA for 10 minutes for 4 treatment sessions over a 1-week period.	No significant difference between groups in pain with palpation of the lateral epicondyle, pain with resisted wrist extension, or pain with gripping.
Cleland et al., 2009[100]	Plantar fasciitis	Randomized, clinical trial: iontophoresis with dexamethasone (dose, 40 mAmin) and exercise versus manual physical therapy and exercise. Both groups received 6 treatments over a 4-week period.	The manual physical therapy and exercise group showed greater improvement on the Lower Extremity Functional Scale (LEFS), the Foot and Ankle Ability Measure (FAAM), and the Numeric Pain Rating Scale (NPRS) compared to the iontophoresis and exercise group at 4 weeks and 6 months.

Table 13•9 **Literature Using Iontophoresis for Pain Modulation—cont'd**

| Osborne and Allison, 2006[139] | Plantar fasciitis | Double-blind, randomized, placebo controlled trial of LowDye taping plus either 0.4% dexamethasone, placebo (0.9% NaCl), or 5% acetic acid iontophoresis for 6 treatments over a 2-week period to the site of maximum tenderness on the plantar aspect of the foot. | All groups showed a significant improvement in morning pain, average pain, and morning stiffness. Acetic acid yielded a greater improvement in morning pain than dexamethasone. Long-term treatment effects on pain only remained significant for acetic acid and taping and dexamethasone and taping. Only acetic acid maintained treatment effect for morning stiffness. |

CASE STUDY 13•3 PLANTAR HEEL PAIN (PLANTAR FASCIITIS/FASCIOSIS)—IONTOPHORESIS

A 38-year-old male runner is referred for left medial plantar heel pain. Pain is worst first thing in the morning, after walking prolonged distances, and is recreated with palpation of the proximal insertion of the plantar fascia into the calcaneus.

CLINICAL DECISION-MAKING

1. Does the patient have a dysfunction, limitation, or problem that can be improved with the use of iontophoresis?

   Answer: Yes, iontophoresis can be used for the transdermal delivery of medication to reduce pain and inflammation.

2. Is the patient appropriate for iontophoresis (i.e., do any of the general precautions or contraindications to electrical stimulation apply to the patient, or are there any specific considerations regarding application of iontophoresis to this patient)?

   Answer: Yes, as long as sensation is in tact, none of the generalized precautions or contraindications apply, and there are no drug allergies.

3. What are the specific goals to be achieved with the use of iontophoresis?

   Answer: To decrease pain and allow patient to reduce/eliminate compensations during gait.

4. What type of stimulation and specific iontophoretic medications would be appropriate for the patient?

   Answer: A direct current stimulator is needed for the transdermal delivery of medication. Dexamethasone sodium phosphate, a glucocorticoid, would be appropriate for chronic inflammation. Acetic acid could also be used if heel spurs were present to help reduce soft tissue calcifications.

5. Can you select the specific parameters of iontophoresis that are appropriate for the patient?

   Answer: The following parameters are appropriate for iontophoresis:

Type of device: Portable direct current generator specifically used for iontophoresis.

Current dosage: 40 to 80 ma · min.

Amplitude: Should be set to patient tolerance. Most units have a maximum output of 4 mA.

Duration: Calculated by the unit to deliver the set current dosage once the amplitude has been determined.

6. What are the proper application procedures for iontophoresis?

   Answer:

Instruct the patient: Inform the patient of the purpose and procedure, including the anticipated sensation and effect of the stimulation.

Preinspection: Inspect the area to be treated for skin compromise and assess for intact sensation.

Electrode application: The skin should be gently cleaned with soap and water over the electrode sites. Attach the negative lead (cathode) to the delivery electrode filled to capacity with dexamethasone sodium phosphate. The medication should be absorbed within the electrode, and the contact surface of the electrode should be wet before applying the delivery electrode to the left medial plantar surface of the heel. Attach the positive lead (anode) to the dispersive or reference electrode and place on the lower leg over the gastrocnemius muscle belly.

Patient position: The patient should be positioned prone or supine to allow access to the plantar surface of the heel.

Postinspection: Remove the electrodes and inspect the skin for any signs of skin irritation or adverse effects. If redness occurs, explain to the patient that this is not uncommon and should disappear in less than 24 hours.

Associated Impairments

Many factors can contribute to a patient's perception of pain. Some of these include the following:

- Joint stiffness due to arthritis or injury
- Muscle weakness due to immobilization or a central nervous system lesion, such as a cerebrovascular accident
- Edema
- Open or closed wounds

Interstitial edema can contribute to pain by increasing pressure on mechanoreceptors or by affecting chemical mediators located within the inflammatory exudate that sensitize or activate nociceptors. Choosing a modality may depend on the presence of other impairments. For example, if acute edema is present, using a heating agent may not be the best choice to promote pain modulation because the increased blood flow within the target area could increase the amount of edema and subsequently increase pain.

The use of electrical stimulation using NMES parameters to strengthen weak shoulder girdle muscles has been successful in reducing shoulder pain in patients following stroke (e.g., cerebrovascular accident).[106,107] Chantraine and colleagues[106] reported that pain measures (VAS and presence of pain with motion) were lower in subjects with shoulder pain following hemiplegia with subluxation who received NMES to shoulder girdle muscles than in the control group, which used an upper extremity orthotic. Yu and associates[107] reported similar findings of pain reduction in a multicenter, single-blinded, randomized clinical trial that used intramuscular or percutaneous neuromuscular electrical stimulation.

Use of Modalities to Increase Motion

The use of modalities to reduce tissue contractures and restore ROM and function is well documented. Both superficial and deep heating modalities (e.g., hot packs, short-wave diathermy, and ultrasound) are commonly used adjuncts to treatment in preparation for joint mobilization (Fig. 13-5) and passive stretch

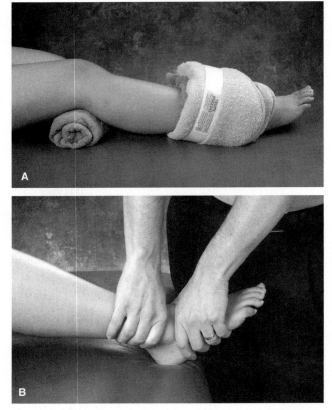

Fig 13•5 (A) Use of moist heat packs around the ankle joint. (B) Prior to joint mobilization of the ankle.

(Fig. 13-6). Electrical muscle stimulation can also be used to facilitate gains in ROM.

Heating modalities alter both collagen viscoelasticity and extensibility, allowing for tissue elongation and plastic deformation. *Plastic deformation* refers to the permanent change or elongation in tissues that occurs when a sufficient stress is applied. Because heating increases collagen elasticity, greater changes in tissue length can occur. Early studies in both frog and rat tendons suggest that tissue temperatures of greater than 40°C (104°F) are necessary to induce permanent changes.[108–111]

Deep-heating modalities may be more effective than superficial heating modalities at elevating tissue temperatures to the appropriate level.[112] Deep-heating modalities are capable of raising tissues temperatures by 4°C to 4.6°C (7.2°F to 8.3°F),[113,114] whereas superficial heating modalities can raise tissue temperature by only 1°C (1.8°F) at a 3-cm depth.[115] However, the use of hot pack application in combination with ultrasound can also raise tissue temperatures above 4°C (7.2°F).[116]

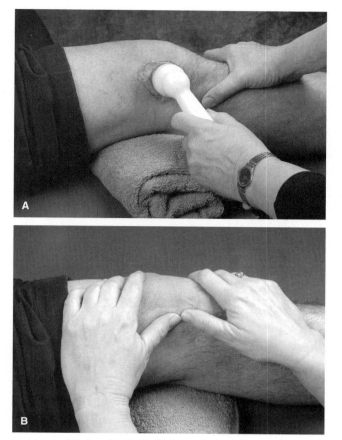

Fig 13•6 (A) Application of ultrasound to the lateral retinaculum of the knee. (B) Prior to passive stretch of the lateral retinaculum.

Joint mobilization or stretching should be done immediately after the application of a heat modality to take advantage of the "stretch window." Tissue temperatures can remain elevated for approximately 3.3 minutes following the application of 3 MHz US to 5°C (9°F).[117] The stretch window is longer if the stretch is applied during the application of the modality. The application of 1 MHz US to target deeper structures may also increase the stretch window, because deeper structures are higher in temperature and the superficial structures serve as a barrier to heat loss.[117]

The duration of tissue stretch is also an important consideration in the management of joint contractures. To have a permanent effect on remodeling of connective tissue, the application of a low-load force should be applied over an extended period of time (e.g., minutes, hours, or days, depending on the severity of contracture). Studies have shown that heat in conjunction with short-duration stretching (e.g., 30-second duration) is

no more effective than short-duration stretching alone.[118] However, heat in conjunction with prolonged stretching (e.g., 10-minute duration) can induce changes in muscle flexibility.[119] Short-wave diathermy and long-duration stretching have been shown to have a positive effect on both hamstring and gastroc-soleus flexibility more than prolonged stretching alone.[119,120]

When considering the use of heat to elevate tissue temperature, the modality must be able to affect the intended tissue. Several recent studies on normal subjects have shown that diathermy and ultrasound in combination with stretch can be more effective in increasing hamstring length or dorsiflexion ROM more than just stretch alone.[119–121] In one study, Draper and associates[119] determined that there was a cumulative effect of consecutive treatments of diathermy and stretch applied to shortened hamstring muscle.

Pulsed short-wave diathermy offers advantages over ultrasound for heating tissues prior to stretching.[113] Short-wave diathermy units can heat a much larger tissue area than ultrasound devices in the same amount of time. In addition, tissue temperatures remain elevated three times longer when heated with pulsed short-wave diathermy.[113] Similar to short-wave diathermy, superficial hot packs can heat a larger volume of tissue; however, the depth of heating is only 1 to 2 cm, so hot packs can target only superficial tissues.

Many of the studies using heat modalities and stretch to enhance motion have been done in normal subjects. We can extrapolate information from these studies to apply to a patient population, but we are still in need of well-designed clinical trials to clarify the candidates and dosages for these techniques. Michlovitz and colleagues[122] performed a systematic review of techniques to restore joint motion in patients following upper extremity injuries and found no studies in the literature that examined the contribution of modalities. Techniques that had moderate evidence in the literature of increasing motion after joint contracture included joint mobilization, a supervised exercise program, and the use of splinting and casting. Heat may be used to precondition the tissue prior to stretch or lengthening techniques. A number of intervention strategies are used to increase the length of adaptively shortened tissues (Box 13-4).

Box 13•4	**Management of Joint Contractures**

- Heat in conjunction with or followed by "stretch" via:
  - Joint mobilization
  - Passive ROM exercises
- Splinting or casting at end ROM
- Surgically lengthening muscles and tendons
- Surgically releasing joint capsule
- Gradual stretching provided by external fixation

In addition to heat decreasing the pain associated with stretching, elevating the temperature of adaptively shortened and contracted structures to high but tolerable levels results in tissue being stretched so that ROM can improve. The stretch should begin after temperature levels have reached their maximum, and a slow, prolonged stretch should be held throughout the period necessary for the tissues to cool back to preheated values. This increased tissue "length" should be maintained over a long duration—that is, up to hours. Devices such as splints and casts can be used to maintain motion increases obtained by facilitating increases in ROM.[122]

Contractures From Burn Scar

Two reports have examined the use of heating modalities and their effect on burn contractures. Burns and Conin[123] advocated the use of paraffin wax daily for 2 to 3 weeks (on average). The paraffin was applied and left on for 15 to 20 minutes, and the patient's limb was held in a position of maximum stretch using some other form of restraint, often a 500-g (1-pound) weight. Their recommendation was to apply the wax to a larger area than necessarily required in order to lubricate the surrounding skin and therefore ease the discomfort of the tight skin and scars that result from burns.

Head and Helms[124] described a similar intervention protocol utilizing paraffin wax and sustained stretch to treat burn contractures. Patients whose joint ROM had plateaued were chosen for this intervention regimen. The temperature of the wax was lowered to 33°C (91.4°F) to accommodate decreases in skin sensitivity and the decreased viability of any newly healed skin. A variety of body parts and joints were treated either by the wax dip method or the wax paint method. The area was covered by a sheet of plastic, and several layers of toweling were used to maintain the heat for 20 to 30 minutes. In a review of 20 patients, joint ROM measurements taken immediately upon removal of the wax demonstrated an increase of 2° to 20°, averaging 8°. The skin appeared softer and was more pliable and more comfortable to the patient. Patients also reported a decrease in joint pain following the wax intervention.

Further Clinical Considerations: Contraindications and Precautions

A comprehensive patient history and physical examination will identify the presence of precautions or contraindications and must be completed prior to modality application. Impaired sensation or circulation will limit the use of heat and cold modalities for pain modulation because of diminished temperature-regulation capabilities. In this situation, electroanalgesia may be the best choice for pain modulation. Before using electrotherapy, however, the practitioner should consider the patient's skin condition and whether active muscle contraction is contraindicated. The skin's condition will influence electrode selection and placement. If muscle contraction must be avoided, then only sensory or noxious levels of electroanalgesia can be used. There are many scenarios that are patient-specific. Earlier chapters in this text provide details regarding the contraindications to and precautions for the use of each of the modalities.

Home Use Versus Clinic Use of Modalities for Pain Control and Loss of Motion

Initial modality selection will most likely occur in the clinic; therefore, selection will be based on equipment availability. Budgetary demands of the clinic limit equipment expenditures, so purchasing decisions are frequently based on evidence of best practice. Because there is a paucity of literature to support the use of specific modalities for specific conditions, there is likely to be a variety of modalities available; however, it is highly likely that certain modalities will not be available for some conditions. Based on sound clinical reasoning, practitioners will select an appropriate modality from the available equipment. Most of the equipment is line-powered, so appropriate electrical outlets must be convenient to patient treatment areas.

The use of modalities at home will also be dependent on:

- Equipment availability
- Ease of application
- Nature of the patient's pain condition
- Patient's cognitive status or availability of caregiver

Practitioners who provide in-home services rely on the use of portable ultrasound and electrotherapy devices. The availability of the equipment in this method of service delivery is similar to that of clinical use previously discussed, except that some of the devices have a battery power source.

Modalities may be incorporated into a home program for pain control and for improving flexibility of soft tissues. Ultrasound units and iontophoresis devices are not available for home use without a practitioner's supervision, so they are excluded from the selection process. If a portable electrotherapy device such as a TENS unit is indicated for pain modulation, then the patient's insurance coverage needs to be considered. These devices may be rented to purchase price or purchased for a patient who requires long-term use. Medical insurance may cover a portion or all of the costs. Practitioners considering this for a patient must determine whether the patient has durable medical equipment (DME) coverage within an insurance plan. Patients most likely will not know this without checking with their insurance provider. Another aspect to determine is whether DME coverage is for the device only or if supplies such as electrodes are also covered.

Practitioners may also have a limited selection of electrotherapy devices to choose from, depending on whether the insurance provider requires that the device come from a specific vendor. A prescription from the patient's physician is often required, along with a letter of medical necessity from either the practitioner or the physician. There are many considerations for the use of electrotherapy in the home setting related just to obtaining the device. If the patient does not have the necessary insurance coverage or is unable to pay for either the device or supplies, an alternative pain control technique must be selected.

Commercial heat and cold modalities are readily available for home use, so these are frequently used for at-home pain modulation. They are also easy for the patient or practitioner to apply in the home setting. Practitioners need to be diligent with patient instructions to ensure safe use at home (Box 13-5). It is strongly recommended that the initial heat or cold application occur in the clinic where the practitioner can observe for harmful signs, such as intolerance to heat or cold sensitivity, respectively. Patients and practitioners should also use caution when using homemade methods of cold or heat applications. It may be perfectly safe to use a bag of frozen vegetables (with a moist towel interface between the bag and the skin) in place of a commercial cold pack. However, the use of a homemade paraffin bath using a double boiler or electric pot may lead to a burn or an electrical shock; therefore, commercial brands of paraffin baths are recommended, not the home-concocted versions.

Selection of the Appropriate Modality for Pain Modulation or Loss of Motion

The practitioner should consider the physiological rationale, biophysical properties, proposed mechanisms of pain modulation or loss of motion, and precautions or contraindications for each modality to ensure the safe and effective use. Selection of a particular modality will depend on the source of pain mediation, location of the target tissue, and the presence of other impairments such as edema or loss of motion. Earlier chapters in this text provide details of these considerations. Modality selection may be influenced by the availability of equipment and supplies. Finally, modality selection should be based on evidence of best practice as reported in the peer-reviewed literature and systematic reviews.

Box 13•5 | **Items to Include in Instructions for Home Use of Modality**

- Duration of application
- Frequency of application
- Timing of application: before or after exercise
- Observation of harmful signs
- Contact number for practitioner

Documentation Tips

When applying modalities to reduce pain or improve range of motion, documentation of the following should be included:

1. Pain
   a. Type, intensity, frequency, and location before and after application
   b. Functional ability before and after application of modality
2. ROM
   a. Before and after application
3. Specific parameters of selected modality (refer to specific chapters for selected modality)
4. Position of patient
5. Integrity of skin before and after application
6. Duration of application
7. Patient response to treatment

☐ REFERENCES

1. Mersky H, Bogduk N, eds. *Classification of Chronic Pain: Descriptions of Chronic Pain Syndromes and Definitions of Pain Terms*. Seattle: IASP Press; 1994.
2. Gifford LS, Butler DS. The integration of pain sciences into clinical practice. *J Hand Ther*. 1997;10:86–95.
3. Urban MO, Gebhart GF. Central mechanisms in pain. *Med Clin North Am*. 1999;83(3):585–596.
4. Hardy MA, Hardy SG. Reflex sympathetic dystrophy: the clinician's perspective. *J Hand Ther*. 1997;10(2):137–150.
5. Walsh MT, Muntzer E. Therapist's management of complex regional pain syndrome (reflex sympathetic dystrophy). In: Mackin E, Callahan AD, Osterman AL, et al, eds. *Rehabilitation of the Hand and Upper Extremity*. St Louis, MO: Mosby; 2002:1707–1724.
6. Fields HL. *Pain*. New York: McGraw-Hill; 1987.
7. Goodman CC, Fuller C, Boissanault W. *Pathology: Implications for the Physical Therapist*. Philadelphia: WB Saunders; 2002.
8. Cyr LM, Ross RG. How controlled stress affects healing tissues. *J Hand Ther*. 1998;11:125–130.
9. O'Rourke D. The measurement of pain in infants, children, and adolescents: from policy to practice. *Phys Ther*. 2004;84(6):560–570.
10. Meghani SH, Cho E. Self-reported pain and utilization of pain treatment between minorities and nonminorities in the United States. *Public Health Nurs*. 2009;26(4):307–316.
11. Spadoni GF, Stratford PW, Solomon PE, Wishart LR. The evaluation of change in pain intensity: a comparison of the P4 and single-item numeric pain rating scales. *J Orthop Sports Phys Ther*. 2004;34(4):187–193.
12. Turk DC, Melzak RM, eds. *Handbook of Pain Assessment*. New York: Guilford Press; 1992.
13. Turk DC, Okifuji A. Assessment of patients' reporting of pain: an integrated perspective. *Lancet*. 1999;353(9166):1784–1788.
14. Finch E, Brooks D, Stratford PW, Mayo NE. *Physical Rehabilitation Outcome Measures: A Guide to Enhance Clinical Decision Making*. Baltimore: Lippincott Williams & Wilkins; 2002.
15. Ecternach JL. Clinical evaluation of pain. *Phys Ther Pract*. 1993;2:14–19.
16. Jensen MP, Karoly P, Braver S. The measurement of clinical pain intensity: a comparison of six methods. *Pain*. 1986;27(1):117–126.
17. Scudds RA. Pain outcome measures. *J Hand Ther*. 2001;14(2):86–90.
18. Melzack R. The McGill Pain Questionnaire: major properties and scoring methods. *Pain*. 1975;1(3):277–299.
19. Morsi E. Continuous-flow cold therapy after total knee arthroplasty. *J Arthroplasty*. 2002;17(6):718–722.
20. Hochberg J. A randomized prospective study to assess the efficacy of two cold-therapy treatments following carpal tunnel release. *J Hand Ther*. 2001;14(3):208–215.
21. Ohkoshi Y, Ohkoshi M, Nagasaki S, Ono A, Hashimoto T, Yamane S. The effect of cryotherapy on intraarticular temperature and postoperative care after anterior cruciate ligament reconstruction. *Am J Sports Med*. 1999;27(3):357–362.
22. Barber FA, McGuire DA, Click S. Continuous-flow cold therapy for outpatient anterior cruciate ligament reconstruction. *Arthroscopy*. 1998;14(2):130–135.
23. Lessard LA, Scudds RA, Amendola A, Vaz MD. The efficacy of cryotherapy following arthroscopic knee surgery. *J Orthop Sports Phys Ther*. 1997;26(1):14–22.
24. Brandner B, Munro B, Bromby LM, Hetreed M. Evaluation of the contribution to postoperative analgesia by local cooling of the wound. *Anaesthesia*. 1996;51(11):1021–1025.
25. Whitelaw GP, DeMuth KA, Demos HA, Schepsis A, Jacques E. The use of the Cryo/Cuff versus ice and elastic wrap in the postoperative care of knee arthroscopy patients. *Am J Knee Surg*. 1995;8(1):28–30; discussion 30–31.
26. Norkin CC, White DJ. *Measurement of Joint Motion: A Guide to Goniometry*. Philadelphia: FA Davis; 2003.
27. Magee D. *Orthopedic Physical Assessment*. Philadelphia: WB Saunders; 2002.
28. McOwan CG, MacDermid JC, Wilton J. Outcome measures for evaluation of scar: a literature review. *J Hand Ther*. 2001;14(2):77–85.
29. Melzack R, Wall PD. Pain mechanisms: a new theory. *Science*. 1965;150(699):971–979.
30. Knutsson E, Mattsson E. Effects of local cooling on monosynaptic reflexes in man. *Scand J Rehabil Med*. 1969;1(3):126–132.
31. Eldred E, Lindsley DF, Buchwald JS. The effect of cooling on mammalian muscle spindles. *Exp Neurol*. 1960;2:144–157.
32. Newton MJ, Lehmkuhl D. Muscle spindle response to body heating and localized muscle cooling: implications for relief of spasticity. *Phys Ther*. 1965;45:91–105.
33. Mense S. Effects of temperature on the discharges of muscle spindles and tendon organs. *Pflugers Arch*. 1978;374(2):159–166.
34. Harris GR, Susman JL. Managing musculoskeletal complaints with rehabilitation therapy: summary of the Philadelphia Panel evidence-based clinical practice guidelines on musculoskeletal rehabilitation interventions. *J Fam Pract*. 2002;51(12):1042–1046.
35. Saeki Y. Effect of local application of cold or heat for relief of pricking pain. *Nurs Health Sci*. 2002;4(3):97–105.
36. Algafly AA, George KP. The effect of cryotherapy on nerve conduction velocity, pain threshold and pain tolerance. *Br J Sports Med*. 2007;41(6):365–369; discussion 369.
37. Saito N, Horiuchi H, Kobayashi S, Nawata M, Takaoka K. Continuous local cooling for pain relief following total hip arthroplasty. *J Arthroplasty*. 2004;19(3):334–337.

38. Singh H, Osbahr DC, Holovacs TF, Cawley PW, Speer KP. The efficacy of continuous cryotherapy on the postoperative shoulder: a prospective, randomized investigation. *J Shoulder Elbow Surg.* 2001;10(6):522–525.

39. Gallo JA, Draper DO, Brody LT, Fellingham GW. A comparison of human muscle temperature increases during 3-MHz continuous and pulsed ultrasound with equivalent temporal average intensities. *J Orthop Sports Phys Ther.* 2004;34(7): 395–401.

40. Miller MD, Wirth MA, Rockwood CA Jr. Thawing the frozen shoulder: the "patient" patient. *Orthopedics.* 1996;19(10):849–853.

41. Ayling J, Marks R. Efficacy of paraffin wax baths for rheumatoid arthritic hands. *Physiotherapy.* 2000;86:190–201.

42. Cetin N, Aytar A, Atalay A, Akman MN. Comparing hot pack, short-wave diathermy, ultrasound, and TENS on isokinetic strength, pain, and functional status of women with osteoarthritic knees: a single-blind, randomized, controlled trial. *Am J Phys Med Rehabil.* 2008;87(6):443–451.

43. McGray RE, Patton NJ. Pain relief at trigger points: a comparison of moist heat and short-wave diathermy. *J Orthop Sports Phys Ther.* 1984;5:175–178.

44. Williams J, Harvey J, Tannenbaum H. Use of heat versus ice for the rheumatoid arthritic shoulder: a pilot study. *Physiother Canada.* 1986;38:8–13.

45. Eyring EJ, Murray WR. The effect of joint position on the pressure of intra-articular effusion. *J Bone Joint Surg Am.* 1964; 46:1235–1241.

46. Michlovitz S, Hun L, Erasala GN, Hengehold DA, Weingand KW. Continuous low-level heat wrap therapy is effective for treating wrist pain. *Arch Phys Med Rehabil.* 2004;85(9): 1409–1416.

47. Nadler SF, Steiner DJ, Erasala GN, et al. Continuous low-level heat wrap therapy provides more efficacy than Ibuprofen and acetaminophen or acute low back pain. *Spine* (Phila Pa 1976). 2002;27(10):1012–1017.

48. Nadler SF, Steiner DJ, Erasala GN, Hengehold DA, Abeln SB, Weingand KW. Continuous low-level heat wrap therapy for treating acute nonspecific low back pain. *Arch Phys Med Rehabil.* 2003;84(3):329–334.

49. Nadler SF, Steiner DJ, Petty SR, Erasala GN, Hengehold DA, Weingand KW. Overnight use of continuous low-level heat wrap therapy for relief of low back pain. *Arch Phys Med Rehabil.* 2003;84(3):335–342.

50. Gam AN, Johannsen F. Ultrasound therapy in musculoskeletal disorders: a meta-analysis. *Pain.* 1995;63(1):85–91.

51. Robertson VJ, Baker KG. A review of therapeutic ultrasound: effectiveness studies. *Phys Ther.* 2001;81(7):1339–1350.

52. van der Windt DA, van der Heijden GJ, van den Berg SG, ter Riet G, de Winter, AF, Bouter LM. Ultrasound therapy for musculoskeletal disorders: a systematic review. *Pain.* 1999;81(3): 257–271.

53. Welch V, Brosseau L, Peterson J, Shea B, Tugwell P, Wells G. Therapeutic ultrasound for osteoarthritis of the knee. *Cochrane Database Syst Rev.* 2001;(3):CD003132.

54. Philadelphia Panel evidence-based clinical practice guidelines on selected rehabilitation interventions for knee pain. *Phys Ther.* 2001;81(10): 1675–1700.

55. Brosseau L, Casimiro L, Robinson V, et al. Therapeutic ultrasound for treating patellofemoral pain syndrome. *Cochrane Database Syst Rev.* 2001;(4):CD003375.

56. Casimiro L, Brosseau L, Robinson V, et al. Therapeutic ultrasound for the treatment of rheumatoid arthritis. *Cochrane Database Syst Rev.* 2002;(3):CD003787.

57. Almeida TF, Roizenblatt S, Benedito-Silva AA, Tufik S. The effect of combined therapy (ultrasound and interferential current) on pain and sleep in fibromyalgia. *Pain.* 2003;104(3): 665–672.

58. Muche JA. Efficacy of therapeutic ultrasound treatment of a meniscus tear in a severely disabled patient: a case report. *Arch Phys Med Rehabil.* 2003;84(10):1558–1559.

59. Ebenbichler GR, Resch KL, Nicolakis P, et al. Ultrasound treatment for treating the carpal tunnel syndrome: randomised "sham" controlled trial. *BMJ.* 1998;316(7133):731–735.

60. Klaiman MD, Shrader JA, Danoff JV, Hicks JE, Pesce WJ, Ferland J. Phonophoresis versus ultrasound in the treatment of common musculoskeletal conditions. *Med Sci Sports Exerc.* 1998;30(9):1349–1355.

61. Craig JA, Bradley J, Walsh DM, Baxter GD, Allen JM. Delayed onset muscle soreness: lack of effect of therapeutic ultrasound in humans. *Arch Phys Med Rehabil.* 1999;80(3):318–323.

62. Gam AN, Warming S, Larsen LH, et al. Treatment of myofascial trigger-points with ultrasound combined with massage and exercise—a randomised controlled trial. *Pain.* 1998; 77(1):73–79.

63. Falconer J, Hayes KW, Chang RW. Effect of ultrasound on mobility in osteoarthritis of the knee. A randomized clinical trial. *Arthritis Care Res.* 1992;5(1):29–35.

64. Binder A, Hodge G, Greenwood AM, Hazleman BL, Page Thomas DP. Is therapeutic ultrasound effective in treating soft tissue lesions? *Br Med J.* 1985;290:512–514.

65. van der Heijden GJMG, Leffers P, Wolters P, et al. No effect of bipolar interferential electrotherapy and pulsed ultrasound for soft tissue shoulder disorders: a randomised controlled trial. *Ann Rheum Dis.* 1999;58(9):530–540.

66. American Physical Therapy Association (APTA). *Electrotherapeutic Terminology in Physical Therapy.* Alexandria, VA: APTA; 1990.

67. Carroll D, Moore RA, McQuay HJ, Fairman F, Tramer M, Leijon G. Transcutaneous electrical nerve stimulation (TENS) for chronic pain. *Cochrane Database Syst Rev.* 2001;(3):CD003222.

68. Deyo RA, Walsh NE, Martin DC, Schoenfeld LS, Ramamurthy S. A controlled trial of transcutaneous electrical nerve stimulation (TENS) and exercise for chronic low back pain. *N Engl J Med.* 1990;7(23):1627–1634.

69. Chesterton LS, Foster NE, Wright CC, Baxter GD, Barlas P. Effects of TENS frequency, intensity and stimulation site parameter manipulation on pressure pain thresholds in healthy human subjects. *Pain.* 2003;106(1-2):73–80.

70. Meyler WJ, de Jongste MJ, Rolf CA. Clinical evaluation of pain treatment with electrostimulation: a study on TENS in patients with different pain syndromes. *Clin J Pain.* 1994;10(1):22–27.

71. Khadilkar A, Odebiyi DO, Brosseau L, Wells GA. Transcutaneous electrical nerve stimulation (TENS) versus placebo for chronic low-back pain. *Cochrane Database Syst Rev.* 2008;(4):CD003008.

72. Rizk TE, Christopher RP, Pinals RS, Higgins AC, Frix R. Adhesive capsulitis (frozen shoulder): a new approach to its management. *Arch Phys Med Rehabil.* 1983;64(1):29–33.

73. Mannheimer C, Carlsson CA. The analgesic effect of transcutaneous electrical nerve stimulation (TENS) in patients with rheumatoid arthritis. A comparative study of different pulse patterns. *Pain.* 1979;6(3):329–334.

74. Mannheimer C, Lund S, Carlsson CA. The effect of transcutaneous electrical nerve stimulation (TENS) on joint pain in patients with rheumatoid arthritis. *Scand J Rheumatol.* 1978; 7(1):13–16.

75. Kumar VN, Redford JB. Transcutaneous nerve stimulation in rheumatoid arthritis. *Arch Phys Med Rehabil.* 1982;63(12): 595–596.

76. Lewis B, Lewis D, Cumming G. The comparative analgesic efficacy of transcutaneous electrical nerve stimulation and a

non-steroidal anti-inflammatory drug for painful osteoarthritis. *Br J Rheumatol.* 1994;33(5):455–460.

77. Rutjes AW, Nuesch E, Sterchi R, et al. Transcutaneous electrostimulation for osteoarthritis of the knee. *Cochrane Database Syst Rev.* 2009;(4):CD002823.

78. Enwemeka CS, Parker JC, Dowdy DS, Harkness EE, Sanford LE, Woodruff LD. The efficacy of low-power lasers in tissue repair and pain control: a meta-analysis study. *Photomed Laser Surg.* 2004;22(4):323–329.

79. Michener LA, Walsworth MK, Burnet EN. Effectiveness of rehabilitation for patients with subacromial impingement syndrome: a systematic review. *J Hand Ther.* 2004;17(2):152–164.

80. Sauers EL. Effectiveness of rehabilitation for patients with subacromial impingement syndrome. *J Athl Train.* 2005;40(3): 221–223.

81. Saunders L. The efficacy of low-level laser therapy in supraspinatus tendinitis. *Clin Rehabil.* 1995;9:126–134.

82. England S, Farrell AJ, Coppock JS, Struthers G, Bacon PA. Low power laser therapy of shoulder tendonitis. *Scand J Rheumatol.* 1989;18(6):427–431.

83. Papadopoulos ES, Smith RW, Cawley MID, Mani R. Low level laser therapy does not aid in the management of tennis elbow. *Clin Rehabil.* 1996;10:9–11.

84. Stasinopoulos DI, Johnson MI. Effectiveness of low-level laser therapy for lateral elbow tendinopathy. *Photomed Laser Surg.* 2005;23:425–430.

85. Basford JR, Sheffield CG, Cieslak KR. Laser therapy: a randomized, controlled trial of the effects of low intensity Nd:YAG laser irradiation on lateral epicondylitis. *Arch Phys Med Rehabil.* 2000;81(11):1504–1510.

86. Brosseau L, Robinson V, Wells G, et al. Low level laser therapy (Classes I, II and III) for treating rheumatoid arthritis. *Cochrane Database Syst Rev.* 2005;(4):CD002049.

87. Oken O, Kahraman Y, Ayhan F, Canpolat S, Yorgancioglu ZR, Oken OF. The short-term efficacy of laser, brace, and ultrasound treatment in lateral epicondylitis: a prospective, randomized, controlled trial. *J Hand Ther.* 2008;21(1):63–67; quiz 68.

88. Hegedus B, Viharos L, Gervain M, Galfi M. The effect of low-level laser in knee osteoarthritis: a double-blind, randomized, placebo-controlled trial. *Photomed Laser Surg.* 2009; 27(4):577–584.

89. Shirani AM, Gutknecht N, Taghizadeh M, Mir M. Low-level laser therapy and myofacial pain dysfunction syndrome: a randomized controlled clinical trial. *Lasers Med Sci.* 2009; 24(5):715–720.

90. Yousefi-Nooraie R, Schonstein E, Heidari K, et al. Low level laser therapy for nonspecific low-back pain. *Cochrane Database Syst Rev.* 2008;(2):CD005107.

91. Santamato A, Solfrizzi V, Panza F, et al. Short-term effects of high-intensity laser therapy versus ultrasound therapy in the treatment of people with subacromial impingement syndrome: a randomized clinical trial. *Phys Ther.* 2009;89(7):643–652.

92. Kahn J. Iontophoresis and ultrasound for postsurgical temporomandibular trismus and paresthesia. *Phys Ther.* 1980; 60(3):307–308.

93. Banta CA. A prospective, nonrandomized study of iontophoresis, wrist splinting, and antiinflammatory medication in the treatment of early-mild carpal tunnel syndrome. *J Occup Med.* 1994;36(2):166–168.

94. Bélanger, A. *Evidenced-Based Guide to Therapeutic Physical Agents.* Philadelphia: Lippincott Williams & Wilkins; 2002.

95. Bertolucci LE. Introduction of antiinflammatory drugs by iontophoresis: double blind study. *J Orthop Sports Phys Ther.* 1982;4(2):103–108.

96. Harris PR. Iontophoresis: clinical research in musculoskeletal inflammatory conditions. *J Orthop Sports Phys Ther.* 1982;4(2):109–112.

97. Delacerda FG. A comparative study of three methods of treatment for shoulder girdle myofascial syndrome. *J Orthop Sports Phys Ther.* 1982;4(1):51–54.

98. Kaya A, Kamanli A, Ardicoglu O, Ozgocmen S, Ozkurt-Zengin F, Bayik Y. Direct current therapy with/without lidocaine iontophoresis in myofascial pain syndrome. *Bratisl Lek Listy.* 2009;110(3):185–191.

99. Reid KI, Dionne RA, Sicard-Rosenbaum L, Lord D, Dubner RA. Evaluation of iontophoretically applied dexamethasone for painful pathologic temporomandibular joints. *Oral Surg Oral Med Oral Pathol.* 1994;77(6):605–609.

100. Cleland JA, Abbott JH, Kidd MO, et al. Manual physical therapy and exercise versus electrophysical agents and exercise in the management of plantar heel pain: a multicenter randomized clinical trial. *J Orthop Sports Phys Ther.* 2009; 39(8):573–585.

101. Nirschl RP, Rodin DM, Ochiai DH, Maartmann-Moe C. Iontophoretic administration of dexamethasone sodium phosphate for acute epicondylitis. A randomized, double-blinded, placebo-controlled study. *Am J Sports Med.* 2003;31(2):189–195.

102. Demirtas RN, Oner C. The treatment of lateral epicondylitis by iontophoresis of sodium salicylate and sodium diclofenac. *Clin Rehabil.* 1998;12(1):23–29.

103. Gudeman SD, Eisele SA, Heidt RS Jr, Colosimo AJ, Stroupe AL. Treatment of plantar fasciitis by iontophoresis of 0.4% dexamethasone. A randomized, double-blind, placebo-controlled study. *Am J Sports Med.* 1997;25(3):312–316.

104. Li LC, Scudds RA, Heck CS, Harth M. The efficacy of dexamethasone iontophoresis for the treatment of rheumatoid arthritic knees: a pilot study. *Arthritis Care Res.* 1996;9(2): 126–132.

105. Baskurt F, Ozcan A, Algun C. Comparison of effects of phonophoresis and iontophoresis of naproxen in the treatment of lateral epicondylitis. *Clin Rehabil.* 2003;17(1):96–100.

106. Chantraine A, Baribeault A, Uebelhart D, Gremion G. Shoulder pain and dysfunction in hemiplegia: effects of functional electrical stimulation. *Arch Phys Med Rehabil.* 1999; 80(3):328–331.

107. Yu DT, Chae J, Walker ME, et al. Intramuscular neuromuscular electric stimulation for poststroke shoulder pain: a multicenter randomized clinical trial. *Arch Phys Med Rehabil.* 2004;85(5):695–704.

108. Gersten JW. Effect of ultrasound on tendon extensibility. *Am J Phys Med.* 1955;34(2):362–369.

109. Rigby BJ. The effect of mechanical extension upon the thermal stability of collagen. *Biochim Biophys Acta.* 1964;79:634–636.

110. Warren CG, Lehmann JF, Koblanski JN. Heat and stretch procedures: an evaluation using rat tail tendon. *Arch Phys Med Rehabil.* 1976;57(3):122–126.

111. Lehmann JF, Masock AJ, Warren CG, Koblanski JN. Effect of therapeutic temperatures on tendon extensibility. *Arch Phys Med Rehabil.* 1970;51(8):481–487.

112. Robertson VJ, Ward AR, Jung P. The effect of heat on tissue extensibility: a comparison of deep and superficial heating. *Arch Phys Med Rehabil.* 2005;86(4):819–825.

113. Garrett CL, Draper DO, Knight KL. Heat distribution in the lower leg from pulsed short-wave diathermy and ultrasound treatments. *J Athl Train.* 2000;35(1):50–55.

114. Draper DO, Knight K, Fujiwara T, Castel JC. Temperature. *Sports Phys Ther.* 1999;29(1):13–8; discussion 19–22.

115. Minton J. 1992 student writing contest—1st runner-up: a comparison of thermotherapy and cryotherapy in enhancing supine, extended-leg, hip flexion. *J Athl Train.* 1993;28(2):172–176.

116. Draper DO, Harris ST, Schulthies S, Durrant E, Knight KL, Ricard M. Hot-pack and 1-MHz ultrasound treatments have an additive effect on muscle temperature increase. *J Athl Train.* 1998;33(1):21–24.

117. Draper DO, Ricard MD. Rate of temperature decay in human muscle following 3 MHz ultrasound: the stretching window revealed. *J Athl Train.* 1995;30(4):304–307.

118. Draper DO, Miner L, Knight KL, Ricard MD. The carry-over effects of diathermy and stretching in developing hamstring flexibility. *J Athl Train.* 2002;37(1):37–42.

119. Draper DO, Castro JL, Feland B, Schulthies S, Eggett D. Short-wave diathermy and prolonged stretching increase hamstring flexibility more than prolonged stretching alone. *J Orthop Sports Phys Ther.* 2004;34(1):13–20.

120. Peres SE, Draper DO, Knight KL, Ricard MD. Pulsed short-wave diathermy and prolonged long-duration stretching increase dorsiflexion range of motion more than identical stretching without diathermy. *J Athl Train.* 2002;37(1):43–50.

121. Knight CA, Rutledge CR, Cox ME, Acosta M, Hall SJ. Effect of superficial heat, deep heat, and active exercise warm-up on the extensibility of the plantar flexors. *Phys Ther.* 2001;81(6):1206–1214.

122. Michlovitz SL, Harris BA, Watkins MP. Therapy interventions for improving joint range of motion: A systematic review. *J Hand Ther.* 2004;17(2):118–131.

123. Burns S, Conin T. The use of paraffin wax in the intervention of burns. *Physiother Can.* 1987;39:258.

124. Head MD, Helms PA. Paraffin and sustained stretching in the treatment of burn contractures. *Burns.* 1977;4:136.

125. Barber FA. A comparison of crushed ice and continuous flow cold therapy. *Am J Knee Surg.* 2000;13(2):97–101; discussion 102.

126. Fountas KN, Kapsalaki EZ, Johnston KW, Smisson HF 3rd, Vogel RL, Robinson JS Jr. Postoperative lumbar microdiscectomy pain. Minimalization by irrigation and cooling. *Spine* (Phila Pa 1976). 1999;24(18):1958–1960.

127. Kullenberg B, Ylipaa S, Soderlund K, Resch S. Postoperative cryotherapy after total knee arthroplasty: a prospective study of 86 patients. *J Arthroplasty.* 2006;21(8):1175–1179.

128. Sellwood KL, Brukner P, Williams D, Nicol A, Hinman R. Ice-water immersion and delayed-onset muscle soreness: a randomised controlled trial. *Br J Sports Med.* 2007;41(6):392–397.

129. Mayer JM, Mooney V, Matheson N, et al. Continuous low-level heat wrap therapy for the prevention and early phase treatment of delayed-onset muscle soreness of the low back: a randomized controlled trial. *Arch Phys Med Rehabil.* 2006;87(10):1310–1317.

130. Dogru H, Basaran S, Sarpel T. Effectiveness of therapeutic ultrasound in adhesive capsulitis. *Joint Bone Spine.* 2008;75(4):445–450.

131. Ainsworth R, Dziedzic K, Hiller L, Daniels J, Bruton A, Broadfield J. A prospective double blind placebo-controlled randomized trial of ultrasound in the physiotherapy treatment of shoulder pain. *Rheumatology (Oxford).* 2007;46(5):815–820.

132. Giombini A, Di Cesare A, Safran MR, Ciatti R, Maffulli N. Short-term effectiveness of hyperthermia for supraspinatus tendinopathy in athletes: a short-term randomized controlled study. *Am J Sports Med.* 2006;34(8):1247–1253.

133. Ebenbichler GR, Erdogmus CB, Resch KL, et al. Ultrasound therapy for calcific tendinitis of the shoulder. *N Engl J Med.* 1999;340(20):1533–1538.

134. D'Vaz AP, Ostor AJ, Speed CA, et al. Pulsed low-intensity ultrasound therapy for chronic lateral epicondylitis: a randomized controlled trial. *Rheumatology (Oxford).* 2006;45(5):566–570.

135. Ozgonenel L, Aytekin E, Durmusoglu G. A double-blind trial of clinical effects of therapeutic ultrasound in knee osteoarthritis. *Ultrasound Med Biol.* 2009;35(1):44–49.

136. Johansson KM, Adolfsson LE, Foldevi MO. Effects of acupuncture versus ultrasound in patients with impingement syndrome: randomized clinical trial. *Phys Ther.* 2005;85(6):490–501.

137. Kurtais Gursel Y, Ulus Y, Bilgic A, Dincer G, van der Heijden GJ. Adding ultrasound in the management of soft tissue disorders of the shoulder: a randomized placebo-controlled trial. *Phys Ther.* 2004;84(4):336–343.

138. Runeson L, Haker E. Iontophoresis with cortisone in the treatment of lateral epicondylalgia (tennis elbow)—a double-blind study. *Scand J Med Sci Sports.* 2002;12(3):136–142.

139. Osborne HR, Allison GT. Treatment of plantar fasciitis by LowDye taping and iontophoresis: short term results of a double blinded, randomised, placebo controlled clinical trial of dexamethasone and acetic acid. *Br J Sports Med.* 2006;40(6):545–549; discussion 549.

140. Dincer U, Cakar E, Kiralp MZ, Kilac H, Dursun H. The effectiveness of conservative treatments of carpal tunnel syndrome: splinting, ultrasound, and low-level laser therapies. *Photomed Laser Surg.* 2009;27(1):119–125.

141. Yeldan I, Cetin E, Ozdincler AR. The effectiveness of low-level laser therapy on shoulder function in subacromial impingement syndrome. *Disabil Rehabil.* 2009;31(11):935–940.

chapter 14

Therapeutic Modalities for Tissue Healing

Ed Mahoney, PT, DPT, CWS

Effective tissue healing requires that the practitioner have a thorough understanding of the normal healing process along with well-developed diagnostic skills and appropriate interventions. When used as part of a treatment plan based on an accurate assessment of the patient's condition, modalities can be effective in promoting healing or reducing the effects of pathology. This chapter provides an overview of modalities used in rehabilitation practice, along with information regarding the most appropriate uses of each modality.

The Normal Healing Process

Understanding the normal healing process will facilitate proper use of a given modality. There are three basic phases of wound healing: inflammation, proliferation, and remodeling. The inflammatory response is the body's nonspecific defense mechanism and begins almost immediately following injury. Inflammation can be triggered by a variety of causes, including trauma, disease, invading pathogens, or allergic reactions. Acute inflammation is characterized by varying degrees of redness, warmth, pain, swelling, and loss of function.

During the inflammatory phase, hemostasis occurs first. It begins almost immediately after injury and is responsible for stopping bleeding at the injury site. The most important cellular component is the platelet, which responds to the injured area, adheres to exposed collagen, and forms a clot that stops the bleeding. In addition, platelets play a role in later stages of healing because of the growth factors that they produce. After the bleeding has been stopped, edema continues to accumulate in the injured area due to extravasation, which is movement of fluid from the blood vessels into the extravascular space. This excess fluid results in swelling, redness, and elevated local temperature. In addition, distention of the tissues and irritation of the nerve ends in the area result in pain. Although inflammation is usually perceived as being negative, a healthy inflammatory process is critical to successful healing. The tissue distention allows for increased space for the influx of phagocytic cells and proteins that set the stage for later phases of healing. These cells, specifically neutrophils and macrophages, are responsible for cleaning the wounded area of nonviable material so the proliferative phase can begin.

The inflammatory phase leads to the proliferative phase, in which fibroblasts and keratinocytes predominate. The function of this phase is to repair the defect. It can last several weeks, depending on the injury. Fibroblasts are attracted to the wound by macrophages in the inflammatory phase and typically arrive in the area 48 to 72 hours after injury. They lay down collagen and elastin, which replace the tissue that was damaged in the initial injury or removed during the inflammatory process. If the injury resulted in a break in the skin, keratinocytes will also be important to cover the wound with a new layer of epithelium.

The final stage is remodeling. During this phase, the newly formed collagen matrix is rearranged and continues to gain tensile strength. This stage is by far the longest and can last in excess of 1 year.

Tissue healing can become problematic at any phase. Tissues may remain chronically inflamed or may fail to regenerate as needed to heal the defect. In an effort to maximize healing, modalities have been used in all phases of wound healing. The remainder of this chapter focuses on common physical modalities and their effect on tissue healing. A more encompassing discussion of the healing process itself is available elsewhere.[1]

Conventional Ultrasound: Therapeutic Ultrasound at 1 and 3 MHZ

Ultrasound (US) at 1 and 3 MHz frequency, which we will call *conventional US*, uses sound energy to promote tissue healing. The physics relating to the generation and transmission of US are discussed in Chapter 4.

This section will focus on how the physical properties of US contribute to tissue healing. When continuous-wave (100% duty cycle) ultrasound at a sufficient intensity is used, tissue temperatures are elevated as acoustic energy is transferred to the tissues in the form of heat. This thermal effect has been shown to reduce pain and muscle spasms in chronic injuries but has not been shown to affect tissue healing directly. Most of the beneficial effects in regard to tissue healing stem from the proposed nonthermal effects of ultrasound, often delivered with a 20% duty cycle pulsed mode.

Pulsed ultrasound transfers energy to the tissues in the same manner that continuous ultrasound does, but the off-time of each pulse period allows the thermal energy to dissipate, so the net tissue temperature is not elevated. A principle nonthermal physiological effect of pulsed US is cavitation. When high-intensity ultrasound is applied, gas bubbles form in the tissue that expand and compress in response to the vibration caused by ultrasound. If the ultrasound intensity is too high, the bubbles will burst and damage the tissue. At therapeutic intensities, the bubbles may expand and contract to a smaller extent without bursting. This is referred to as *stable cavitation* and is not by itself clinically significant.

The stable vibration of the gas bubbles does set the stage for the remaining nonthermal effects, namely acoustic streaming and microstreaming. The vibration of gas bubbles leads to pressure differences within the tissue. The pressure differences cause a circular flow of cellular fluids; this is known as *acoustic streaming*. Acoustic streaming is thought to be responsible for transporting materials within the ultrasound field, which can be used to alter cellular activities. The same general process is occurring at a cellular level and is called *microstreaming*. These microscopic currents are thought to assist with moving ions that have accumulated next to the cell membrane, which will improve the cell's activity. The use of ultrasound shortly after injury has been shown to accelerate the inflammatory process.[2] Since applying ultrasound during the inflammatory phase causes mast cells to release histamine, it is hypothesized that ultrasound may also cause the release of other chemical mediators that are stored in mast cells, which would lead to wound healing.[3]

Several studies have demonstrated that pulsed ultrasound can affect different aspects of cellular metabolism in vitro, including alterations in the amount of calcium uptake and growth factor production.[3-5] Many clinicians recommend ultrasound in the inflammatory phase because these factors can lead to a rapid onset of the proliferative phase of wound healing. In the proliferative phase, pulsed ultrasound increases collagen synthesis by human fibroblasts in vitro.[6] Another proposed mechanism by which pulsed ultrasound promotes tissue healing in the proliferative phase is by increasing the rate that capillary beds and blood vessels form; this has been demonstrated in ischemic muscle.[7] Animal studies examining the role of ultrasound in the remodeling phase of healing are largely inconclusive and appear to support the belief that ultrasound is most effective if begun within the week following injury.

More recent clinical studies have produced variable results when investigating the effects of ultrasound on wound healing. It is difficult to synthesize all the data pertaining to tissue healing to determine if ultrasound is effective because many of the studies lack control groups or are designed with different parameters. Even in studies with similar populations and methods, results are often inconclusive. A meta-analysis by Johannsen et al.[8] reviewed the available literature pertaining to ultrasound in the treatment of chronic leg ulcers. Results showed that US significantly reduced wound size at 4 weeks and 8 weeks compared to controls but did not demonstrate a statistical improvement in the percentage of ulcers that healed completely. Another meta-analysis reported evidence that ultrasound has a mild positive effect in healing venous ulcerations, but the authors point out that the studies were poor-quality research with limited sample sizes.[9] For pressure ulcers, pooled results of randomly controlled trials do not support the use of conventional ultrasound for wound healing.[10] Despite the evidence supporting ultrasound for wound healing in vitro, the results in human wounds are equivocal at this point. More well-designed, controlled trials with larger patient samples are required to determine the true effectiveness of therapeutic ultrasound. Table 14-1 lists contraindications and precautions to US (Table 14-1).

Low-Frequency Ultrasound

The use of low-frequency ultrasound for wound care has recently gained popularity. Low-frequency ultrasound

Table 14•1 Contraindications and Precautions to Therapeutic Ultrasound
Neoplasm
Pregnancy or using US over reproductive tissue
Circulatory impairment
Over eyes
Implants
Over epiphyseal plates in children
Sensory impairment
Bleeding/acute trauma
Over neural tissue
Infection

shares many of the same principles of conventional ultrasound but has a frequency in the 20 to 40 kHz range (i.e., 20,000 to 40,000 Hz), compared to 1 to 3 MHz (1 million to 3 million Hz) for conventional ultrasound. Low-frequency US is further divided into low-intensity and high-intensity forms. The low-intensity form uses a fine saline mist to transmit the ultrasonic energy to the tissues (Fig. 14-1). This form is nonthermal and is used to promote wound healing by cleansing the wound and performing maintenance debridement.

Two randomized studies by Ennis et al. and Kavros et al., combined with five retrospective studies and one prospective controlled study, have shown this form of ultrasound to be effective. Ennis et al.[11] reported that

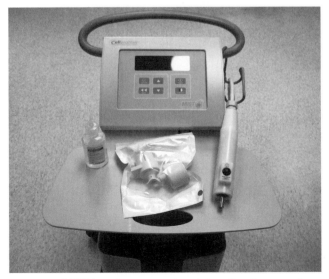

Fig 14•1 MIST low-frequency, low-intensity ultrasound device. *(Courtesy of Celleration, Inc., Eden Prairie, MN.)*

40.7% of diabetic foot ulcers healed within 12 weeks when treated with ultrasound, compared to 14.3% that were treated with a sham device. Kavros et al.[12] reported a 63% reduction in wound size compared to a 29% reduction in the control group.

The second form of low-frequency US involves a higher intensity and is delivered through a probe that is in direct contact with the tissue and causes tissue heating. This is the newest form of US on the market. It is best described as *ultrasound guided debridement* (Fig. 14-2).

Randomized, controlled studies have not been performed to verify low-frequency US to promote wound healing, but numerous case studies and in vitro evidence demonstrate effectiveness in the removal of nonviable tissue and the destruction of bacteria. In vitro, ultrasonic debridement was found to reduce bacterial colonization by greater than 1 $\log_{10}$ compared to irrigation with saline[13] and was shown to increase the periwound skin perfusion pressure.[14]

KEY POINT! High-intensity, low-frequency ultrasound is intended to be used as a debridement agent and therefore should be administered only if debridement is indicated.

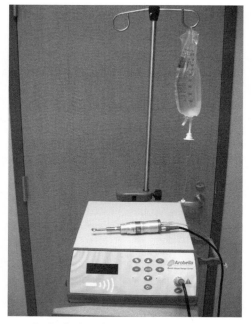

Fig 14•2 Arobella low-frequency, high-intensity US device. *(Courtesy of Arobella, Inc., Minnetonka, MN.)*

Ultraviolet Light

Ultraviolet (UV) radiation has a shorter wavelength (100 to 400 nm) than visible light and lies between the violet end of the visible spectrum and x-rays on the electromagnetic spectrum. UV is a form of light energy and can be further divided into ultraviolet light A (UVA), ultraviolet light B (UVB), and ultraviolet light C (UVC). All are produced naturally by the sun, but UVC is blocked by the ozone layer. As a result, the ambient sunlight we receive contains primarily UVA, small amounts of UVB, and no UVC.

KEY POINT! Although UVC light is blocked by the ozone layer, therapeutic UVC is administered to the tissue via specialized lamps.

In terms of wavelength and energy, UVA is closest to visible light and is the longest (i.e., wavelength) and least energetic, while UVC is the shortest and most powerful, lying closest to x-rays on the light spectrum. That ultraviolet light has been shown to stimulate skin pigmentation, cell proliferation, and epidermal thickness; to enhance blood flow in cutaneous capillaries; to facilitate wound debridement; and to kill bacteria, which supports its use for healing.[15–20]

Because of the vastly different effects of UVA and UVB versus UVC, each will be discussed separately. The most common use for UVA and UVB is the treatment of skin disorders, including psoriasis, vitiligo, lichen planus, dermatitis, and more. When UVA is used to treat skin problems, a skin-sensitizing agent, such as psoralen, is typically applied first to maximize the amount of energy delivered to the tissue. UVB is delivered as broadband or narrowband ultraviolet energy. Broadband UVB (BB-UVB) encompasses the wavelengths of 290 to 320 nm. The lower end of this range (between 290 and 310 nm) has been associated with nontherapeutic responses, such as burning and premature aging, because those wavelengths carry more energy than higher wavelengths do.

In attempts to eliminate the undesirable effects of these lower wavelengths, narrowband UVB (NB-UVB) has been developed. NB-UVB, with a wavelength of 311 to 313 nm, has spread in popularity as the preferred treatment for skin conditions because it avoids the burns and carcinogenic risks associated with

CASE STUDY 14•1 LOW-FREQUENCY ULTRASOUND

A 58-year-old patient with sensory neuropathy developed a heel ulcer due to driving a taxicab for an extended shift. The ulcer presents with a thick layer of adhered fibrinous slough with a moderate odor. Posterior tibial and dorsalis pedis pulses are palpable.

CLINICAL DECISION-MAKING

1. Does the patient have a problem that can be improved with the use of low-frequency ultrasound?
   Answer: Yes, low-frequency ultrasound is intended for the debridement of nonviable tissue, such as slough and eschar.

2. Is the patient appropriate for application of low-frequency ultrasound (i.e., do any of the general precautions or contraindications to low-frequency ultrasound apply, or are there any specific considerations regarding application of low-frequency ultrasound to this patient)?
   Answer: Yes, this patient could benefit from ultrasound since he does not have any hardware in the area or vascular compromise that could be made worse by debridement.

3. What are the specific goals to be achieved with the use of low-frequency ultrasound?
   Answer: Remove nonviable tissue from the wound bed and reduce the risk of infection associated with the presence of that nonviable tissue.

4. What specific low-frequency ultrasound would be appropriate for the patient?
   Answer: Low-frequency, high-intensity ultrasound would be most appropriate to debride extensive

nonviable tissue rapidly. This is not a pain-free procedure, but given the patient's neuropathy, that should not be a factor.

5. What specific parameters of low-frequency ultrasound would be appropriate for this patient?
   Answer: Duty cycle: Continuous
   Frequency: 22.5 to 35 kHz (dependent upon the brand; the frequency is preset)
   Intensity: 100% (reduce if uncomfortable)
   Duration: Depends on the size of the wound. Typically less than 10 minutes

6. What are the proper application procedures for low-frequency ultrasound related to this case?
   Answer:
   - Remove any excess exudate and loosely adhered slough from the wound surface.
   - Examine the wound for any contraindications to ultrasound therapy.
   - Explain the procedure to the patient and position the patient prone if possible to allow for optimal viewing of the heel ulcer.
   - Drape the wound and don personal protective equipment (i.e., gloves, gown, mask) to avoid splash-back.
   - Treat the wound by placing the probe in direct contact with the wound surface and moving it slowly, as in conventional ultrasound.
   - Continue treating as long as a visible reduction in wound bioburden is occurring.

BB-UVB and does not have the side effects of oral psoralen. Because NB-UVB eliminates the lower wavelengths that are primarily responsible for producing erythema, positive results for the treatment of skin conditions have been achieved with fewer burning episodes.[21] Wavelengths longer than NB-UVB do not have an effect on psoriasis and vitiligo. Shorter wavelengths produce more burning, which could potentially be more carcinogenic.[22] NB-UVB was found to have comparable healing results with fewer burns and has longer duration of remission of psoriasis compared to those treated with broadband therapy.[23] Because of the lower energy emitted, larger starting doses are needed compared to broadband and more lamps are needed because of the reduced power.

The evidence for ultraviolet light as an effective modality for treating skin disorders is overwhelmingly positive. Two of the most common disorders treated are vitiligo and psoriasis. The application of NB-UVB or psoralens and UVA (PUVA) are considered to be the most important treatments for patients with vitiligo that affects more than 10% to 20% of the skin surface.[24] Several articles have demonstrated NB-UVB to be superior to PUVA treatment as assessed by stability of the disease after treatment and color match of the repigmented skin for generalized vitiligo.[25–27]

It is proposed that repigmentation occurs when NB-UVB is applied to vitiligo because it stimulates proliferation and migration of melanocytes, which are the cells responsible for skin pigment.[28] This has been shown in vitro but has not been demonstrated in vivo to this point. The results of NB-UVB in the treatment of psoriasis are also very positive. Narrowband therapy has been shown to produce similar responses compared to broadband therapy, with a lower risk of burn, and has demonstrated a longer period of remission between flare-ups.[23]

In addition to its effectiveness, UVB has proved to be a safe treatment option. There is a low incidence of acute adverse events, and it can be used effectively at suberythemogenic doses, which eliminates the discomfort associated with burns and reduces the risk of cancer.[22,29] However, there is conflicting evidence regarding the cancer risk associated with UVB treatment. In animal studies, narrowband therapy has been implicated with DNA damage typically seen in cancer, and some human studies report a higher carcinogenesis of narrowband compared to broadband.[30] There are also studies reporting no evidence for increased skin cancer risk with UVB treatment.[31] Ultimately, a greater long-term risk is expected with higher doses. As a result, the smallest amount of UVB exposure necessary to achieve results should be used. Equivocal results have been shown in the treatment of psoriasis when NB-UVB was administered twice per week or four times per week.[32] Based on this, two times per week as opposed to four may be the preferred treatment frequency.

Clinical Controversy

Exposure to ultraviolet light is associated with certain cancers. However, it is an effective treatment for several skin diseases. Due to this conflict, it is recommended that the smallest effective dose be utilized to minimize the cumulative effects of ultraviolet light.

Unlike UVA and UVB, UVC is effective at reducing bacterial colonization in wounds and has been used for that purpose for the better part of a century. During the middle of the last century, its use fell out of favor as new antibiotics came into use and the effects of long-term radiation became apparent. However, there has been a resurgence in the use of UV as bacteria continue to develop resistance to antibiotics and clinicians revert to previous methods to eradicate them.

UVC radiation has wavelengths between 200 and 280 nm and is typically delivered from a lamp in the 250 nm wavelength range. At this wavelength, the erythemal effectiveness peaks but rarely causes burning as UVB and UVA do, even at high doses.[18] This is due to the poor penetration of UVC, as it is almost completely absorbed by the epidermis. In addition, it is thought that UVC is less carcinogenic because any mutations it may cause will be sloughed off by the constantly changing epidermis.[33]

UVC has repeatedly exhibited effectiveness against bacteria, including those that are resistant to antibiotics. Both in vivo and in vitro studies have impressive outcomes. In vivo results have demonstrated 100% kill rates of methicillin-resistant staphylococcus aureus at 180 seconds. In vitro studies have demonstrated effectiveness in reducing bacteria in artificially inoculated animal wounds.[34,35] The total exposure time to eradicate bacteria from chronic wounds is longer; this is due to several factors, including increased amounts of bacteria and bacteria that have invaded the tissue. Studies of a 3-minute exposure time of UVC to wounds of various etiologies showed greatly reduced numbers of bacteria, but the bacteria were not completely eradicated from the wound (Fig. 14-3). Colonized superficial wounds respond well, but results are not as strong for heavily infected wounds or deep wounds.[36]

For any ultraviolet treatment, the proper dose needs to be calculated. The power of the lamp, the distance the lamp is held from the skin, the patient's previous

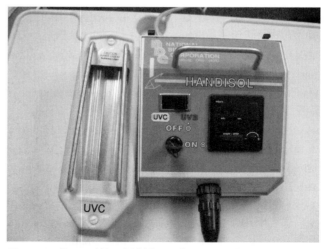

Fig 14•3 DermaWand UVC applicator and control unit. Wand can be changed to provide UVB as well. *(Courtesy of National Biological Corporation, Twinsburg, OH.)*

exposure to ultraviolet energy, and any medications that may sensitize the patient to UV light must all be recorded. The most important factor that needs to be determined is treatment duration, which ultimately depends on the patient's skin color. Individuals with light skin will burn faster than those with darker skin and must be treated with a smaller dose. As the amount of pigment increases in the skin, the amount of UV therapy applied will have to be raised to get the desired benefit. This is the same thing that occurs at the beach when fair-skinned people burn easily but those with a tan do not. Dosing for UV therapy is determined by performing a minimal erythema dose (MED) test. In this test, the smallest amount of time needed to produce a mild sunburn is calculated (Box 14-1).

Electrical Stimulation

A review of the general principles of electrotherapy is suggested prior to reading this section. For an in-depth discussion on the basics of electrotherapy, refer to Chapters 9 and 10 of this text.

Electrical stimulation (ES) for tissue healing is intended to accentuate the normal healing process that occurs when skin is injured. Foulds and Barker[37] identified a separation of charge between the interior and exterior of the human skin. Based on these findings, they were able to determine that the skin's exterior has a negative polarity relative to the skin's interior. This difference creates potential energy in the same way that a battery stores energy; thus, it is referred to as a human skin battery (see Chapter 9). A primary factor in the production of the negative external polarity is the movement of sodium (Na+) along its concentration gradient from the external skin surface into the epithelial cells. When there is a break in the skin, the interior of the wound is positively charged compared to the periwound area, which creates a voltage difference at the wound margin. This difference in electrical charges drives the healing process—as cells and ions are drawn to areas of opposite polarity and repelled from areas with the same polarity.

When ES is applied to the skin to promote tissue healing, it produces current flow in the tissues that mimics the natural skin battery. The two most com-

monly used waveforms to promote tissue healing are high-volt pulsed current (HVPC) and low-intensity direct current (LIDC, or microcurrent; for a review of the specifics of these current types, see Chapter 9). HVPC and LIDC are both monophasic currents that result in a net flow of charged particles, which in turn yields the desired effects of wound healing. The process of attracting charged cells to an electric field of opposite polarity is known as *galvanotaxis*. When a positively charged electrode (anode) is placed over a wound, cells and ions that are negatively charged will be drawn toward the electrode. Cells and ions that are positively charged will be repelled.

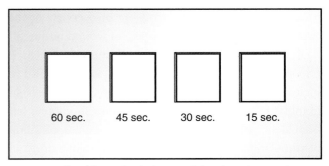

60 sec.   45 sec.   30 sec.   15 sec.

Fig 14•4 Card for calculating a minimal erythema dose.

CASE STUDY 14•2 ULTRAVIOLET LIGHT

An 80-year-old female is referred for treatment of an infected venous ulceration on the medial lower leg. Upon removal of the dressing, you note a strong, foul odor with a green tint to the drainage.

CLINICAL DECISION-MAKING

1. Does the patient have a problem that can be improved with the use of ultraviolet light?
   Answer: Yes, this patient could benefit from ultraviolet C (UVC) in order to reduce the bacterial colonization of the wound.

2. Is the patient appropriate for application of ultraviolet light (i.e., do any of the general precautions or contraindications to ultraviolet light apply, or are there any specific considerations regarding application of ultraviolet light to this patient)?
   Answer: If cancer, acute psoriasis, herpes simplex, or eczema is not present in the periwound skin, then the patient is appropriate for UVC therapy.

3. What are the specific goals to be achieved with the use of ultraviolet light?
   Answer: Eradicate bacteria from the wound, which will reduce wound odor.

4. What specific ultraviolet light would be appropriate for the patient?
   Answer: UVC radiation (200 to 280 nm wavelength) is most effective for reducing bacterial loads on a wound.

5. What specific parameters of ultraviolet light would be appropriate for this patient?
   Answer: Treatment with UVC ranging from 250 to 280 nm is most effective for destroying bacteria. A minimal erythema dose is not typically performed with UVC. Therapy for infection is typically 180 seconds daily.

6. What are the proper application procedures for ultraviolet light related to this case?
   Answer:
   - Cleanse the wound and pat it dry.
   - Apply sun protectant or layer of petrolatum to any periwound skin that may be exposed.
   - Both the patient and therapist should wear eye protection.
   - Allow the lamp to warm up prior to treatment.
   - Position the patient so the UVC lamp can be held 1 inch from the wound surface, and treat for 180 seconds daily.

KEY POINT! When the electrodes are placed close together in a direct current circuit, an increased amount of charge builds up because there is less area for it to disperse. This can be damaging to the skin and must be monitored carefully.

Studies pertaining to the effects of galvanotaxis on different cell types have led to a general understanding of which electrode setup will be most effective during different stages of healing. For example, if the goal of stimulation is to produce granulation tissue, the cathode is placed over the wound to attract fibroblasts that are positively charged. (See Table 14-2 for an overview of the appropriate polarity for each aspect of wound healing.)

In addition to the effects of galvanotaxis, which is responsible for cell migration, ES has also been shown to increase cellular proliferation (the creation of new cells) in fibroblasts. An increase in DNA and protein synthesis has been identified in several studies involving the application of stimulation.[39–42] In one study by Bourguignon,[43] an increase in calcium uptake and an upregulation of insulin receptors was reported. These changes led to an increase in protein and DNA synthesis, which is important for the production of granulation tissue.

None of the cellular mechanisms that occur in response to ES would be of any significance if they did not translate into improved clinical outcomes. There is an abundance of clinical evidence supporting both the LIDC and high-voltage approaches to tissue healing. (See Table 14-3 for a brief summary of the effects of LIDC on tissue healing in humans.)

Table 14•2 Choosing the Appropriate Current Based on the Goal of Treatment

Treatment Goal	Cells Recruited	Polarity of Current
Debridement	Macrophages	(+)
	Neutrophils	(+)
Infection	Activated neutrophils	(−)
Granulation	Fibroblasts	(−)
Wound contraction	Myofibroblasts	(−)
Epithelialization	Keratinocytes	(−)
	Epidermal cells	(+)

Adapted from Kloth, 2005.[38]

CASE STUDY 14•3 ELECTRICAL STIMULATION

A 74-year-old male sustained a skin tear to his left upper arm as a result of a fall in his bathroom. The wound has not responded to 6 weeks of conservative therapy and remains red with no signs of new skin growth.

CLINICAL DECISION-MAKING

1. Does the patient have a problem that can be improved with the use of electrical stimulation?
   Answer: Yes, impaired wound healing can be addressed through the application of electrical stimulation.

2. Is the patient appropriate for application of electrical stimulation (i.e., do any of the general precautions or contraindications to electrical stimulation apply, or are there any specific considerations regarding application of electrical stimulation to this patient)?
   Answer: As long as there is no cancer in the wound or osteomyelitis in the arm and the electrodes are not placed over the neck or thorax, the patient is appropriate for electrical stimulation.

3. What are the specific goals to be achieved with the use of electrical stimulation?
   Answer: Promotion of epithelial growth to close the wound.

4. What specific electrical stimulation would be appropriate for the patient?
   Answer: Monophasic current applied as either microampere direct current, or high-voltage pulsed current.

5. What specific parameters of electrical stimulation would be appropriate for this patient?
   Answer: Low-intensity direct current (LIDC) applied between 100 and 800 µA or high-voltage pulsed current (HVPC) between 75 and 150 V with the positive pole at the wound site to promote skin growth. Apply directly over the wound to avoid damaging fragile periwound skin. Duration is ideally 60 minutes daily.

6. What are the proper application procedures for electrical stimulation related to this case?
   Answer:
   • Cleanse the skin to remove oil and dry skin that will impair electrical current.
   • Select a device capable of producing a low-intensity direct current or pulsed monophasic current waveform.
   • In the case of dry, reusable electrodes, apply gel or hydrogel moistened gauze to the entire electrode surface. Gel is not needed for adhesive electrodes (see photo).

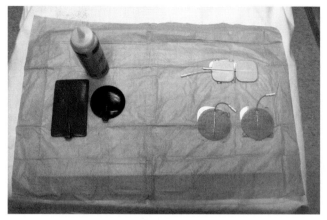

Example electrodes used for electrical stimulation. Nonadhesive electrodes and conducting gel are on the left, and adhesive electrodes are on the right.

• Select the desired polarity of the treatment electrode based on the desired effect; in this case, positive for epithelialization.

Positive	Negative
Epithelialization	Granulation
Autolysis/debridement	Infection
Promote inflammation	Edema reduction

• Place desired electrode over treatment area and a larger dispersive electrode 15 to 30 cm away. If an open wound is present, the treatment electrode may be placed directly over the wound or adjacent to it.
• Voltage: Will be dependent upon waveform used.
   • HVPC: Should be set to a strong tingling paresthesia in patients with intact sensation. If patient is insensate, voltage can be increased until slight muscle twitching is evident and then reduced until twitching stops. This voltage range is typically between 75 and 150 V with HVPC.
   • LIDC: This form of electrical stimulation will be subsensory, so feedback from the patient is not possible. Positive effects of this form of stimulation have been reported with current ranging from less than 100 µA to 800 µA.
• Duration: Ideally, 60 minutes per day, 7 days per week.

Clinical evidence for the use of high-voltage pulsed current is also strong and corroborates the findings in animal and in vitro models. In human studies, HVPC has led to improved blood flow,[52,53] faster healing rates,[54] and higher percentages of wounds that heal versus a control group.[54] A meta-analysis by Gardner et al.[54] examined the effects of various forms of ES on chronic wound healing. Based on data from the 15 studies reviewed—consisting of 591 ulcers in the treatment group and 212 in the control group—the authors found a significant increase in the overall healing rates when ES was used compared to the control group. A statistical difference was not obtained when healing rates for different forms of ES were compared. Other forms of ES have been successfully used in wound care, but a discussion of them is beyond the scope of this chapter.

Infrared Energy

Initially, infrared energy was used for its local heating (i.e., thermal effect), but this is no longer a common practice for most clinicians. Currently, the primary use for infrared energy is to restore protective sensation, which is often lost in diseases that affect the peripheral nerves, most notably diabetes, and is a primary risk factor in the development of foot ulcers.[55] Many practitioners have used monochromatic infrared energy (MIRE) to restore sensation to affected limbs. The MIRE device delivers an 890 nm wavelength of infrared energy that is transmitted directly to the skin via pads containing 60 diodes each.[56] (Figs. 14-5 and 14-6).

MIRE was initially approved by the FDA for increasing circulation and reducing pain.

KEY POINT! The proposed mechanism of action is the stimulation of nitric oxide (NO) release from hemoglobin into the circulation when hemoglobin absorbs the infrared energy. Since NO is a strong vasodilator, increased amounts of it under the diodes will lead to improved circulation in that area.[56]

The current use of MIRE is to improve sensation and is thought to work in the same manner, with increased circulation leading to healthier nerves and a return of sensation.

Experimentally, results from studies using MIRE to improve sensation are equivocal. A number of studies report that MIRE had a positive effect on loss of protective sensation, ranging from mild improvement to complete resolution.[57–61] Conversely, there are independent studies that did not find MIRE to be beneficial for

---

Table 14•3 Low-Intensity Direct Current and Tissue Healing in Humans

Author	Study Type and Population	Parameters	Polarity	Results
Junger et al., 1997[44]	15 pt case series; venous ulcers	630 µA at 128 pps with pulse duration of 140 µs with for 30 min/day	(−) for 7–14 d, then (+) for 7–10 d, then (−)	Improved capillary density; ulcer size reduced 63%
Assimacopoulos, 1968[45]	Three case reports; venous ulcers	50–100 µA continuously	(−)	All healed within 42 days
Wolcott et al., 1969[46]	5 pts in a clinical trial; venous ulcers	200–800 µA for ≥ 2 hr/d	(−)	Higher rate of healing than control
Wolcott et al., 1969[46]	75 ulcers in a clinical trial; ischemic ulcers	200–800 µA for ≥ 2 hr/d	(−)	40% healed in treatment group; 0% of controls healed
Gault et al., 1976[47]	Controlled trial; 106 ulcers in 76 patients; ischemic ulcers	200–800 µA for 6 hr/d	(−) for 3 days or until 3 days after infection cleared, then (+)	48% healed and another 11% improved > 95%; no control ulcers healed
Wolcott et al., 1969[46]	6 pts in a clinical trial; multiple pressure ulcers	200–800 µA for ≥ 2 hr/d	(−)	5/6 of wounds treated with stimulation healed; 0/6 of controls healed
Barron et al., 1985[48]	Prospective study; 6 pts with nonhealing pressure ulcers (retrospective)	600 µA, 3x/wk for 3 weeks	Biphasic	5/6 healed in 1 month; 95% average area of reduction
Wood et al., 1993[49]	Double-blind, controlled study; 74 pts with chronic stage II and III pressure ulcers	600 µA pulsed current 3x/wk for 8 weeks	(−)	Treatment: 58% healed; 72.9% reduced > 80%; 0 increased in size

Control: 3% healed; 12.9% reduced > 80%; 32.3% increased in size |
| Huckfeldt et al., 2007[50] | RCT; 30 pts with full thickness burns | 50–100 µA dependent upon wound resistance | (+) | 36% faster healing in treatment group |
| Carley et al., 1985[51] | 30 pt clinical trial with wound of various etiologies | 300–700 µA depending on innervation of skin | (−) for first 3 days, then reversed | Treatment group healed 1 to 2.5x faster than paired controls after 3 weeks of stimulation |

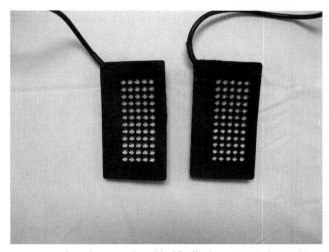

Fig 14•5 Anodyne pads with 60 diodes per pad used to deliver MIRE. *(Courtesy of Anodyne Therapy, LLC, Tampa, FL.)*

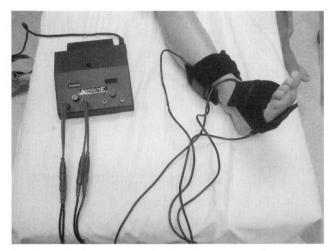

Fig 14•6 Pad placement for MIRE treatment of neuropathy: two pads on lower leg and one each on the plantar and dorsal aspects of the foot.

treating impaired sensation when compared to control groups.[62–64] The authors of many studies point out that small sample sizes may limit the power of the study, making it difficult to identify a difference between the control and treatment group.

Clinical Controversy

In addition to the controversy over MIRE's effectiveness, there is also disagreement pertaining to the duration of effect, if any, once the modality is discontinued.

CASE STUDY 14•4 INFRARED

A 60-year-old patient with diabetes is referred for the treatment of an open, noninfected foot ulcer. Examination results reveal strong pulses with decreased sensation on the plantar aspect of both feet.

CLINICAL DECISION-MAKING

1. Does the patient have a problem that can be improved with the use of infrared energy?
   Answer: Some evidence exists that infrared energy can be beneficial in reversing sensory loss associated with diabetes. This may be helpful in healing the foot ulcer, as the patient would become more aware of how often he is walking on it.

2. Is the patient appropriate for application of infrared energy (i.e., do any of the general precautions or contraindications to infrared energy apply, or are there any specific considerations regarding application of infrared energy to this patient)?
   Answer: Yes, the patient does not have any condition that would preclude the use of infrared energy.

3. What are the specific goals to be achieved with the use of infrared energy?
   Answer: Improve sensation to the feet for the purpose of increasing the patient's awareness of his foot and weight-bearing activities.

4. What specific infrared energy would be appropriate for the patient?
   Answer: Monochromatic infrared energy (MIRE) applied at 890 nm through multiple diode pads that are secured to the skin.

5. What specific parameters of infrared energy would be appropriate for this patient?
   Answer: Specific data regarding optimal duration and frequency have not been determined for the use of MIRE.

6. What are the proper application procedures for infrared energy related to this case?
   Answer:
   • Cleanse the skin to remove any dirt, oil, dry skin, and so on.
   • MIRE diodes can be applied directly to the skin or over a plastic covering to avoid contamination.
   • The diodes are secured in place to achieve optimal contact with the skin but should not be so tight that they cause indentations or cut off circulation.
   • The machine is turned on and the area is treated for 20 to 30 minutes per day, 3 to 7 days per week.[56]

At present, there are still many unexplored factors that may play a role in the effectiveness of MIRE therapy. Severity of neuropathy at the initiation of therapy appears to be related to the effectiveness of MIRE.[59] In addition, there is no clearly defined frequency and duration of treatment in the literature that offers the best evidence for successful outcomes. To truly determine the effectiveness of MIRE, well-designed, double-blind studies with larger sample sizes need to be performed. There is currently no consistent body of evidence supporting MIRE as a modality for the treatment of sensory neuropathy.

Intermittent Pneumatic Compression

This section will focus on the physiological effects of compression therapy that promote wound healing. The use of intermittent pneumatic compression (IPC) is covered in more detail in Chapter 8.

Despite the wide use of intermittent compression, no single theory has been proven regarding the exact mechanism of action. Proposed effects of IPC can be mechanical or chemical in nature. The mechanical effects, as identified in a study by Khanna et al.,[65] include improved vascularity, cyclical loading, and a redirection of blood flow. When IPC is applied, it squeezes the limb, which compresses blood vessels and causes blood to move forward through the vessel (Fig. 14-7). The increased force leads to an increased peak flow velocity, which is thought to reduce the

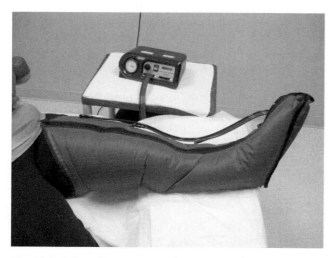

Fig 14•7 Intermittent pneumatic compression applied to treat an ulceration caused by venous insufficiency. (*Courtesy of Bio Compression Systems, Inc., Moonachie, NJ.*)

amount of blood that pools in the sinuses around the valves.[66] When the pooling of blood is reduced in the veins, the pressure there will also be reduced. This creates a larger pressure gradient between the arterial system and the venous system, which leads to increased blood flow to the affected limb. With more oxygenated blood in the vessels, there is more blood available for tissue healing, including soft tissue and bone.[67,68] The theory that increased blood flow caused by compression will bring nutrients to tissues to assist with the healing process seems to be supported by the studies discussed in Chapter 8.

The other proposed mechanical effects pertain specifically to injured bone. Applying IPC to muscles proximal to a fracture site has been shown to increase cyclical loading in the bones of sheep. It is hypothesized that the same effect would be achieved in humans, leading to increased bone formation at the fracture site.[69] The third proposed mechanical effect is a redirection of blood flow that occurs when the venous system is compressed. When compression is applied to the leg, raising the pressure in the venous system, venous channels in the long bones are recruited to assist with venous circulation. Ultimately, adding IPC increases blood flow to the bone in the area being compressed, which is thought to assist with bone healing. Significant increases in blood flow to the periosteum following IPC have been demonstrated in rabbits.[67] In humans, adding IPC to one limb following the injection of a radiopharmaceutical agent led to significantly increased uptake by the long bones, indicating that more blood was being delivered to the bones under compression.[70]

One of the proposed chemical effects of IPC is an increased production of nitric oxide. This effect has been demonstrated experimentally in cultured endothelial cells by exposing them to a cyclic strain at 60 cycles per minute and in rats following 30 minutes of IPC.[71,72] It is thought that nitric oxide is produced in response to the shear stresses on the endothelium of the blood vessels created by compression.[73] Since nitric oxide is a vasodilator, it is believed that an increase in nitric oxide will lead to increased blood flow to the area. A second chemical effect of pneumatic compression is an increase in certain proinflammatory agents. The proposed benefit of this relates to the secondary effect of these agents. In addition to their role in promoting inflammation, chemical mediators, such as substance P and calcitonin gene-related peptide, play a role in the early phase of tissue healing.[74] An investigation by Dahl et al.[68] identified increased levels of these mediators, along with elevated sensory neuropeptides following daily compression therapy given to rats with imposed Achilles tendon injuries. The increased levels of mediators were accompanied by increased production of fibroblasts and a higher blood vessel density in the area of treatment.

Clinical Controversy

Despite the widely held belief that arterial compromise is a contraindication to compression therapy, there is evidence that high pressures applied for short durations may promote healing when ischemia is present.[75]

Superficial Heating Modalities

There are several modalities available to the practitioner that are designed to produce superficial heating through conduction. The primary indications for superficial heating are to reduce pain, promote tissue distensibility, and relieve muscle spasms. However, heating injured tissues does have a theoretical benefit in regard to healing, so the proposed mechanisms for how this may occur with superficial heat will be addressed briefly.

The superficial heating modalities most commonly used are hot packs and paraffin wax. Hot packs can be divided into disposable and reusable varieties as well as moist and dry. The disposable hot packs are rarely used in clinical practice because of the excessive cost and waste associated with them. When a hot pack is heated in a microwave or hydrocollator or through an exothermic reaction (in the case of a disposable pack), the pack absorbs heat. The hot pack is then placed on the skin over a protective layer of towels to prevent burning. The heat will be transferred from the hot pack to the skin, with a 1 cm to 2 cm layer of towels acting as insulation to prevent the skin temperature from rising too high. This layer is critical since hydrocollator temperatures are typically set between 70°C and 80°C (158°F and 176°F), and the desired skin temperature achieved is approximately 40°C (104°F).

KEY POINT! Tissue temperature will increase faster when superficial heat is applied under compression therapy. If compression must be applied (e.g., with a patient lying on a hot pack), extra layers of towels should be placed over the hot pack to avoid tissue trauma.

Similarly, paraffin wax transfers heat to the skin through conduction. To accomplish this, the affected extremity is repeatedly dipped in wax until a layer of wax 2 mm to 3 mm thick is produced. It is then wrapped to provide insulation. Wax can be comfortably applied at temperatures of 50°C because the wax will cool and solidify when it contacts the skin. The wax is typically left in place for 15 to 20 minutes, at which point it is adding a small amount of heat to the tissue and providing insulation that greatly reduces the amount of heat loss. This is a common superficial heating modality in the treatment of rheumatoid arthritis and burns in areas of potential contracture formation, most notably the hands.

Although studies using superficial heat to promote tissue healing are lacking, superficial heating is known to raise the local skin temperature and lead to vasodilation.[76,77] An elevated local metabolism and increased blood flow accompanying increases in temperature also assist tissue healing. A second proposed mechanism by which superficial heat could promote healing is the reduction of muscle spasms, which can lead to local ischemia. Wright and Sluka[78] describe the role that heating could play on reducing ischemia by increasing the firing of the type Ib Golgi tendon organ afferent fibers. This reduces the firing of the agonist muscles, which would reduce muscle spasms and, in turn, reverse localized ischemia. Despite the documented local improvement in blood flow that could potentially contribute to tissue healing, there is a lack of evidence that supports superficial heat as a primary modality to promote tissue healing.

If superficial heating is used, either as a primary modality to increase blood flow or in conjunction with another modality, several concerns need to be addressed. The skin should always be inspected prior to initiating therapy with a hot pack. The clinician should assess for skin sensitivity to hot and cold and arterial perfusion, and he or she should perform a thorough history to identify any condition or medication that may make the tissue intolerant to heat. Because metal conducts heat faster than soft tissue, caution must be taken when applying heat to any area with implants.

A 49-year-old male with a history of peripheral vascular disease presents with a painful lesion to the dorsum of the foot. The limb is cool to the touch, and he reports hanging the foot off the side of the bed to get minor pain relief.

CLINICAL DECISION-MAKING

1. Does the patient have a problem that can be improved with the use of superficial heat?

   Answer: Although the application of superficial heat would cause vasodilation and theoretically increase blood flow to the ischemic leg, it would not be a safe option when applied with a hot pack.

2. Is the patient appropriate for application of superficial heat (i.e., do any of the general precautions or contraindications to superficial heat apply, or are there any specific considerations regarding application of superficial heat to this patient)?

   Answer: At this point, the patient is not appropriate for the application of superficial heat due to the lack of blood flow to the leg. Heat applied at temperatures typical of hot packs and paraffin wax could cause further damage, as there is no mechanism to dissipate the heat.

3. What are the specific goals to be achieved with the use of superficial heat?

   Answer: Low-level warming should take place to prevent vasoconstriction.

4. What specific superficial heat would be appropriate for the patient?

   Answer: Conservative mechanisms would be more appropriate to provide warmth to the foot, such as a lamb's wool boot or similar device.

5. What specific parameters of superficial heat would be appropriate for this patient?

   Answer: Superficial heat should not be applied to the ischemic area of this patient. Little evidence exists pertaining to the effectiveness of heat applied more proximally.

6. What are the proper application procedures for superficial heat related to this case?

   Answer: Avoid excessive heating mechanisms. Keep limb covered and warm with boot, socks, blankets, and so on.

Superficial heating should be avoided in cases of poor vascularity because the lack of blood flow will impair heat dissipation via convection. Finally, because heating leads to vasodilation and increased blood flow to the area, it is contraindicated in the presence of cancer and is generally harmful in the presence of heavily draining wounds, as drainage will increase. Even if there are no contraindications, the patient should still be frequently reassessed during the treatment. The patient should be given some mechanism, such as a bell, to call for the therapist if the heat source is getting too hot.

Cryotherapy

Because of its role in reducing edema, cryotherapy, in the form of ice or cold packs, is a common treatment during the initial inflammatory process following soft tissue injuries. As the cold pack is placed on the skin, energy is transferred between the two through conduction, leading to warming of the ice pack and cooling of the tissue. As tissues cool, blood vessels in the area constrict and microvascular permeability decreases.[79,80] Despite the wide use of cold therapy, few studies have been performed to determine the optimal parameters of treatment (i.e., duration and frequency of treatment and temperature of the cold pack at the beginning of treatment).

A study by Enwemeka et al.[81] investigated the effects of cold pack therapy at different tissue depths. For superficial tissues (1 cm deep) in healthy individuals, a significant drop in temperature was observed following 8 minutes of cold pack therapy. Although there was a rapid change superficially, 20 minutes of cold pack therapy did not reduce the temperature of tissues deeper than 2 cm. Interestingly, the authors noted a temperature reduction in the deeper tissues after the cold pack was removed. One factor that may play a role in this is the shunting of blood from the superficial vessels to the deep vessels due to vasoconstriction followed by a reversed flow of blood from the deep to superficial vessels to reheat the tissue. The effective depth of penetration depends on the amount of circulation in the area as well as the type and amount of tissue that is present. Ice used to lower the temperature of deeper tissues will be impaired by adipose tissue because of its insulating qualities.

KEY POINT! With the exception of ice massage, ice should never be placed directly on the skin due to the risk of frostbite.

Due to different quantities of adipose tissue between species, it is difficult to base recommendations for treatment duration and frequency of cryotherapy on animal studies, but the physiological changes may be the same. Closed tissue injuries in rats responded favorably to the application of cryotherapy. Improvements in functional capillary density, decreased intramuscular pressures, reduced number of granulocytes, and reduced tissue damage were all noted with cryotherapy.[82]

These findings support the use of ice in the inflammatory phase to reduce edema, which can speed up the healing process. Although ice is commonly used in all phases of rehabilitation to manage pain and muscle spasms, there is no evidence that it promotes healing beyond the inflammatory phase. A systematic review of randomized controlled trials showed ice to be more effective than heat or alternating heat and cold on edema management.[83] This review pointed out the lack of consistent protocols, making an evidence-based recommendation for treatment duration difficult. A general consensus is that 15 to 20 minutes is an acceptable time frame because it is long enough to decrease tissue temperature but is not likely to cause tissue damage.[81,83–85] The majority of studies involve superficial injuries to ankles and knees, so caution must be taken when attempting to extrapolate these findings to deeper injuries, such as a hamstring tear.

Investigations into the most effective temperature for cryotherapy are predominantly related to the acute treatment of burns. Although a specific temperature has not been identified as most effective, cold tap water at 12°C to 18°C (54°F to 64°F) has proven to be more effective than ice in reducing the amount of tissue damage following a burn.[86] In fact, the application of ice caused more tissue damage to burned tissue than no treatment at all.[86,87]

CASE STUDY 14•6 CRYOTHERAPY

A 14-year-old girl sprained the extensor ligaments of her wrist when she fell during a high school field hockey game. Her goal is to return to the team as soon as the ligaments are healed.

CLINICAL DECISION-MAKING

1. Does the patient have a problem that can be improved with the use of cryotherapy?
   Answer: Yes, in the acute stages of healing, cryotherapy can be beneficial to reduce edema.

2. Is the patient appropriate for application of cryotherapy (i.e., do any of the general precautions or contraindications to cryotherapy apply, or are there any specific considerations regarding application of cryotherapy to this patient)?
   Answer: Cryotherapy would be an appropriate method to reduce edema, thus speeding up the inflammatory process, as she has no contraindications and the area is superficial.

3. What are the specific goals to be achieved with the use of cryotherapy?
   Answer: Reduce edema in the injured area to assist with the transition out of the inflammatory phase.

4. What specific form of cryotherapy would be appropriate for the patient?

Answer: An ice pack or crushed ice because it can conform to the wrist.

5. What specific parameters of cryotherapy would be appropriate for this patient?
   Answer: No specific parameters have shown to be most effective. Ice packs and gel packs are typically stored in −10°C to −20°C (−50°F to −68°F) ranges.

6. What are the proper application procedures for cryotherapy related to this case?
   Answer:
   • Assess for adequate circulation to the area to be treated.
   • Assess for hot/cold sensation.
   • Cover cold pack in a pillowcase or place ice in a plastic bag and wrap loosely to hold in place on skin.
     • Note: Compression, from wrapping too tight or lying on the ice pack, will increase the rate of cooling and can produce burns.
   • Duration: Treat for 15 to 20 minutes.
   • Frequency: There is no evidence to support how often treatment should occur, but the effect from cryotherapy has been demonstrated to last up to 4 hours in some investigations and as little as 18 minutes for superficial tissue in others.[81]

Hydrotherapy

Hydrotherapy, in the form of whirlpools, has been a mainstay in wound care for decades. Initially used in burn units to assist with removing adhered dressings, whirlpool use expanded in some clinics to cleaning the majority of wounds, not just burns. Since that time, the use of whirlpools has been curtailed due to concerns over cross-contamination and the development of new methods to deliver hydrotherapy to wounds (Fig. 14-8).

The primary indication for hydrotherapy in wound healing is mechanical debridement (Table 14-4). Loosely adhered necrotic tissue and slough, exudate, dirt, and contaminants in and around the wound are removed by the movement of the water.[88] The use of whirlpools for wound cleansing has several proposed benefits. First is the reduction in pain associated with dressing removal because it soaks the bandage and allows it to come off slowly. The warm water in a whirlpool can also improve blood flow to the immersed area, potentially improving healing. In the past, whirlpool use in addition to standard dressing changes showed improved wound healing in stage III and IV pressure ulcers compared to standard dressing changes alone.[89] However, when a RevMan analysis was performed on this data, no significant differences were found.[90] The mechanisms by which whirlpool therapy improves wound healing have not been analyzed in any form of a controlled study. Proposed methods include reducing bacterial colonization and increasing the tissue temperature due to the warm water.

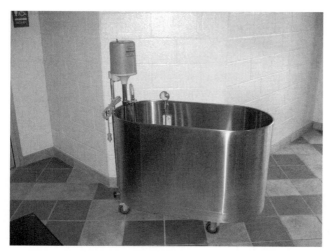

Fig 14•8 Whirlpool tank with agitator. *(Courtesy of Whitehall, City of Industry, CA.)*

Table 14•4 Hydrotherapy Indications	
Whirlpool	**Pulsed Lavage**
• Stage III or IV pressure ulcers with heavy amounts of necrotic tissue • Burns • Removal of adherent dressings • Greater than 50% necrotic tissue	Variety of wound types including: • Pressure ulcers • Diabetic foot ulcers • Venous insufficiency ulcers • Deep or tunneling wounds • Infected surgical sites • Heavily contaminated wounds • Burns • Multiple wounds

Despite the proposed benefits, there are also many potential side effects associated with whirlpool therapy. This modality has the potential to transmit bacteria from one patient to another as well as from an infected wound to a noninfected wound on the same patient if both wounds are immersed in water.[91] This risk can be reduced by cleansing the whirlpool effectively, which can be time-consuming, and by adding antimicrobial agents to the water, which can be hazardous to healthy tissues.[92–94] Prolonged immersion in water also has the potential of macerating the periwound skin and increasing edema when positioned in a dependent position. This is particularly problematic for venous ulcers of the lower limb.[95] Another issue with whirlpools is that it is difficult to control the pressure of the water at the wound's surface. When whirlpool is used, it is typically used for 20 to 30 minutes, three to five times per week. The use of whirlpool should be discontinued once the wound has a healthy bed of granulation.

In response to many of the problems inherent in whirlpool therapy, newer, more directed approaches to debridement have been developed. Pulsed lavage or pulsed lavage with suction (PLWS) have become increasingly popular as alternatives to whirlpool therapy for the treatment of open wounds (Box 14-2). Pulsed lavage involves irrigating (typically with saline) the wound at a set pressure (Fig. 14-9).

The recommended water pressure range is 4 to 15 psi. Pressures less than this have proved to be ineffective for removing debris, and pressures higher than this range are implicated in tissue damage and possibly a spread of bacteria.[96] Not only has pulsed lavage been shown to be effective for debridement, but it also increases the rate of granulation tissue formation compared to whirlpool.[97] PLWS is not without risk of

Box 14•2 | Proper Use of Pulsed Lavage

- Coordinate therapy with patient's medication schedule to maximize comfort.
- Position the patient comfortably with treatment area exposed and easily accessible.
- Assemble sterile, single-patient pulsed lavage unit, including irrigants, suction canister, and lavage gun. (Note: It may be beneficial to warm the irrigants under warm running water prior to therapy.)
- Ensure that the patient is appropriately draped and that the therapist is wearing personal protective equipment (i.e., gloves, mask, gown) to avoid backsplash. The lavage gun should be covered with a plastic barrier to reduce aerosolization.
- Treat wound at 4 to 15 psi to remove nonviable material.
- Treatment duration will vary based on wound size, patient tolerance, and amount of nonviable tissue.
- At the completion of treatment, the unit is disposed of in accordance with facility policy; in some cases, the device may be saved for subsequent use on the same patient.

contamination, as aerosolization of particles may occur, but this risk can be minimized by treating the patient in a private room and using a plastic shield to protect the area. Different attachments are also available to assist with the treatment of open tracts and tunnels. As with whirlpool, the use of pulsed lavage should be discontinued once a clean wound is achieved.

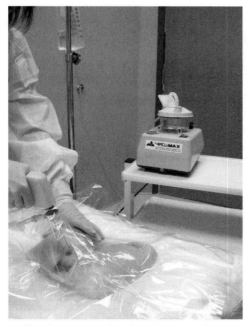

Fig 14•9 Simulated use of pulsed lavage with suction on a sacral ulcer. Note the plastic splash protector. *(Courtesy of Davol, Inc., Cranston, RI.)*

Opinions on the use of whirlpool therapy are varied (Box 14-3). Many wound care clinicians feel there are very rare instances in which a whirlpool is appropriate, given other methods to cleanse the wound, while other clinicians use whirlpool at the majority of patient visits (Tables 14-5, 14-6, and 14-7).

Box 14•3 | Proper Use of Whirlpool

- Assess patient and patient's record for any contraindications or concerns regarding whirlpool therapy.
- Coordinate therapy with patient's medication schedule to maximize comfort.
- Set the water temperature to 35.5°C to 39°C (96° to 102°F) for most wound care applications. For total immersion, the temperature should be at the lower end of the range; higher temperatures are okay for local immersion.
- Remove clothing from the area to be treated and immerse patient in water.
- Turn on agitators after patient is safely positioned.
- Typical treatments last approximately 20 minutes.
- The whirlpool is cleansed and disinfected after each use.

Table 14•5 Contraindications and Precautions for Full-Body Immersion in Whirlpool Therapy

Contraindication	Rationale
Cardiac dysfunction	Inability to regulate temperature/dissipate heat if submerged in warm water
Bowel incontinence	Contamination of wound and whirlpool
Impaired consciousness	Risk of drowning
Severe peripheral vascular disease	Inability to dissipate heat may lead to tissue damage
Infectious conditions that can spread in water	Risk of contamination
Multiple sclerosis	Hot water contraindicated
Uncontrolled bleeding	Risk of hemorrhage
Pregnant women	Risk of injury to fetus with high temperatures
Granulating wounds	No need for debridement
Precautions	
Confusion	Risk of drowning
Urinary incontinence	Contamination
Hydrophobia	
Certain medications	Reduced tolerance to heat

Laser Therapy

The use of lasers in tissue healing remains controversial because of conflicting results. On the positive side, a meta-analysis performed by Enwemeka and colleagues[98]

Table 14•6	Contraindications and Precautions for Local Immersion in Whirlpool Therapy

Contraindication	Rationale
Uncontrolled bleeding	Increases blood flow to area; risk of hemorrhage
Maceration	Weakens skin; may increase risk of skin infection
Venous insufficiency ulcers	Prolonged dependent positions and warm environment will exacerbate edema
Granulating wounds	No need for debridement
Precautions	
Infections that can spread in water	Risk of contamination
Impaired cognition	Potential injury from falling; contact with turbine
Recent skin grafts	Graft destruction

Table 14•7	Contraindications and Precautions for Pulsed Lavage

Contraindication	Rationale
Uncontrolled bleeding; blood vessels in the wound	May exacerbate the problem
Granulating wounds	No need for debridement
Precautions	
Recent skin grafts in area	Potential to disrupt graft

examined the effects of low-level laser therapy (LLLT) on in vivo tissue repair in animals and humans. Their results revealed a positive effect of laser therapy on tissue repair and revealed specific indices of tissue repair, including collagen formation, rate of healing, tensile stress, strength, and overall flap survival. Several other studies on diabetic rats, which were not included in Enwemeka's analysis, produced similar results. Wound collagen content was stimulated and a reduction in wound area was noted with laser therapy compared to control groups.[99,100] In the inflammatory stage of healing, reduced edema, reduced number of inflammatory cells, increased phagocytosis by white blood cells, and proliferation of inflammatory cells have all been attributed to laser therapy.[101–103] The effects continued to be positive in the proliferative phase with an increased number of myofibroblasts, collagen deposition, and epithelial cells observed.[103,104]

CASE STUDY 14•7 HYDROTHERAPY

A 54-year-old female with a history of venous insufficiency and diabetes presents with an open, infected Charcot foot ulcer to the plantar midfoot.

CLINICAL DECISION-MAKING

1. Does the patient have a problem that can be improved with the use of hydrotherapy?
   Answer: Yes, the wound could be effectively cleaned with hydrotherapy.

2. Is the patient appropriate for application of hydrotherapy (i.e., do any of the general precautions or contraindications to hydrotherapy apply, or are there any specific considerations regarding application of hydrotherapy to this patient)?
   Answer: The patient is appropriate for the application of hydrotherapy. Prolonged dependent positions and warm water may exacerbate swelling associated with venous insufficiency. Excessive moisture can lead to maceration and weakening of skin in diabetics.

3. What are the specific goals to be achieved with the use of hydrotherapy?
   Answer: Removal of loosely adhered nonviable tissue as well as bacteria that may be causing a localized infection.

4. What specific hydrotherapy would be appropriate for the patient?
   Answer: Pulsed lavage with suction (PLWS) would be the best choice, as it can limit maceration, does not require the limb to be soaking in water in a dependent position, and reduces the risk of cross-contamination.

5. What specific parameters of hydrotherapy would be appropriate for this patient?
   Answer: PLWS between 4 and 15 psi, typically toward the higher range for heavily contaminated/infected wounds. Suction is usually set to 60 to 100 mm Hg.

6. What are the proper application procedures for hydrotherapy related to this case?
   Answer: A sterile lavage gun is used for each treatment. Ensure that the lavage gun is in contact or in close proximity to the wound before pulling the trigger to avoid water spraying in all directions.

In addition to the multitude of studies that have demonstrated positive outcomes using LLLT, there are many studies that did not find an effect of laser therapy.[105–111] A literature review by Posten et al.[112] pointed out many positive effects that have been observed with laser therapy but concluded that there is not an adequate body of literature to support widespread use of lasers in wound healing. Flemming and Cullum[113] performed a Cochrane review that examined laser's effects on venous ulcer healing and did not find any benefit. Factors that are thought to contribute to the discrepancy between studies with positive and negative findings include the duration and frequency of laser therapy, the wavelength of the laser, and the species of animal being studied.

Currently, not enough research has been performed to determine the most beneficial parameters for laser therapy. Positive results have been demonstrated with different forms of laser, including helium neon (632.8 nm) and gallium arsenide (904 nm), with helium neon having the largest body of evidence.[114] Based on the current literature, there appears to be a positive effect of laser on cellular activities. However, the evidence that this translates into wound healing in humans is lacking. Table 14-8 lists contraindications and precautions for LLLT (Table 14-8).

Negative-Pressure Wound Therapy

Negative-pressure wound therapy (NPWT) involves the application of subatmospheric pressure to wound tissues. The concept of using negative pressure is not new. It has been used in drains to remove body fluids for much of the last century.[115] Within the last

---

Table 14•8 Contraindications to Low-Level Laser Therapy

- Exposure to eyes
- Over cancer
- Pregnancy

CASE STUDY 14•8 LASER THERAPY

A 27-year-old female is referred for treatment to address a partial tear of the Achilles tendon sustained in a soccer injury.

CLINICAL DECISION-MAKING

1. Does the patient have a problem that can be improved with the use of laser therapy?
   Answer: Yes, laser therapy can be used to assist with tendon healing because of its role in stimulating collagen synthesis.

2. Is the patient appropriate for application of laser therapy (i.e., do any of the general precautions or contraindications to laser therapy apply, or are there any specific considerations regarding application of laser therapy to this patient)?
   Answer: This patient is appropriate for laser therapy. Eye protection should be worn during treatment to avoid inadvertent exposure.

3. What are the specific goals to be achieved with the use of laser therapy?
   Answer: Promote tendon repair by increasing collagen formation at the site of injury.

4. What specific laser therapy would be appropriate for the patient?

   Answer: Gallium/aluminum arsenide laser would be most appropriate because it has a deeper penetration than helium-neon lasers.

5. What specific parameters of laser therapy would be appropriate for this patient?
   Answer: Gallium/aluminum arsenide laser is applied at a 904 nm wavelength at an intensity ranging from 1 to 48 J/cm^2.

6. What are the proper application procedures for laser therapy related to this case?
   Answer: The patient should be treated in a private room to minimize the risk of exposing others to the laser. Position the patient so that laser therapy can be comfortably applied to the Achilles area. The laser probe is applied to the skin before turning the machine on and is held in direct contact with the skin. Treatment occurs in a grid pattern with a laser spot applied in each square over the entire treatment area. At this time, there is no set data on duration or frequency of laser therapy; however, it is typically applied three to five times per week.

20 years, there has been a dramatic increase in the use of negative pressure therapy in wound care (Tables 14-9 and 14-10).

NPWT is currently available in several different forms, all of which involve using a power source that is connected to a dressing on the wound. The power source, either battery or line power, creates suction that pulls fluid from the wound into a collection canister or, in some cases, into the absorbent dressing. The dressing is left in place for from 1 to several days, depending on wound characteristics, but therapy can be adjusted so that negative pressure is applied continuously or intermittently (e.g., 5 minutes on and 2 minutes off).

Clinical Controversy

A major difference between NPWT devices is the contact layer, which can be foam, gauze, or absorbent dressings. Controversy exists regarding the proposed risks and benefits associated with using different materials with negative pressure.

Table 14•9 Indications for Negative-Pressure Wound Therapy[120]

Acute Wounds	Chronic Wounds
• Traumatic and surgical wounds	• Stage III and IV pressure ulcers
• Dehisced wounds	• Diabetic foot ulcers
• Skin grafts and graft substitutes	• Arterial ulcers (post- revascularization)
• Fasciotomy	and venous ulcers
• Partial thickness burns	
• Flap salvage	

Table 14•10 Contraindications and Precautions for Negative-Pressure Wound Therapy[121]

Contraindications	Precautions
• Exposed vital organs	• Active bleeding
• Inadequately debrided wounds	• Anticoagulant medications
• Untreated osteomyelitis or sepsis in the vicinity of the wound	• Exposed blood vessels
• Presence of untreated coagulopathy	
• Necrotic tissue with eschar	
• Malignancy in the wound	
• Non-enteric and unexplored fistulas	
• Allergy to any component of the device	

The first of the subatmospheric devices designed specifically for wound care was the VAC device; as a result, a large proportion of negative-pressure studies were performed with this device (Fig. 14-10). Based on the outcomes of VAC therapy, several proposed mechanisms of action have developed, including removal of wound exudate and bioburden, edema reduction, improved blood flow, and a promotion of fibroblasts in the wound.[116] Although all of these may contribute to wound healing, microdeformation is thought to be the primary means by which NPWT influences wound healing. Microdeformation is the mechanical deformation of cells in response to a stimulus—in this case, the application of subatmospheric pressure. This theory has been supported by studies that identified increased cellular proliferation and angiogenesis in response to mechanical stress on tissues.[117,118]

Negative-pressure wound therapy has changed the way wound care is performed in many facilities. An important benefit of negative pressure is the ability to leave the dressing in place for several days, compared to twice-daily dressing changes that were typical of wet to moist dressings. The ability for a dressing to remain in place has several positive effects, including cost and time for health-care professionals to change the dressing and, most importantly, less pain for the patient due to the reduced frequency of dressing changes.[119]

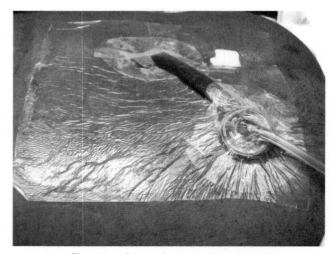

Fig 14•10 The use of negative pressure to manage a dehisced abdominal wound. *(VAC device shown courtesy of Kinetic Concepts, Inc., San Antonio, TX.)*

CASE STUDY 14•9 NEGATIVE-PRESSURE WOUND THERAPY

A 21-year-old female is referred for treatment of a dehisced surgical wound following a cesarean section. Sutures were removed 2 days ago due to infection, and the wound has been packed with moistened gauze.

CLINICAL DECISION-MAKING

1. Does the patient have a problem that can be improved with the use of NPWT?

   Answer: Yes, this open postsurgical wound could benefit from the application of subatmospheric pressure to remove exudates and facilitate approximation of the wound margins.

2. Is the patient appropriate for application of NPWT (i.e., do any of the general precautions or contraindications to NPWT apply, or are there any specific considerations regarding application of NPWT to this patient)?

   Answer: As long as there is no malignancy and the patient's bleeding is controlled, this patient would be appropriate for NPWT.

3. What are the specific goals to be achieved with the use of NPWT?

   Answer: Promote removal of exudates, control bacterial bioburden in the wound, and promote wound contraction and proliferation of granulation tissue in the wound. A secondary goal is improved pain due to the less frequent dressing changes.

4. What specific NPWT would be appropriate for the patient?

   Answer: An approved device intended specifically for providing NPWT should be used. Wall suction is not recommended because the pressure at the wound surface cannot be regulated, and there is no alarm system to signify a problem.

5. What specific parameters of NPWT would be appropriate for this patient?

   Answer: For the initiation of therapy, 125 mm Hg of negative pressure applied continuously is recommended. After that, evidence suggests that intermittent therapy (5 minutes on and 2 minutes off) is more beneficial. If it is difficult to obtain a seal, continuous therapy may continue to be the best option.

6. What are the proper application procedures for NPWT related to this case?

   Answer:
   - Review patient history to rule out any contraindications/precautions to NPWT.
   - Cleanse wound and debride necrotic tissue, if applicable.
   - Apply skin protectant to periwound to reduce risk of breakdown from maceration.
   - Cut foam or adjust gauze to fit inside wound to maximize contact with wound bed while avoiding contact with intact skin.
   - Obtain a seal and connect tubing to dressing.
   - Set parameters to 125 mm Hg continuous therapy for initiation of therapy.
   - Ensure that suction is achieved with no leaks.
   - Recommended frequency of dressing change is every 48 hours for most wounds, every 24 hours in the presence of infection, and up to 5 to 7 days over skin grafts.

KEY POINT! When applied correctly, the contact layer of the dressing should touch the entire wound bed but should not connect with intact skin. In cases of wounds with any sort of tunneling or depth, all areas should be filled in loosely. A common mistake is overpacking the wound with the contact dressing.

Evidence has demonstrated positive clinical outcomes with NPWT, including improved healing times, shorter hospital stays, reduced infection rates, and increased survival of flaps and grafts. NPWT is typically not intended to be used until complete wound closure; rather, it is used as a method to prepare the wound bed for definitive closure.[120] For a thorough review of expert guidelines pertaining to the use of negative pressure, refer to the guidelines document by Bollero and colleagues.[120]

Clinical Controversy

Despite the moderate to strong evidence that NPWT promotes healing, the majority of the wounds treated have been acute/postsurgical, so controversy still exists concerning its effectiveness compared to other therapies in chronic wounds.

Documentation Tips

- Tissue area stimulated
- Stimulation settings
  - Polarity, type, and placement of electrodes
  - Type and size of electrodes

(continued next page)

- Waveform type (i.e., high volt, direct current, etc.)
- Purpose (i.e., epithelialization, debridement, etc.)
- Patient position
- Duration and frequency of stimulation
- Response to treatment (i.e., inspection of tissue area)
- Any skin irritation post-treatment.

☐ REFERENCES

1. Dunn S. The wound healing process. In: McCulloch J, Kloth L. *Wound Healing: Evidence-Based Management.* 4th ed. Philadelphia: F.A. Davis; 2010:9–34.
2. Dyson M. Mechanisms involved in therapeutic ultrasound. *Physiotherapy.* 1987;73:116–120.
3. Fyfe M, Chahl I. Mast cell degradation: a possible mechanism of action of therapeutic ultrasound. *Ultrasound Med Biol.* 1982;1 Suppl:62.
4. Mortimer A, Dyson M. The effect of therapeutic ultrasound on calcium uptake in fibroblasts. *Ultrasound Med Biol.* 1988; 14(6):499–506.
5. Harvey W, Dyson M, Pond JB, et al. The stimulation of protein synthesis in human fibroblasts by therapeutic ultrasound. *Rheumatol Rehabil.* 1975;14(4):237.
6. Webster DF, Pond JB, Dyson M, et al. The role of cavitation in the in vitro stimulation of protein synthesis in human fibroblasts by ultrasound. *Ultrasound Med Biol.* 1978;4(4):343–351.
7. Hogan RD, Burke KM, Franklin TD. The effect of ultrasound on microvascular hemodynamics in skeletal muscle: effects during ischemia. *Microvasc Res.* 1982;23(3):370–379.
8. Johannsen F, Gam AN, Karlsmark T. Ultrasound therapy in chronic leg ulceration: a meta-analysis. *Wound Repair Regen.* 1998;6(2):121–126.
9. Cullum N, et al. Therapeutic ultrasound for venous leg ulcers (review). *Cochrane Database Syst Rev.* 2010;6:CD001180.
10. Akbari Sari A, et al. Therapeutic ultrasound for pressure ulcers. *Cochrane Database Syst Rev.* 2006(3):CD001275.
11. Ennis WJ, Foremann P, Mozen N. Ultrasound therapy for recalcitrant diabetic foot ulcers: results of a randomized, double-blind, controlled, multicenter study. *Ostomy Wound Manage.* 2005;51(8):24–39.
12. Kavros SJ, Miller JL, Hanna SW. Treatment of ischemic wounds with noncontact, low frequency ultrasound: the Mayo Clinic experience, 2004–2006. *Adv Skin Wound Care.* 2007; 20(4):221–226.
13. Jacobson MJ, Piper KE, Kavros SJ. In Vitro Activity of the Arobella Acoustic Curette Against Planktonic and Biofilm Bacteria. Presented at American Society for Microbiology. Philadelphia; 2009.
14. Suzuki K, Cowan L, Aronowitz, J. Low-Frequency Ultrasound Therapy of Lower Extremity Wounds Significantly Increases the Peri-wound Skin Perfusion Pressure. Diabetic Foot Global Conference. Los Angeles; 2009.
15. Eaglstein WH, Weinstein GD. Prostaglandin and DNA synthesis in human skin; possible relationship to ultraviolet light effects. *J Invest Dermatol.* 1975;64(6):386–389.
16. Agin PP, Rose AP III, Lane CC, et al. Changes in epidermal forward scattering absorption after UVA-UVB irradiation. *J Invest Dermatol.* 1981;76(3):174–177.
17. Greeves MW, Sondergaard J. Pharmacological agents released in ultraviolet inflammation studied by continuous skin perfusion. *J Invest Dermatol.* 1970;54(5):365–367.
18. Nussbaum EL, Blemann I, Mustard B. Comparison of ultrasound/ultraviolet-C and laser for treatment of pressure ulcers in patients with spinal cord injury. *Phys Ther.* 1994; 74(9):812–825.
19. High AS, High JP. Treatment of infected skin wounds using ultraviolet radiation: an in-vitro study. *Physiotherapy.* 1983; 69(10):359–360.
20. Burger A, Jordan AJ, Schoombee GE. The bactericidal effect of ultraviolet light on infected pressure sores. *SAJPA.* 1985; 41(2):55–57.
21. Shelk J, Morgan P. Narrow-band UVB: A practical approach. *Dermatol Nurs.* 2000;12(6):407–411.
22. Walters IB, Burack LH, Coven TR. Suberythemogenic narrow-band UVB is markedly more effective than conventional UVB in treatment of psoriasis vulgaris. *J Am Acad Dermatol.* 1999; 40(6 pt. 1):893–900.
23. Green C, Ferguson J, Lakshmitpathi T, et al. 311 nm UVB phototherapy—an effective treatment for psoriasis. *Br J Dermatol.* 1988;119(6):691–696.
24. Falabella R, Barona MI. Update on skin repigmentation therapies in vitiligo. *Pigment Cell Melanoma Res.* 2008;22(1):42–65.
25. Parsad D, Kanwar AJ, Kumar B. Psoralen-ultraviolet A vs. narrow-band ultraviolet B phototherapy for the treatment of vitiligo. *J Eur Acad Dermatol Venereol.* 2006;20(2):175–177.
26. Forschner T, Buchholtz S, Stockfleth E. Current state of vitiligo therapy—evidence-based analysis of the literature. *J Dtsch Dermatol Ges.* 2007;5(6):467–475.
27. Bhatnagar A, Kanwar AJ, Parsad D. Psoralen and ultraviolet A and narrow-band ultraviolet B in inducing stability in vitiligo, assessed by vitiligo disease activity score: an open prospective comparative study. *J Eur Acad Dermatol Venereol.* 2007; 21(10):1381–1385.
28. Wu CS, Yu CL, Wu CS. Narrow-band ultraviolet-B stimulates proliferation and migration of cultured melanocytes. *Exp Dermatol.* 2004;13(12):755–763.
29. Martin JA, Laube S, Edwards C. Rate of acute adverse events for narrow-band UVB and Psoralen-UVA phototherapy. *Photodermatol Photoimmunol Photomed.* 2007;23(2-3):68–72.
30. Kunisada M, Kumimoto H, Ishikazi K, et al. Narrow-band UVB induces more carcinogenic skin tumors than broad-band UVB through the formation of cyclobutane pyrimidine dimer. *J Invest Dermatol.* 2007;127(12):2865–2871.
31. Weischer M, Blum A, Eberhard F, et al. No evidence for increased skin cancer risk in psoriasis patients treated with broadband or narrowband UVB phototherapy: a first retrospective study. *Acta Derm Venereol.* 2004;84(5):370–374.
32. Leenutaphong V, Mimkulrat P, Sudtim S. Comparison of phototherapy two times and four times a week with low doses of narrow-band ultraviolet B in Asian patients with psoriasis. *Photodermatol Photoimmunol Photomed.* 2000;16(5):202–206.
33. Sterenborg H, van der Putte SC, van der Leun JC. The dose-response relationship of tumorigenesis by ultraviolet radiation of 254 nm. *Photochem Photobiol Sci.* 1988;47(2):245–253.
34. Connor-Kerr TA, Sullivan PK, Gaillard J, et al. The effects of ultraviolet radiation on antibiotic-resistant bacteria in vitro. *Ostomy Wound Manage.* 1998;44(10):50–56.
35. Connor-Kerr TA, Sullivan PK, Keegan BS, et al. UVC reduces antibiotic-resistant bacterial numbers in living tissue. *Ostomy Wound Manage.* 1999;45(4):84.
36. Thai TP, Keast DH, Campbell KE. Effects of ultraviolet light C on bacterial colonization in chronic wounds. *Ostomy Wound Manage.* 2005;51(10):32–45.
37. Foulds IS, Barker AT. Human skin battery potentials and their possible role in wound healing. *Br J Dermatol.* 1983; 109(5):515–522.

38. Kloth LC. Electrical stimulation for wound healing: a review of evidence from in vitro studies, animal experiments, and clinical trials. *Int J Low Extrem Wounds.* 2005;4(1):23–44.

39. Bassett C, Herrmann I. The effect of electrostatic fields on macromolecular synthesis by fibroblasts in vitro (abstract). *J Cell Biol.* 1968;39(9a).

40. Bourguignon GJ, Bourguinon LYW. Effect of high voltage pulsed galvanic stimulation on human fibroblasts in cell culture (abstract). *J Cell Biol.* 1986;Supplement:344a.

41. Bourguignon GJ, Bourguignon LYW. Electric stimulation of protein and DNA synthesis in human fibroblasts. *FASEB J.* 1987;1(5):398–402.

42. Cheng N, van Hoof H, Bockx E, et al. The effects of electric currents on ATP generation, protein synthesis, and membrane transport in rat skin. *Clin Orthop Relat Res.* 1982;171:264–272.

43. Bourguinon GJ, Jy W, Bourguignon LY. Electric stimulation of human fibroblasts causes an increase in Ca2+ influx and the exposure of additional insulin receptors. *J Cell Physiol.* 1989;140(2):379–385.

44. Junger M, Zuder D, Steins A, et al. Treatment of venous ulcers with low frequency pulsed current (Dermapulse): effects on cutaneous microcirculation. *Hautartz.* 1997;48(12):879–903.

45. Assimacopoulos D. Low intensity negative electric current in the treatment of ulcers of the leg due to chronic venous insufficiency. *Am J Surg.* 1968;115(5):683–687.

46. Wolcott LE, Wheeler PC, Hardwicke HM, et al. Accelerated healing of skin ulcers by electrotherapy: preliminary clinical results. *South Med J.* 1969;62(7):795–801.

47. Gault WR, Gates PF. Use of low intensity direct current in management of ischemic skin ulcers. *Phys Ther.* 1976;56(3):265–269.

48. Barron JJ, Jacobson WE, Tidd G. Treatment of decubitus ulcers: a new approach. *Minn Med.* 1985;68(2):103–106.

49. Wood JM, Evan PE III, Schallreuter KU, et al. A multicenter study on the use of pulsed low-intensity direct current for healing chronic stage II and stage III decubitus ulcers. *Arch Dermatol.* 1993;129(8):999–1009.

50. Huckfeldt R, Flick AB, Mikkelson D, et al. Wound closure after split-thickness skin grafting is accelerated with the use of continuous direct anodal microcurrent applied to silver nylon wound contact dressings. *J Burn Care Res.* 2007;28(5):703–707.

51. Carley PJ, Wainapel SF. Electrotherapy for acceleration of wound healing: low intensity direct current. *Arch Phys Med Rehabil.* 1985;66(7):443–446.

52. Goldman R, Brewley B, Zhou L, et al. Electrotherapy reverses inframalleolar ischemia: a retrospective, observational study. *Adv Skin Wound Care.* 2003;16(2):79–89.

53. Goldman RJ, Brewley BI, Golden MA. Electrotherapy reoxygenates inframalleolar ischemic wounds on diabetic patients: a case series. *Adv Skin Wound Care.* 2002;15(3):112–120.

54. Gardner SE, Frantz RA, Schmidt FL. Effect of electrical stimulation on chronic wound healing: a meta-analysis. *Wound Repair Regen.* 1999;7(6):495–503.

55. Steeper R. A critical review of the aetiology of diabetic neuropathic ulcers. *J Wound Care.* 2005;14(3):101–103.

56. Burke TJ. 5 questions—and answers—about MIRE treatment. *Adv Skin Wound Care.* 2003;16(7):369–371.

57. Harkless LB, DeLillis S, Carnegie DH, et al. Improved foot sensitivity and pain reduction in patients with peripheral neuropathy after treatment with monochromatic infrared photo energy—MIRE. *J Diabetes Complications.* 2006;20(2):81–87.

58. Kochman AB, Carnegie DH, Burke TJ. Symptomatic reversal of peripheral neuropathy in patients with diabetes. *J Am Podiatr Med Assoc.* 2002;92(3):125–130.

59. Leonard DR, Farooqi MH, Myers S. Restoration of sensation, reduced pain, and improved balance in subjects with diabetic peripheral neuropathy. *Diabetes Care.* 2004;27(1):316–321.

60. Prendergast JJ, Miranda G, Sanchez M. Improvement of sensory impairment in patients with peripheral neuropathy. *Endocr Pract.* 2004;10(1):24–30.

61. DeLellis SL, Carnegie DH, Burke TJ. Improved sensitivity in patients with peripheral neuropathy: effects of monochromatic infrared photo energy. *J Am Podiatr Med Assoc.* 2005;95(2):143–147.

62. Clifft JK, Kasser RJ, Newton TS, et al. The effect of monochromatic infrared energy on sensation in patients with diabetic peripheral neuropathy. *Diabetes Care.* 2005;28(12):2896–2900.

63. Franzen-Korzendorfer H, Blackinton M, Rone-Adams S, et al. The effect of monochromatic infrared energy on transcutaneous oxygen measurements and protective sensation: results of a controlled, double-blind, randomized clinical study. *Ostomy Wound Manage.* 2008;54(6):16–31.

64. Lavery LA, Murdoch DP, Williams J, et al. Does Anodyne light therapy improve peripheral neuropathy in diabetes? *Diabetes Care.* 2008;31(2):316–321.

65. Khanna A, Gougoulias N, Maffulli N. Intermittent pneumatic compression in fracture and soft-tissue healing. *Br Med Bull.* 2008;88(1):147–156.

66. Dai G, Gertler JP, Kamm RD. The effects of external compression on venous blood flow and tissue deformation in the lower leg. *J Biomech Eng.* 1999;121(6):557–564.

67. Park S, Silva M. Intermittent pneumatic soft tissue compression: changes in periosteal and medullary blood flow. *J Orthop Res.* 2008;26(4):570–577.

68. Dahl J, Li J, Bring DK, et al. Intermittent pneumatic compression enhances neurovascular ingrowth and tissue proliferation during connective tissue healing: a study in the rat. *J Orthop Res.* 2007;25(9):1185–1192.

69. Challis MJ, Welsh MK, Jull GA, et al. Effect of cyclic pneumatic soft tissue compression on simulated distal radius fractures. *Clin Orthop Relat Res.* 2005;(433):183–188.

70. Morris RJ, Elsaid M, Elgazzar AH, et al. The effect of intermittent pneumatic compression on the bone uptake of (99m) Tc-labelled methylene diphosphonate in the lower limb. *Arch Orthop Trauma Surg.* 2005;125(5):348–354.

71. Awolesi MA, Sessa WC, Sumpio BE. Cyclic strain upregulates nitric oxide synthase in cultured bovine aortic endothelial cells. *J Clin Invest.* 1995;96(3):1449–1454.

72. Liu K, Chen LE, Seaber, AV, et al. Intermittent pneumatic compression of legs increases micro-circulation in distant skeletal muscles. *J Orthop Res.* 1999;17(1):88–95.

73. Lefer AM, Tsao PS, Lefer DJ, et al. Role of endothelial dysfunction in the pathogenesis of reperfusion injury after myocardial ischemia. *FASEB J.* 1991;5(7):2029–2034.

74. Schaffer M, Beiter T, Becker HD, et al. Neuropeptides: Mediators of inflammation and tissue repair? *Arch Surg.* 1998;133(10):1107–1116.

75. Kavros SJ, Delis KT, Turner NS, et al. Improving limb salvage in critical ischemia with intermittent pneumatic compression: a controlled study with 18-month follow-up. *J Vasc Surg.* 2008;47(3):543–549.

76. Petrofsky JS, Bains S, Raju C, et al. The effect of the moisture content of a local heat source on the blood flow response in the skin. *Arch Dermatol Res.* 2009;301(8):581–585.

77. Oosterveld FG, Rasker JJ, Jacobs JW,, et al. The effect of local heat and cold therapy on the intraarticular and skin surface temperature of the knee. *Arthritis Rheum.* 1992;35(2):146–152.

78. Wright A, Sluka K. Nonpharmacological treatments for musculoskeletal pain. *Clin J Pain.* 2001;17(1):33–46.

79. Taber C, Contryman K, Fahrenbruch J, et al. Measurement of reactive vasodilation during cold gel pack application to nontraumatized ankles. *Phys Ther.* 1992;72(4):294–299.

80. Deal DN, Tipton J, Rosencrance E, et al. Ice reduces edema. A study of microvascular permeability in rats. *J Bone Joint Surg Am.* 2002;84-A(9):1573–1578.

81. Enwemeka CS, Allen C, Avila P, et al. Soft tissue thermodynamics before, during, and after cold pack therapy. *Med Sci Sports Exerc.* 2002;34(1):45–50.

82. Schaser KD, Disch AC, Stover JF, et al. Prolonged superficial local cryotherapy attenuates microcirculatory impairment, regional inflammation, and muscle necrosis after closed soft tissue injury in rats. *Am J Sports Med.* 2007;35(1):93–102.

83. Bleakley C, McDonough S, Macauley D. The use of ice in the treatment of acute soft-tissue injury: a systematic review of randomized controlled trials. *Am J Sports Med.* 2004;32(1): 251–261.

84. Drez D, Faust DC, Evans JP. Cryotherapy and nerve palsy. *Am J Sports Med.* 1981;9(4):256–257.

85. Lee JM, Warren MP, Mason SM. The effects of ice on nerve conduction velocity. *Physiotherapy.* 1978;64(1):2–7.

86. Venter TH, Karpelowsky JS, Rode H. Cooling of the burn wound: the ideal temperature of the coolant. *Burns.* 2007; 33(7):917–922.

87. Sawada Y, Urushidate S, Yotsuyanagi T, et al. Is prolonged and excessive cooling of a scalded wound effective? *Burns.* 1997;23(1):55–58.

88. Niederhuber SS, Stribley RF, Koepke GH. Reduction of skin bacterial load with use of therapeutic whirlpool. *Phys Ther.* 1975;55(5):482–486.

89. Burke DT, Ho CH, Saucier MA, et al. Effects of hydrotherapy on pressure ulcer healing. *Am J Phys Med Rehabil.* 1998; 77(5):394–398.

90. Moore Z, Cowman S. A systematic review of wound cleansing for pressure ulcers. *J Clin Nurs.* 2008;17(15):1963–1972.

91. Embil JM, McLeod JA, Al-Barrak AM, et al. An outbreak of methicillin resistant Staphylococcus aureus on a burn unit: potential role of contaminated hydrotherapy equipment. *Burns.* 2001;27(7):681–688.

92. Cardany CR, Rodeheaver GT, Horowitz JH, et al. Influence of hydrotherapy and antiseptic agents on burn wound bacterial contamination. *J Burn Care Rehabil.* 1985;6(3):230–232.

93. Lineaweaver W, Howard R, Soucy D, et al. Topical antimicrobial toxicity. *Arch Surg.* 1985;120(3):267–270.

94. Rodeheaver G, Bellamy W, Kody M, et al. Bactericidal activity and toxicity of iodine-containing solutions in wounds. *Arch Surg.* 1982;117(2)181–186.

95. McCulloch J, Boyd V. The effects of whirlpool and the dependent position on lower extremity volume. *J Orthop Sports Phys Ther.* 1992;16(4):169–172.

96. Bergstrom N, Allman R, Alvarez O, et al. Treatment of pressure ulcers: clinical practice guideline No. 15. Rockville, MD: AHCPR Publication No. 95-0652; December 1994.

97. Haynes LJ, Brown MH, Handley BC, et al. Comparison of Pulsavac and sterile whirlpool regarding the promotion of tissue granulation (abstract). *Phys Ther.* 1994;74(5 Suppl):S4.

98. Enwemeka CS, Parker JC, Dowdy DS, et al. The efficacy of low-power lasers in tissue repair and pain control: a meta-analysis study. *Photomed Laser Surg.* 2004;22(4):323–329.

99. Al-Watban FA, Zhang XY, Andres BL, et al. Low-level laser therapy enhances wound healing in diabetic rats: a comparison of different lasers. *Photomed Laser Surg.* 2007;25(2): 72–77.

100. Reddy GK, Stehno-Bittel L, Enwemeka CS. Laser photostimulation accelerates wound healing in diabetic rats. *Wound Repair Regen.* 2001;9(3):248–255.

101. Karu TI, Ryabykh TP, Fedoseyeva GE, et al. Helium-neon laser induced respiratory burst of phagocytic cells. *Lasers Surg Med.* 1989;9(6):585–588.

102. Ohta A, Abergel RP, Uitto J. Laser modulation of human immune system: inhibition of lymphocyte proliferation by a gallium-arsenide laser at low energy. *Lasers Surg Med.* 1987;7(2):199–201.

103. Medrado AR, Pugliese LS, Reis SR, et al. Influence of low level laser therapy on wound healing and its biological action upon myofibroblasts. *Lasers Surg Med.* 2003;32(3):239–244.

104. Yu HS, Chang KL, Yu CL, et al. Low-energy helium-neon laser irradiation stimulates interleukin-1 alpha and interleukin-8 release from cultured human keratinocytes. *J Invest Dermatol.* 1996;107(4):593–596.

105. Abergel RP, Lyons RF, Castel JC, et al. Biostimulation of wound healing by lasers: experimental approaches in animal models and in fibroblast cultures. *J Dermatol Surg Oncol.* 1987;13(2):127–133.

106. Pereira AN, Eduardo Cde. P, Matson E, et al. Effect of low-power laser irradiation on cell growth and procollagen synthesis of cultured fibroblasts. *Lasers Surg Med.* 2002;31(4): 263–267.

107. Allendorf JD, Bessler M, Huang J, et al. Helium-neon laser irradiation at fluences of 1, 2, and 4 J/cm^2 failed to accelerate wound healing as assessed by both wound contracture rate and tensile strength. *Lasers Surg Med.* 1997;20(3): 340–345.

108. Smith RJ, Birndorf M, Gluck G, et al. The effect of low-energy laser on skin flap survival in the rat and porcine animal models. *Plast Reconstr Surg.* 1992;89(2):306–310.

109. Cambier DC, Vanderstraeten GG, Mussen MJ, et al. Low-power laser and healing of burns: a preliminary assay. *Plast Reconstr Surg.* 1996;97(3):555–558.

110. Walker MD, Rumpf S, Baxter GD, et al. Effect of low-intensity laser irradiation (660 nm) on a radiation-impaired wound healing model in murine skin. *Lasers Surg Med.* 2000;26(1): 41–47.

111. Hunter J, Leonard L, Wilson R, et al. Effects of low energy laser on wound healing in a porcine model. *Lasers Surg Med.* 1984;3(4):285–290.

112. Posten W, Wrone DA, Dover JS, et al. Low-level laser therapy for wound healing: mechanism and efficacy. *Dermatol Surg.* 2005;31(3):334–340.

113. Flemming K, Cullum N. Laser therapy for venous leg ulcers. Cochrane Library. Cochrane Database Syst Rev. 2000;(2): CD001182 .

114. Albaugh K. What else can we do? Therapeutic interventions (MIRE, ES, and LASER). 11th Annual Wound Care Congress. Houston, TX; 2007.

115. Fox JW, Goden GT. The use of drains in subcutaneous surgical procedures. *Am J Surg.* 1976;132(5):673-674.

116. Miller MS, Lowery CA. Negative pressure wound therapy: "A rose by any other name." *Ostomy Wound Manage.* 2005; 51(3):44–49.

117. Iwasaki H, Eguchi S, Ueno H, et al. Mechanical stretch stimulates growth of vascular smooth muscle cells via epidermal growth factor receptor. *Am J Physiol Heart Circ Physiol.* 2000;278(2):H521–H529.

118. Cherry GW, Austed E, Pasyk K, et al. Increased survival and vascularity of random-pattern skin flaps elevated in controlled, expanded tissue. *Plast Reconstr Surg.* 1983;72(5): 680–687.

119. Apelqvis J, Armstrong DG, Lavery LA, et al. Resource utilization and economic costs of care based on a randomized trial of vacuum-assisted closure therapy in the treatment of diabetic foot wounds. *Am J Surg.* 2008;195(6):782–788.

120. Bollero D, Driver V, Glat P, et al. The role of negative pressure wound therapy in the spectrum of wound healing: a guidelines document. *Ostomy Wound Manage.* 2010;56(5 Suppl):1–18.

121. Agency for Healthcare Research and Quality. (n.d.). Negative pressure wound therapy devices: Technology assessment report. Available at http://www.ahrq.gov/clinic/ta/hegpresswtd/. Accessed April 19, 2011 http://www.ahrq.gov/clinic/ta/negpresswtd/

Alternative Modalities and Electrophysiologic Testing

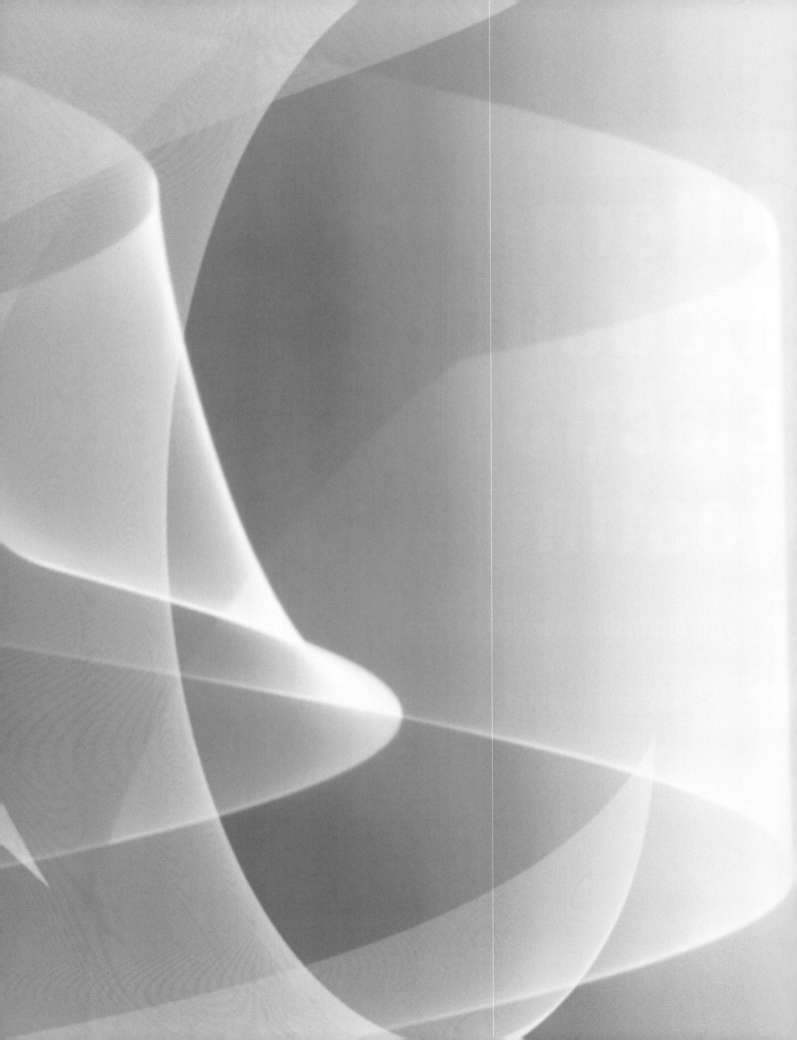

chapter 15

Alternative Modalities for Pain and Tissue Healing

Thomas P. Nolan Jr., PT, DPT, OCS | Susan L. Michlovitz, PT, PhD, CHT

We have chosen to operationally define alternative modalities as "technologies that have become popularized for treatment of conditions involving chronic pain and delayed tissue healing." There are many thoughts about why these techniques may be of interest to the therapist and the patient. Our patients want to get better. We want our patients to get better. For a variety of reasons, previous interventions may have been unsuccessful—thus the search for another option. In many cases of chronic pain and delayed tissue healing, attempts may be made to maximize recovery of function at any cost. In this chapter, we discuss the use of magnet therapy, monochromatic infrared therapy (MIRE), hyperbaric oxygen therapy (HBOT), and extracorporeal shock wave therapy (ESWT). The popularity of these interventions may not parallel their published effectiveness. Magnet therapy, MIRE, and HBOT are within the scope of practice of non-physician practitioners; ESWT is used by physicians and surgeons.

Magnet Therapy

The use of magnets for therapeutic purposes dates back 2,000 years.[1,2] Greek healers in AD 200 used magnetic rings as a treatment for arthritis. During the emergence of complementary/alternative medicine (CAM) in the late twentieth and early twenty-first centuries, there has been increasing interest in the use of magnets for therapeutic benefit.[3] The use of pulsed electromagnetic fields (PEMF) for promotion of fracture healing and other orthopedic problems, such as osteoarthritis, has been commonplace during this time.[4]

Physical Principles of Magnets

Magnets are metals such as iron that exhibit an attractive or repulsive force. This force can be represented by field lines drawn around a magnet (Fig. 15-1). The force one magnet exerts on another magnet can be described as the interaction between the magnetic fields of each magnet. The number of lines per unit area representing the magnetic field is proportional to the magnitude of the field. The direction of the magnetic field at a given point is defined as the direction that the north pole of a compass needle would point when placed at that position. The pole of a freely suspended magnet that points north is the north pole. The other pole, which points south, is called the south pole. The earth acts as a huge magnet with a magnetic field and north and south poles.[5] For thousands of years, voyagers have used compasses for navigation; these devices are attracted to the earth's north pole by the earth's magnetic field.

KEY POINT! Magnets used for therapeutic effects are known as *static* or *permanent magnets*. The strength of the magnetic field produced by a permanent magnet is expressed in units known as teslas (T) or gauss (G). The relationship of tesla to gauss is 1 G = 10^{-4} T.

The magnetic field of the earth at its surface is about 0.5 G—or 0.5 × 10^{-4} T.[5] Most magnets marketed for therapeutic effects have an advertised strength of 500 to 1,000 G compared to the 15,000 G produced by magnetic resonance imaging (MRI) devices.[6] Blechman and colleagues[7] used a gaussmeter to determine the field flux density in gauss for magnets marketed for medical use. Field flux density helps determine the magnetic field's tissue penetration, which can be considered its "effective dosage." The gauss listed by the distributors or suppliers of four out of five magnets they measured differed significantly from the measurements taken with the gaussmeter.

KEY POINT! All magnets have two poles. However, the application of magnets for therapeutic purposes can be unipolar or bipolar. Unipolar magnets are arranged so that only one pole is facing or touching the skin, usually the north pole. The south pole of the magnet is facing away from the skin. Bipolar magnets are arranged so that both the north and south poles are facing the skin or in contact with it, usually using multiple magnets.[6,8]

Pulsed Magnetic Fields

Movement of charges in an electric current will produce a magnetic field. The magnetic field produced by a current in a straight wire is represented by lines in the form of circles, with the wire at the center (Fig. 15-2).[5] There are electrical devices that can create strong magnetic fields in a coil into which a body part can be placed. Other devices that create a weaker magnetic field use a flat coil placed in contact with the body part. Therapeutic application of a pulsed electromagnetic field (PEMF) is also known as *magnetotherapy*. The physiological effect of pulsed magnetic fields is likely secondary to induction of currents in the tissues exposed to the fields, resulting in movement of ions across cell membranes and stimulation of DNA transcription.[4,9]

Proposed Physiological Effects of Magnets

For many years, there has been speculation on the physiological effects of magnets. Most manufacturers' claims for the therapeutic effects of magnets and PEMF have

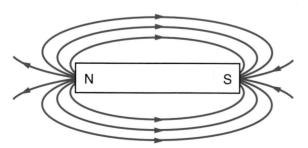

Fig 15•1 Magnetic field lines drawn around a bar magnet having north (N) and south (S) poles.

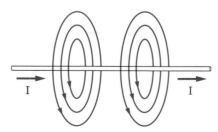

Fig 15•2 Magnetic fields generated around a live electric wire. Arrows represent the direction of current.

not been substantiated.[6,9] However, there is an abundance of experimental and clinical data demonstrating that magnetic fields may have a profound effect on biological tissues at the cellular level. Magnetic fields are capable of inducing selective changes in the microenvironment around and within the cell, including the cell membrane. Modifications of cellular activity may occur with exposure of the cell to magnetic fields, and these modifications may correct certain pathological states. These modifications appear to strongly depend on the parameters of the applied magnetic field. Practitioners need to consider that the known effects of magnetic fields on the cellular level may not translate into therapeutic effects at the clinical level.[10]

Review of the Literature on Magnet Therapy

Table 15-1 reviews some of the relevant literature on magnet therapy. An analysis of these studies allows for the following conclusions:

- Some evidence exists that static magnetic fields of 300 to 500 G will decrease pain associated with postpolio syndrome[23] and diabetic neuropathy.[11,20,21]
- Magnets may not be effective for chronic low back pain.[18]
- The evidence for use of static magnets for osteoarthritis is insufficient to demonstrate a clinically important benefit.[12]

- Magnets with a static magnetic field greater than 500 G were not shown to be more effective than placebo in decreasing pain following intense exercise and for chronic neck and shoulder pain;[22,25] however, a device with four static magnets arranged in alternating polarity with a strength of 1,900 G and a control device with one magnet at 720 G were both shown to significantly decrease knee pain in patients with rheumatoid arthritis.[17]
- Static magnets measured at less than 500 G do not appear to have any effect on the cardiovascular system, including heart rate and blood pressure,[3] blood flow,[13] and surface and intramuscular temperature.[16]
- There is no effect on muscle force production when static magnets are applied to the skin overlying the muscle.[19,22]
- The effect of magnetic fields on nerve excitability and conduction velocity is insignificant.[24,25]
- "Repetitive magnetic stimulation" to trigger points may decrease pain and improve cervical spine range of motion (ROM) more effectively than TENS and placebo for patients who have myofascial pain.[26]
- Pulsed magnetic fields (PEMF) were not effective for treating subacromial impingement syndrome;[27] however, some studies have demonstrated effectiveness in the treatment of lateral epicondylitis,[28] cervical osteoarthritis,[29] and pain and swelling associated with distal radius fractures.[30]

Table 15•1	Selected Literature Review: Magnet Therapy			
Author and Year	**Patient Population**	**Intervention(s)**	**Results**	**Conclusions**
Harlow et al, 2004[31]	OA of hip or knee (n = 194)	Wore standard strength, weak, or dummy magnetic bracelets for 12 weeks	Pain decreased more in subjects who wore standard-strength bracelets.	Uncertain whether results were secondary to effects of magnets or to placebo effect
Weintraub et al., 2003[11]	Diabetic peripheral neuropathy (n = 375)	Wore magnetized insoles or sham continuously for 4 months	Significant decrease in symptoms during months 3 and 4 in group that wore magnetized insoles	Static magnetic fields penetrate up to 20 mm and analgesia is achieved over time.
Hinman et al., 2002[3]	Chronic knee pain (n = 43)	Wore pads with magnets or placebos on knees for 2 weeks	Significant improvement in pain, physical function, and gait speed in magnet group compared to placebo group	Suggests that application of static magnets over painful knee joints reduces pain and enhances functional movement
Martel, et al., 2002[13]	Young, healthy males (n = 20)	Wore static magnets or placebos on anterior surface of forearms for 30 minutes	Average blood flow not significantly different between groups	Static magnets do not result in significant alterations in resting blood flow.
Hinman, 2002[14]	Adults without symptoms of cardiovascular disease or cardiac problems (n = 75)	Subjects lay on mattress with 42 magnets or a placebo for 15 minutes.	No "clinically meaningful" changes in heart rate or blood pressure	Results support the safe use of unipolar static magnetic fields < 1,000 G.

Continued

Table 15•1 **Selected Literature Review: Magnet Therapy—cont'd**

Author and Year	Patient Population	Intervention(s)	Results	Conclusions
Jacobson et al., 2001[15]	Patients (n = 176) with diagnosis of knee pain 2° to osteoarthritis	Exposed to magnetic fields for 48 minutes or a placebo (magnetic field off) for eight sessions in 2 weeks	Significantly greater relief of pain in treatment group compared to control	Low-amplitude, extremely low-frequency magnetic fields are safe and effective for patient with osteoarthritis and chronic knee pain.
Sweeney et al., 2001[16]	Healthy student volunteers (n = 13)	Single 5 × 11 cm magnet or sham applied to anterior thigh for 60 minutes	No difference in skin or intramuscular temperatures measured at 20, 40, and 60 minutes of application	Flexible therapeutic magnets were not effective for increasing skin or deep temperatures.
Segal et al., 2001[17]	Patients with rheumatoid arthritis and persistent knee pain (n = 64)	Four quadripolar static magnet devices (MagnaBloc) or control devices with one magnet were attached around the knees and worn for 1 week.	Average changes in pain intensity were significant for both groups; not significant between groups for percentage pain reduction.	Both MagnaBloc and control devices were significantly efficacious in decreasing pain from baseline.
Collacott et al., 2000[18]	Stable low back pain (n = 20), mean duration 19 years	Bipolar permanent magnets and sham applied to the low back for total of 18 hours for both groups (1 week with magnets and 1 week with shams)	No significant differences between real and sham magnets for pain and lumbosacral spine ROM	Application of one variety of permanent magnet had no effect on a small group of subjects with chronic low back pain.
Tis et al., 2000[19]	Knee surgery or knee injury in past 6 months (n = 20)	Application of pad with seven bar magnets, placebo magnet, or no magnet to anterior thigh for 10 minutes prior to isokinetic exercise	No significant difference in isokinetic force production among all three groups	Application of magnetic pad to quadriceps muscle does not appear to increase isokinetic force production.
Weintraub, 1999[20]	Diabetic (n = 9) patients and non-diabetic patients with neuropathic pain (n = 9)	Wore magnetic foot insoles for one foot and sham on other foot for 30 days; then sides of magnets and sham were switched for 4 weeks; then subjects wore new magnet insoles on both feet for 8 weeks.	Ninety percent decrease in pain in diabetic patients and 33% in nondiabetic patients after 4 months	Magnetotherapy may be a safe and unique therapy in neuropathic foot pain.
Weintraub, 1998[21]	Diabetic neuropathy (n = 8) and nondiabetic neuropathy (n = 6)	Wore magnetic footpad insoles for 24-hour periods up to 4 months. No control group.	Seventy-five percent of diabetic patients and 50% of nondiabetic patients had reduction of symptoms; 64% of all patients experienced a clinical benefit.	Results suggest that wearing magnetic footpads may be a modifiable factor in intractable peripheral neuropathy.
Borsa and Liggett, 1998[22]	Induced biceps brachii muscle microinjury following intense exercise (n = 10)	Application of flexible magnet, sham, or nothing over biceps brachii after exercise for 72 hours	No significant differences between groups for pain, upper arm girth, ROM, and static muscle force production	No significant therapeutic effects on pain control and muscular dysfunction were observed in subjects wearing flexible magnets.
Vallbona et al., 1997[23]	Postpolio syndrome and muscular or arthritic-like pain (n = 50)	Application of active or placebo magnetic devices to the affected area for 45 minutes	Active device group who reported a pain score decrease greater than the average placebo effect was 76%, compared to 19% in the placebo device group.	Application of static magnetic fields of 300 to 500 G over pain trigger point led to significant and prompt relief of pain in postpolio subjects.
Hong, 1987[24]	Normal volunteers (n = 10)	Six-inch round electromagnet placed perpendicularly over peroneal nerve and median and ulnar nerves for 15 sec; no control group.	No significant change in nerve conduction velocities (NCV) of median and peroneal nerves; significant increase in excitability for all nerves measured at 5-, 10-, and 15-sec exposure	Excitability of motor nerve increased when exposed to static magnetic field with density of 1 T.
Hong et al., 1982[25]	Chronic neck and shoulder pain (n = 52), and without pain or neurological signs (n = 49)	Subjects wore either static magnetic field necklace or nonmagnetic necklace 24 hr/day for 3 weeks.	Intensity and frequency of pain significantly reduced in both magnetic and nonmagnetic groups	Wearing magnetic necklace had no significant therapeutic effect on patients with chronic neck and shoulder pain and stiffness.

Clinical Applications of Magnet Therapy

Magnet therapy may be an alternative intervention for pain control in patients with postpolio syndrome or peripheral neuropathy. Patients with pain in the knees associated with rheumatoid arthritis may also benefit from magnet therapy. However, the effectiveness of long-term use of magnets for these applications has not been determined. At this time, magnet application for any other intervention is not supported by the literature.

Static magnets are readily available and relatively inexpensive. Patients can wear static magnets during the day, without the need for direct clinician supervision. Precautions and contraindications for static magnets are not currently known; some possible precautions and contraindications are listed in Box 15-1. Adverse effects from exposure to static magnets are unlikely because of the relatively weak magnetic fields generated by these devices (usually less than 1,000 G). Previous concerns about possible harmful effects from exposure to electromagnetic fields, such as increased risk of cancer, neurobehavioral dysfunction, and reproductive dysfunction, have largely been discounted by recent epidemiological studies.[1,2,10]

Pulsed magnetic fields are primarily used to promote healing of delayed-healing or nonhealing bone fractures. The clinical use of PEMF for other musculoskeletal problems is rather limited despite some studies that have shown effective outcomes. More studies are needed to demonstrate comparative effectiveness of PEMF with other therapeutic modalities, including treatment cost comparisons.

Box 15•1	**Magnet Therapy: Precautions and Contraindications**

- Do not use magnets near cardiac pacemakers, defibrillators, insulin pumps, or any other internal or external electronic devices, because magnets may interfere with their function.
- Do not place magnets over the low back or pelvic region of a pregnant woman because the effect on the fetus is unknown.
- Avoid placing magnets over or near cancerous tissues to prevent the possibility of facilitating growth or spread of the cancer by magnetic fields.
- A protective barrier between the skin and the magnet may help to prevent skin irritation.
- There are some reports of dizziness, light-headedness, discomfort, and malaise after exposure to magnetic fields, so monitor patients closely during and after treatment.

Monochromatic Infrared Photo Energy

During the last century, the use of infrared radiation lamps to heat biological tissues was a common clinical practice.[32] Today, the use of infrared lamps as superficial heating agents has largely been replaced by hot packs because of the increased risk of burns from the constant heating effect of these lamps. Recently the emergence of devices that provide monochromatic infrared energy emitted from diodes has reintroduced the use of infrared radiation to clinical practice. These devices, known as *monochromatic infrared energy*, or MIRE, are thought to work by influencing vasoactive mediators rather than by heating tissues.

Physical Principles of MIRE

MIRE devices produce energy waves from the near-infrared portion of the electromagnetic spectrum. This portion of the spectrum has wavelengths ranging from 780 to 1,500 nm, which are the infrared wavelengths closest to visible light. Devices that produce near-infrared radiation are known as *luminous devices* because the light produced is visible.[6] MIRE devices generate monochromatic near-infrared photo energy at 890 nm from a series of 60 gallium aluminum arsenide diodes on a flexible pad.[33–35] Figure 15-3 shows a MIRE device. Horwitz et al.[36] used a photodiode to measure the uniform average power over a MIRE pad with a surface of 22.5 cm² and found that the diode array on the pad produced 9.0 mW/cm². Each pad had a total energy density of 43.2 J/cm² per 30-minute treatment.

Another device reported in the literature that produces near-infrared radiation uses a superiodine lamp for light generation and an optical fiber for the light path to emit a near-infrared ray.[37] This device produces

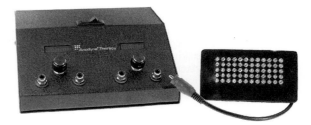

Fig 15•3 MIRE device with diode arrays on flexible pad. *(Courtesy of Anodyne Therapy, LLC, Tampa, FL.)*

a linear polarized near-infrared ray and is similar to low-level laser devices.

Proposed Physiological Effects of MIRE

The physiological effects of MIRE on biological tissue are believed to occur primarily by photochemical reactions rather than by thermal effects. Leonard and colleagues[35] found that MIRE treatments were more effective in improving sensation in patients with peripheral neuropathy than in patients who received placebo pads that emitted a comparable thermal effect. Horwitz and colleagues[36] reported that applying MIRE to the skin for 30 minutes increased plasma nitric oxide (NO). Photo energy releases NO from red blood cells, which is believed to result in vasodilation and increased circulation in the treated tissues. NO is believed to promote vascular perfusion by dilating arterioles, resulting in enhanced tissue oxygenation, nutrient delivery, and removal of waste products of metabolism.[33,36] Human blood lymphocytes irradiated with MIRE had an increased level of ATP in cells.[38] These effects may explain the enhancement of wound healing in patients treated with MIRE.[36] Improving circulation and thus oxygenating tissues treated by MIRE may promote nerve growth in patients with peripheral neuropathy.

Several studies have reported improved sensation in patients with peripheral neuropathy who were treated with MIRE.[33,35,39,40,42,43] However, in a randomized, double-blind, placebo-controlled study, Clifft and colleagues[41] found that 30 minutes of active MIRE applied 3 days per week for 4 weeks was no more effective than placebo MIRE in increasing sensation in 39 subjects with diabetic peripheral neuropathy.

Review of the Literature on MIRE

Table 15-2 provides a review of the relevant literature on MIRE. An analysis of these studies allows for the following conclusions:

- MIRE may reduce the pain and spasm associated with temporomandibular joint (TMJ) dysfunction.[34,37]
- MIRE may promote healing of chronic venous ulcers, diabetic ulcers and wounds, and ulcers associated with scleroderma.[36]
- There is some evidence that MIRE can improve plantar sensation,[33,35,39,40,42,43] although one study failed to show improvement.[41]
- MIRE may help improve balance and reduce falls in patients with peripheral neuropathy. [35,39,42,43]

Table 15•2 **Selected Literature Review: Monochromatic Infrared Energy (MIRE)**

Author and Year	Patient Population	Intervention(s)	Results	Conclusions
Clifft et al., 2005[41]	Diabetic peripheral neuropathy (n = 39)	Active or placebo MIRE 3x/week for 4 weeks	No significant difference between subjects who received active or placebo MIRE	MIRE may not be any more effective than placebo in improving plantar sensation.
DeLellis et al., 2005[42]	Medical records of 1,047 patients with peripheral neuropathy	Association between treatment with MIRE and increased foot sensitivity	Seventy-one percent decrease in insensate sites on both feet; only 43.9% of patients had persistent lack of protective sensation.	MIRE seems to be associated with significant clinical improvement in foot sensation.
Powell et al., 2004[43]	Diabetic peripheral neuropathy, over age 64 (n = 68)	Questionnaire to determine relationship between improved foot sensitivity following MIRE and incidence of new foot wounds	One out of 68 patients who completed the questionnaire developed a new foot wound.	Improved foot sensitivity following MIRE treatments appears to be associated with a lower incidence of new foot wounds in patients with diabetes.
Kochman, 2004[39]	Diabetic peripheral neuropathy (n = 27), polyneuropathy secondary to alcohol abuse (n = 6); decreased sensation secondary to peripheral vascular disease (PVD) (n = 5)	MIRE daily for 30 to 40 minutes using two pads, one each placed medially and laterally on lower leg. No control group.	All patients had restoration of protective sensation measured by SWM, and significantly higher Tinetti scores, reduced Tinetti fall risk category by one level, and average falls per patient reduced by 93% for 3 months after treatment.	Comprehensive therapy intervention that includes infrared photo energy has potential to improve sensation and balance and to decrease fall frequency.

Table 15•2	Selected Literature Review: Monochromatic Infrared Energy (MIRE)—cont'd			
Author and Year	**Patient Population**	**Intervention(s)**	**Results**	**Conclusions**
Prendergast et al., 2004[40]	Peripheral neuropathy (n = 27)	MIRE pulsed at 292 per second and duty cycle on time 50%, power density 8 mW/cm^2, applied for 10 treatments over a 2-week period. No control group.	Significant improvement in sensory impairment based on scores of current perception thresholds taken by neurometer; 16/27 (59%) patients had a score of 0, which indicates normal sensory responses in all nerve fiber subpopulations.	MIRE seems to be safe and effective in reducing sensory impairment associated with peripheral neuropathy due to diabetes and other causes.
Leonard et al., 2004[35]	Diabetic peripheral neuropathy (n = 27)	Subjects received 12 MIRE treatments to one leg and sham devices (created heat but no IR) to the other leg.	Significant decrease in average sites insensitive to 5.07 SWM in subjects who had not progressed to profound sensory loss (almost 50% improvement in restoration of protective sensation); substantial improvement in self-reported balance after six treatments.	MIRE treatments improve sensation in the feet of subjects with diabetic peripheral neuropathy, improve balance, and reduce pain.
Kochman et al., 2002[33]	Diabetic peripheral neuropathy (n = 49)	MIRE pads on foot and lower leg; total of four pads with diode arrays, 30 minutes for 12 treatments. No control group.	Eighty-five percent improvement in sensory perception documented by Semmes-Weinstein monofilaments.	Results suggest that in an outpatient setting, MIRE consistently improves neural function in patients with diabetes.
Horwitz et al., 1999[36]	Lower extremity venous ulcers (n = 3), diabetes and wound dehiscence (n = 1), scleroderma with an ulcer on the hand (n = 1)	MIRE at home for 30 minutes, frequency of treatment varied; one subject with ulcer treated in clinic once per week initially, then every other week. No control group.	All subjects with ulcers had healing of ulcers; subject with wound dehiscence had complete closure of wound; subject with scleroderma had healing of ulcer.	Additional research is needed to show whether MIRE is independently responsible for wound healing in these patients.
Thomasson, 1996[34]	Patients with tendonitis/tendinosis, (n = 102) with TMJ capsulitis (n = 100), with myofascial pain and spasm (n = 361)	MIRE in clinic 9.0 mw/cm^2 for 45 minutes for 3 sessions; at-home device 7.5 mw/cm^2 for 30 minutes daily for 1 week. No control group.	Patients rated percentage of relief of pain or spasm: 88% total/excellent relief for tendonitis/tendinosis; 88.7% total/excellent relief for TMJ capsulitis; 89.8% total/excellent relief for myofascial pain and spasm	MIRE can be considered a first line of physiotherapeutic treatment for soft-tissue disorders encountered in pain management.

Clinical Applications of MIRE

The FDA has approved the use of MIRE for enhancing circulation and reducing pain.[36] Currently, clinical devices are marketed for use by inpatient or outpatient facilities and portable devices for at-home use. The wavelength of these devices is set at 890 nm. The flexible pads containing the diode arrays are placed on the skin. This allows for hands-free application of treatment—an advantage over low-level laser, which requires hands-on treatment. When placing over an open wound, a transparent dressing such as OpSite can be situated over the wound to prevent contamination.[36] Most of the success reported with MIRE has occurred with 30- to 40-minute treatments performed daily or several times a week. One study reported a topical burn

on the dorsal aspect of the foot after a patient fell asleep for several hours with a MIRE device.[43] No other harmful effects of MIRE have been reported in the literature. See Box 15-2 for a list of precautions and contraindications for MIRE.

Hyperbaric Oxygen Therapy

The use of hyperbaric oxygen chambers to treat divers who have decompression sickness (the "bends") has been a common practice for many years. Other uses of hyperbaric oxygen therapy (HBOT) approved by the Undersea and Hyperbaric Medical Society include treatment for air or gas embolism, carbon monoxide poisoning, refractory osteomyelitis, delayed radiation

Box 15•2	Monochromatic Infrared Energy: Precautions and Contraindications

- Do not perform MIRE over the low back or pelvic region of a pregnant woman because the effect on the fetus is unknown.
- Avoid placing MIRE pads over or near cancerous tissues to prevent the possibility of facilitating growth or spread of the cancer by the effects of the infrared radiation.
- Goggles are not required during treatment because the flexible pads containing the diode arrays block the infrared radiation from the eyes; however, avoid placing the pads over the eyes.

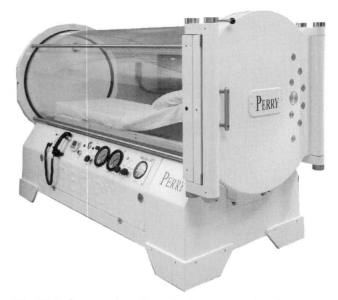

Fig 15•4 A monoplace hyperbaric oxygen chamber.
(Courtesy of Perry Biomedical, Riviera Beach, FL.)

injury, compromised skin grafts and flaps, and thermal burns. It is also approved to enhance wound healing. Recently there has been increased interest in the therapeutic effects of HBOT for musculoskeletal problems such as delayed-onset muscle soreness and fibromyalgia.[44]

Physical Principles of HBOT

HBOT involves inhaling 100% oxygen in a pressurized hyperbaric chamber at a pressure greater than 1 absolute atmosphere (ATA), which is the atmospheric pressure at sea level (1 ATA = 760 mmHg). Typically, HBOT is administered at 2 to 3 ATA for a duration of 30 to 120 minutes. HBOT can be administered to a single patient using a monoplace chamber in which oxygen pressure is raised to 100% or to more than one patient in a multiplace chamber where each person breathes oxygen through a mask.[45] Patients lie supine in monoplace chambers, which are typically 22 inches in diameter and constructed of Plexiglas with metal ends (Fig. 15-4). Multiplace chambers are typically found only at major medical centers and teaching institutions. These chambers can accommodate 12 or more patients who are either sitting in chairs or lying on gurneys.[46]

Proposed Physiological Effects of HBOT

HBOT increases the amount of physically dissolved oxygen in plasma, resulting in immediate hyperoxygenation and hyperoxia. At 2 ATA, there is a 10-fold increase in oxygen tension in blood.[47] The increase in dissolved oxygen in the plasma provides tissues with a readily available supply of oxygen so they do not have to rely on hemoglobin-bound oxygen, which is less accessible to tissues injured by sympathetically-induced

vasoconstriction caused by inflammation.[48] The beneficial effects of hyperoxia occur primarily through improved oxygen delivery to tissues. The result is preservation of tissue viability in ischemic areas, provided there is no occlusion of major arterial vessels. Hyperoxia enhances wound healing by increasing the diffusion distance of oxygen through tissues fluids, which improves oxygen delivery to ischemic and hypoxic tissues. Collagen production by fibroblasts is enhanced, resulting in increased collagen synthesis and angiogenesis, which promotes wound closure rate in hypoxic tissues.

Hyperoxia also enhances oxygen-dependent intracellular killing mechanisms of leukocytes and prevents infection from anaerobic microorganisms by producing toxic oxygen radicals that kill them.[47] Elevating tissue oxygen enhances the "oxidative burst" that ultimately dispatches ingested pathogens, helping to clear bacteria from infected tissues that are suboptimally supplied with oxygen. Hyperoxia will also enhance antibiotic uptake in infected tissues and will improve its effectiveness.[46] Hyperoxygenation has a direct vasoconstricting effect, resulting in decreased capillary transudation flow rates that inhibit edema formation and a reduction of vasogenic edema in patients with compartment syndrome. Hyperoxygenation also enhances microcirculation by reducing local interstitial pressure.[47]

Review of the Literature on HBOT

Table 15-3 provides a review of selected studies and reviews of HBOT use. An analysis of these studies and reviews allows for the following conclusions:

- There is some evidence to support HBOT use for the following conditions: complex regional pain syndrome (CRPS), refractory osteomyelitis, wounds and ulcers, fibromyalgia, myofascial pain syndrome, migraine and cluster headaches, ischemic leg pain, radiation injury, compromised skin grafts and flaps, and thermal burns.

- No evidence from randomized trials supports or refutes the use of HBOT for preventing or treating poorly healing broken bones.
- Insufficient evidence exists to establish the effects of HBOT on ankle and knee sprains and on experimentally induced delayed-onset muscle soreness. Some evidence shows that HBOT may increase interim pain in delayed-onset muscle soreness.
- HBOT may be a cost-effective modality that significantly reduces length of hospital stay, amputation rate, and wound care expenses.

Table 15·3 Selected Literature Review: Hyperbaric Oxygen Therapy

Author and Year	Patient Population	Intervention(s)	Results	Conclusions
Goldman, 2009[49]	Systematic review of 45 studies of at least five subjects	HBOT	High level of evidence for decreasing risk of amputation and healing of wounds. Moderate level of evidence for healing of arterial ulcers and refractory osteomyelitis. Low to moderate level of evidence for healing of ablative or reconstructive surgery and salvage of flaps or grafts.	Safe technique for treatment of refractory osteomyelitis, wounds, and ulcers. Medicare-approved for diabetic foot ulcers (Wagner grades III, IV, and V).
Yildiz et al., 2006[45]	Literature review	HBOT	Studies reviewed found HBOT to be effective for fibromyalgia, chronic regional pain syndrome, myofascial pain syndrome, migraine and cluster headaches, and ischemic leg pain.	Evidence for effectiveness for musculoskeletal conditions listed; optimal treatment protocols need to be established.
Bennett et al., 2005[50]	Cochrane review of randomized controlled trials that compared effects of HBOT to no HBOT (sham or control) on healing of fractures	HBOT	No studies met inclusion criteria.	No evidence from randomized trials to support or refute the use of HBOT for preventing poor healing or treating poorly healing broken bones.
Bennett et al., 2005[1]	Cochrane review of randomized controlled trials of effects of HBOT on delayed-onset muscle soreness and closed soft tissue injury	HBOT	Nine small trials involving a total of 219 subjects were reviewed. No significant difference found between groups that received HBOT and control or sham HBOT for ankle and knee sprains and delayed-onset muscle soreness and no difference in groups for long-term pain scores, swelling, or muscle strength.	Insufficient evidence to establish the effects of HBOT on ankle and knee sprains and on experimentally induced delayed-onset muscle soreness. Some evidence that HBOT may increase interim pain in delayed-onset muscle soreness.
Kranke et al., 2004[52]	Cochrane review of randomized controlled trials of effects of HBOT on healing of lower leg chronic wounds	HBOT	Four trials with a total of 147 patients with diabetic foot ulcers showed a reduction in risk of major amputation; 1 trial with 16 patients with venous ulcers showed significant reduction in ulcer area at 6 weeks.	HBOT seems to reduce the number of major amputations in people with diabetes who have chronic foot ulcers and may reduce the size of wounds caused by disease to the veins of the leg.
Kilralp et al., 2004[53]	Patients with chronic regional pain syndrome (CRPS), $n = 71$ avg. age 29.4	Thirty-seven received HBOT, 34 normal air (control) during fifteen 90-minute sessions in hyperbaric chamber at 2.4 ATA (5 days a week, 1 session per day)	Significant difference in pain, wrist flexion, and wrist circumference for the HBOT group	HBOT is an effective and well-tolerated treatment for reducing pain and edema and increasing wrist motion in patients with CRPS.

Continued

Table 15•3	Selected Literature Review: Hyperbaric Oxygen Therapy—cont'd			
Author and Year	**Patient Population**	**Intervention(s)**	**Results**	**Conclusions**
Greensmith, 2004[46]	Literature review	Reviewed basic research and clinical studies of HBOT	Indications for HBOT include crush injury, compartment syndrome, acute traumatic peripheral ischemia, wound healing, refractory osteomyelitis, radiation injury, compromised skin grafts and flaps, thermal burns.	An expensive, technology-intensive therapy. More research is needed to determine optimal indications, timing, and dosing protocols.
Wang et al., 2002[54]	Literature review	HBOT	Indications for HBOT include refractory osteomyelitis, nonhealing wounds, non- or delayed-union fractures, radiation-induced tissue injury, thermal burns, acute traumatic ischemia, compromised skin and bone grafts, and muscle flaps.	HBOT is a cost-effective modality that significantly reduces length of hospital stay, amputation rate, and wound care expenses.
Staples et al., 1999[48]	"Untrained" male university students, $n = 66$, ages 18–35	Exercise-induced delayed-onset muscle soreness treated with HBOT (100% O_2 1 hour/day at 2 ATA) or sham HBOT (21% O_2 1 hour/day at 1.2 ATA)	Significant difference in recovery of eccentric torque compared to sham group; no significant difference in pain scores.	Exposure to 1 hour of HBOT initiated within 20 minutes after exercise for 3 to 5 days enhances muscle torque recovery but does not significantly affect delayed-onset muscle soreness.
Borromeo et al., 1997[55]	Patients with lateral ankle sprains, $n = 32$, average age 24.2	All subjects sat in pressurized hyperbaric chamber for 90 minutes (first session) and 60 minutes (last 2 sessions); treatment group received 100% O_2 at 2 ATA, control received normal air at 1.1 ATA, for 3 sessions within 7 days.	No significant difference in dependent variables: perceived pain, edema, active and passive ROM, function, and time to return to preinjury activity level	Analysis of objective measures of ankle function showed no difference between subjects who received normal air and those who received HBOT.
Bouachour et al., 1996[47]	Patients with crush injuries, 24 hours after surgery, $n = 32$	Blindly assigned to HBOT at 100% O_2 at 2.5 ATA or placebo at 21% O_2 at 1.1 ATA for 90 minutes 2x/day for 6 days	Complete wound healing without tissue necrosis requiring surgical excision occurred in 17 patients in HBOT group vs. 10 patients in placebo group.	HBOT is a useful therapeutic adjunct in managing severe trauma of the limbs in older people. HBOT improves wound healing and reduces repetitive surgery.

More studies are needed to establish optimal treatment parameters, such as duration and frequency of treatment and dosing protocols.

Clinical Applications of HBOT

In the United States, HBOT is approved by Medicare for treating diabetic foot ulcers (Wagner grades III, IV, and V).[49]

HBOT is considered a relatively safe treatment modality. However, Goldman[49] identified several possible side effects of treatment: increased cardiovascular afterload because of the peripheral vasoconstrictive effect of oxygen; oxygen toxicity that can affect CNS, pulmonary, and ocular function; barotrauma to the inner ear, sinuses, and dental and pulmonary tissues; hypoglycemia; and confinement anxiety. See Box 15-3 for a list of contraindications and precautions.

KEY POINT! The use of HBOT is limited by the cost and availability of hyperbaric chambers. A used monoplace chamber may cost $150,000, and a multiplace chamber may cost several million.[46]

Extracorporeal Shock Wave Therapy

The concept of using high-energy shock waves is not new to us. Most are familiar with the use of lithotripsy for kidney stones. Extracorporeal shock wave therapy (ESWT) is used to treat conditions such as calcific tendonitis, other tendinopathies, and plantar fasciitis. This modality is used exclusively by physicians and surgeons and is not currently available to other health-care practitioners. It is important, though, for practitioners to be familiar with this novel application of sound waves, because our patients may ask us about this as a treatment option.

Box 15•3	HBOT Contraindications and Precautions[46,54]

Contraindications	Precautions
• Undrained hemothorax or untreated pneumothorax	• COPD or asthma
• Currently receiving chemotherapy or radiation	• Seizure disorders
• Pressure-sensitive implanted medical device	• Claustrophobia
• Patients taking certain antineoblastic antibiotics, such as Bleomycin or Doxorubicin, or the antineoplastic heavy metal compound Cisplatin	• Chronic sinusitis or upper respiratory infection • Fever and/or dehydration • History of spontaneous pneumothorax

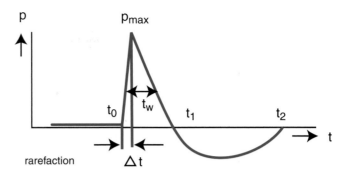

Fig 15•5 A single shock wave used for extracorporeal shock wave therapy. Note parameters of focused shock wave. T, change in time; P_{max}, pressure maximum; Δt, pressure rise time; t_w, half width time; Pr, negative peak pressure. *(Diagram courtesy of Sonorex, Inc., Fayetteville, NC.)*

Physical Principles of ESWT

ESWT uses single-impulse, focused acoustical sound waves that have a rapid rise in pressure. There are several methods by which the shock waves are generated:

- Reverse piezoelectric (electrical to mechanical energy)
- Electromagnetic
- Electrohydraulic

The energy is transmitted from the device through coupling cushions that can transmit acoustical energy. The treatment region must be targeted via ultrasound or fluoroscopic x-ray imaging devices to ensure that the energy is accurately focused to a precise location. The duration of treatment may be up to 30 minutes. Energy for ESWT is described in joules per area (mJ/mm^2) and is characterized as high or low.[56]

These shock waves have high-pressure amplitudes and are of very short duration (Fig. 15-5). ESWT single pulses are at 1 to 4 per second (at a potential frequency of 1,000 to 4,000 shock-wave pulses). The total energy of a treatment includes the number of shock impulses and the energy density together.

Proposed Physiological Effects of ESWT

Shock waves transmit through and are absorbed by soft tissue and are reflected at interfaces of tissues with different densities. The biophysical and physiological effects proposed for this energy include ability to disintegrate calcium deposits, hyperstimulation analgesia,

neovascularization, and changes in cell permeability.[57] The latter two effects have been reported in studies on animal models.

Review of the Literature on ESWT

Table 15-4 provides a review of selected articles on ESWT. In addition, an excellent systematic review of ESWT use for calcific and noncalcific rotator cuff tendonitis (RCT) has been published in the *Journal of Hand Therapy*.[57]

An analysis of these studies allows for the following conclusions:

- There is some support for the use of ESWT for plantar fasciitis.
- There is some support for the use of ESWT for calcific tendonitis of the rotator cuff in the shoulder, although disintegration of calcium deposits may not correlate with improvements in pain and function.[66]
- There is little support for the use of ESWT for noncalcific tendonitis of the rotator cuff and subacromial pain syndrome.
- There is little support for the use of ESWT for lateral epicondylitis.
- A single treatment with high-energy ESWT may be a safe and effective procedure for chronic non-insertional Achilles tendonopathy.[64]

Certainly the addition of new studies to the literature to support the use of this modality for managing chronic tendinopathies and fasciopathies would be welcome.

Table 15•4	Selected Literature Review: Extracorporeal Shock Wave Therapy			
Author(s) and Year	**Patient Population**	**Intervention(s)**	**Results**	**Conclusions**
Engebretsen et al., 2009[63]	Subacromial pain syndrome	Radial ESWT 12-8 Hz, 2,000 pulses per session, pressure between 2.5 and 4 Bar once per week for 4 to 6 weeks or supervised exercise program twice a week for 12 weeks	Treatment effect favored supervised exercise group at 6, 12, and 18 weeks.	Supervised exercise program better than radial ESWT for pain and disability related to subacromial pain syndrome.
Furia, 2008[64]	Chronic noninsertional Achilles tendinopathy	Single dose of high-energy ESWT, 3,000 shocks at 0.21 mJ/mm^2 for a total energy flux density of 604 mJ/mm^2 or traditional forms of nonoperative therapy for 6 months.	Statistically greater percentage of patients who had ESWT had improvement in Roles and Maudsley scores (patient assessment of pain and limitations of activity) compared to control group.	Single treatment of high-energy ESWT is a safe and effective procedure for chronic noninsertional Achilles tendinopathy.
Wilner and Strash, 2004[65]	Chronic proximal plantar fasciopathy (plantar fasciitis)	ESWT using 1,800 shocks at 18 kilovolts and 4 Hz/sec (under general anesthesia)	More than 2 years after treatment, patients rated level of improvement: excellent/good 87%; fair 11%; no improvement 2%	ESWT is an effective and safe noninvasive intervention for chronic plantar fasciitis.
Pleiner et al., 2004[66]	Symptomatic calcific tendonitis of the shoulder for greater than 6 months	ESWT 2 x 2,000 impulses at 0.28 mJ/mm^2 at an interval of 2 weeks or < 0.07 mJ/mm^2 (control group)	Shoulder function significantly improved compared to control; calcifications completely resolved in 19% compared to 8% in control; significant decrease in pain at 1 week but not at 3 and 7 months.	ESWT can significantly improve shoulder function and may help disintegrate calcific deposits but may not result in reduction in pain.
Chung and Wiley, 2004[67]	Lateral epicondylitis of at least 3 weeks but less than 1 year duration	ESWT delivered one session per week for 3 weeks at 2,000 pulses and energy flux density 0.03–0.17 mJ/mm^2 or sham ESWT	Success rates based on level of pain, use of pain meds, quality of life (EuroQoL questionnaire), and grip strength were 39% for ESWT and 31% for sham.	No meaningful difference in pain scores, grip strength, or quality of life between patients who received ESWT and those who received sham ESWT.
Pan et al., 2003[69]	Continuous shoulder pain for at least 6 months with verified calcific tendonitis	ESWT 2,000 shocks at 2 Hz, energy level .26 to .32 mJ/mm^2 for two sessions (14 days apart) or TENS	Subjects who received ESWT had greater functional improvement and pain reduction than those who received TENS.	ESWT is more effective than TENS for relieving pain and improving function for patients with calcific tendonitis of the shoulder.
Gerdesmeyer et al., 2003[59]	Chronic calcific tendonitis of shoulder	High-energy ESWT; low-energy ESWT placebo (sham)	ESWT showed significant improvement in 6-month mean Constant Morrey scale score compared with sham treatment; diminished size of calcifications.	High-energy more effective than low-energy, but both better than placebo
Speed et al., 2003[62]	Plantar fasciitis for at least 3 months	ESWT 0.12 mJ/mm^2 or sham ESWT therapy once a month for 3 months	Both groups improved; no difference between groups.	No treatment effect of moderate-dose ESWT
Buchbinder et al., 2002[58]	Plantar fasciitis	Ultrasound-guided ESWT total dose ($n = 81$) of at least 1,000 mJ/mm^2; placebo to a total dose of 6.0 mJ/mm^2 ($n = 85$)	Improvement in both groups in pain (morning and activity), walking ability, and SF-36 scores	No difference following treatment between groups at 6 to 12 weeks
Speed et al., 2002[60]	Noncalcific tendonitis of the shoulder	Fifteen hundred pulses ESWT at 0.12 mJ/mm^2 or sham ESWT treatment, monthly for 3 months	VAS for night pain (SPADI) scores improved for both groups at 1 and 3 months, both treatments.	No difference between groups
Speed et al., 2002[61]	Chronic lateral epicondylitis	ESWT at 1,500 pulses, ESWT at 0.12 mJ/mm^2 vs. sham ESWT once a month for 3 months	Both groups improved in pain, day and night. No significant differences between groups.	No better than sham therapy

Clinical Applications of ESWT

The FDA has approved the use of certain devices for ESWT. The manufacturer of such devices will have evidence of FDA approval.

The most common applications for ESWT have included management of chronic plantar fasciitis (with or without a heel spur), tendonitis of the shoulder, and tendonitis of the elbow (Fig. 15-6). Another indication for use is in the management of nonunion fractures. Some side effects can occur after treatment, including hematoma, reddening, petechia, and transient pain. Contraindications for ESWT are outlined in Box 15-4.

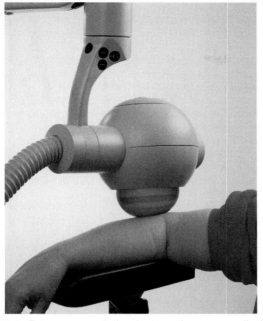

Fig 15•6 Extracorporeal shock wave therapy applied to the lateral elbow for tendonitis. *(Courtesy of Sonorex, Inc., Fayetteville, NC.)*

| **Box 15•4** | **Extracorporeal Shock Wave Therapy: Contraindications** |

- Bleeding conditions
- Pacemakers
- Medications that prolong blood clotting
- Children
- Pregnancy
- Acute injuries

☐ REFERENCES

1. Basford JR. A historical perspective of the popular use of electric and magnetic therapy. *Arch Phys Med Rehabil.* 2001; 82:1261–1269.
2. Macklis RM. Magnetic healing, quackery, and the debate about the health effects of electromagnetic fields. *Ann Int Med.* 1993;118:376–383.
3. Hinman MR, Ford J, Heyl H. Effects of static magnets on chronic knee pain and physical function: a double-blind study. *Altern Ther Health Med.* 2002;8:50–55.
4. Trock DH, Bollet AJ, Markoll R. The effect of pulsed electromagnetic fields in the treatment of osteoarthritis of the knee and cervical spine. Report of randomized, double blind, placebo controlled trials. *J Rheumatol.* 1994;21:1903–1911.
5. Giancoli DC. *Physics: Principles with Applications.* 5th ed. Upper Saddle River, NJ: Prentice Hall; 1998.
6. Starkey C. *Therapeutic Modalities.* 3rd ed. Philadelphia: FA Davis; 2004.
7. Blechman AM, Oz M, Nair V, Ting W. Discrepancy between claimed field flux density of some commercially available magnets and actual gaussmeter measurements. *Altern Ther Health Med.* 2001;7:92–95.
8. Ratterman R, Secrest J, Norwood B, Ch'ien AP. Magnet therapy: what's the attraction? *J Am Acad Nurse Pract.* 2002;14:347–353.
9. Robertson V, Ward A, Low J, Reed A. *Electrotherapy Explained, Principles and Practice.* 4th ed. London: Elsevier; 2006.
10. Markov MS, Colbert AP. Magnetic and electromagnetic field therapy. *J Back Musculoskel Rehabil.* 2001;15:17–29.
11. Weintraub MI, Wolfe GI, Barohn RA, et al. Static magnetic field therapy for symptomatic diabetic neuropathy: a randomized, double-blind, placebo-controlled trial. *Arch Phys Med Rehabil.* 2003;84:736–746.
12. Pittler MH, Brown EM, Ernst E. Static magnets for reducing pain: systematic review and meta-analysis of randomized trials. *Can Med Assoc J.* 2007;177:736–742.
13. Martel GF, Andrews SC, Roseboom CG. Comparison of static and placebo magnets on resting forearm blood flow in young, healthy men. *J Orthop Sports Phys Ther.* 2002;32:518–524.
14. Hinman MR. Comparative effect of positive and negative static magnetic fields on heart rate and blood pressure in healthy adults. *Clin Rehabil.* 2002;16:669–674.
15. Jacobson JI, Gorman R, Yamanashi WS, et al. Low-amplitude, extremely low frequency magnetic fields for the treatment of osteoarthritic knees: a double-blind clinical study. *Altern Ther Health Med.* 2001;7:54–69.
16. Sweeney KB, Merrick MA, Ingersoll CD, Swez JA. Therapeutic magnets do not affect tissue temperatures. *J Athl Train.* 2001;36:27–31.
17. Segal NA, Toda Y, Huston J, et al. Two configurations of static magnetic fields for treating rheumatic arthritis of the knee: a double-blind clinical trial. *Arch Phys Med Rehabil.* 2001; 82:1453.
18. Collacott EA, Zimmerman JT, White DW, Rindone JP. Bipolar permanent magnets for the treatment of chronic low back pain: a pilot study. *JAMA.* 2000;283:1322–1325.
19. Tis LL, Trinkaus MD, Higbie EJ, et al. Effects of magnets on concentric and eccentric isokinetic force production of the quadriceps group. *Isokinet Exerc Sci.* 2000;8:217–221.
20. Weintraub MI. Magnetic bio-stimulation in painful diabetic peripheral neuropathy: a novel intervention—a randomized, double-placebo crossover study. *Am J Pain Manage.* 1999;9: 8–17.
21. Weintraub MI. Chronic submaximal magnetic stimulation in peripheral neuropathy: is there a beneficial therapeutic relationship? *Am J Pain Manage.* 1998;8:12–16.
22. Borsa PA, Liggett CL. Flexible magnets are not effective in decreasing pain perception and recovery time after muscle microinjury. *J Athl Train.* 1998;33:150–155.
23. Valbonna C, Hazlewood CF, Jurida G. Response of pain to static magnetic fields in postpolio patients: a double-blind pilot study. *Arch Phys Med Rehabil.* 1997;78:1200–1203.
24. Hong C-Z. Static magnetic field influence on human nerve function. *Arch Phys Med Rehabil.* 1987;68:162–164.
25. Hong C-Z, Lin JC, Bender LF, et al. Magnetic necklace: its therapeutic effectiveness on neck and shoulder pain. *Arch Phys Med Rehabil.* 1982;63:462–466.
26. Smania N, Corato E, Fiaschi A, Pietropoli P, Aglioti SM, Tinazzi M. Repetitive magnetic stimulation: a novel therapeutic approach for myofascial pain syndrome. *J Neurol.* 2005; 252:307–314.
27. Aktas I, Akgun K, Cakmak B. Therapeutic effect of pulsed electromagnetic field in conservative treatment of subacromial impingement syndrome. *Clin Rheumatol.* 2007;26:1234–1239.
28. Uzunca K, Birtane M, Tastekin N. Effectiveness of pulsed electromagnetic field therapy in lateral epicondylitis. *Clin Rheumatol.* 2007;26:69–74.
29. Sutbeyaz ST, Sezer N, Koseoglu BF. The effect of pulsed electromagnetic fields in the treatment of cervical osteoarthritis: a randomized, double blind, sham-controlled trial. *Rheumatol Int.* 2006;26:320–324.

30. Cheing GLY, Wan JWH, Lo SK. Ice and pulsed electromagnetic field to reduce pain and swelling after distal radius fractures. *J Rehabil Med.* 2005;37:372–377.

31. Harlow T, Greaves C, White A, Brown L, Hart A, Ernst E. Randomising controlled trial of magnetic bracelets for relieving pain in osteoarthritis of the hip and knee. *Br Med J.* 2004;329:1450–1454.

32. Kahn J. *Principles and Practice of Electrotherapy.* 4th ed. Philadelphia: Churchill Livingstone; 2000.

33. Kochman AB, Carnegie DH, Burke TJ. Symptomatic reversal of peripheral neuropathy in patients with diabetes. *J Am Podiatr Med Assoc.* 2002;92:125–130.

34. Thomasson TL. Effects of skin-contact monochromatic infrared irradiation on tendonitis, capsulitis, and myofascial pain. *J Neurol Orthop Med Surg.* 1996;16:242–245.

35. Leonard DR, Farooqi MH, Myers S. Restoration of sensation, reduced pain, and improved balance in subjects with diabetic peripheral neuropathy. *Diabetes Care.* 2004;27:168–172.

36. Horwitz LR, Burke TJ, Carnegie D. Augmentation of wound healing using monochromatic infrared energy. *Adv Wound Care.* 1999;12:35–40.

37. Yokoyama K, Oku T. Rheumatoid arthritis-affected temporomandibular joint pain analgesia by linear polarized near infrared irradiation. *Can J Anesth.* 1999;46:683–687.

38. Vladimirov YA, Osipov AN, Klebanov GI. Photobiological principles of therapeutic applications of laser radiation. *Biochemistry (Moscow).* 2004;69:81–90.

39. Kochman A. Restoration of sensation, improved balance and gait reduction in falls in elderly patients with use of monochromatic infrared photo energy and physical therapy. *J Geriatr Phys Ther.* 2004;27:16–19.

40. Prendergast JJ, Miranda G, Sanchez M. Improvement of sensory impairment in patients with peripheral neuropathy. *Endocr Pract.* 2004;10:24–30.

41. Clifft JK, Kasser RJ, Newton TS, Bush AJ. The effect of monochromatic infrared energy on sensation in patients with diabetic peripheral neuropathy. *Diabetes Care.* 2005;28:2896–2900.

42. DeLellis SL, Carnegie DH, Burke TJ. Improved sensitivity in patients with peripheral neuropathy. *J Am Podiatr Med Assoc.* 2005;95:143–147.

43. Powell MW, Carnegie DE, Burke TJ. Reversal of diabetic peripheral neuropathy and new wound incidence: the role of MIRE. *Adv Skin Wound Care.* 2004;17:295–300.

44. Semon A, Lehr ME. Hyperbaric oxygen therapy in the treatment of musculoskeletal disorders: a literature review. *Ortho Phys Ther Prac.* 2009;21:96–99.

45. Yildiz S, Uzun G, Kiralp MZ. Hyperbaric oxygen therapy in chronic pain management. *Curr Pain Headache Rep.* 2006;10:95–100.

46. Greensmith JE. Hyperbaric Oxygen Therapy in Extremity Trauma. *J Am Acad Ortho Surg.* 2004;12:376-384.

47. Bouachour G, Cronier P, Gouello JP, Toulemonde JL, Talha A, Alquier P. Hyperbaric oxygen therapy in the management of crush injuries: a randomized double-blind placebo-controlled clinical trial. *J Trauma.* 1996;41:333–339.

48. Staples JR, Clement DB, Taunton JE, McKenzie DC. Effects of hyperbaric oxygen on a human model of injury. *Am J Sports Med.* 1999;275:600–605.

49. Goldman RJ. Hyperbaric oxygen therapy for wound healing and limb salvage: a systematic review. *Phys Med Rehabil.* 2009;1:471–489.

50. Bennett MH, Stanford RE, Turner R. Hyperbaric oxygen therapy for promoting fracture healing and treating fracture nonunion. *Cochrane Database Syst Rev.* 2005;1:CD004712.

51. Bennett MH, Best TM, Babul-Wellar S, Taunton JE. Hyperbaric oxygen therapy for delayed onset muscle soreness and closed soft tissue injury. *Cochrane Database Syst Rev.* 2005;4:CD004713.

52. Kranke P, Bennett M, Roeckl-Wiedmann I, Debus S. Hyperbaric oxygen therapy for chronic wounds. *Cochrane Database Syst Rev.* 2004;2:CD004123.

53. Kilralp MZ, Yildiz S, Vural D, Keskin I, Ay H, Dursun H. Effectiveness of hyperbaric oxygen therapy in the treatment of complex regional pain syndrome. *J Int Med Res.* 2004;32:258–262.

54. Wang J, Li F, Calhoun JH, Mader JT. The role and effectiveness of adjunctive hyperbaric oxygen therapy in the management of musculoskeletal disorders. *J Post Graduate Med.* 2002;48:226–231.

55. Borromeo CN, Ryan JL, Marchetto PA, Peterson L, Bore AA. Hyperbaric oxygen therapy for acute ankle sprains. *Am J Sports Med.* 1997;25:619–625.

56. Loew M, Daecke W, Kusnierczak D, et al. Shock wave therapy for chronic calcifying tendonitis of the shoulder. *J Bone Joint Surg (Br).* 1999;81:863–867.

57. Harmiman E, Carette, Kennedy C, Beaton D. Extracorporeal shockwave therapy for calcific and noncalcific tendinitis of the rotator cuff: a systematic review. *J Hand Ther.* 2004;17:132–151.

58. Buchbinder R, Ptasznik R, Gordon J. Ultrasound-guided extracorporeal shock wave therapy for plantar fasciitis: a randomized controlled trial. *JAMA.* 2002; 288:1364–1372.

59. Gerdesmeyer L, Wagenpfeil S, Haake M, et al. Extracorporeal shock wave therapy for the treatment of chronic calcifying tendonitis of the rotator cuff: a randomized controlled trial. *JAMA.* 2003;290:2573–2580.

60. Speed CA, Richards C, Nichols D, et al. Extracorporeal shockwave therapy for tendonitis of the rotator cuff: a double-blind, randomised, controlled trial. *J Bone Joint Surg (Br).* 2002; 84:509–512.

61. Speed CA, Nichols D, Richards C, et al. Extracorporeal shock wave therapy for lateral epicondylitis—a double blind randomised controlled trial. *J Orthop Res.* 2002;20:895–898.

62. Speed CA, Nichols D, Wies J, et al. Extracorporeal shock wave therapy for plantar fasciitis: a double blind randomised controlled trial. *J Orthop Res.* 2003;21:937–940.

63. Engebretsen K, Grotle M, Bautz-Holter E, et al. Radial extracorporeal shockwave treatment compared with supervised exercises in patients with subacromial pain syndrome: single blind randomised study. *BMJ.* 2009;339:b3360.

64. Furia JP. High-energy extracorporal shock wave therapy as a treatment for chronic noninsertional Achilles tendinopathy. *Am J Sports Med.* 2008;36:502–508.

65. Wilner JM, Strash WW. Extracorporal shockwave therapy for plantar fasciitis and other musculoskeletal conditions utilizing the Ossatron—an update. *Clin Podiatr Med Surg.* 2004;21:441–447.

66. Pleiner J, Crevenna R, Langenberger H, et al. Extracorporeal shockwave treatment is effective in calcific tendonitis of the shoulder. A randomized controlled trial. *Wien Klin Wochenschr.* 2004;116:536–541.

67. Chung B, Wiley JP. Effectiveness of extracorporeal shock wave therapy in the treatment of previously untreated lateral epicondylitis: A randomized controlled trial. *Am J Sports Med.* 2004;32:1660–1667.

68. Pan PJ, Chou CL, Chiou HJ, Ma HL, Lee HC, Chan RC. Extracorporeal shock wave therapy for chronic calcific tendinitis of the shoulders: a functional and sonographic study. *Arch Phys Med Rehabil.* 2003;84:988–993.

chapter 16

Electrophysiological Testing of Nerves and Muscles

Arthur J. Nitz, PT, PhD I James W. Bellew, PT, EdD

What Is Electroneuromyography?

Clinical electroneuromyography includes observing, analyzing, and interpreting the bioelectrical activity of muscles and nerves as they respond to electrical stimulation, needle provocation, and voluntary activation. Most often, the testing consists of a combination of nerve conduction studies (NCS) and electromyography (EMG), although additional tests may occasionally be appropriate. These may include somatosensory-evoked potentials (SSEPs or SEPs), brainstem auditory evoked potentials (BAEPs), visual-evoked potentials (VEPs), intraoperative monitoring, and repetitive stimulation (RS). Of these additional electrophysiological tests, somatosensory-evoked potentials and repetitive stimulation are more commonly accomplished on a routine basis. However, the focus of this overview will be on clinical NCS and EMG studies.

Anatomy and Physiology Review

Peripheral Nerve Structure

The anatomic unit of the nervous system is the *neuron,* with its various processes or nerve fibers.[1] By contrast, the functional unit of the neuromuscular system is the *motor unit,* consisting of the anterior horn cell, the nerve root, the plexus, individual nerve fibers, the neuromuscular junction, and all the muscle fibers innervated by that axon (Fig. 16-1).

ENMG testing assesses various aspects of the neuron and the motor unit. EMG testing examines the delineated components of the motor unit, allowing the practitioner to determine the location of a neuromuscular impairment.

Results of ENMG testing cannot be used to identify the actual cause of a nerve or muscle impairment, although it is often assumed to do so. For instance, if testing reveals that a patient has slowed neural conduction in the median nerve across the carpal tunnel of the wrist and the opponens pollicis muscle demonstrates evidence of denervation with EMG examination, we would refer to this condition as carpal tunnel syndrome. However, the ENMG testing identifies only the location (carpal tunnel) and severity (mild, moderate, severe) of the condition, not its cause. The cause could be an abnormally thickened flexor tendon putting pressure on the nerve, a thickened transverse carpal ligament (flexor retinaculum), a bony impingement from advanced arthritis or from a fracture, or a temporary generalized edema accumulation such as can occur during the second and third trimesters of pregnancy. Imaging studies (radiograph, MRI, etc.) may be able to identify the anatomical or structural cause of a condition, but ENMG is restricted to identifying the location of a neuromuscular impairment.

Peripheral nerves are composed of a variety of elements and cell types. One naturally thinks of the axon, which is composed of neurofilaments and microtubules along with mitochondria interspersed in the cytoplasm (Fig. 16-2). Myelinated nerve fibers are surrounded by layers of lipoprotein sheets (myelin) produced by the Schwann cells that lie on the outside of the axon. Periodic interruption of myelin occurs where longitudinally sequential Schwann cells meet, forming the node of Ranvier—an area of relatively decreased resistance to ionic exchange—and more easily permitting depolarization (Fig. 16-3). In large myelinated nerve fibers, this depolarization "jumps" from node to node, thereby accelerating the speed of conduction while simultaneously reducing the space needed for a nerve with this conduction speed. This diminishes the energy needs for depolarization because it is occurring only at the nodes of Ranvier and not along the entire course of the nerve.

Nerves are comprised of numerous unmyelinated fibers, mast cells, fibroblasts, blood vessels, and extensive connective tissue elements. In fact, as seen in Figure 16-4, connective tissue surrounds the entire nerve (epineurium), the fascicles (perineurium), and the individual axons (endoneurium).

Peripheral Nerve Function

As ENMG testing is primarily a functional assessment of the neuromuscular system, a discussion of a few key

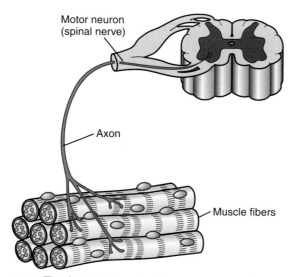

Fig 16•1 The functional unit of the neuromuscular system is the motor unit, which consists of the anterior horn cell, the nerve root, the brachial or lumbosacral plexus, individual nerve fibers, the neuromuscular junction, and all the muscle fibers innervated by that axon.

Motor neuron (spinal nerve)
Axon
Muscle fibers

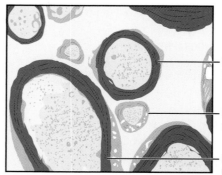

Small diameter myelinated axon
Small diameter unmyelinated axon
Large diameter myelinated axon

Fig 16•2 Electron micrograph cross-section of a peripheral nerve with axons of various diameter. Note that some axons are surrounded by myelin while others are unmyelinated. Axons typically consist of numerous subcellular organelles such as microtubules, neurofilaments, connective tissue, and mitochondria, which reflect the complexity of nerves.

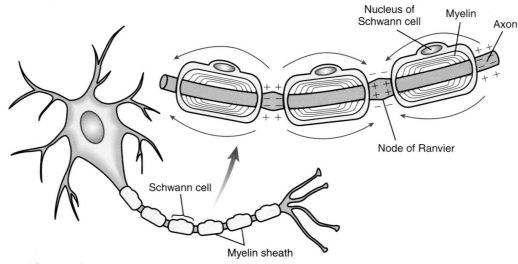

Fig 16•3 Node of Ranvier for a typical myelinated nerve fiber. Absence of myelin at the node facilitates the propagation of neural impulses via "saltatory" conduction. Saltatory conduction increases speed of conduction, decreases space needs, and reduces the amount of energy expenditure required for impulse propagation. For myelinated nerve fibers, depolarization occurs only at the node of Ranvier.

features of nerve physiology is appropriate. The principal basis for the production and conduction of electrical signals in biological tissue is the separation of charge across the cell membrane of the major ions—potassium (K+), sodium (Na+), and chloride (Cl−). The cell membrane is designed to permit selective permeability of these ions so that at rest the inside of the nerve and muscle cells are electrically negative (assisted by the sodium-potassium pump). This electronegativity is referred to as the *resting membrane potential* and establishes the excitability of nerve cells.

When a stimulus of sufficient amplitude occurs, the voltage across the nerve cell membrane will exceed a threshold value, producing an "all-or-none," self-perpetuating action potential (Fig. 16-5). The all-or-none feature of nerve physiology is especially important in nerve conduction testing, because it helps the practitioner determine how much stimulus to apply to the nerve during the procedure. It is necessary to apply a strong enough stimulus to exceed the nerve's threshold, thereby achieving a self-propagating action potential. Once this level of stimulus is reached, no amount of additional stimulus strength will increase the response. Either the nerve (or muscle fiber) depolarizes or it does not—that is, all or none.

Finally, an important feature of excitable tissue related to electrophysiological testing is volume conduction. Nerve and muscle are electrically excitable, whereas skin, subcutaneous fat, connective tissue, bone,

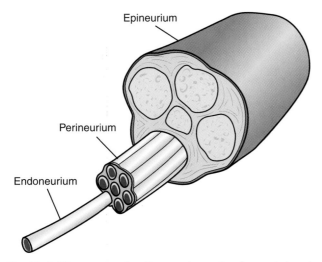

Fig 16•4 The connective tissue elements of a peripheral nerve are extensive and include the epineurium surrounding the entire nerve, the perineurium encircling the fascicles, and the endoneurium around each axon.

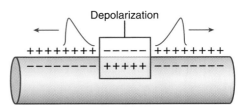

Fig 16•5 The wave of depolarization proceeds in two directions and is self-propagating once a threshold stimulus is reached. When a threshold stimulus occurs, the axon responds completely (the "all-or-none" feature).

blood vessels, and other tissues are not. Because of this, electrical stimulation can be applied transcutaneously, and the practitioner can be assured that the stimulus will excite only the tissue laden with electrolytes—nerve and muscle. As a result, direct visualization and stimulation of the muscle and nerve are not necessary and can be accomplished relatively comfortably.

A final important feature of neural conduction worth considering is referred to as *saltatory* (literally "jumping") *conduction* (see Fig. 16-3). This property of neural conduction results from the resistance to depolarization produced by the presence of myelin derived from the Schwann cells associated with many axons. Consequently, the "path of least resistance" becomes the nonmyelinated node of Ranvier. Therefore, depolarization along a myelinated axon "jumps" from node to node, rather than being propagated along the entire length of the fiber in a sequential or contiguous fashion.

Saltatory conduction has at least three benefits for nerve conduction. First, the speed of saltatory conduction is substantially higher than nonsaltatory conduction. Second, the amount of energy needed to propagate a nerve response by saltatory conduction is considerably less, since depolarization and the ATP-driven sodium-potassium pump is necessary only at the nodes of Ranvier, where the "action" is occurring. Finally, the relative physical space needed for a nerve that can conduct at the speeds necessary to achieve physiological normalcy (velocities of 40 to 70 meters per second) are markedly less for myelinated nerves than for unmyelinated fibers.

Equipment to Conduct ENMG

An EMG machine permits visualization and recording of human bioelectric signals so that nerves, muscles, and the neuromuscular junction can be objectively evaluated. However, the signals are ordinarily so small that they must be filtered and amplified in order to be processed, measured, and displayed on an oscilloscope or a computer screen. Simultaneously, the signal is sent to speakers that allow the examiner and the patient to "hear" the muscle or nerve response to activation, serving as a form of biofeedback—especially for the patient. Electrodes attached to the patient allow the equipment to record the signal. As seen in Figure 16-6, there are

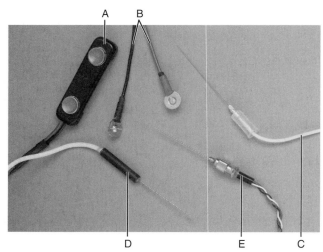

Fig 16•6 Standard EMG/NCS electrodes used in everyday practice. (A) Surface ("bar") electrode for NCS. (B) Surface disk electrodes for NCS and some EMG applications. (C) Monopolar needle electrode for EMG. (D) Concentric needle electrode for EMG. (E) Bipolar needle electrode for EMG.

surface electrodes for nerve conduction studies (NCS and some aspects of EMG) and needle electrodes (most EMG and occasional application for NCS). Nerve conduction testing requires an adjustable stimulator to trigger a stimulus that depolarizes the nerve, whose response is captured on the oscilloscope (Fig. 16-7). These responses can be physically manipulated with the dials or controlled with computer software in order to obtain a variety of measurement properties of the waveform, including latency, amplitude, and area under the curve. Nerve conduction velocity (NCV) can be calculated from these responses by dividing the latency

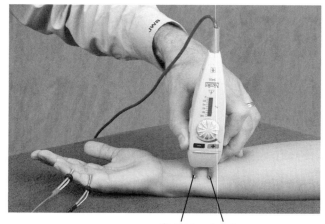

Cathode   Anode

Fig 16•7 A stimulator and recording ring electrodes for nerve conduction velocity testing.

difference between two spatially separated waveforms into the distance between the two stimulation sites (Fig. 16-8). A more detailed description of this process is presented later in the chapter.

Indications: Who Needs ENMG Testing?

Patients with signs and symptoms of neuromuscular disorder can usually benefit from the information obtained from ENMG testing. Although there are occasional exceptions, patients who complain of numbness, tingling, and pain involving the sensory division of the peripheral nervous system (PNS) and weakness (implicating the motor division of the PNS) are usually referred for ENMG testing. Because complaints and objective findings of sensory and motor impairment may arise from central nervous system (CNS) disorders, one feature of electrophysiological

testing is to delineate such complaints as deriving from either the PNS or the CNS. ENMG testing is a particularly sensitive procedure for directly evaluating PNS complaints while CNS disorders are primarily established by inference from relatively normal findings with this form of testing and, more commonly, from imaging studies such as MRI. One notable exception would be the patient who has a disease of the anterior horn cells—such as amyotrophic lateral sclerosis (ALS, or Lou Gehrig's disease)—that are located in the spinal cord (CNS) but are functionally part of the lower motor neuron. In the case of ALS, the peripheral nerve responses to electrical stimulation are altered during motor nerve conduction studies. Needle EMG examination of the muscles supplied by the axons deriving from the affected nerve cells will show evidence of an unstable membrane (denervation). Nevertheless, ENMG testing is usually conducted when PNS—not CNS—disorders are suspected.

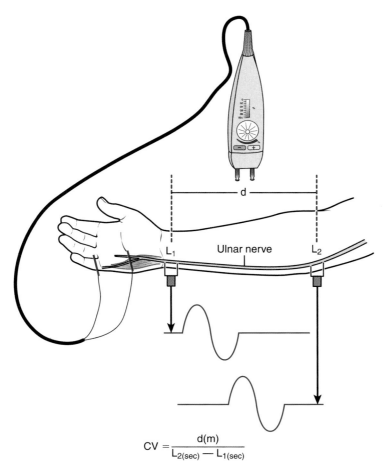

$$CV = \frac{d(m)}{L_{2(sec)} - L_{1(sec)}}$$

Fig 16•8 Motor nerve conduction for the ulnar nerve: Recording electrode is on the abductor digiti minimi muscle, and stimulation is applied just proximal to the wrist to obtain the distal motor latency (L_1). A proximal latency (L_2) is obtained by stimulating the ulnar nerve at the elbow, and the distance between the two sites of stimulation is recorded.

There are two major types of nerve injury—segmental demyelination and axon degeneration—that electrophysiological testing seeks to delineate. The first is *segmental demyelination,* which represents a focal conduction abnormality along the course of an otherwise normal axon and is best detected by nerve conduction study.[2] Unlike the changes noted by needle EMG, conduction abnormalities can be present almost immediately after the disorder begins or after the onset of nerve injury. Usual causes of segmental demyelination include mild to moderate compression, such as seen with carpal tunnel syndrome, or a primary demyelinating condition, as observed after exposure to diphtheria toxin. Regardless of the cause, the effect on the nerve test is slowed conduction velocity.

The second major type of nerve abnormality is *axon degeneration* (axonopathy). It is best detected by needle EMG examination but usually takes about 21 days after injury to be demonstrated.[2] This is the general length of time necessary for Wallerian degeneration to proceed sufficiently to manifest itself as muscle membrane instability, which the needle EMG identifies. Causes of axon loss include severe nerve compression (e.g., nerve root compression from herniated disc) or direct trauma, inflammation, and ischemia of the nerve. Most often, the speed of conduction is preserved (at least early on), but the amplitude of the compound muscle action potential or sensory nerve action potential is reduced. These NCS changes are usually preceded by EMG spontaneous potentials already mentioned.

KEY POINT! Wallerian degeneration is the degeneration of an axon that has been severed from its cell body. The myelin sheath also degenerates, but the neurilemma does not and forms a tube that will direct the growth of the regenerating axon.

Both axonopathy and demyelination seem to have similar clinical manifestations. Both can lead to weakness, and both often produce complaints of pain or other sensory manifestations. Even though there is great value in delineating a condition as primarily arising from one cause or the other, the reality is that many dysfunctions encountered in the peripheral nervous system (PNS) will have both segmental demyelination and axon degeneration characteristics. An example is the patient who has moderate to severe levels of compressive median neuropathy at the wrist (e.g., carpal tunnel syndrome). The NCS will invariably demonstrate clear slowing of conduction across the wrist (demyelination) as well as reduction in amplitude of action potentials—motor and sensory (usually associated with axon injury and loss). In addition, the EMG will often show signs of spontaneous potentials, another indication of axonopathy. Because of this common overlap in demyelination and axon degeneration associated with nerve disorders, it is recommended that ENMG testing include both nerve conduction study and needle EMG to thoroughly examine a patient with PNS complaints.

Clinical Examples of Diagnostic Dilemma for Which ENMG Testing Is Important

A 45-year-old female office worker has had 6 weeks of neck pain and numbness in the left nondominant thumb, index, long, and portions of the ring finger. The numbness regularly awakens her at night, but the cervical spine pain makes it difficult to achieve a position of comfort to fall asleep. An MRI of the cervical spine demonstrates some degenerative disk changes at C6 and C7, with some slight compression of the nerve root in the foramen. No spinal stenosis is identified by the imaging study. Manual cervical spine distraction alleviates much of the neck pain and some, but not the majority, of the hand numbness. Rotation of the head and neck to the left aggravates the radicular symptoms. The patient has a diminished triceps deep-tendon reflex (DTR) and 3/5 muscle weakness of the left triceps muscle, forearm flexors, and extensors. She demonstrates a positive median nerve compression test and a positive Phelan test, both at the left wrist. Muscle testing of the intrinsic muscles of the hand reveals a 3+/5 abductor pollicis brevis voluntary muscle test. The patient's family practice physician has recently informed her that she is "borderline" type 2 diabetic, and this is currently being monitored and managed by diet and exercise. The patient has been referred for physical therapy with the standard "evaluate and treat" prescription.

Reasonable goals for this patient include a reduction in C6–7 radicular signs and symptoms in the left upper extremity, improvement in cervical spine range of motion (ROM), and reduction in sensory symptoms in the median nerve distribution. Hopefully, this approach will result in less sleep disturbance for her. It seems appropriate to include cervical traction and neural glides[3–8] in the treatment procedures for this patient, but there is some uncertainty about this case that suggests that additional information would allow the practitioner to make more informed decisions about management. Specifically:

1. How much of this patient's complaint of numbness is the result of a probable median neuropathy at the wrist (e.g., carpal tunnel syndrome)?
2. How much of the hand numbness is attributed to the radiculopathy that her signs and symptoms suggest?
3. Do any of her complaints relate to the recent onset of type 2 diabetes and its tendency to adversely affect peripheral nerve function?
4. Is it likely that mechanical traction will effectively deal with the patient's radicular complaints? How severely injured is the nerve root?
5. Would this patient benefit from a resting night splint for the wrist along with neural glides, or would this be wasted effort?

Is ENMG testing able to answer these questions so that the intervention can be more focused and a more realistic prognosis can be offered? Here are some reasons that an ENMG examination should be conducted with this patient:

1. ENMG can establish whether she has a compressive neuropathic injury at the wrist and determine its severity.
2. ENMG can determine whether the apparent weakness in the upper extremity is the result of nerve root compression and establish whether the muscle response is still deteriorating or beginning to show signs of recovery.
3. ENMG can explore the motor and sensory responses of several nerves in both arms to see whether the type 2 diabetes has affected neural function, diffusely.

The answers provided by ENMG testing will firmly establish and document the extent of neural injury and involvement in this case and give a much clearer prospect of improvement. Information such as this will help ensure the patient is given the appropriate therapy and will allow the therapist to focus on those aspects of

therapy or interventions likely to result in the most success.[9] Oftentimes this allows the patient to spend time on those aspects of the home program (e.g., home traction or neural glides) that are more likely to reinforce the in-clinic administered therapy and usually result in fewer in-clinic visits to achieve discharge goals.

Another example involves a 64-year-old male who sustained a proximal humeral fracture 6 weeks previously and has now been sent to initiate physical therapy with a request to "concentrate on *active* arm elevation." The initial evaluation reveals 115° of passive flexion but virtually no active flexion or abduction. Furthermore, palpation of the deltoid muscle during the patient's efforts to abduct and flex the glenohumeral joint suggests essentially no discernable muscle activation. There is decreased sensory acuity to crude and light touch over the middle deltoid ("deltoid patch"). Two weeks later, the patient is noted to have 125° of passive flexion but still no active arm elevation. At this point, the therapist must ask whether this patient has a low threshold of pain tolerance, is poorly motivated, has profound "disuse atrophy," or has actually sustained a neural injury (axillary, in this case). A brief needle EMG demonstrates that the deltoid muscle is severely denervated, and the patient essentially is unable to volitionally activate a sufficient number of motor units to elevate the arm—the patient has sustained an axillary nerve injury.

With this information, the focus of therapy efforts, temporarily, must be to protect the limb until reinnervation occurs and concentrate on those muscles that have normal or near normal innervation (i.e., interscapular stabilizers and serratus anterior and upper trapezius muscles). In this way, the therapist minimizes the likelihood of harming the patient by directing therapeutic efforts to those structures that have the potential to benefit from exercise and stimulation.[10–12] Additional therapeutic activity for those muscles that are denervated should be withheld until the lengthy process of reinnervation nears completion, at which point more aggressive exercise can begin.

There are numerous similar clinical scenarios in which such questions arise during the delivery of care and the standard clinical examination does not sufficiently delineate the most appropriate treatment direction. Additional information about the status of the neuromuscular system is needed, and ENMG testing can often provide just such data to guide clinical decisions.

Precautions

Patients with pacemakers represent a precaution for conducting ENMG testing because the nerve stimulator may interfere with the pacemaker signal. This concern is especially relevant for the NCS and less so for the EMG portion of the study. Individuals taking blood thinners (anticoagulants) are another group that need to be monitored carefully during and after the needle EMG to be certain that excessive bleeding does not occur. In patients who have blood-transmittable diseases (e.g., HIV, hepatitis, Jakob-Creutzfeldt disease), all universal precautions should be taken (i.e., latex gloves, eye protection, gown) to protect the examiner from possible infection during the ENMG testing procedure.[13]

Nerve Conduction Studies

Nerve conduction studies assess motor and sensory nerve function by recording the evoked response produced by electrical stimulation of the nerve. A number of important clinical questions can be answered by NCS and include the following:[13]

1. Is the peripheral nervous system involved in the patient's condition?
2. What is the location of the peripheral nerve condition, and is more than one nerve involved?
3. Is the peripheral nerve condition mild, moderate, or severe (conduction block partial or complete)?
4. Does the condition appear to be focal or diffuse (systemic disorder)?
5. Does the condition primarily involve motor fibers or sensory fibers, or are they equally affected by the nerve condition?

With these questions in mind, an attempt to adhere to certain NCS principles should be made. These principles include:[13]

1. Examine motor and sensory fibers whenever possible.
2. Test several segments of nerve suspected to be involved.

3. Be prepared to test upper and lower limbs if the preliminary findings warrant this approach.
4. Test when likely to obtain optimal "diagnostic yield." Because NCS findings can demonstrate abnormality almost immediately after the onset of a condition, there is no "bad time" to conduct this test. This is not true for the EMG examination, where it may take approximately 3 weeks for abnormalities to manifest.

General Influencing Factors

A variety of factors may significantly impact NCS results. The examiner must remain alert to their influence on the testing procedures listed here:[14,15]

1. Upper vs. lower limb study
2. Age
3. Limb length (height)
4. Limb temperature
5. Anomalous innervation patterns.

Upper extremity nerve conduction velocity is, on average, 5 to 10 meters per second faster than the lower extremity nerves. This may be because the lower extremity is longer than the upper extremity, so the cell bodies for lower extremity nerves are farther away—which may make the lower extremity axons less nutritionally competent. Presumably this has the effect of slightly slowing down conduction velocity.

Age has an influence on latency, amplitude, and conduction velocity values. Nerve conduction velocity does not achieve the normal adult values until age 7, although some elements of the PNS may not fully mature until age 14 to 18. Prior to age 7 (when myelination is not yet complete), NCV values are roughly half of adult velocities. This chapter will not provide special information on conducting NCS with pediatric clients.

The relationship of aging on conduction velocity has been extensively studied, but there remains some debate on the precise effect of age on nerve values. It is generally accepted that beyond the age of 60, values decline 1 to 2 meters per second for each decade (over 60). Some authors contend that this decline actually begins after age 40, but that has been refuted by other investigators. In any event, even with this slight slowing that may occur with age, the conduction velocity should not drop below the lower limit of normal, even for those in their 80s.

Height, and consequently limb length, influences nerve conduction velocities. In general, the longer the limb, the slower the conduction velocity. This fact reinforces the importance of comparing conduction velocity values for both extremities to be certain that slowed conduction represents a disease state rather than the normal variation associated with limb length.

Limb temperature has a decided effect on distal latency and nerve conduction values. Because a cool limb conducts electrical signals more slowly than one of normal temperature, skin temperature is measured, recorded, and monitored during the ENMG examination. Upper or lower extremity limbs whose temperatures fall below 30°C (86°F) must be warmed with hot packs or warm towels until this threshold is achieved. Interestingly, sensory action potential amplitudes actually increase with a cool limb and might be a clue to warm the limb. If the latency of a sensory nerve action potential is slowed but the amplitude is higher than would be predicted, the examiner should suspect a cool limb. Efforts should be made to warm the limb to see if both values will return to the normal range.

Anomalous innervation patterns can present a confusing picture to the ENMG examiner, but teasing this possibility out is important to provide a clear picture to the referring individual. Approximately 20% of individuals have an anastomosis (nerve connection) between the median and ulnar nerve in the forearm; this is called a Martin-Gruber anastomosis (Fig. 16-9). The condition is characterized by median nerve fibers that cross over to join the ulnar nerve in the forearm proximal to the stimulation site at the wrist. When stimulation is carried out over the normal median nerve sites at the wrist and at the elbow, this pattern of nerve connection will usually result in abnormally high conduction velocity calculations (e.g., often as high as 100 meters per second). In addition to this abnormally high conduction velocity, there is usually a change in the waveform configuration between the stimulation sites at the wrist and the elbow—another clue that some unusual pattern is present. Being alert to the possibility of this nerve arrangement will limit the likelihood of erroneous interpretation of nerve responses to stimulation.

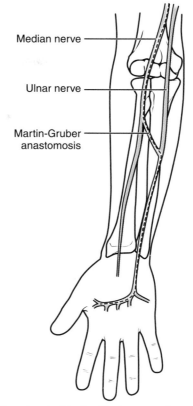

Fig 16•9 The classic Martin-Gruber anastomosis between the median and ulnar nerve is one example of anomalous innervations. Anatomical variances such as this will dramatically affect conduction velocity values.

Motor Nerve Conduction Study

Motor nerve conduction studies are often the first portion of the ENMG test following the patient history and clinical examination and provide information about the function of the axons, myelin, and neuromuscular junction. The physiological response evoked by stimulating the nerve during this portion of the examination is called the *compound muscle action potential* (CMAP) and represents the simultaneous depolarization of all the individual motor units under the recording electrode (Fig. 16-10). The general procedure for obtaining motor nerve conduction and relevant portions of the waveform are described below.

Procedure

Motor conduction studies are generally accomplished by placing a pair of surface electrodes on a distal muscle supplied by the nerve being tested and then stimulating that nerve at various sites along its anatomical

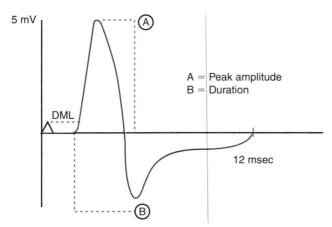

Fig 16•10 Standard compound muscle action potential (CMAP) for a typical motor nerve study following stimulation. The time from stimulus artifact to initial departure from the baseline is the distal motor latency (DML). Other important features of this response include the peak latency, duration of the waveform, its shape, and the area under the curve.

course. More specifically, the "active" electrode (of the pair) is placed as close to the anatomical motor point as possible while the "reference" electrode is placed over the nonexcitable tendon of that muscle. These two electrodes together are referred to as the *recording electrodes*. A ground electrode is also placed on nonexcitable tissue, often over a bony prominence, ideally between the stimulating and recording electrodes (Fig. 16-11).

The mixed peripheral nerve is electrically stimulated at some set distance from the active electrode in an

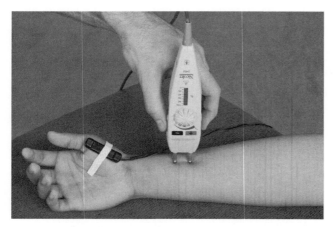

Fig 16•11 Standard setup for median nerve motor conduction study: A ground electrode is placed over the bony aspect of the dorsum of the hand, the black recording electrode is placed on the middle of the abductor pollicis brevis muscle, and the red reference electrode is placed on the volar surface of the thumb metacarpal phalangeal joint.

effort to obtain a CMAP response. For upper extremity nerves, this distance is usually 8 centimeters from the cathode of the stimulating device. For lower extremity nerves, it may vary between 8 and 12 centimeters. The stimulator's cathode is oriented so that it is closest to the muscle to be depolarized.

The key point here is to be consistent in electrode placement and distal stimulation distance. The intensity of stimulation should be advanced incrementally until a maximal CMAP is obtained; this response represents the *distal motor latency* (DML, also termed the *M-wave*) and is a reflection of the ability of the fastest conducting axons to conduct the electrical stimulation to the neuromuscular junction (NMJ), bridge the junction, depolarize the muscle fibers that they innervate, and contract the muscle. Because there is no consistent way for clinical ENMG testing to accurately calculate the rate of conduction across and distal to the NMJ, motor conduction velocity measurement requires at least two stimulation sites; the second site is referred to as the *proximal latency* and is generally obtained at some common anatomical site to ensure consistency within the test and between individuals tested.

The examiner measures the linear distance between the two stimulation sites. He or she then subtracts the difference between the two latencies and simply divides the latency difference into the distance between the two stimulation sites to obtain the NCV between the two sites, as noted in the following formula (see Fig. 16-8):

$$\text{Nerve Conduction Velocity (m/sec)} = \frac{\text{Distance Between Proximal and Distal Stimulation Sites (mm)}}{\text{Proximal Latency} - \text{Distal Latency (msec)}}$$

Note that the millimeters and the milliseconds cancel each other out in this calculation, which leaves the unit of conduction velocity as meters per second. Often a third (or even a fourth) stimulation site is warranted to more thoroughly evaluate the motor nerve conduction status; for example, above and below the elbow for the ulnar nerve to identify cubital tunnel syndrome or above and below the fibular head to document fibular nerve compression at this site. Typical values for distal motor latency, motor conduction velocity, and amplitude of the CMAP for commonly studied upper and lower extremity nerves are noted in Table 16-1.

Table 16•1	Normal Motor-Conduction Values of Commonly Tested Nerves in Adults		
Nerve	Distal Latency (msec)	Conduction Velocity (m/sec)	CMAP Amplitude (mV)
Median			
Wrist–APB muscle (8 cm)	< 4.2	> 45	> 4
Elbow-wrist			
Ulnar			
Wrist–ADM muscle (8 cm)	< 4	> 45	> 3.5
Elbow–wrist			
Radial			
Forearm–EIP muscle (8 cm)	< 3.5	> 45	> 2.5
Mid-humerus–forearm			
Fibular (Deep Peroneal) (7 cm)	< 6	> 40	> 3.5
Ankle–EDB muscle			
Above fibular head–ankle			
Tibial (10 cm)			
Ankle–AH muscle	< 6	> 40	> 3
Knee–ankle			

Key: *CMAP, compound motor action potential; APB: abductor pollicis brevis; ADM: abductor digiti minimi; EIP: extensor indicis proprius; EDB: extensor digitorum brevis; AH: abductor hallucis*

What the Findings Mean

Taking a closer look at the distal motor latency CMAP, the ENMG examiner is interested in the time from the stimulus artifact (the instant the signal is delivered to the nerve) to the initial deflection of the waveform from the baseline. As noted previously, this value in milliseconds represents the conduction along the nerve, across the NMJ, and to all the muscle fibers innervated by the axons stimulated. If sufficient demyelination has occurred, this latency value will fall above the upper limit of normal and will be considered slowed or delayed. As such, the latency values reflect the state of the myelin surrounding the largest and fastest conducting axons of the nerve under investigation. Typical DML values for commonly studied upper and lower extremity nerves are noted in Table 16-1.

KEY POINT! Note that an increase in latency reflects a decrease in conduction velocity.

The examiner is also very interested in the amplitude of the evoked response, which is measured in millivolts (mV) and is described as representing the number of functioning motor units innervated by the nerve being studied. Localized nerve compression (e.g., carpal tunnel syndrome) or diffuse disease processes, such as

advanced diabetes, adversely affect the number of functioning motor units in a muscle, thereby leading to a decreased CMAP amplitude. Some computer-based ENMG testing units have software programs that can provide "area under the curve," which is actually a more accurate measure of functioning motor units for any given muscle. However, amplitude is a well-accepted representation of this nerve feature. Lower limit of amplitude values are also shown for upper and lower extremity nerves in Table 16-1.

Duration is the length of time from the initial deflection of the signal from the baseline until it crosses the baseline again. This feature of the nerve response indicates the state of myelination and is excessively prolonged in certain demyelinating disorders. Related to duration is the process called *temporal dispersion,* which represents the electrical activity of individual nerve fibers that may be slower in conducting velocity. The effect of temporal dispersion on the waveform is to spread it out (prolong the duration) and make it less uniform in shape (Fig. 16-12).

Nerve conduction velocity (NCV) values are usually established for each laboratory, although many facilities rely on nationally accepted norms to guide practice and decisions. The examiner generally compares the obtained NCV values from both limbs for internal consistency and against standard laboratory ranges to identify abnormalities. Nerves that have been injured by trauma or disease will not conduct signals at normal speeds. Often the injured segment is identified by carefully comparing sequential segments of each nerve studied.

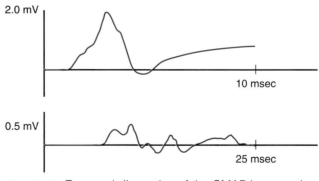

Fig 16•12 Temporal dispersion of the CMAP is caused by the relative difference in velocity of the fastest and slowest conducting fibers. Disproportionate slowing of some fibers occurs when nerves are compressed, and the result is a CMAP that is increased in duration, reduced in amplitude, and less smooth in shape.

KEY POINT! A reduction in NCV of more than 10 meters per second between consecutive segments of the same nerve would indicate a possible nerve injury.

It should be noted that conduction velocities in the upper extremities are roughly 10 meters per second faster than expected in the lower extremity. Velocities in the order of 45 to 50 meters per second are considered the lower limit of normal for upper extremity nerves, while a value of 40 meters per second is considered the lower limit for lower extremity nerves. One reason for the lowered conduction velocity for lower extremity nerves is perhaps related to the sheer length difference between upper and lower extremities, which results in reduced limb temperature, which has a known slowing effect on conduction velocity.

Which Nerves to Study?

Practitioners should be familiar with the routine motor nerve conduction techniques as they are most commonly performed and reported with normal values. The most commonly examined nerves and corresponding muscles are:

- Median nerve—electrodes on the abductor pollicis brevis
- Ulnar nerve—electrodes on the abductor digiti minimi
- Fibular nerve—electrodes on the extensor digitorum brevis
- Tibial nerve—electrodes on the abductor hallucis

Familiarization with the standard normal values for these four nerves will greatly enhance understanding for reading an ENMG report. Other nerves are less commonly studied but might include, among others:

- Radial nerve—electrodes on the extensor indicis proprius
- Axillary nerve—electrodes on the middle deltoid
- Spinal accessory nerve (CN XI)—electrodes on the upper trapezius
- Femoral nerve—electrodes on the vastus medialis
- Fibular nerve—electrodes on the tibialis anterior

Sensory Nerve Conduction Study

Sensory nerve conduction studies are generally performed by placing a surface or ring recording electrode on the skin directly over a nerve trunk and stimulating the nerve to produce a sensory nerve action potential (SNAP; Fig. 16-13). The SNAP is the summated response of all the depolarized sensory fibers in the nerve trunk in much the same way that the CMAP is the summated response of all the motor units responding to maximal electrical stimulation. However, there are some important differences that should be noted. The SNAP is a direct response having no intervening synapse like the NMJ for motor nerve conduction. Thus, a single point of stimulation provides sufficient information to measure a distal latency, obtain an amplitude, and, unlike motor conduction, obtain a sensory conduction velocity.

Secondly, SNAPs are significantly smaller than CMAPs (Table 16-2). A typical CMAP may be on the order of 5 to 10 mV while a normal SNAP response may be as small as 5 to 10 microvolts, or µV (remember that 1 mV = 1,000 µV). This represents a *1,000-fold difference,* so different sensitivity settings are required to obtain the much smaller SNAP response. The profound difference is because the CMAP is the summation of numerous muscle fiber action potentials that comprise several motor units. There are occasions when the sensory response is so diminutive that a special procedure called *signal averaging* is used to summate several responses and depict the summated waveform as a single response. This kind of additional signal

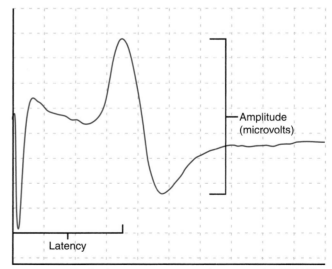

Fig 16•13 Typical sensory nerve action potential (SNAP) showing latency to the "takeoff," latency to the peak and "peak-to-peak" amplitude. The amplitude of the sensory response (measured in microvolts) is significantly smaller than the CMAP amplitudes (measured in millivolts).

Table 16·2 Normal Values of Commonly Tested Sensory Nerves in Adults

Nerve	Distal Latency to peak (msec)	Velocity (m/sec)	SNAP Amplitude (µV)
Median			
Wrist–digit (14 cm)	3.5 ± 0.5	50 ± 10	15–60
Palmar (7–9 mm)	< 2.5	——	> 10
Ulnar			
Wrist–digit (14 mm)	3.0 ± 0.5	50 ± 10	15–50
Palmar (7–9 mm)	< 2.5	——	> 10
Superficial Radial			
Forearm–wrist recording (12 cm)	< 3.0	50 ± 10	10–50
Superficial Fibular (Peroneal; 10–14 cm)	2.5 ± 0.5	45 ± 5	> 10
Sural (14 cm)	3.5 ± 0.5	45 ± 5	> 5

processing is rarely needed for motor stimulation, because the responses are usually large enough that it is unnecessary.

The depolarization produced by sensory nerve stimulation is propagated in both directions. As a result, sensory nerve can be stimulated distally while recording proximally on the nerve trunk (the normal direction of afferent fiber depolarization). This is referred to as *orthodromic stimulation.* Conversely, the nerve can be stimulated at some proximal site, and the recording can be accomplished distally (the reverse of the normal direction of afferent fiber depolarization). This is referred to as *antidromic stimulation.* Both procedures are used by most examiners because the results are nearly identical for the two methods with no distinct advantage for either.

KEY POINT! Orthodromic stimulation refers to propagation of the electrical stimulus in the normal or customary direction. For motor testing, this is proximal to distal yet distal to proximal for sensory.

Procedure

The basic premise and setup for performing a sensory nerve conduction study is much like that of the previously described motor stimulation. Stimulation occurs by means of the adjustable stimulating probe placed over the course of the nerve, with the cathode (negative pole) positioned closest to the recording electrode. Of course, the examiner does need to determine whether

they wish to conduct the signal orthodromically or antidromically—unlike the motor study, which is always conducted orthodromically. The recording electrode pair can come in the form of a ring, often used for upper extremity nerve studies, or typical surface electrodes, used for both upper and lower extremity studies (see Fig. 16-7). The intensity of stimulation necessary to obtain a maximal response is usually less than that necessary in a motor study. For this reason, some examiners prefer to begin with the sensory portion of the NCS, as it introduces the patient to the experience of electrical stimulation a bit more gently than the more intense stimulation necessary for most motor studies.

The parameters of interest with the sensory NCS are, in general, the same as those examined during the motor study and include the following:

1. Distal sensory latency (DSL)—the time from the stimulus artifact to either the onset or peak of the SNAP. As recording equipment has become more sophisticated and sensitive over time, the onset has become a more reliable parameter to measure. This was not true with most of the first- or even second-generation devices. Therefore, many examiners prefer to report both onset and peak latency values for SNAPs in their analysis. The accepted values for these various nerve responses have been established over predetermined distances between stimulation site and recording electrode.

2. Amplitude—a reflection of all the individual SNAPs summated into a compound SNAP. This parameter informs the examiner of the general function of the nerve axons in the segment studied. It is also reflective (by inference) of some important conclusions. Sensory nerve cell bodies are located in the dorsal root ganglion (DRG) within the intervertebral foramen. Lesions located proximal to the ganglion (principally, radiculopathies) do not usually affect the cell body; consequently, the SNAPs are ordinarily normal. By contrast, brachial or lumbar plexopathies and other neuropathic conditions often result in reduced amplitude or absent SNAPs. As such, sensory nerve studies can be useful for delineating proximal or distal causes for sensory complaints. For instance, a lumbar radiculopathy

can cause numbness, but the sural nerve SNAPs are invariably normal because the lesion (usually a disk herniation) is proximal to the DRG; therefore, the intact nerve cell body keeps the nerve and the distal responses normal.

3. Waveform, duration, and nerve conduction velocity are additional parameters that might be evaluated for a sensory nerve study, but practically speaking, the DSL and amplitude are the most commonly reported values for most sensory nerves.

Which Nerves to Study?

Much like the motor conduction studies, there are basic nerves that tend to be studied routinely along with a host of less commonly studied sensory nerves. The more commonly examined sensory nerves include median, ulnar, radial, medial antebrachial cutaneous, sural, superficial peroneal, and saphenous nerves.

Central Conduction and Long-loop Responses (F-wave and H-reflex)

Although motor and sensory nerve stimulation studies as described thus far are the most common procedures undertaken during nerve conduction testing, there are other techniques that have become somewhat routine because they are relatively easy to accomplish and they provide additional information about the status of the nerve complex.

F-wave

With motor conduction studies, we described a procedure whereby the motor nerve is stimulated proximally to obtain an orthodromically derived distal motor latency (DML), also referred to as the *M-wave*. Simultaneously, the nerve conducts an action potential antidromically to the anterior horn cells in the spinal cord that, in turn, send back a small action potential that contracts some of the muscle fibers under the recording electrode on the distal muscle. This delayed, small action potential is referred to as the *F-wave*, so named because it was originally recorded from the foot muscles (Fig. 16-14). F-wave latencies are usually smaller than 500 μV. Because they must traverse the distance of the entire limb length twice, they are much longer than the M-wave latencies (from 20 to 32 msec for upper extremities and 42 to 58 msec for lower extremities). The limb's length clearly will significantly impact this delayed response, so the patient's height (and limb length, itself, in some laboratories) is recorded for reference to normal values for these latencies.

The usual technique for this procedure is virtually identical to that for obtaining the DML, except that the cathode and the anode of the handheld stimulator are reversed so the primary action potential proceeds toward the spinal cord rather than toward the distal muscle. Besides being a much smaller response than the M-wave, the presence and shape of the F-wave is variable. Consequently, it is routine to obtain a number of

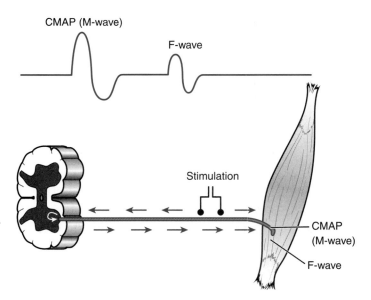

Fig 16•14 The F-wave is a long-loop response produced by stimulating the nerve at a distal site. The stimulus proceeds bidirectionally and produces the M response (DML) and also sends a volley proximally to the spinal cord. There, a number of anterior horn cells are activated that then send a small response back to the distal muscle to be recorded as the F-wave. This response is slowed in conditions that affect the overall conductivity of the nerve (various neuropathies) and may also be slowed with focal demyelination or axonopathy in conditions affecting the nerve roots or the plexus.

F-wave responses (5 to 10, typically) and report the shortest latency as the accepted value. Since the series of 5 to 10 consecutive F-waves are obtained in response to maximal stimulation, this is one procedure that patients often find uncomfortable during the NCS.

The principal purpose for obtaining an F-wave response is to examine nerve conduction in proximal nerve segments for conditions like thoracic outlet syndrome, some radiculopathies, or diffuse demyelinating diseases. For patients who have significant distal neural compression (e.g., carpal tunnel syndrome), a prolonged F-wave does not contribute any specific information regarding the location of compression that is not already demonstrated with the normal DML and NCV testing. However, if a patient demonstrates normal distal latencies and nerve conduction and yet exhibits prolonged F-waves, this strongly suggests that compromise of the neural system is located at a more proximal site, such as the plexus or nerve root.

H-reflex

Sometimes the standard nerve conduction and EMG examination does not identify a clear electrophysiological explanation for a patient's pain or numbness and tingling in a radicular pattern. More subtle tests of neural compromise may be useful at such a time. One such example is the *H-reflex*. This is an action potential response first described by Hoffman in 1922 and later named the "H-reflex" by Magladery and McDougal in 1950. It is most often undertaken for the tibial nerve when an S_1 radiculopathy is suspected, although it is gaining some acceptance for the median nerve when a C7 nerve compression is suspected. A few investigators have described a femoral nerve H-reflex, but it has not become a routine test for ENMG examination.[16]

As noted previously, when an electrical stimulus is applied to a mixed motor and sensory nerve, action potentials are propagated bidirectionally. In the case of the tibial nerve H-reflex, an action potential will travel from the point of stimulation (popliteal space) to the spinal cord, where it synapses with an alpha-motor neuron in the anterior horn. The activated motoneuron results in an action potential propagated back to the peripheral muscle, in this case the medial head of the gastrocnemius, an S_1 innervated muscle (Fig. 16-15). The time from the stimulus artifact to the muscle

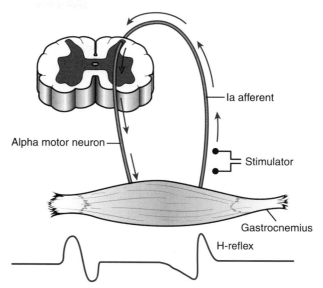

Fig 16•15 The H-reflex is another long-loop response evoked by stimulating the tibial nerve at the popliteal fossa and directing the signal toward the spinal cord. From there, a monosynaptic response sends a signal back to the recording site on the medial gastrocnemius muscle and is recorded as the H-reflex. This response is slowed in S1 radiculopathies, often when no other abnormalities are noted on the nerve conduction study or the EMG.

action potential is the H-reflex and ranges from 26 to 33 milliseconds in most individuals. Like the F-wave, the H-reflex is also a limb length–dependent response. Nomograms are available that factor in age and height (limb length) for this response to see if the values obtained for the patient are falling within a predicted range. The H-reflex is a very consistent reflex and represents the same pathway as the monosynaptic deep tendon reflex for the ankle that is elicited clinically. Although consistent, it is somewhat sensitive to voltage variation and is usually elicited in response to a submaximal, rather than a maximal, stimulation delivery. In fact, in many cases, a delivery of maximal levels of stimulation will cause the H-reflex (elicited by submaximal stimulation) to disappear while the M-wave dominates the screen. This narrow window between achieving threshold for eliciting the H-reflex and obscuring the response by applying stimulation levels that are too high can make obtaining this response a challenge for the examiner. However, the information obtained with this procedure is important for corroborating the presence of conditions such as S_1 and C_7 radiculopathies and is worth the effort in most cases.

To reiterate, the procedure for obtaining a tibial nerve (S₁) H-reflex is as follows:

1. Place the active surface electrode on the medial head of the gastrocnemius muscle belly and place the reference electrode on the tendon of the muscle.
2. Stimulate the tibial nerve at the popliteal space with the cathode pointed toward the spinal cord.
3. Slowly increase the stimulus amplitude until a depolarization response is first noted. Continue increasing the amplitude until a maximal H-reflex is obtained.
4. Compare the obtained H-reflex value to:
   a. The contralateral H-reflex
   b. A predicted H-reflex normalized for age and limb length
5. Determine whether the difference between obtained and predicted H-reflex values exceeds acceptable variation (usually a difference of 1 millisecond is considered the acceptable variation).

Height and limb length are important factors when conducting long-loop latency responses (H-reflex, F-wave). The length of time for an electrical signal to depolarize the nerve in the direction of the spinal cord, synapse with an anterior horn cell that sends a signal back to the peripheral muscle (H-reflex), or activate a group of anterior horn cells to depolarize and send a signal to the peripheral muscle (F-wave) is dependent on the distance the signal must travel to accomplish such electrical events. In fact, nomograms have been devised in which an individual's height or limb length and age can be factored to arrive at a predicted latency value.

Coming to Some Conclusions: What Do We Know So Far?

At this point in the examination process, the motor and sensory conduction studies described above have been completed and the special responses of F-wave and H-reflex have been obtained. It is possible that the findings up till now require other nerves to be examined or even additional limbs (upper or lower, in the case of possible polyneuropathy) to be analyzed. Furthermore, we have not described the needle EMG portion of the examination or the findings from such a study.

In any event, this is a good time to evaluate what we know so far. First of all, beginning the process of analysis and determining an ENMG diagnosis is based on accurate awareness of normal ranges and values for the responses obtained during the NCS. An abridged list of typical latency, nerve conduction velocity, and amplitude, values are noted in Table 16-1. The data collected in the study needs to be compared to these normal values to determine the status of the nerve.

When nerves are injured by disease or compression, their ability to conduct electrical signals is diminished or abolished. This abnormality, referred to as a *conduction block,* is what nerve conduction studies measure. A conduction block is present when the CMAP elicited from a more proximal site has less amplitude than the CMAP elicited at a distal site. This indicates that some of the fibers along the course of the nerve failed to conduct a signal but that the axons and myelin are normal distally. NCS is used to help figure out if a patient's neural complaints are caused primarily from demyelination (e.g., nerve compression or diffuse disease), from axonal degeneration (e.g., dying back neuropathy, severe axon injury from compression), or from some combination of these two processes.

KEY POINT! The primary indicator of demyelination is prolonged distal latencies and slowing of nerve conduction velocity, while the principal feature of axonal degeneration is reduced amplitude and area under the curve of the CMAP or SNAP.

Clinically, the most common categorization scheme for neural injuries was first described by Seddon in 1943 and includes neurapraxia, axonotmesis, and neurotmesis[17] (Fig. 16-16). *Neurapraxia* is the mildest form of peripheral nerve disorder and is characterized by local conduction block without any axonal injury. We have all experienced very transient versions of this category when we have slept on our arm for a short period of time and then were unable to feel or move the limb for several seconds to a couple of minutes while blood flow was reestablished to the nerves and muscles. More serious neurapraxias are caused by sustained or intense nerve pressure, stretching, or focal inflammation that are believed to cause localized demyelination. Strictly speaking, the axons and surrounding connective tissue sheath of the nerve are intact with a neurapraxia.

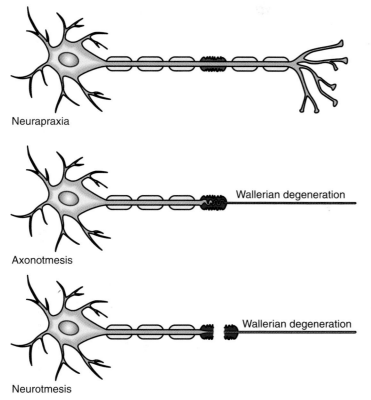

Neurapraxia

Axonotmesis

Wallerian degeneration

Wallerian degeneration

Neurotmesis

Fig 16•16 Standard description of nerve injury categories include neurapraxia (a myelin injury or condition), axonotmesis (axonal degeneration and myelin injury in most cases), and neurotmesis (myelin, axon, and connective tissue injury). Both axonotmesis and neurotmesis result in Wallerian degeneration, but neurotmesis is a far worse injury because the connective tissue sheath injury makes nerve regeneration less likely.

Classic examples of this category of nerve injury are the occasional tourniquet palsy associated with compression during surgery and the ever popular "Saturday night palsy," so named for the compression neuropathy of the radial nerve at the spiral groove of the humerus (usually caused by sustained focal nerve pressure from a long period of sleep secondary to inebriation or drug abuse). The effect on the electrophysiological examination is reduced nerve conduction velocities and proximal CMAPs (those obtained by stimulation above the focal demyelination). In some severe cases, conduction is blocked entirely, resulting in no response to stimulation across the injury site. If a pure neurapraxia has been sustained, the recovery usually takes weeks and occurs when remyelination of the large diameter axons is complete, or nearly so. If recovery takes several months, then it is possible that a second level of nerve injury, axonotmesis, has occurred.

Axonotmesis lesions are caused by more severe nerve pressure, stretching, or inflammation and are the result of a disruption of axonal continuity leading to some level of Wallerian degeneration (axonopathy).

Interestingly, research has shown that this axonal degeneration occurs distal to the lesion and one node of Ranvier proximal to the lesion. However, the connective tissue layers (epineurium, perineurium, endoneurium) remain intact with an axonotmesis, so the opportunity for recovery is possible. The clinical effect of this injury is diminished, or there is loss of sensation if sensory nerves are involved and muscle weakness if motor axons are injured.

Electrophysiologically, the effect of axonotmesis is virtually identical to that of neurapraxia for the first 2 to 5 days following the lesion. Specifically, the NCS is normal below the level of the injury, but there is no response across the axons that have experienced conduction block. After this 2- to 5-day period, axonal degeneration occurs, and the involved axons do not respond to stimulation above or below the lesion. If a sufficient number of axons are involved, the amplitude of motor- and sensory-evoked potentials (CMAP, SNAP) will be reduced, although the conduction velocity will approximate the normal rate because the myelin (especially of the large fibers) is still intact.

KEY POINT! Provided the connective tissue sheathes are intact, the prognosis for recovery from an axonotmesis is reasonably good, although not nearly as hopeful as that for neurapraxia. Recovery usually takes somewhere between 3 and 12 months for an axonotmesis and generally is a very incremental process, proceeding at about 1 mm per day in most cases.

The most severe category of nerve injury is referred to as a *neurotmesis* and involves not only axonal degeneration, but also injury to some aspect of the connective tissue sheath around the nerve. The electrophysiological effects of a neurotmesis are indistinguishable from an axonotmesis with immediate loss of conduction ability across the lesion and loss of distal excitability over a 2- to 5-day period following the injury. What distinguishes neurotmesis from axonotmesis is the fact that the former shows no improvement with follow-up (serial) testing over time, indicating the absence of reinnervation of the injured neural structure. Because

reinnervation by normal nerve regeneration processes is so tenuous for neurotmesis lesions, surgical exploration and repair may be necessary to extend any hope of recovery. Fortunately, most neural injuries do not fall into this category, so the prognosis for recovery is fair or good for most patients.

Additional techniques can identify within 1 cm the precise location of the conduction block, which is valuable information for the surgeon if surgical exploration and compression relief is contemplated. One such procedure is called the *inching technique* and involves the same setup as described for the motor conduction study but with additional stimulation sites at every centimeter from primary sites below and above the elbow. For a 12 cm segment, as noted in this brief case, the examiner would have 12 separate responses to stimulation to evaluate.

This case also underscores the limitation of the nerve conduction study, as the presence of axonal degeneration

---

CASE STUDY 16•1 NERVE CONDUCTION VELOCITY

JD is a 48-year-old male training for his first triathlon. For 6 weeks, he has had increasing right dominant elbow pain and numbness in the ulnar nerve distribution. He especially notices these symptoms when he is training for long periods of time on his bike. In addition, JD mentions that doing the buttons on his shirt has become difficult because of numbness and clumsiness with his hands. He has no family history of nerve disorders, is not diabetic, and is 6 feet tall.

Clinical exam shows decreased two-point discrimination in the ulnar nerve distribution, a positive Tinel sign over the ulnar nerve in the cubital tunnel, and a mildly positive Wartenberg's sign (indicative of weakness of ulnar-innervated hand intrinsics). Further, he demonstrates tenderness over Guyon's canal in the hand, which is the area on which he rests his weight during long training bike rides. Cervical spine screening exam is unremarkable. Thoracic outlet tests do not provoke any diminution in radial pulse.

RATIONALE FOR NERVE CONDUCTION STUDY
This patient has signs and symptoms of ulnar nerve compression at the elbow (i.e., cubital tunnel syndrome), although compression of the ulnar nerve at Guyon's canal, fairly common in competitive cyclists, may also explain the hand symptoms and intrinsic muscle weakness. Obtaining information from a nerve

conduction of the upper extremities will help to localize the source of the problem more definitively, rule out the possibility of co-morbidities (e.g., simultaneous ulnar nerve compression at the elbow and the wrist), and provide a more sound basis for therapeutic intervention and advising the patient about future effects of training.

NCS PLAN
Conduct bilateral upper extremity nerve conduction studies; this includes motor, sensory, and long-loop responses (F-waves, H-reflexes) for the median and ulnar nerves.

FINDINGS
1. Median motor and sensory latencies and conduction values, F-wave, and H-reflexes are normal bilaterally.
2. Left ulnar nerve motor and sensory conduction values are normal.
3. Right ulnar nerve distal motor and sensory latencies are normal, and the conduction velocity from below the cubital tunnel to the wrist is also normal.
4. Right ulnar nerve conduction velocity across the elbow drops to 35 meters per second, which is below the lower limit of normal for conduction (45 meters per second); amplitude of the CMAP

CASE STUDY 16-1 cont. from p. 420

drops from 8 mA in the wrist and forearm response to 3 mA for the across-the-elbow segment; right ulnar nerve F-wave is mildly prolonged.

5. Right ulnar nerve sensory conduction across the elbow is 27 meters per second, well below the lower limit of normal.

INTERPRETATION

1. Findings are consistent with ulnar nerve compression at the elbow; moderate severity.
2. The nerve conduction slowing and reduced amplitude of the CMAP across the elbow indicates involvement of myelin (neurapraxia), but definitive evidence of coincidental axonotmesis (axonal degeneration) is not established on the basis of nerve conduction findings alone. Proximal neural compression (nerve root compression, brachial plexopathy) does not seem likely on the basis of these findings but cannot be strictly excluded without additional testing.

PROCEDURES

The portion of the NCS that provided the most useful diagnostic information was the conduction study of the right ulnar nerve. As noted in the illustration, the recording electrode is placed on the abductor digiti minimi muscle, and nerve stimulation is carried out at a minimum of four locations:

1. Wrist: proximal to Guyon's canal
2. Distal to the elbow (just below the cubital tunnel)
3. Proximal to the elbow (just proximal to the cubital tunnel)
4. Axilla

A latency is obtained at each stimulation site, and the distance between the contiguous sites is measured with a tape measure. In addition, the amplitude and shape of the CMAP is noted and recorded at each stimulation site. For the sake of simple computation,

the distal motor latency (the one obtained by stimulating the ulnar nerve at the wrist) is 3 msec, and the latency just distal to the elbow is recorded as 7 msec—a difference of 4 msec; the distance between these two sites is 24 centimeters (240 millimeters). So according to the formula, our conduction velocity is obtained by dividing the difference (4 msec) between the two latencies into the distance between the two sites (240 mm), which yields a value of 60 meters per second—well within the normal range of 45 to 70 m/sec. The across-the-elbow segment is 12 cm in length (120 mm), and the latency difference between the stimulation sites above and below is 2.92 msec. Dividing 2.92 msec into 120 mm yields a conduction value of 35 m/sec—well below the lower limit of the acceptable range (45 m/sec). In addition, the amplitude dropped precipitously from 8 milliamps (mA) below the elbow to 3 millivolts (mV) at above the elbow site—evidence of partial conduction block.

The final segment of the motor study involves stimulating the ulnar nerve in the axilla and recording the distance between this new site and the one just above the elbow. Here we obtain a latency difference of 2 msec, and the distance is 12 cm (120 mm) once again. This results in a return to normal conduction of 60 m/sec, but the amplitude remains at 3 millivolts (mV) because the signal must go past the area of compression to reach the target organ where the recording electrodes are located (ADM muscle of the hypothenar eminence).

The F-wave for the right ulnar nerve is 38 msec—prolonged for a 6-foot individual and significantly longer than the ipsilateral median nerve F-wave value of 29.8 msec. The sensory conduction for ulnar nerve follows a similar course with normal distal values (below the level of the compression) and slowed and reduced amplitude responses across the elbow—lending further evidence to the conclusion that the ulnar nerve is compressed at the cubital tunnel.

---

is not clearly determined unless an EMG is also conducted to identify signs of abnormality associated with axonotmesis.

Clinical Electromyography (EMG)

There are certain features of the second part of the ENMG—the needle EMG—that provide important

complementary information for clinical decision-making. Up to this point, the nerve has been artificially stimulated in order to evoke certain motor and sensory potentials, but now the interest is to monitor and explore the muscle-nerve complex without this externally applied stimulus. Although it is possible to examine basic muscle contractility by means of surface EMG electrodes, this technique provides very little diagnostic information about the motor unit. By contrast, a pin electrode inserted directly into the muscle belly yields a wealth of information, especially about the status of the motor unit. The one big disadvantage of needle EMG, of course, is the typical discomfort associated with the examination. Patients are sometimes comforted by being informed that the electrode is very thin (28 gauge in the case of many monopolar needles) and is coated by Teflon so it moves as smoothly as possible through the muscle. Nevertheless, this portion of the exam is somewhat uncomfortable but is generally very tolerable when conducted well.

The basic equipment needed to conduct an EMG examination is the same as that used for the NCS, except that no externally applied electrical stimulation is involved during EMG testing. There are a variety of needle types that can be used, such as a concentric, bipolar, or single-fiber needle, but the Teflon-coated monopolar electrode is by far the most common (see Fig. 16-6). There are specific reasons to use the previously mentioned electrodes, but we will restrict our discussion to the typical findings using the Teflon electrode, because that is the choice of most practitioners conducting ENMG examinations.

What Can Be Learned by Needle EMG That Has Not Already Been Determined by the NCS?

Although the NCS can reveal a demyelinating lesion, such as a focal nerve compression of the fibular nerve at the fibular head, NCS cannot determine the particular status of the motor units. Specifically, the NCS cannot accurately tell whether some axons have been injured in addition to the focal demyelination. Clinical testing is often not sensitive enough to identify subtle neural injury that may be causing symptoms.

This presents a conundrum that EMG examination is able to elucidate because the intramuscular nature of the study allows it to depict the discrete characteristics of individual motor units. On rare occasion, a patient with various forms of denervation develops fasciculations that are visible to the naked eye.

KEY POINT! It has been estimated that a patient with 50% loss of motor units can still provide two or three contractions graded as "normal" by voluntary muscle testing, although the patient often complains of fatigue or weakness.

To assess the integrity of the motor unit, it is necessary to examine the muscle with an electrode in very close proximity to the injured motor units. This can only be done with a needle electrode. Furthermore, in many conditions affecting the neuromuscular system, the nerve conduction study does not identify a clear location of the problem, nor does it accurately delineate the cause of the complaints. For instance, a lumbar radiculopathy often results in complaints of pain, numbness, and tingling. The clinical exam demonstrates subtle motor weakness in the lower extremity. Unfortunately, the motor and sensory NCS is invariably normal and sheds no delineating light on the location of the problem. However, the needle EMG exam can often identify patterns of partial denervation that correspond to a nerve root.

KEY POINT! The pattern of EMG muscle involvement confirms the probable location of the problem, identifies the severity of individual muscle involvement, and provides a hint at the prognosis.

To summarize the kind of information the needle EMG examination provides, we will provide standard clinical questions answered by the procedure. Robinson and Kellogg[13] have identified several such questions, including:

1. Is the muscle normally innervated, partially innervated (which means, if true, it is also partially denervated), or completely denervated?
2. Is there evidence of motor unit recovery, which means reinnervation is taking place?
3. Do the specific findings tend to be more consistent with a neuropathic or myopathic disorder (often determined by the nature of the motor unit recruitment pattern)?
4. Is the pattern of EMG abnormality most consistent with involvement of:
   a. Anterior horn cell (polio, ALS)
   b. Nerve root (herniated nucleus pulposus, tumor)
   c. Plexus (stretch, compression, tumor)
   d. Mixed nerve (cubital tunnel syndrome)
   e. Neuromuscular junction disease (myasthenia gravis)
   f. Myopathic disorder (facioscapulohumeral muscular dystrophy)

5. If a neuropathic condition is suspected, what is the location of the lesion?

6. Finally, does the pattern of muscle involvement correspond to a posterior primary rami distribution (paraspinal muscles), an anterior primary rami (extremity muscles), a combination of both, or is there cranial nerve involvement (such as seen with anterior horn cell disease like ALS)?

Just as certain principles guided the nerve conduction study, similar principles guide the EMG examination. These principles are predicated on the examiner having committed to memory which nerve root levels and specific nerves innervate individual muscles in the limb. The specific principles include the following:

1. Examining several muscles above and below the suspected site of the pathology. The muscles studied during an EMG examination are chosen for their likelihood of contributing information to the eventual or suspected diagnosis. If a nerve root injury is suspected, then the practitioner is required to choose muscles that would confirm and disprove this possibility. Alternatively, if a peripheral nerve lesion is anticipated, muscles supplied by other peripheral nerves than the one suspected must be examined along with muscles supplied by the nerve root levels that contribute to the peripheral nerve in question. This ensures the examiner's conclusion from the EMG study is correct. In other words, the planning of the EMG exam (just as the planning of the NCS) must be done to avoid errors of clinical reasoning.

2. Examining muscles innervated by other nerves in the same extremity (as explained in no. 1 above).

3. Sampling several sites in each muscle tested (to obtain accurate representation). This sounds more uncomfortable than it actually is. The sampling should be done so that several motor unit regions can be accessed by means of redirecting the tip of the needle electrode to various depths in the muscle (Fig. 16-17).

4. Preparing to examine muscles in the contralateral extremity or upper/lower extremity. If the findings during the EMG examination indicate a more pervasive explanation for the patient's

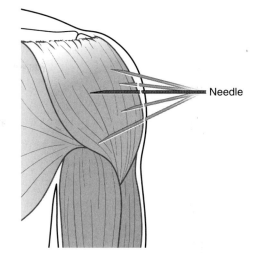

Fig 16•17 An example of examining various "quadrants" of the same muscle belly region through one insertion site. This limits the number of times the highly innervated investing deep fascia must be pierced in order to conduct a thorough EMG examination.

symptoms than was first suspected (e.g., a polyneuropathic process rather than a mononeuropathic lesion), then the examiner should extend the testing to include other limbs in the study to confirm or rule out this possibility.

5. Recalling proper time frame to conduct study to maximize information provided by the exam.

This last point needs some elaboration, because it is often not well understood by referring sources for patients with apparent neuromuscular involvement. If a patient has a sudden onset of hand numbness and is referred for "EMG/NCS" just days after the first presenting symptoms occur, it is possible the NCS may show some early signs of neural injury, but the EMG is not showing abnormality until approximately 3 weeks. The time-honored standard time frame for signs of denervation to develop is 21 days following onset of symptoms. This is an average value because it is entirely possible for muscles in very close proximity to the site of a nerve injury to demonstrate EMG abnormalities as early as 10 to 14 days following onset of symptoms (e.g., paraspinal muscles with a nerve root compression). It is usually best to delay either the entire test or at least the EMG portion of the study until more accurate results are likely to be obtained.

Because the needle EMG study is not entirely pleasant, it is preferable not to conduct this portion of the exam when little or no diagnostic information is likely to be gained. By the same token, ENMG studies conducted many months after the onset of symptoms and signs of neural involvement may yield little helpful information to guide the practitioner's clinical decision-making. The reason for this is that a neural injury is generally followed by attempts at neural repair, which eventually clouds the electrophysiological picture. For instance, 4 months after a disk herniation in the lumbar spine, the electrical evidence of denervation (spontaneous potential) has largely dissipated and been replaced by more subtle changes in motor recruitment characteristics. These alterations in recruitment profile are much harder to quantify and often do not proceed at the same rate in the various muscles that were formerly denervated. Meanwhile, the patient continues to have complaints of numbness, tingling, and pain in a radicular pattern. Although there are good clinical reasons to conduct ENMG examinations even at a late date, the clearest information provided by this test is obtained when the examination is performed in the optimal time frame.

There is a peculiar feature of EMG testing that is not considered during the NCS portion of the examination—the *sound* of the responses. There is a very distinct sound of the responses to needle provocation and voluntary activation. The characteristic sounds are associated with each of the four segments of the EMG examination described here, listed in the order in which they are ordinarily conducted in a typical patient testing session:

1. Insertion
2. Rest
3. Minimal activation
4. Maximal activation (recruitment)

Insertion

When a needle electrode is first inserted into the muscle, there is a brief burst of electrical activity that corresponds to the electrode's movement; this is a normal response. Ironically, this activity has historically been referred to as *injury potentials,* although now the most common designation is *insertional activity.* It should last between 50 and 300 msec, although some practitioners doing this test include as much as 500 msec in the normal range. In any event, normal insertional activity ends abruptly when the electrode movement ceases. If the muscle membrane is more irritable than it

should be, there will be prolonged depolarization that can continue far beyond this upper limit of 500 msec.

In cases of severe denervation in which the muscle membrane is extremely unstable, the insertional activity (membrane depolarization) will continue unabated. By contrast, sometimes the insertional activity is diminished or nearly absent. In most cases, this is the result of long-standing denervation and represents the effect on electrical activity of connective tissue or fatty infiltration into the muscle. Terms used to delineate the characteristics of the insertional activity include *normal, increased, sustained, decreased,* or *absent.* Abnormalities in insertional activity are not pathognomonic of any particular neural condition; they simply indicate an abnormality of the muscle membrane stability.

Most patients find the EMG examination uncomfortable because a needle electrode is used to obtain the signals. Nevertheless, to obtain a representative sample of the muscle's state, several sections of each muscle included in the study should be examined. In addition, three to four levels of depth should be explored by the examiner with each section of the muscle to be studied. The discomfort associated with the sheer number of needle sticks required to obtain reliable and representative information using these sampling criteria would be overwhelming for a majority of patients. Fortunately, multiple sections (quadrants) of the muscle can be accessed through a single needle insertion by carefully directing and redirecting the tip of the electrode to various regions to obtain a valid sample (see Fig. 16-17).

Rest

After assessing the insertional activity of a muscle quadrant, the examiner will "rest" (cease needle movement) to see if the muscle will return to electrical silence or whether spontaneous potentials will appear. At rest, the normal state of the motor unit and muscle fibers is complete electrical silence. One form of spontaneous electrical activity is entirely normal and is thought to occur when the tip of the electrode is near the neuromuscular junction and is producing a localized, transient depolarization. These rapidly firing potentials (2,000 to 3,000 Hz) are of very low amplitude (10 to 50 μV) and are characterized by an initial upward directed spike (negative); they are referred to as *miniature end-plate potentials* (MEPPs; Table 16-3).

The sound produced by this spontaneous activity is much like that heard when holding a large seashell to the ear. These potentials occur only in the endplate zone, which is usually found in the middle of the muscle belly, the prime target area for needle examination.

KEY POINT! Note this oddity of EMG convention: For ENMG signals, upward deflections are designated as negative and those that are directed downward are considered positive. Although this is not in keeping with the usual designation in other areas of scientific exploration (usually we think of up as positive and down as negative), it has been the practice for more than 60 years of ENMG history and is not likely to change in the near future.

Another form of normal spontaneous potential is referred to as *end-plate spikes,* or *end-plate noise* (see Table 16-3). Like the MEPPs, the initial deflection for these potentials is generally upward (negative), although they are much larger, ranging from 100 to 200 µV. They are very short duration (1 to 4 msec) and usually fire at a slightly higher rate (100 to 300 Hz) than the abnormal wave with which they are most often confused: fibrillation potentials. The distinguishing difference is the initial upward deflection for end-plate spikes in contrast to the downward deflection for fibrillation potential. A peculiar feature of end-plate spikes is that they are invariably painful; fortunately, a very slight adjustment of the needle electrode tip will relieve the symptoms and usually oblate the end-plate signal.

Common forms of abnormal spontaneous potentials include:

- Positive sharp waves
- Fibrillations
- Fasciculations
- Complex repetitive discharges
- Myotonic discharges
- Myokymic discharges

As their name suggests, *positive sharp waves* (PSWs) are positive-directed potentials, although this initial phase is followed by a low-amplitude, comparatively long-duration negative phase (see Table 16-3). The amplitude range noted in the literature is from as little as 10 µV to as high as 1,000 µV (1,000 µV = 1 mV), and the rate of discharge is regular and ranges from 1 to 200 Hz. PSWs have a characteristic sound like a dull thud, much like that of a motor boat engine at low idle. Positive sharp waves result from an abnormally sensitive muscle membrane and probably represent the depolarization of a single muscle fiber, although their exact etiology has not been completely delineated. A motor unit firing from some distance may initially appear as a positive sharp wave, but three clues should alert the examiner to avoid this error in interpretation:

1. There is no negative initial deflection with a PSW, although this is often the case with a distant firing motor unit.
2. A motor unit's rate of firing is usually quite a bit lower in frequency compared to a PSW and is fairly rhythmic.
3. With effort, a volume-conducted motor unit (coming from a distance away) can be eliminated with sufficient patient relaxation, which is not the case for true spontaneous potentials. Often PSWs appear with other forms of spontaneous potentials, such as fibrillations and complex repetitive discharges and are seen with both neuropathic and myopathic conditions and with anterior horn cell disease.

Fibrillations are common spontaneous potentials with an initial positive deflection and are of very short duration (usually less than 5 msec). Reported amplitudes for fibrillations range from 20 µV to over 1 mV, and they generally discharge somewhat irregularly at rates between 1 and 30 Hz (see Table 16-3). As with PSWs, fibrillations are the firing of individual muscle fibers because of membrane instability and hypersensitivity to acetylcholine. The typical sound of fibrillation potentials has been described as "rain on a tin roof" when projected through the EMG speaker. Together, PSWs and fibrillations have been called denervation potentials, because the most common cause of these spontaneously firing potentials is muscle denervation. Strictly speaking, however, this designation is not correct because myopathic processes and anterior horn cell disease can generate these abnormal potentials. The presence of positive sharp waves and fibrillations are usually graded from 0 to 4. Findings of 3 to 4+ PSWs and fibrillations indicate more severe muscle membrane instability than a 1 to 2+ designation. Consequently,

Table 16•3 Characteristics of Normal and Abnormal Potentials During Electromyography

	Wave	Image	Amplitude	Rate	Duration	Sound	Characteristics
Normal Potentials	Miniature end-plate potentials		10–50 µV	2,000–3,000 Hz	0.5 to 1 msec	Large seashell held to the ear	Normally occurring insertional activity. Found only in the end-plate zone. Initial upward directed spike (negative).
	End-plate spikes		100–200 µV	100–300 Hz	1–4 msec	Low-level murmur	Normally occurring insertional activity. Initial deflection upward (negative).
	Motor unit potential		250 µV to 5 mV	Onset of 5 to 15 Hz up to 60 Hz	5 to 15 msec	Sharp, crisp discharge	bi- or triphasic waves
Abnormal Spontaneous Potentials	Positive sharp waves		10 µV to as high as 1,000 µV	1–200 Hz	< 10 Hz up to 100 msec	Dull thud like motor boat engine	Biphasic initially positive with long, low amplitude negative phase
	Fibrillations		20 µV to > 1 mV	1–30 Hz	< 5 msec	Rain on a tin roof	Initial positive deflection

		Amplitude	Frequency	Duration	Sound	Description
Fasciculations		Similar to normal motor unit potentials	1Hz to 1 every few sec	Similar to normal motor unit potentials	Popping sound	Considered to be a involuntary motor unit firing. May be normal but considered abnormal if attended by other forms of spontaneous potentials.
Complex repetitive discharges		Few to several hundred µV	20 Hz to 100 Hz	10–50 msec	Machine gun firing	High-frequency polyphasic potentials initiated by needle movement or tapping, waning to low frequency. Not specific to particular condition but usually associated with chronic neuropathic processes
Myotonic discharges		10 µV to 1 mV (1,000 µV)	20–150 Hz	1–5 msec	Dive-bomber or chainsaw	Rhythmically waxing and waning potentials initiated by needle movement or tapping. Biphasic initially downward.
Myokymic discharges		250 µV to 2 mV	2–60 Hz	Rapid, staccato discharge	Marching sound	Consecutively firing potentials that do not wax and wane; not specific to particular condition but clearly are associated with an unstable muscle membrane.

their prognosis for recovery is less. This method of quantification of spontaneous potentials is useful when serial or repeat studies are undertaken. Progression from one grade to another over time is a means to gauge improvement (or lack of it) and provides objective documentation for making predictions regarding recovery from neuromuscular injury or disease.

Another spontaneous potential that may occur during the "rest" segment of the study is a *fasciculation*, considered to be a nonvoluntary motor unit firing. Most people have experienced an involuntary twitch of the eyelid muscle. This is a benign, albeit annoying, form of fasciculation. Fasciculations have the appearance of normal motor units, but their sound is unique, probably because they are activated in relative isolation. They are characterized by a popping sound. If there is another motor unit fasciculating at some distance from the tip of the needle electrode, it will produce a dull thud sound. Together, the sound is typified by a random sequence of *pop, pop, thud, pop, pop, thud* sounds. Fasciculations may occur in otherwise normal individuals, but they are often observed in patients with anterior horn cell disease; if attended by other forms of spontaneous potentials, they are considered an abnormal waveform. They may also be present in other disorders, such as entrapment neuropathies and radiculopathies. Unlike PSWs and fibrillations, there is no attempt to grade fasciculations; simply noting their presence is the accepted standard.

Complex repetitive discharges (CRDs) are spontaneous potentials that are not specific to any particular condition but are usually associated with chronic neuropathic processes (see Table 16-3). These were formerly called *bizarre high-frequency discharges*. These waves may vary in shape from linked PSWs or fibrillations to multiple polyphasic-like waveforms (a phase is measured as each time the motor unit signal crosses the baseline). They usually fire initially at a high frequency (up to 100 Hz), are evoked by movement of the electrode's tip, and then wane down to a lower frequency of 20 to 30 Hz. CRDs tend to start and stop abruptly and sound like a machine gun firing. Although CRDs are not specific to any particular condition, they are usually associated with chronic neuropathic processes.

Myotonic discharges are rhythmic spontaneous potentials often initiated by needle movement or tapping

(see Table 16-3). The initial frequency of firing for these potentials is very high—as much as 150 Hz—and then fade to a rate of 20 to 30 Hz over a period of a couple of seconds. Myotonic discharges differ from CRDs in that in addition to waning in frequency, they will also resume a higher frequency—waxing. This characteristic waxing and waning sound reminded early ENMG examiners of WWII dive-bomber sounds; at one time, these potentials were referred to as *dive-bomber potentials*. Usually the waveform for myotonic discharges corresponds to that of sharp waves or fibrillations. These spontaneous potentials are noted in patients with myotonic dystrophy and myotonia congenita but have also been observed in patients with chronic radiculopathies.

A final spontaneous potential to be mentioned is the *myokymic discharge*. Myokymia is a muscle disorder that produces wormlike contractions of long sections of muscle. The electrical representation of this disorder appears like consecutively firing fasciculation potentials and produces an unmistakable marching sound. Unlike myotonic discharges, myokymia does not wax and wane. In fact, volitional activity does not seem to alter these abnormal potentials, and they have even been observed during sleep. Myokymic discharges appear most often in chronic conditions, radiation plexopathies, Bell's palsy, and the facial muscles of patients with multiple sclerosis. Like positive sharp waves and fibrillations, they are not specific to any particular neuromuscular disease but clearly are associated with an unstable muscle membrane.

Minimal Activation

Up to this point in the EMG examination, the patient has been asked only to tolerate the procedure and remain as relaxed as possible, because insertional activity and spontaneous activity at rest are entirely passive electrical phenomena. However, during the third segment of the EMG, the patient's full cooperation is needed to accomplish the goal. Segment three is referred to as *minimal activation*. The primary goal is to assess the motor units volitionally recruited by the patient. A normal motor unit potential (MUP) has a duration of 5 to 15 msec, an amplitude of 250 μV to 5 mV, and an onset firing frequency of 5 to 15 per second (upper range less than 60 Hz; Fig. 16-18). The typical configuration of an MUP is biphasic or triphasic, although up to four phases is still considered normal. More than four phases constitutes a "polyphasic" motor unit. Although generally considered an abnormal MUP, normal, young to middle-aged individuals are "allowed" to have up to 15% of their volitionally recruited motor units appear as polyphasics. The proportion of polyphasic motor units increases with age and is considered a normal variation when up to 30% of the recruited motor units are polyphasic in those 60 years or older.

A polyphasic motor unit is one that has five or more phases (Fig. 16-18). Although these abnormal motor units can occur during the process of denervation, small, low-amplitude, long-duration polyphasics usually indicate a recent attempt to reinnervate an injured or diseased motor unit. They have been given a special name—*nascent (polyphasic) potentials*—and are seen only during the early stages of reinnervation. When collateral or terminal sprouting by an injured or diseased axon occurs, the configuration of the motor unit changes because of the poorly synchronized conduction of its distal branches. As a result, the normal biphasic or triphasic configuration gives way to the polyphasic form. By contrast to the nascent polyphasic motor units, large-amplitude polyphasics are often observed in patients who have chronic neuropathies. Small-amplitude, short-duration polyphasics are believed to be a hallmark sign of myopathic disease.

One principle of volitional motor unit activation is that the first MUPs recruited are those with the lowest threshold. These tend to be the smallest motor units that are innervated by small-diameter alpha (α) motoneurons and are comprised primarily of slow-oxidative, fatigue-resistant muscle fibers. When greater levels of motor contraction are needed, these motor units increase their firing frequency and more motor units are also recruited to meet this demand. Then, as still greater contraction strength is needed, larger motor units comprised of fast-twitch, fatigue-resistant muscle fibers are activated. Finally, when very strong muscle contractions are called for, the slow (red muscle fiber) motor units and the fastest-twitch, readily fatigable motor units are recruited at even faster frequencies. This process of recruiting motor units according to size and frequency in response to imposed demand is referred to as *rate coding*; it can be identified to a certain extent by electrophysiological assessment during the minimal activation portion of the examination. The size of the motor units (amplitude) and their frequency will characterize the recruited potentials as large or small, although this is often an academic point without a great deal of clinical utility.

Maximal Activation (Recruitment)

The final segment of the EMG examination is to evaluate the recruitment or interference pattern of each muscle. We have mentioned the process of motor unit recruitment, but here we are not interested in the characteristics of the discrete units. Rather, the focus is to observe the orderly recruitment of MUPs and the ability to "fill the screen" with electrical activity while the patient begins with a minimal contraction and builds to a maximal contraction (Fig. 16-19). With full muscle

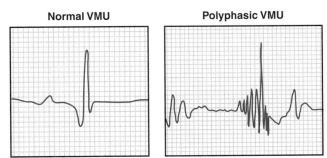

Normal VMU   **Polyphasic VMU**

Fig 16•18 A normal motor unit is usually biphasic or triphasic, has a duration of 5 to 15 msec, an amplitude of 250µV to 5 mV, and an onset frequency of 5 to 15 per second. A polyphasic motor unit is characterized by five or more phases and may be small during initial attempts at reinnervation or large in patients with chronic neuropathies.

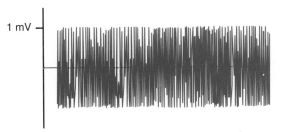

1 mV

Fig 16•19 Full-screen interference indicates normal recruitment of motor units. The baseline is no longer visible because the electrical activity associated with depolarization of the large number of normal units has obscured it.

contraction, the examiner should no longer be able to identify the baseline, as the entire screen will be filled with summated motor units with amplitudes of roughly 4 mV from peak to peak (top of the positive phase to the bottom of the negative phase). The extent of electrical activity from maximal activity should "interfere" with the baseline. Many examiners refer to this pattern of activity as the *interference pattern*. Abnormalities noted during this segment of the study include the following:

- Neuropathic recruitment pattern
- Myopathic recruitment pattern
- Decreased activation

A neuropathic recruitment pattern is characterized by decreased recruitment for the entire muscle, because a significant number of motor units have been lost through denervation (Fig. 16-20). Somewhat counterintuitively, any individual motor unit (whether healthy or diseased) in a muscle that has an overall decreased recruitment pattern will actually fire at a faster than normal frequency; this is usually referred to as *rapid firing rate* and is a classic sign of lower motor neuron injury or disease. The sound made by motor units exhibiting decreased recruitment and increased firing frequency is like that made by a playing card against moving bicycle spokes or rapidly running a stick along a picket fence. The rapid firing rate of the still-viable motor units in a muscle that is partially denervated is one good indication that a patient is fully cooperating during the examination. Failure to see an increased firing frequency in a muscle exhibiting weakness may suggest less-than-complete patient effort from pain, volition, or CNS involvement.

A myopathic recruitment pattern (Fig. 16-21) is characterized by small-amplitude, short-duration polyphasic motor units that appear almost immediately with little effort. In fact, it is almost impossible to isolate individual motor units in patients who have myopathic processes, because they recruit their existing motor units so readily. Although this may initially appear as an actual increase in number of motor units recruited, the fact that it appears with almost no effort and that it is often attended by clinical weakness suggests that the muscle itself is diseased.

Decreased activation of motor units is an abnormality noted during recruitment, although it is often the examiner's subjective sense that leads to this designation. In the presence of organic lower motor neuron disease or injury, motor units may be decreased in number but will fire more rapidly to accomplish a task such as maximal muscle contraction. If the practitioner asks the patient to give greater effort during a muscle contraction and the firing frequency remains unchanged, several explanations may apply. First, the patient may be experiencing pain that is prohibiting him or her from cooperating fully, resulting in the expected increase in activation frequency. If this is the case, slightly adjusting the needle's tip may circumvent the problem, reduce the patient's discomfort, and allow a more robust contraction (characterized by the expected frequency of motor unit firing). This is a fairly common occurrence during a typical EMG examination.

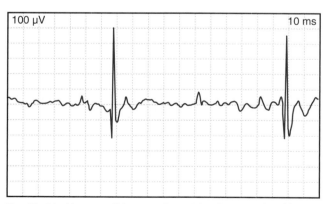

Fig 16•20 Neuropathic recruitment is characterized by a decreased number of motor units firing; those that are activated usually fire at a faster-than-normal rate—called *rapid firing rate.*

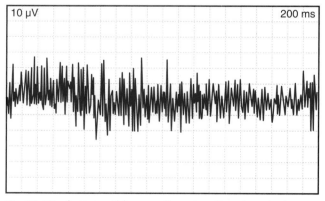

Fig 16•21 A myopathic recruitment pattern is noted for rapidly filling the screen with small-amplitude, short-duration polyphasic motor units accomplished with little effort.

Alternatively, a patient may not be giving full effort for reasons other than pain, such as secondary gain or symptom magnification. In this case, the decreased activation and failure to increase the motor unit firing frequency is entirely voluntary. It should be noted in the interpretation report that the motor unit firing is less than expected based on other findings. Results inconsistent with a failure to increase the frequency of motor unit firing and achieve full recruitment include the absence of any muscle atrophy, normal motor and sensory nerve conduction values, and no evidence of other electrophysiological abnormalities generally associated with denervation, such as positive sharp waves or fibrillation potentials (Fig. 16-22).

Finally, when a central nervous system injury has resulted in motor weakness, a diminished number of motor units firing at a set frequency is the result of impaired signal to the anterior horn cells from higher centers. The patient may very well give the best effort, but the CNS lesion will prevent the lower motor neuron (anterior horn cells) from being activated, resulting in an increased firing rate. EMG of patients with CNS lesions is generally not recommended, as it is not good at identifying the location and extent of such an injury. A summary of general EMG findings is noted in Table 16-4.

Interpretation of Electrophysiological Evaluation Findings

When the information from the NCS and the EMG examination has been obtained, the examiner must provide the referring practitioner with a summary of the findings and an interpretation that can answer the following primary questions:

1. Is this a normal or abnormal study?
2. If abnormal, are the findings more consistent with a neuropathic or a myopathic disorder?

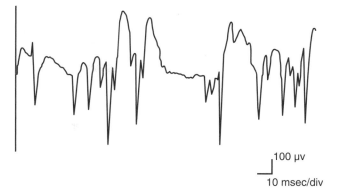

Fig 16•22 Positive sharp waves and fibrillation potentials are seen during EMG examination when axonal degeneration (denervation) has occurred. The extent of abnormal waves of this nature are usually graded from 1 to 4, depending on severity of involvement.

3. If the examiner determines that the findings are most consistent with a neuropathic condition, does the lesion seem to affect the myelin or the axon preferentially?
4. If the lesion is neuropathic in its primary effect, does it appear to be focal (discrete site) or systemic?
5. Does the condition appear to be mild, moderate, or severe? Often the terminology used is *partial* or *complete,* which may refer to the extent of conduction block on NCS or spontaneous potentials (denervation-like potentials) on EMG. There is no certain way to distinguish between the denervation associated with an axonotmesis compared to a neurotmesis, outside of serial studies conducted over several months after finding a lesion.
6. Is there any hint that recovery might be occurring (e.g., presence of small-amplitude, polyphasic motor unit potentials on EMG for a neuropathic disorder)?

If ENMG examination provides answers to these questions, clinically useful information can be ascertained to

Table 16•4	Summary of EMG Findings			
Testing Category	**Normal Muscle**	**Peripheral Nerve Disorder**	**Myopathic Process**
Insertional activity	Brief	Increased or prolonged	Brief or increased
Spontaneous activity	None	Present	Usually present
Minimal motor unit activation	Normal	Polyphasics, increased duration, large or small amplitude	Polyphasics, decreased duration, small amplitude
Maximal motor unit activation	Full interference	Reduced	Full with nominal activity

establish the presence and severity of disease, chart a patient's course of care, and serve as an important indicator for prognosis.

Again, the questions used to construct and qualify the examination findings are time-dependent—that is, in the first few weeks that a disorder affecting the muscle and nerve is present, the abnormal findings (if there are any) would be primarily noted during the NCS. At the 3- to 4-week mark, abnormalities consistent with neurapraxia and axonotmesis would be present during the NCS *and* the EMG. The EMG changes, in particular, would be consistent with a recent-onset condition, because the Wallerian degeneration and consequent muscle membrane instability associated with a neural injury are most prevalent in the 3- to 6-week mark. As time progresses, the NCS begins to return to some semblance of normalcy, and the acute changes associated with denervation (e.g., spontaneous potentials on the EMG) begin to give way to chronic motor unit recruitment findings. The full process of reinnervation may take several months to complete and often results in large-amplitude polyphasic motor units during recruitment, but little else will indicate presence of a neural insult. This is why an ENMG is especially useful for identifying abnormalities during the early stages of a neuromuscular disorder.

CASE STUDY 16•2 EMG STUDY

TM is a 59-year-old female who works as a forklift operator for a local bottling company. She has had a 2-month history of low back pain, left lower extremity pain, and paresthesias to the lateral side of the foot. She especially notices the discomfort and numbness in the foot after sitting for 30 minutes or longer at work. TM denies any history of recent trauma, but her physician has told her that she is "borderline diabetic," and she has been advised to control this condition with diet and exercise. Most troubling for TM is that she recently began a walking program to lose weight and is noticing a bandlike feeling around her ankle and a sense of weakness after walking for 10 minutes or more.

Clinical examination shows signs of neural tension in the left lower extremity with straight leg raise test and slump testing. Both of these tests refer pain from the lumbar spine into the lateral aspect of the gastrocnemius muscle. Sensory testing reveals diminished sensory acuity to crude and light touch in the S_1 distribution and muscle weakness at 3+/5 in the gastrocsoleus complex, the tibialis posterior, and the fibularis longus. Great toe extensors are graded at 4/5, as is the tibialis anterior and the tensor fascia lata muscle. The deep tendon reflexes are normal at the knee, and the right ankle jerk is graded as 2+, but the left ankle DTR is absent. Exquisite palpation tenderness is noted in the midline at L5S1. The pain provocation tests for the SI joint are normal, and the hip exam does not reveal any joint restriction.

SUMMARY OF NCS FINDINGS
Bilateral nerve conduction studies included the fibular and tibial motor nerves and F-waves, sural nerve sensory latencies, and the H-reflexes. The motor and sensory nerve conduction studies were normal, but the tibial nerve F-wave on the left side was mildly prolonged. In addition, the left H-reflex was significantly prolonged when compared to her uninvolved right side H-reflex.

RATIONALE FOR EMG
The NCS failed to identify a localized conduction block or area of segmental demyelination to explain TM's symptoms. The mildly prolonged F-wave and markedly prolonged H-reflex on the right side are certainly suggestive of a neural problem, but there is no definitive indication as to the severity or location of the problem. An EMG of the left lower extremity and paraspinal muscles should provide evidence of ongoing axonal degeneration, should it be present. Recruitment characteristics of the muscles examined will also provide some information for clinical decisions regarding intervention.

EMG PLAN
Monopolar needle EMG examination of the left and right T12–S1 paraspinals and the following lower extremity muscles will be conducted: tensor fascia lata, medial and lateral hamstrings, quadriceps femoris, tibialis anterior, tibialis posterior, fibularis longus, medial head of the gastrocnemius, and the soleus. These muscles will help to show whether the patient's complaints are arising from a radiculopathic process, a lumbosacral plexopathy, or some other cause.

FINDINGS
Monopolar needle EMG study of the left L5S1 paraspinals and the lateral hamstrings, tensor fascia lata, medial gastrocnemius, tibialis posterior, and

CASE STUDY 16-2 cont. from p. 432

fibularis longus revealed sharp waves and fibrillation potentials, indicating ongoing axonal injury. Motor recruitment in these muscles was impaired, but early signs of recovery potentials (small amplitude polyphasic motor units) were noted. Muscles examined without any electrical evidence of abnormality included the T12–L4 paraspinals, quadriceps, tibialis anterior, and soleus muscles. The muscles examined revealed no evidence of myopathic motor units, and no fasciculation potentials were noted at rest. No abnormality was identified in any of the similar muscles examined on the right side.

INTERPRETATION

1. Findings are consistent with a moderately severe radiculopathic process primarily affecting the (L5) S1 innervated muscles of the left lower extremity. Findings of similar abnormality in the left lumbar paraspinals clearly implicate the location of the neural injury to the level of the nerve root.

2. Early signs of reinnervation (small amplitude polyphasic motor units) indicate some attempt at neural recovery is ongoing and is likely to proceed over time.

3. No indication of abnormality is noted in the right paraspinals or lower extremity.

SUMMARY

EMG findings are best explained by a nerve root compression; correlation with clinical exam findings and any imaging studies is recommended to identify the cause of the compression (herniated nucleus pulposus, tumor, etc). The indication of ongoing reinnervation suggests that conservative management is appropriate for this patient, but vigilance should be maintained to detect any signs of progressive neurological deficit.

Reporting Results

After the examiner completes the technical aspect of data collection for the ENMG and has come to a conclusion after interpreting the information, the next task is to communicate the results to the referring physician in a manner that is readily understandable and usable.

KEY POINT! To arrive at the diagnosis, the information from the ENMG testing must be used in light of the clinical and historical information obtained from the patient. Imaging studies or other specialist test procedures (blood analysis) are also complementary in this process.

Summarizing the test results is the final step in the evaluation process. A sufficient history and brief details of a clinical examination should be given to justify the need for the ENMG testing. Then the data from the NCS are usually depicted in tabular form so the nerves studied and the numerical results are clearly identified (Table 16-5). Many current EMG machines can generate reports that include the values obtained during the study and a comparison list of normal values. The normal values usually are obtained from a national database and the current literature and are programmed

into the computer. Examiners should verify with their own laboratory that these values are appropriate for their particular setting; if not, more clinically applicable values should be used for comparison.

KEY POINT! A categorical statement should not be made about the cause of the findings since the ENMG cannot actually determine this.

Information from the needle EMG portion of the exam would follow and is usually presented in tabular format to include muscles studied and the response of each muscle to insertion, rest, minimal activation, and maximal activation (interference pattern with recruitment). The interpretation often presents, in list form, the abnormal findings from the study, an impression as to whether the findings are most consistent with segmental demyelination or axonal degeneration, and a concluding remark about the likely location of the lesion should the ENMG identify one. It is common for a referring clinician to call after receiving the report to seek clarification regarding prognosis based on the findings and to obtain counsel about the potential benefit of conservative management of a patient's neuromuscular disorder. Clinical experience with such cases gained over the years may

Table 16•5 **Sample Report Following ENMG Study**

Muscle	Insertional Activity	Spontaneous Activity	Motor Units	Interference Pattern
Cervical paraspinals (C3–T1) R and L	Brief	None	Full	Not tested
Deltoid: R and L	Brief	None	Full	Full
Biceps: R and L	Brief	None	Full	Full
Triceps: R and L	Brief	None	Full	Full
Flexor carpi radialis: R and L	Brief	None	Full	Full
Flexor digitorum sublimis: R and L	Brief	None	Full	Full
Extensor digitorum communis: R and L	Brief	None	Full	Full
(L) Abductor pollicis brevis and opponens pollicis	Brief	None	Full	Full
(L) First dorsal interosseous	Brief	None	Full	Full
(R) Abductor pollicis brevis and opponens pollicis	Prolonged	1+ sharp waves and numerous fibrillations	Shows partial interference pattern with motor unit dropout and rapid firing rate	Shows partial interference pattern with motor unit dropout and rapid firing rate
(R) First dorsal interosseous	Prolonged	1+ sharp waves and numerous fibrillations	Shows partial interference pattern with motor unit dropout and rapid firing rate	Shows partial interference pattern with motor unit dropout and rapid firing rate
(R) Extensor pollicis longus	Brief	None	Full	Full
(R) Abductor digiti minimi	Prolonged	Occasional to 1+ sharp wave and fibrillations	Mixed polyphasic and normal	Showed slight motor unit dropout and slight rapid firing rate

R & L = right and left

allow the ENMG examiner to provide additional useful information and recommendations based on the results of the testing and brief clinical exam.

Does ENMG Bear Any Relationship to EMG Biofeedback?

EMG biofeedback (i.e., surface EMG), discussed in Chapter 11, uses electrical signals of muscle depolarization in much the same way that diagnostic EMG does, but with two important distinctions. First, EMG biofeedback is an entirely therapeutic procedure for the purpose of helping a patient increase or decrease skeletal muscle activity. There is little diagnostic element to the biofeedback procedure. Second, EMG biofeedback almost always uses surface EMG electrodes (not needles), and the equipment is usually smaller and more portable than diagnostic EMG units. Nevertheless, there is a connection between the two procedures, because although ENMG is a

diagnostic test, its purpose is to answer a clinical question that leads to a more informed therapeutic intervention.

Consider this example: A patient who has had total knee arthroplasty (TKA) 3 weeks previous has been sent to the clinic to begin outpatient physical therapy. On clinical examination, you note that the patient has a 3/5 muscle contraction of the quadriceps, and this finding represents a barrier to the normal course of exercise intervention. Although you are aware that pain, inhibition, and preoperative disuse atrophy can contribute to such a finding, you are also familiar with the literature that indicates that up to 70% of TKA patients have a femoral nerve injury produced by the compression of the pneumatic tourniquet used during the surgery to control excessive bleeding in the surgical field. Since you are not certain what exactly caused this muscle impairment, you proceed with brief needle EMG of the quadriceps and other thigh muscles. You find that the patient has no increase in insertional activity and no spontaneous potentials at rest (i.e., no positive sharp waves or fibrillations). The motor units appear to be primarily biphasic and triphasic, although they are decreased in number. Efforts to recruit a full interference pattern are compromised initially by pain, but with continued effort, a full pattern is achieved. From this information, you conclude that the patient has *not* sustained a neural injury but is, indeed, suffering from postoperative pain, inhibition, and typical muscle atrophy. This patient has plenty of viable motor units to recruit and thus is an ideal candidate for both EMG biofeedback as a primary adjunct to therapeutic exercise and high-amplitude neuromuscular electrical stimulation. Often, after three to five sessions of EMG biofeedback, the patient has mastered the ability to recruit available motor units without causing significant pain or experiencing inhibition. At that point, the biofeedback procedures can be discontinued and the patient can concentrate on therapeutic exercise activities. This is an example of how ENMG testing leads to a therapeutic intervention that makes primary use of EMG biofeedback to optimize outcome without tissue irritation or injury.

Documentation Tips

When documenting the procedures and results of an ENMG, the following should be presented:

- Medical screening/history findings
- Clinical exam findings
  - Neuro exam
  - Musculoskeletal screening exam
  - Height
  - Age
  - Surface temperature of the extremity
- Nerve conduction study
  - Nerve segment distance
  - Latency (motor, sensory)
  - Amplitude (motor, sensory)
  - Duration of the action potential
  - Shape (configuration) of the waveform
  - Nerve conduction velocity (motor, sensory)
- EMG
  - Needle type (e.g., monopolar Teflon, concentric, bipolar, etc.)
  - Muscles examined
    - Specific nerve supply
    - Nerve root derivation
  - Key findings
    - Insertion
    - Rest
    - Minimal activation
    - Maximal activation
  - List of abnormal findings
  - Interpretation/impression

Clinical Controversies

- Some controversy exists regarding the use of antidromic vs. orthodromic sensory latency and conduction values. Orthodromic technique is certainly more consistent with the anatomical and physiological direction of impulse propagation (afferent: distal to proximal); however, antidromic technique is easier to use in many cases, and the amplitude of response is often larger than orthodromically obtained responses and is therefore easier to see and record.
- Many practitioners often identify a neural lesion as a "neurapraxia" or an "axonotmesis," but caution should be used here. Most neural lesions are a combination of myelin and axon involvement. Although it is true that a neural injury may be primarily myelin or axonal, they are rarely one or the other. Caution should be exercised in describing them as such.
- Currently, 48 states and the District of Columbia allow physical therapists to evaluate patients without a prior physician's referral, and 44 states and the District of Columbia further improve accessibility by allowing physical therapists to evaluate and treat, under certain conditions, patients without a referral from a physician.

☐ REFERENCES

1. Clark RG. *Manter and Gatz's Essentials of Clinical Neuroanatomy and Neurophysiology.* 5th ed. FA Davis, Philadelphia; 1975:1.
2. Chémali KR, Tsao B. Electrodiagnostic testing of nerves and muscles: when, why, and how to order. *Cleveland Clin J of Med.* 2005;72(1):37–48.
3. Coppieters MW, Hough AD, Dilley A. Different nerve-gliding exercises induce different magnitudes of median nerve longitudinal excursion: an in vivo study using dynamic ultrasound imaging. *J Orthop Sports Phys Ther.* 2009;39(3):164–171.
4. Burke FD, Ellis J, McKenna H, Bradley MJ. Primary care management of carpal tunnel syndrome. *Postgrad Med J.* 2003;79:433–437.
5. Coppieters MW, Alshami AM. Longitudinal excursion and strain in the median nerve during novel nerve gliding

exercises for carpal tunnel syndrome. *J Orthop Res.* 2007; 25:972–980.

6. Michlovitz SL. Conservative interventions for carpal tunnel syndrome. *J Orthop Sports Phys Ther.* 2004;34:589–600.

7. Muller M, Tsui D, Schnurr R, Biddulph-Deisroth L, Hard J, MacDermid JC. Effectiveness of hand therapy interventions in primary management of carpal tunnel syndrome: a systematic review. *J Hand Ther.* 2004;17:210–228.

8. Rozmaryn LM, Dovelle S, Rothman ER, Gorman K, Olvey KM, Bartko JJ. Nerve and tendon gliding exercises and the conservative management of carpal tunnel syndrome. *J Hand Ther.* 1998;11:171–179.

9. Chang CW, Wang YC, Chang KF. A practical electrophysiolgic guide for non-surgical and surgical treatment of carpal tunnel syndrome. *J Hand Surg (Eur).* 2008;33E(1):32–27.

10. Brown MC, Ironton R. Suppression of motor nerve terminal sprouting in partially denervated mouse muscle. *J Physiol.* 1977;272(1):70P–71P.

11. Sanes JR, Covault J. Axon guidance during reinnervation. *Trends Neurosci.* 1985;8:523–528.

12. Johnson EW, Braddom R. Over-work weakness in fascioscapulohumeral muscular dystrophy. *Arch Phys Med Rehabil.* 1971;52:333–336.

13. Robinson AJ, Kellogg R. *Clinical Electrophysiologic Assessment in Clinical Electrophysiology: Electrotherapy and Electrophysiologic Testing.* 2nd ed. by AJ Robinson and Lynn Snyder-Mackler, Baltimore: Williams & Wilkins;1995:415–416.

14. Halle J, Scoville C, Greathouse D. Ultrasound's effect on the conduction latency of the superficial radial nerve in man. *Phys Ther.* 1981;61:345–350.

15. Oh S, ed. Physiological factors affecting nerve conduction. In: *Clinical Electromyography—Nerve Conduction Studies.* 2nd ed. Baltimore: Williams & Wilkins; 1993:297–313.

16. Sabbahi MA, Khalil M. Segmental H-reflex studies in upper and lower limbs of healthy subjects. *Arch Phys Med Rehabil.* 1990;71:216–222.

17. Seddon H. Three types of nerve injury. *Brain.* 1943;66: 237–288.

Glossary

Absolute atmosphere (ATA) The atmospheric pressure at sea level, equal to 1 ATA (760 mm Hg).

Acoustic impedance A material's ability to transmit sound; related to the molecular density and structure of the material. Impedance is inversely related to transmission.

Allodynia Pain produced by an otherwise non-noxious stimulus, such as light touch of the skin following sunburn; a form of hyperalgesia.

Alpha motoneuron The large, lower motor neurons of the brain and spinal cord that innervate skeletal muscle.

Alternating current (AC) The uninterrupted bidirectional flow of ions or electrons that must change direction at least one time per second.

Ampere (A; amp) The unit of electrical current reflecting the volume of current (electrons) passing a given point in a given time; 1 amp = 1 coulomb/sec.

Amplification The act of repeatedly bouncing light between two parallel reflectors arranged at opposite ends of a lasing chamber, causing the excitation of more photons.

Analgesia The decrease or absence of pain.

Ankle-Brachial Index (ABI) A method used to determine the presence and severity of peripheral arterial disease, calculated as the ratio of ankle systolic blood pressure to the arm systolic blood pressure.

Anode A point or region of a circuit that has a deficiency of electrons; also referred to as the *positive pole.*

Antidromic Conduction along a nerve in the direction opposite of normal; for example, proximal to distal for sensory and distal to proximal for motor axons.

Aquatic therapy A therapeutic intervention, usually performed in a pool that uses water to facilitate physiological effects or exercise programs.

Asymmetrical Condition when the amplitude and duration characteristics between the two phases of the biphasic waveform differ in any manner.

Attenuation A measure of the decrease in sound energy either by absorption, reflection, or refraction.

Axonotmesis Axonal degeneration and myelin sheath disruption that occurs distal to and one node of Ranvier proximal to the nerve lesion.

Balanced When the area under the curve of the first phase (i.e., phase charge) of a biphasic pulse is equal to that of the second phase.

Beam nonuniformity ratio (BNR) The ratio between spatial peak intensity and spatial average intensity of an ultrasound beam.

Beat frequency The frequency at which peak constructive or destructive interference occurs for interferential current; calculated as the difference in frequency between the currents interfered.

Bipolar An electrode configuration in which all the electrodes of a single electrical circuit are placed over the treatment area.

Body mass index (BMI) A value that represents a measure of mass, calculated as body mass (in kg) divided by height (in meters) squared (kg/m^2).

Buoyancy A force on a body immersed in a fluid that is equal to the weight of the fluid displaced by that object.

Burst   A series of pulses or brief periods of alternating current delivered consecutively and separated from the next series or period.

Burst frequency   The frequency at which bursts are generated.

Capacitance   The amount of charge that a material can hold for a given voltage imposed upon it.

Capacitive or electric field method (diathermy)   An applicator system that requires making the patient's tissues part of the dielectric of a capacitor.

Carrier frequency   The frequency of the alternating current or pulse train that is interrupted into bursts.

Cathode   A point or region of a circuit that has an excess of electrons; also referred to as the *negative pole*.

Causalgia   Type 2 complex regional pain syndrome identified as painful burning sensations in an extremity that usually occurs along the distribution of a nerve.

Cavitation   Pulsation of gas bubbles in biological tissues in response to the passage of ultrasound.

Charge (*Q*)   Electrical state obtained by the addition or removal of electrons; charge is measured in coulombs (C) or microcoulombs (μC).

Chemical mediators   Substances located in inflammatory cells that attract and activate fibroblasts to the site of an injury; for example, histamines, cytokines, and leukotrienes.

Chronaxie   The duration of a stimulus that is two times the rheobase amplitude and capable of eliciting a minimally detectable motor response. Chronaxie is used to assess the integrity of tissue, as healthy innervated tissue should have a chronaxie less than 1 msec.

Chronic venous insufficiency (CVI)   Vascular disease that begins at the junction of superficial and deep vein systems and creates valvular incompetence.

Chronic wound   A wound that deviates from the expected sequence of repair in terms of time, appearance, and response to aggressive and appropriate treatment.

Classification system for pain   Developed by the International Association for the Study of Pain; it includes definitions for pain terms and descriptions of pain syndromes.

Claudication pain   Pain in the calves when walking, brought on by muscle ischemia; the cardinal symptom of peripheral arterial disease.

Cold bath   Immersion of distal extremities in a tub or basin with circumferential contact of the cooling agent.

Cold packs   Flexible frozen ice, gel, or liquid packs used for cryotherapy.

Cold urticaria   Hypersensitivity to cold that results in a vascular skin reaction in response to cold exposure; typically characterized by smooth, itchy, elevated red patches.

Comorbidity   Any existing medical illnesses concurrent with a primary disorder.

Complex regional pain syndrome (CRPS)   Categorized as either type 1 (RSD) or type 2 (causalgia). Both types are forms of pain in the sympathetic nervous system, either with or without known involvement of the peripheral nerves.

Complex repetitive discharges   Abnormal spontaneous electrical potentials not specific to any particular condition but usually associated with chronic myopathic or neuropathic processes.

Compound motor action potential   The summated response of all the depolarized motor units in a nerve.

Compression sleeve   Sleeve donned on a limb with inflatable chambers to provide a compression force to the limb.

Condensations   Areas of compression or increased molecular density in biological tissues in response to the passage of ultrasound.

Conduction   A method of heat transfer between objects in direct contact with each other, where the kinetic motion of atoms and molecules of one object of higher energy (i.e., temperature) is passed to the other object of lesser energy.

Conductor   A material that permits the flow of electrical current.

Constant current (CC)   Related to Ohm's law (I = V/R) where flow of current is directly related to voltage; constant current devices maintain a constant current (I) by continually adjusting voltage (V).

Constant voltage (CV)   Related to Ohm's law (V = IR); CV devices maintain a constant voltage (V) by continually changing current (I).

Continuous mode   (1) Therapeutic ultrasound delivered without interruption at 100% duty cycle for the entire treatment period; (2) the uninterrupted delivery of pulsed electrical current.

Controlled–cold compression unit   A device that alternately pumps cold water and air into a sleeve that is wrapped around a patient's limb to provide cold therapy and compression.

Convection   A method of heat transfer in which the heated molecules move or circulate from one place to another, such as the movement of water in a whirlpool.

Cosine law   Maximum absorption of radiant energy occurs when the source is at a right angle to the absorbing surface; when the source is not at a right angle to the absorbing surface, the angle formed by the source and perpendicular to the absorbing surface determines the effect of the energy.

Coulomb   The unit of measure of electrical charge; equal to 6.24151×10^{18} electrons.

Cryoglobulinemia   A disorder characterized by the presence of an abnormal blood protein that, when exposed to cold temperatures, results in agglutination of serum proteins that can impair circulation, resulting in ischemia or gangrene.

Cryotherapy   The use of cold modalities (e.g., ice, cold packs, cold compression devices, vapocoolant sprays) for therapeutic purposes.

Current   The movement of ions or electrons in a conductor in response to a voltage force; represented by I (in amperes).

Current density   A measure of the electrical charge per unit area of an electrode's cross-sectional area (mA/cm^2 or mm^2). Current density is inversely proportional to electrode size. Also referred to as *charge density*.

Cytokines   Chemical mediator protein molecules that allow for receptor-mediated communication between cells to trigger cell transformation, secretion, migration, proliferation, and death.

Deep vein thrombosis (DVT)   The presence of a thrombosis within the venous system.

Denervation   Loss of nerve supply to muscles or other tissues.

Diabetic polyneuropathy   The consequence of a diabetic vasculopathy, presented as multiple areas of nerve damage.

Diathermy   A therapeutic modality device that produces radiofrequency radiation, usually used to heat through biological tissues.

Dielectric constant   The ratio of the capacity of a material (tissue) to that of free space.

Diode   A two-terminal electronic component that conducts electric current in only one direction.

Diplode   A hinged drum connected to a diathermy device that enables one or more body-part surfaces to be treated simultaneously.

Direct current   The continuous unidirectional flow of charged particles (electrons or ions) for at least 1 second.

Dosage   (1) The total amount of energy or force delivered by a therapeutic modality to a patient during a treatment session; (2) the intensity or amplitude of electrical stimulation required to generate a specific muscular force or torque.

Duty cycle   The percentage of the on-time to the total time (on-time plus off-time) of electrical current, multiplied by 100%.

Edema   Presence of excess fluid in the interstitial space.

Effective radiating area (ERA)   A measure of the actual cross-sectional area of the ultrasound beam as it exits the metal end plate of the transducer, expressed in square centimeters (cm^2).

Electroanalgesia   The modulation of pain through the use of electrical stimulation.

Electrode   The interface relaying current between an electrical stimulation device and the patient.

Electromigration   Movement of charged particles in response to an applied voltage.

Electroneuromyography   The recording of nerve and muscle activity in response to an electrical stimulus.

Electroosmosis   Bulk or volume fluid flow in response to a voltage difference imposed across a charged membrane, such as the skin.

Electroporation   The increase in the porosity of the superficial skin in response to electrical stimulation.

Endogenous opiates   Hormones released into the blood as a part of the response to stressful stimuli that inhibit the perception and experience of pain.

End plate spikes   Normal nonpropagated spontaneous electrical potentials observed when the tip of the EMG needle electrode is near a motor end plate. End plate spikes are induced by the release of acetylcholine from the presynaptic axon terminal in response to an action potential.

Enkephalin   Inhibitory neuropeptide that is widely distributed in the central and peripheral nervous systems.

Evidence-based practice   The clinical practice of basing patient-management decisions and interventions on evidence of effectiveness found in the scientific literature, patient values, and expert opinion.

Examination   A sequential, iterative process that consists of three parts: history, systems review, and specific tests and measures.

Extracorporeal shock wave therapy (ESWT) Application of single-impulse, focused acoustical sound waves with a rapid rise in pressure to biological tissues.

Fall time The time required for the trailing edge of a single phase to return to the isoelectric line.

Fasciculations Repetitive twitchlike spontaneous electrical potentials that reflect discharge of single or multiple motor units.

FDA Food and Drug Administration (USA).

FES Functional electric stimulation, usually indicating the use of neuromuscular electrical stimulation in substitution for an orthotic device.

Fibrillations Abnormal spontaneous electrical potentials indicative of unstable muscle membrane; thought to represent depolarization of a single muscle fiber.

Fluidotherapy A dry-heat modality that transfers heat energy by forced convection.

Frequency In electrotherapy, the number of cycles per second (Hz or cps) for an alternating current or the number of pulses per second (pps) for a pulsed current.

Functional limitations The inability to carry out specific functional activities.

F-wave An action potential produced by an antidromically directed motor stimulus that is part of neurodiagnostic testing used to examine conduction problems in the proximal and distal region of peripheral nerves.

Gauss (G) Unit used to express strength of a magnetic field; the relationship of the gauss and the tesla is $1 \text{ G} = 10^{-4} \text{ T}$.

Granulation tissue New tissue that grows inward from surrounding healthy connective tissue; it is filled with new capillaries and is surrounded by fibroblasts and macrophages.

Gridding Treatment performed by a series of vertical and horizontal strokes with a laser applicator over the length and width of an area of skin.

Ground substance Amorphous gel that forms the extracellular matrix within a wound.

Growth factors Factors that stimulate cellular proliferation and tissue growth and repair.

High-voltage pulsed current (HVPC) A twin-peaked monophasic pulsed current with voltage up to 500 volts and very short pulse duration resulting in a current with a relatively low average current yet high peak voltage.

H reflex An action potential produced by an orthodromically directed sensory stimulus that is part of neurodiagnostic testing that assesses the monosynaptic stretch reflex.

Hunting response Cold-induced vasodilation following the initial period of vasoconstriction, resulting in cyclic periods of vasodilation and vasoconstriction and in cyclic warming and cooling of the skin of the face, hands, fingers, feet, and toes.

Hydrostatic pressure Force exerted by water on a body or body part immersed in water.

Hydrotherapy Therapeutic use of water and water-based modalities.

Hyperalgesia Increased sensitivity to pain.

Hyperbaric oxygen therapy (HBOT) Inhalation of 100% oxygen in a pressurized hyperbaric chamber at a pressure greater than 1 absolute atmosphere (ATA).

Hyperemia Increased blood flow caused by a tissue temperature elevation.

Hyperstimulation A form of noxious-level stimulation often using monophasic currents of long pulse durations or direct current.

Hypertrophic scar Excessive collagen synthesis resulting in a raised scar that remains within the original boundaries of the wound.

Ice massage A cryotherapy technique in which ice is rubbed over a small area of the skin to produce rapid analgesia.

Impedance Frequency-dependent resistance to the flow of alternating current.

Inductive or magnetic field method (diathermy) Use of an inductive applicator in which an oscillating magnetic field produces "eddy" currents in the treated tissues, usually resulting in a tissue temperature rise.

Insertional activity Normal brief electrical activity noted upon insertion of EMG needle electrode within a muscle.

Insulator A material in which the movement of current (i.e., electrons or ions) is opposed or not free to move.

Interference pattern Visual disruption of the isoelectric line during electromyographic examination reflecting electrical potentials of multiple motor units during maximal voluntary muscle contraction. Individual motor units cannot be identified when a patient demonstrates a full interference pattern.

Interferential current   An amplitude modulated form of alternating current commonly used for pain modulation (i.e., electroanalgesia).

Intermittent pneumatic compression (IPC)   A modality that applies compressive force to a limb through a sleeve garment that alternately fills and empties with air pumped into the garment by an air compressor.

Intermittent traction   A mechanical device that alternately applies and releases traction to the neck or back at preset intervals.

Interphase interval   The time between successive phases of a single pulse.

Interpulse interval   The time between successive pulses.

Intrapulse interval   See *Interphase interval.*

In vitro studies   Studies performed outside of a living organism.

In vivo studies   Studies performed within a living organism.

Ionohydrokinesis   See *Electroosmosis.*

Iontophoresis   Use of direct current to induce the transcutaneous movement of ions across the skin into target tissues.

Keloid   Raised scar that extends beyond the original boundaries of the wound and can invade surrounding tissue.

Laser   Light amplification by stimulated emission of radiation.

Latency   Time between an electrical stimulus and the initial deflection of the compound sensory or motor action potential.

Light   Electromagnetic energy that is transmitted through space either as a propagated wave or as small parcels of energy called *photons.*

Longitudinal waves   Ultrasound waves that are parallel to the direction of the sound beam.

Low-intensity direct current (LIDC)   See *Microcurrent.*

Lymphedema   Swelling of an extremity brought on by decreased ability of the lymph system to transport fluid, resulting in an increase in protein-rich fluid that damages artery and venous systems.

Magnetic field   The attractive or repulsive force represented by field lines drawn around a magnet.

Magnet therapy   The use of magnets for therapeutic purposes.

Manual traction   Traction applied to a body part by the hands of a therapist or other health-care provider.

Mechanical traction   Traction applied to the neck or back for a period of time via the use of an electrical or mechanical motor unit.

Microcurrent   Current with a peak amplitude less than 1 mA.

Microstreaming   Flux of ions present within and around cells; intracellular and extracellular fluids in tissue exposed to ultrasound energy.

Miniature end plate potentials   Normal spontaneous electrical potentials observed when the tip of the EMG needle electrode is near a neuromuscular junction, producing a localized, transient depolarization initiated by the spontaneous release of individual acetylcholine quanta from the presynaptic axon terminal.

Minimal erythema dose (MED)   The smallest dose of ultraviolet light that produces an erythema that appears within 1 to 6 hours and fades without a trace within 24 hours.

Modulation   The changing or alteration of specific parameters of an electrical stimulus, such as the frequency and amplitude.

Monochromatic infrared energy (MIRE)   Refers to devices used to produce energy from the near-infrared portion of the magnetic spectrum for therapeutic purposes.

Monochromatic light   Light that has a singular wavelength and therefore is one color.

Monode   A drum attached to a diathermy device that is used to treat a single body surface.

Monophasic pulsed current   The repeated delivery of monophasic pulses produced by intermittently interrupting a DC current source.

Monopolar   An electrode configuration in which at least one electrode of a single circuit is placed over the intended treatment area with another electrode placed in a nontreatment area. Monopolar electrode placement is most commonly used with DC and monophasic pulsed currents and maintains a constant anode and cathode.

Motor unit   An alpha motoneuron and all muscle fibers it innervates.

Myofascial pain syndrome   Pain or autonomic phenomena referred from active myofascial trigger points with associated dysfunction.

Myokymic discharges Abnormal consecutively firing spontaneous electrical potentials that do not wax and wane and that are followed by a short period of electrical silence.

Myotonic discharges Abnormal rhythmic spontaneous electrical potentials initiated by movement or by tapping the inserted EMG needle electrode due to independent, repetitive discharges of single muscle fibers.

Neurapraxia The mildest form of peripheral nerve disorder characterized by local conduction failure or block across the affected segment without any axonal injury.

Neurolemma The outermost layer of the nerve membrane.

Neuropeptide Substance secreted at perivascular terminals of noradrenergic and cholinergic fibers; it has been shown to affect cellular events in all three phases of healing.

Neurotmesis Nerve injury characterized by disruption of the axon with damage to the associated connective tissue layers of the nerve.

NMES Neuromuscular electrical stimulation.

Nociception Response to noxious stimuli that results in perception of pain; the neural mechanism involved in detecting tissue damage.

Nociceptor Receptors located in tissues that are stimulated by noxious chemical, mechanical, or thermal stimuli associated with inflammation and tissue healing.

Nonionizing radiation Radiation with insufficient energy concentration to dislodge orbiting electrons from atoms.

Numerical pain rating scale A scale used by an individual to rate pain. It is most often marked 0 to 10 from one end to the other.

Ohm's law The relationship between resistance (R) and the flow of current (I), where current is directly proportional to the voltage force (V) and inversely proportional to resistance (I = V/R).

Orthodromic Conduction along a nerve in the normal direction of propagation; proximal to distal for motor and distal to proximal for sensory axons.

Paraffin wax A conductive thermal modality consisting of a mixture of seven parts wax to one part mineral oil.

Paresthesia An abnormal sensation often associated with pain localized to the nerve root or peripheral nerve sensory distribution.

Paroxysmal cold hemoglobinuria Release of hemoglobin into the urine from lysed red blood cells in response to local or general exposure to cold.

Pathology A wide variety of diseases that arise from different etiologies, including infection, trauma, and degenerative processes.

Peak pulse power The power (in watts) delivered during a pulse of ultrasound.

Percutaneous electrodes Thin wires implanted near the motor point of a muscle.

Period The inverse of frequency (*f*) calculated as 1/*f*. *Period* is the duration of one cycle in a repeated event such as alternating current.

Peripheral arterial disease (PAD) Obstructive atherosclerosis or arteriosclerosis obliterans.

Phase Flow of current in one direction from the iso-electric line; commonly expressed in microseconds.

Phase duration The time from the beginning of one phase to the end of that phase.

Phonophoresis The use of ultrasound to enhance the delivery of topically applied medications through the skin.

Photobiostimulation Application of laser light on biological tissues, causing photochemical interactions between photons and cells that result in increased cellular activity.

Piezoelectricity The phenomenon in which a crystal generates an electric voltage when mechanically compressed.

Polarity The property of having charge—either positive or negative.

Positive sharp wave Abnormal spontaneous electrical potentials usually initiated by needle movement within the muscle thought to represent an unstable muscle membrane.

Power The rate at which energy is being produced; measured in watts.

Pressure sores Tissue necrosis that occurs when external forces are applied for a prolonged period of time. Compression of the integumentary tissue between the external force and a bony prominence, which results in a skin wound.

Prognosis A prediction of the time required to achieve the goals of therapeutic interventions.

Proinflammatory Effects of ultrasound that augment both the quantity and quality of the healing process.

Proteinases Cellular enzymes necessary for pathogen control, cellular migration, and tissue remodeling.

Pulse An isolated electrical event separated from the next by a finite period of time.

Pulsed current The uni- or bidirectional flow of ions or electrons, which periodically ceases for a short period of time before the next electrical event.

Pulsed electromagnetic field (PEMF) A field that produces an electric current by inducing the movement of ions in body fluids.

Pulsed lavage with concurrent suction (PLWCS) Form of mechanical debridement that applies a stream or spray under controlled pressure to remove loosely adherent necrotic tissue or foreign material.

Pulsed radio frequency radiation (PRFR) Pulses of electromagnetic energy from the radiofrequency part of the spectrum.

Pulsed ultrasound Noncontinuous or interrupted ultrasound.

Pulse duration Time from the beginning to the end of all phases of a single pulse, including any interphase interval.

Pulse period The pulse on-time plus the pulse off-time.

Pulse train See *Train*.

Quadrant testing Examination of motor units in multiple regions via single needle insertion completed by redirecting the needle tip without completely removing it from the muscle.

Quadripolar An electrode configuration in which the electrodes of two separate circuits are placed on the treatment area with intention for the currents to intersect; used with quadripolar interferential current.

Radiation The process by which energy is propagated through space.

Radio frequency (RF) radiation Propagating waves between the frequencies of 10 kilohertz (kHz) and 300 gigahertz (GHz) on the electromagnetic spectrum.

Ramp-down The time it takes for the current to decrease from peak amplitude to zero amplitude during any one on-time period.

Ramp-up The time it takes for the current to increase from zero amplitude to peak amplitude for any one on-time period.

Rarefactions Areas of decreased molecular density in tissues in response to the passage of ultrasound.

Raynaud's phenomenon A vasospastic disorder resulting in paroxysmal digital cyanosis with cold exposure.

Reflection The change in the path of propagation of a beam of energy occurring at a discontinuity in the acoustical impedance.

Reflex sympathetic dystrophy (RSD) Type 1 complex regional pain syndrome that is identified when it is unknown whether there is any peripheral nerve involvement.

Refraction The bending of waves as they pass from one medium to another, proportional to the difference in acoustic impedance.

Resistance Opposition to current flow.

Rheobase The minimum strength of an electrical stimulus of infinite duration that is capable of eliciting a minimally detectable motor response.

Rise time The time required for the leading edge of a single phase to reach peak amplitude.

Russian current A burst-modulated form of alternating current that is commonly used for activation of skeletal muscle.

Saltatory conduction The propagation of action potentials along myelinated axons between nodes of Ranvier.

Sarcolemma The cell membrane of a muscle cell.

Scan See *Vector scan*.

Segmental demyelination A focal conduction abnormality characterized by the intermittent absence of myelin along normally myelinated axons.

Sensory-level stimulation The threshold at which an electrical stimulus elicits a sensory response.

Sensory nerve action potential (SNAP) The summated response of all the depolarized sensory fibers in a nerve.

Sonic Accelerated Fracture Healing System (SAFHS) Specific ultrasound units designed to deliver fixed parameters—20% duty cycle, 1.5 MHz, $I_{SATA} = 30$ mW/cm^2 for 20 minutes—for the purpose of promoting fracture healing.

Spasticity Velocity-dependent increase in resistance to passive stretch associated with exaggerated deep tendon reflexes.

Spatial average intensity (I_{SA}) A measure of the average acoustic power of ultrasound across the ERA of the transducer; expressed in watts per square centimeter (W/cm²).

Spatial average temporal average intensity (I_{SATA}) An intensity value calculated by multiplying I_{SATP} by the duty cycle of the applied ultrasound.

Spatial average temporal peak intensity (I_{SATP}) The spatial average intensity of an ultrasound beam between interruptions during pulsed ultrasound.

Spatial peak intensity (I_{SP}) The acoustic power of an ultrasound beam at its highest point.

Specific gravity The ratio of the density of a substance to the density of water at 4°C (39.2°F).

Specific heat A measure of the amount of energy (heat) required to heat a material and thus the amount of energy (heat) stored in a material.

Standing wave When waves are in phase with each other, their energies are added together, creating an area of more intense energy in the tissue.

Static magnets Magnets used with constant poles for therapeutic purposes.

Streamline or laminar flow Occurs when each particle of the fluid follows a smooth path without crossover of paths.

Strength-duration curve A plot of the range of combinations of current amplitude and pulse duration that result in depolarization of sensory or motor nerves.

Suberythemal dose (SED) The situation in which none of the ultraviolet light exposure spots on the skin produces a minimal erythemal dose.

Suprathreshold stimulus An electrical stimulus exceeding the minimal threshold stimulus required to elicit depolarization.

Sustained (static) traction Form of traction applied continuously to a body part by an electrical or mechanical device.

Sweep Modulation of the beat frequency of interferential current.

Swing Denotes the temporal characteristics of the sweep of interferential current.

Symmetrical Condition when the amplitude and duration characteristics of the two phases of the biphasic waveform are identical.

TENS Transcutaneous electrical nerve stimulation.

Tesla (T) Unit used to measure the strength of a magnetic field. The relationship of tesla to gauss is $1\ G = 10^{-4}\ T$.

Therapeutic modalities Devices or techniques applied to a patient as part of a plan of care for a therapeutic purpose.

Thermal conductivity A measure of the efficiency of a material or tissue in conducting heat.

Thermal medium The product of thermal conductivity, density, and specific heat.

Thermoreceptors Receptors in the skin that respond to changes in temperature.

Thermotherapy Modalities primarily used to cause an increase in tissue temperature.

Traction The process of drawing or pulling apart a body part, usually a joint or joints.

Train The uninterrupted generation of pulses at a fixed frequency or a brief period of alternating current.

Transducer The part of an ultrasound device that houses a piezoelectric crystal where high-frequency electrical energy is converted to ultrasound energy.

Transverse waves Ultrasound waves perpendicular to the direction of the sound beam.

Trigger point A palpable band or nodule within the muscle or connective tissue that refers pain, elicits a local twitch response when pressed, and is generally hypersensitive.

Turbine A motor that agitates water in a whirlpool tank to create a "whirlpool" effect.

Turbulent flow The flow of fluids in erratic, small, whirlpool-like circles called *eddy currents* or *eddies*.

Ultraviolet An electromagnetic energy, invisible to the human eye, that lies between visible light and X-ray on the electromagnetic spectrum.

Ultraviolet light A (UVA) Also known as long-wave UV, it is non-ionizing and produces fluorescence in many substances.

Ultraviolet light B (UVB) Also known as middle-wave UV, it is non-ionizing and produces most skin erythema.

Ultraviolet light C (UVC) Ultraviolet light defined as the wavelength 180–250 nm.

Unbalanced When the area under the curve of the first phase (i.e., phase charge) of a biphasic pulse is unequal to that of the second phase; the result is a net charge, either positive or negative.

Urine incontinence Inability to control bladder function.

Vapocoolant spray A cold therapy delivery method in which one sprays rapidly evaporating chemicals on the skin; used for temporary pain relief and for preparation prior to stretching muscles with active trigger points.

Vasoconstriction Contraction of vascular smooth muscle, which results in decreased diameter of blood vessels and decreased blood flow.

Vasodilation Relaxation of vascular smooth muscles, which results in increased diameter of blood vessels and increased blood flow.

Vector scan The modulation of the amplitude of one or both currents of interferential current, which results in a rhythmic change in position of the interference pattern or vector.

Venous ulcers Chronic venous insufficiency that leads to the formation of a chronic wound.

Viscosity The internal friction present in liquids secondary to the cohesive forces between the molecules.

Visual analog scale (VAS) A scale using visual input for an individual to rate pain, most often a scale 10 cm in length.

Voltage An electrical force capable of moving charged particles through a conductor between two regions or points secondary to a potential difference between the points.

Wallerian degeneration Axon degeneration distal to the site of nerve transaction.

Waveform A description or visual representation of the characteristics of an electrical current, including shape, magnitude, and duration, depicted on an amplitude–time plot.

Zero net DC A state of no net charge between phases of a bi- or polyphasic waveform.

Index

Note: Page numbers followed by *f* indicate figures; *t*, tables; *b*, boxes.